Advances in Experimental Medicine and Biology

Volume 1189

Series Editors
Wim E. Crusio, *CNRS and University of Bordeaux UMR 5287, Institut de Neurosciences Cognitives et Intégratives d'Aquitaine, Pessac Cedex, France*
John D. Lambris, *University of Pennsylvania, Philadelphia, PA, USA*
Nima Rezaei, *Children's Medical Center Hospital, Tehran University of Medical Sciences, Tehran, Iran*

More information about this series at http://www.springer.com/series/5584

Miyuki Azuma • Hideo Yagita
Editors

Co-signal Molecules in T Cell Activation

Immune Regulation in Health and Disease

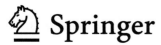

Editors
Miyuki Azuma
Department of Molecular Immunology
Graduate School of Medical and Dental
Sciences
Tokyo Medical and Dental University
Tokyo, Japan

Hideo Yagita
Department of Immunology
Juntendo University School of Medicine
Tokyo, Japan

ISSN 0065-2598   ISSN 2214-8019 (electronic)
Advances in Experimental Medicine and Biology
ISBN 978-981-32-9719-7   ISBN 978-981-32-9717-3 (eBook)
https://doi.org/10.1007/978-981-32-9717-3

© Springer Nature Singapore Pte Ltd. 2019
This work is subject to copyright. All rights are reserved by the Publisher, whether the whole or part of
the material is concerned, specifically the rights of translation, reprinting, reuse of illustrations, recitation,
broadcasting, reproduction on microfilms or in any other physical way, and transmission or information
storage and retrieval, electronic adaptation, computer software, or by similar or dissimilar methodology
now known or hereafter developed.
The use of general descriptive names, registered names, trademarks, service marks, etc. in this publication
does not imply, even in the absence of a specific statement, that such names are exempt from the relevant
protective laws and regulations and therefore free for general use.
The publisher, the authors, and the editors are safe to assume that the advice and information in this book
are believed to be true and accurate at the date of publication. Neither the publisher nor the authors or the
editors give a warranty, expressed or implied, with respect to the material contained herein or for any
errors or omissions that may have been made. The publisher remains neutral with regard to jurisdictional
claims in published maps and institutional affiliations.

This Springer imprint is published by the registered company Springer Nature Singapore Pte Ltd.
The registered company address is: 152 Beach Road, #21-01/04 Gateway East, Singapore 189721,
Singapore

Contents

Part I Basic Understanding of Co-signal Molecules in T Cell Activation

1 **Co-signal Molecules in T-Cell Activation** 3
   Miyuki Azuma

2 **The CD28–B7 Family of Co-signaling Molecules**. 25
   Shigenori Nagai and Miyuki Azuma

3 **The TNF–TNFR Family of Co-signal Molecules** 53
   Takanori So and Naoto Ishii

4 **Signal Transduction Via Co-stimulatory
   and Co-inhibitory Receptors** 85
   Shuhei Ogawa and Ryo Abe

5 **Molecular Dynamics of Co-signal Molecules
   in T-Cell Activation** 135
   Takashi Saito

6 **Role of Co-stimulatory Molecules in T Helper
   Cell Differentiation** 153
   Michelle Schorer, Vijay K. Kuchroo, and Nicole Joller

7 **Control of Regulatory T Cells by Co-signal Molecules** 179
   James Badger Wing, Christopher Tay, and Shimon Sakaguchi

Part II Co-signal Molecules in Health and Disease

8 **Stimulatory and Inhibitory Co-signals in Autoimmunity** 213
   Taku Okazaki and Il-mi Okazaki

9 **Co-signaling Molecules in Neurological Diseases**. 233
   Pia Kivisäkk and Samia J. Khoury

10 Costimulation Blockade in Transplantation 267

Melissa Y. Yeung, Tanja Grimmig, and Mohamed H. Sayegh

11 Cancer Immunotherapy Targeting Co-signal Molecules 313

Masao Nakajima and Koji Tamada

Part I
Basic Understanding of Co-signal Molecules in T Cell Activation

Chapter 1
Co-signal Molecules in T-Cell Activation

Historical Overview and Perspective

Miyuki Azuma

Abstract The two-signal model of T-cell activation, proposed approximately four decades ago, has undergone various refinements while maintaining its principal doctrine. Since the discovery of CD28, a variety of co-signal molecules, including co-stimulatory and co-inhibitory receptors and ligands, have been identified. These molecules fine-tune various immune responses both in the primary or secondary lymphoid tissues and in the peripheral tissues. Most co-signal receptors are expressed and induced on T cells during distinct stages (naïve/resting, activating, memory, and exhausting). These co-signaling pathways play critical and diverse roles in maintaining T-cell tolerance and eliciting T-cell immune responses in health and disease. This introductory chapter provides a historical overview of the key findings that have led to our current view of T-cell co-stimulation.

Keywords Co-signals · Co-stimulation · Co-inhibition · T-cell activation · Two-signal model · Tolerance

1.1 Historical Overview

1.1.1 Classical Two-Signal Model of Lymphocyte Activation

Our immune system needs to eliminate harmful microbes and substances, but at the same time must also tolerate beneficial microbes and harmless substances. Since the1960s, immunologists have tried to understand how the immune system controls the magnitude and type of immune response on encountering antigens. T and B

M. Azuma (✉)
Department of Molecular Immunology, Graduate School of Medical and Dental Sciences,
Tokyo Medical and Dental University, Tokyo, Japan
e-mail: miyuki.mim@tmd.ac.jp

© Springer Nature Singapore Pte Ltd. 2019
M. Azuma, H. Yagita (eds.), *Co-signal Molecules in T Cell Activation*,
Advances in Experimental Medicine and Biology 1189,
https://doi.org/10.1007/978-981-32-9717-3_1

lymphocytes, which possess diverse antigen-specific receptors, have two possible outcomes: induction (activation) or tolerance (paralysis or inactivation).

The "two-signal" model of lymphocyte activation tries to answer the question of why lymphocytes become unresponsive, or only partially activated, after exposure to an antigen, and it has evolved considerably over the past 50 years (Baxter and Hodgkin 2002). In 1970, Bretscher and Cohn revised their old model of B-cell antibody responses and proposed a two-signal model for B-cell stimulation (Bretscher and Cohn 1970) (Fig. 1.1a). Antigen recognition by B lymphocytes provides signal

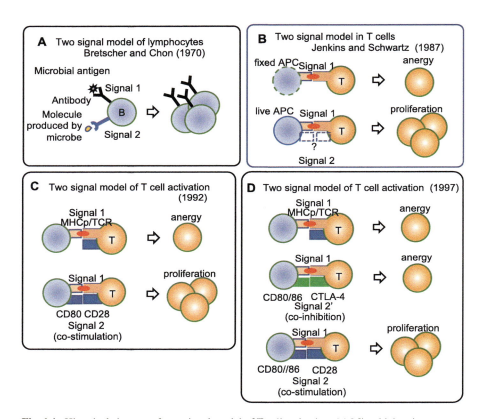

Fig. 1.1 Historical changes of two-signal model of T-cell activation. (a) Microbial antigen recognition by B lymphocytes provides signal 1, and molecules produced by microbes provide "signal 2." Both signals are required for B-cell activation (antibody response), and signal 1 alone induces unresponsiveness. (b) Chemically fixed antigen-presenting cells (APCs) induce an unresponsive state in T cells. The live cell–cell interaction between an APC and a T cell provides additional signals (signal 2) required for optimal T-cell activation. (c) Optimal T-cell activation requires both signal 1 and signal 2. Signal 1 is provided by the binding of MHC–peptide to the CD3–TCR complex, and signal 2 is provided by the CD28–CD80-mediated co-stimulation. Signal 1 without co-stimulation induces antigen-specific unresponsiveness (anergy) in T cells. (d) Signal 2 is not only co-stimulatory. Co-stimulatory (signal 2) and co-inhibitory (signal 2′) signals are provided by the cognate interaction with an APC and a T cell. When a T cell encounters antigens under the lack of CD28 co-stimulation or the presence of CTLA-4 co-inhibition, T cell will become anergy

1 Co-signal Molecules in T-Cell Activation 5

1 for the activation of the lymphocytes, and components of microbes or substances produced during innate immune responses to microbes provide signal 2. Later, Lafferty and Cunningham modified Bretscher and Cohn's model to include T-cell responses (Cunningham and Lafferty 1977; Lafferty and Cunningham 1975).The updated two-signal model explains why lymphocytes may only be partially activated, or even unresponsive, after exposure to signal 1 alone. Signal 2 is provided by stimulator cells, and this was later termed co-stimulation. The discovery of interleukin (IL)-2 as a critical T-cell growth factor permitted the prolonged culture of T lymphocytes and the establishment of T-cell clones. In 1987, Jenkins and Schwartz found that chemically fixed antigen-presenting cells (APCs) induced an unresponsive state in T cells even when they received signal 1 via the major histocompatibility complex (MHC)/antigen (Jenkins et al. 1987; Jenkins and Schwartz 1987; Schwartz 1990). Thus, they speculated that signal 2 might be provided by the live cell–cell interaction between an APC and a T cell (Fig. 1.1b). Identification of signal 2 on the molecular level was not accomplished until the discovery of the interaction between CD28 on T cells and CD80 (B7) on activated B cells (Linsley et al. 1991a).

1.1.2 Two-Signal Model of T-Cell Activation

1.1.2.1 Homologous CD28 and CTLA-4 Receptors

Before identification of the binding of CD80 to CD28, most studies of T-cell activation were performed using monoclonal antibodies (mAbs). CD28 was first discovered as a 44 kDa homodimeric glycoprotein expressed on roughly 80% of human peripheral blood T cells utilizing mAb 9.3 (Damle et al. 1981; Lesslauer et al. 1986). Cross-linking CD28 with anti-CD28 mAb stimulated with alloantigen, mitogen (PHA), phorbol myristate acetate (PMA), or anti-CD3 mAb greatly enhanced the IL-2 production, proliferative responses, and cytotoxicity of resting T cells (June et al. 1990; Jung et al. 1987; Lesslauer et al. 1986). The CD28 mAb-mediated signal, in cooperation with PMA, induced the activation of protein kinase C, in turn resulting in increased T-cell activation; however, the CD28 signal alone did not induce T-cell proliferation or IL-2 production (Hara et al. 1985). Unlike anti-CD3 stimulation, enhancement of IL-2 transcripts by CD28-mediated signaling was partially resistant to the addition of cyclosporin, which is a calcineurin phosphatase pathway inhibitor (June et al. 1987), suggesting differential activation signaling between CD3 and CD28. CD28-mediated stimulation increased the expression of CD25 (IL-2R-α) and multiple cytokines, including IL-2, interferon (IFN)-γ, tumor necrosis factor (TNF)-α, and granulocyte-macrophage colony-stimulating factor (GM-CSF), through stabilization of mRNA (Lindstein et al. 1989). Molecular cloning revealed that CD28 is a type I transmembrane receptor of the immunoglobulin (Ig) superfamily containing an extracellular region with a V-like domain, a transmembrane region, and an intracellular region (Aruffo and Seed 1987). CD28 exists in both monomeric and homodimeric forms on the surface of T cells.

Unlike CD28, cytotoxic T lymphocyte antigen 4 (CTLA-4, CD152) was initially identified by screening mouse cytotoxic T lymphocyte-derived cDNA libraries (Brunet et al. 1987), followed by identifying and cloning a human homolog (Dariavach et al. 1988). Similar to CD28, CTLA-4 is a member of the Ig superfamily with a single V domain in the extracellular region. The molecular function of CTLA-4 took some time to identify. Based on the close structural relationship, chromosomal location, and mRNA expression levels between CD28 and CTLA-4, it was speculated that these two genes share an evolutionary precursor and possess similar functional properties (Harper et al. 1991; Lafage-Pochitaloff et al. 1990).

1.1.2.2 Two-Signal Model of T-Cell Activation

In 1991, Linsley and Ledbetter found that CD28 was the primary counter receptor for a B-cell activation antigen, CD80 (B7, BB1, B7-1) (Linsley et al. 1991a). Subsequently, they found that CTLA-4 also binds to CD80 and that the CTLA-4Ig fusion protein, comprising the extracellular domain of CTLA-4 and the Fc domain of IgG1, was a potent inhibitor of the cellular responses of T and B cells (Linsley et al. 1991b). Their study was the first to identify co-stimulatory molecules on the cell surface. Subsequently, additional chimeric Ig fusion proteins were generated to characterize their binding properties and functional interactions. Since then, the use of Ig fusion proteins has become a convenient tool for analyzing functional interactions between cell surface receptors and their ligands. Similar to anti-CD28 mAb, CD80-tranfected cells augmented T-cell proliferation and IL-2 production in response to anti-CD3 mAb, PMA, or peptide stimulation, and the enhanced activation was inhibited by the addition of anti-CD80 mAb (Gimmi et al. 1993; Gimmi et al. 1991). Interestingly, the CD28–CD80-mediated signaling prevented the induction of an unresponsive state in T cells (clonal anergy), by receiving signal 1 via the binding of MHC–antigen to the CD3–TCR complex (Gimmi et al. 1993; Harding et al. 1992; Schwartz 1992). In the context of anergy blockade and amplification of signal 1, the CD28–CD80 pathway was distinguishable from adhesion molecules, such as LFA-1 (CD11a/CD18)-ICAMs (CD54, CD102, CD50) and VLA-4-VCAM-1, and represented as a crucial co-stimulatory pathway that provides signal 2 for amplifying T-cell responses. Thus, the molecular basis of the two-signal model of T-cell activation was established (Fig. 1.1c).

1.1.2.3 The CD28–CD86 Co-stimulatory Pathway

The inhibitory effects of CTLA-4Ig and anti-CD28 mAb in T-cell-dependent antibody responses and CD28-dependent natural killer (NK)-like cell-mediated cytotoxicity against B-cell lines clearly differed from the effects of anti-CD80 mAb and the action of CD80-deficient B cells (Azuma et al. 1992b; Freeman et al. 1993b; Linsley et al. 1992b). Eventually, a second ligand for CD28 and CTLA-4, CD86 (B7-2, B70), was identified in humans and mice (Azuma et al. 1993; Freeman et al.

1 Co-signal Molecules in T-Cell Activation 7

1993c). Both CD86 and CD80 are members of the Ig superfamily with a single V and C-like domain in the extracellular region, but their amino acid sequences, cytoplasmic regions, and expression kinetics are quite different. CD86 is constitutively expressed or upregulated quickly after activation of B cells, dendritic cells (DCs), and macrophages (Lenschow et al. 1993). Both CD80 and CD86 induce T-cell activation (Freeman et al. 1993a; Lanier et al. 1995; Nakajima et al. 1995); however, studies on APCs and T-cell-mediated immune responses in vitro and in vivo indicate that CD86 is the dominant ligand in CD28-costimulated T-cell responses (Azuma et al. 1993; Caux et al. 1994; Inaba et al. 1994; Lenschow et al. 1993; Nakajima et al. 1995; Nuriya et al. 1996).

1.1.2.4 CTLA-4 as a Co-inhibitory Receptor

The biological function of CTLA-4 was not elucidated for another half decade because it was difficult to determine whether the use of mAbs had an effect on the experimental results, even when Fab fragments, which do not induce signaling, and cross-linked forms of mAb, which induce agonistic signaling, were used (Kearney et al. 1995; Krummel et al. 1996; Linsley et al. 1992a). The inhibitory role of CTLA-4 was confirmed by the generation of CTLA-4-deficient mice. CTLA-4-deficient mice develop a fatal lymphoproliferative disorder characterized by massive polyclonal T-cell infiltration and tissue destruction in multiple organs (Tivol et al. 1995; Waterhouse et al. 1995). CTLA-4 in the extracellular regions shares an MYPPPY-binding motif with CD28 that targets CD80 and CD86 (Harper et al. 1991), but CTLA-4 binds CD80 and CD86 with much higher affinity than CD28 (Linsley et al. 1991b). Unlike CD28, CTLA-4 is not detected on naïve T cells; instead it is transiently induced on the T-cell surface following TCR stimulation (Linsley et al. 1996; Linsley et al. 1992a). The cytoplasmic tail of CTLA-4 interacts with a clathrin-associated adaptor protein (AP-2) that also regulates tyrosine phosphorylation and trafficking of CTLA-4 (Bradshaw et al. 1997; Shiratori et al. 1997).

Based on the complexed CD28–CTLA-4-CD80–CD86 axis, the detrimental phenotype observed in CTLA-4-deficient mice mostly results from the competitive co-stimulatory action of CD28 (Chambers et al. 1997).The co-inhibitory role of CTLA-4 was confirmed by generating peptide-specific CD4[+] and CD8[+] T cells with MHC class I- or class II-restricted TCRs in the CTLA-4-deficient mice (Chambers et al. 1999; Chambers et al. 1998). The cytoplasmic domain of CTLA-4 lacks immunoreceptor tyrosine-based inhibitory motif (ITIM), which most inhibitory receptors possess, but instead has a YVKM motif. It was speculated that tyrosine phosphorylation of the YVKM motif recruits the Src homology protein 2 (SH2) domain-containing phosphatase-2 (SHP-2) to downregulate early TCR-mediated downstream signaling (Lee et al. 1998; Marengere et al. 1996). The inhibitory function of CTLA-4 involved both cell-intrinsic and cell-extrinsic mechanisms. Extrinsic co-inhibition is the result of ligand-binding competition with an activating receptor CD28 and of reverse signaling via CD80–CD86 in APCs (Grohmann et al. 2002).

1.1.2.5 Revised Two-Signal Model of T-Cell Activation

Verification of CTLA-4-mediated co-inhibitory function and the realization that signal 2 can not only be co-stimulatory but also co-inhibitory led to further modification of the two-signal model (Fig. 1.1d) (Chambers and Allison 1999; Thompson and Allison 1997). When a T cell encounters antigens with high TCR binding affinity and APC expressing CD80–CD86 at high levels, the T cell will be activated by CD28-mediated co-stimulation (signal 2). However, if the T cell encounters antigens with low affinity for the TCR, or is presented with antigens by APCs expressing little or no CD80–CD86, the T cell will become anergy due to the lack of CD28 co-stimulation (signal 2) or the presence of the CTLA-4 co-inhibition (signal 2′).

CTLA-4 is preferentially involved in maintaining peripheral tolerance by naïve CD4$^+$ T cells. Ligand binding is critical for the localization of CTLA-4, but not CD28, at the immunological synapse following TCR engagement (Pentcheva-Hoang et al. 2004). For CTLA-4 localization at the synapse, CD80 is the main ligand, while, for CD28 localization, CD86 is the main ligand. Subsequent studies have revealed that CTLA-4 reverses stop signals that are required for stable conjugate formation between the T cell and the APC, resulting in a heightened signal threshold for T-cell activation (Rudd 2008; Schneider et al. 2006).

1.1.3 Modified Two-Signal Model of T-Cell Activation

1.1.3.1 PD-1-Mediated Peripheral T-Cell Tolerance

Programmed cell death-1 (PD-1, CD279) was identified as a member of the Ig superfamily, which is involved in programed cell death (Ishida et al. 1992) and was eventually recognized as a member of the CD28 and B7 family. Direct involvement of PD-1 in programmed cell death was not confirmed in the subsequent experiments (Agata et al. 1996). PD-1 deficiency demonstrated the role of PD-1 in autoimmunity by resulting in moderate splenomegaly and hyper B-cell activation stimulated with IgM (Nishimura et al. 1998). It also resulted in the development of a variety of strain- and organ-specific autoimmune diseases, such as lupus-like arthritis and glomerulonephritis, in the C57BL/6 background, as well as in dilated cardiomyopathy in BALB/c mice (Nishimura et al. 1999; Nishimura et al. 2001). Although regulatory roles of PD-1 in T- and B-cell-mediated immune responses have been reported, the addition of PD-1 to the CD28–B7 family did not occur until the identification of the PD-1 ligands, PD-L1 (B7-H1, CD174) (Dong et al. 1999; Freeman et al. 2000) and PD-L2 (B7-DC, CD173) (Latchman et al. 2001; Tseng et al. 2001).

Unlike T-cell-restricted expression of CD28 and CTLA-4, PD-1 expression can be induced by stimulation of various immune cells, including CD4$^+$ and CD8$^+$T cells; NK, NKT, and B cells; macrophages; and several subsets of DCs (Agata et al. 1996; Yamazaki et al. 2002). Despite such broad expression, the functional contribution of PD-1-mediated regulation is mostly dominant in CD8$^+$ T-cell responses and the effector phase of T-cell responses in peripheral tissues (Dong et al. 2004; Goldberg et al. 2007; Iwai et al. 2003; Keir et al. 2006). This is because PD-1-mediated inhibition is often overcome by high IL-2 and CD28 co-stimulation in the presence of APCs (Carter et al. 2002; Kuipers et al. 2006). PD-L1 expression on parenchymal tissue cells, rather than on hematopoietic immune cells, is heavily involved in the PD-1-mediated peripheral T-cell tolerance (Dong et al. 2004; Keir et al. 2006; Ritprajak et al. 2010). Studies using neutralizing antibodies against PD-1, PD-L1, and/or PD-L2 demonstrate the involvement of PD-1–PD-L1-mediated regulation in murine models of chronic diseases and peripheral tolerance (Ansari et al. 2003; Fife et al. 2006; Habicht et al. 2007; Salama et al. 2003; Tanaka et al. 2007). PD-L1-expressing peripheral tissue cells lacking class II MHC and high CD80–CD86 expression levels are the most likely cell interacting with PD-1-expressing CD8$^+$T cells to effect immune regulation.

The cytoplasmic domain of PD-1 contains two tyrosine residues, one each in the N-terminal ITIM and the C-terminal immunoreceptor tyrosine-based switch motif (ITSM). While mutation of the ITIM tyrosine had little effect, mutation of the ITSM tyrosine abolished PD-1-mediated signaling in B and T cells (Chemnitz et al. 2004; Okazaki et al. 2001). PD-L1 binding to PD-1 recruits the phosphatase SHP-2, which induces the dephosphorylation of the proximal TCR signaling, thereby resulting in the PD-1-mediated immune regulation (Chemnitz et al. 2004; Sheppard et al. 2004; Yokosuka et al. 2012). Unlike CTLA-4, interactions between PD-1 and PD-L1 promote T-cell tolerance by blocking the TCR-induced stop signal required for close T and APC interaction (Fife et al. 2009).

1.1.3.2 The Extended CD28–B7 Family

During the late1990s to early 2000s, the CD28–B7 family was expanded, and additional co-stimulatory or co-inhibitory receptor–ligand pairs were identified (Fig. 1.2) (Carreno and Collins 2002; Chen 2004; Greenwald et al. 2005). These included inducible co-stimulator (ICOS; AILIM, H4, CD278) (Hutloff et al. 1999) and its ligands (ICOSL, B7-H2, B7h, B7RP-1, CD275) (Mak et al. 2003; Smith et al. 2003; Wang et al. 2000), B7-H3 (B7-RP2, CD276) (Chapoval et al. 2001; Suh et al. 2003; Sun et al. 2002), B7-H4 (B7S1, B7x, *Vtcn1*) (Choi et al. 2003; Prasad et al. 2003; Sica et al. 2003; Zang et al. 2003), and B and T lymphocyte attenuator (BTLA, CD272) (Watanabe et al. 2003).

The ICOS–ICOSL pathway is critical for T-cell-dependent B-cell responses, such as isotype class switching, germinal center formation, and the development of memory B cells (Mak et al. 2003; Smith et al. 2003; Wang et al. 2000). Homozygous mutation of ICOS in human is associated with common variable immunodeficiency (CVID) and adult-onset of hypogammaglobulinemia (Grimbacher et al. 2003). Both B7-H3 and B7-H4 are detectable in various normal tissues at the mRNA level (Chapoval et al. 2001; Sica et al. 2003); however, the functional contribution of cell surface B7-H3 and B7-H4 to T-cell co-stimulation and co-inhibition is still obscure (Schildberg et al. 2016; Yi and Chen 2009).

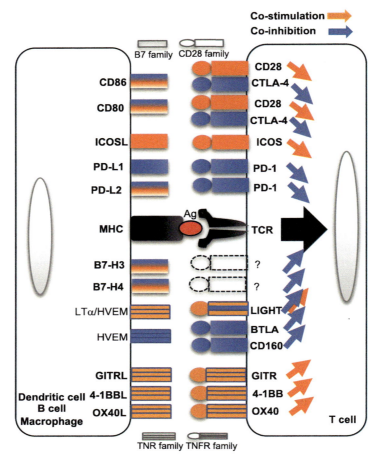

Fig. 1.2 Representative T-cell co-signal molecules at early 2000s. The CD28–B7 family and the tumor necrosis factor superfamily (TNFSF) and TNF receptor superfamily (TNFRSF) are two major co-signal receptors and their ligands in T-cell activation. CD28, ICOS, GITR, 4-1BB, and OX40 pathways co-stimulate T-cell activation. CTLA-4, PD-1, BTLA, and CD160 pathway co-inhibit T-cell activation. Most co-signal ligands are expressed or induced on antigen-presenting cells (APCs), such as dendritic cells (DCs), B cells, and macrophages, while most co-signal receptors on T cells are constitutively expressed or induced after TCR activation

B7-H3 and B7-H4 are generally understood to be co-inhibitory B7 ligands, but their respective inhibitory counter-receptors on T cells have not yet been identified. Triggering receptor expressed on myeloid cell-like transcript 2 (TLT-2), which co-stimulates CD8[+] T-cell responses, has been reported as a counterpart for B7-H3 (Hashiguchi et al. 2008; Kobori et al. 2010).

BTLA was shown to be the third T-cell co-inhibitory receptor with an ITIM motif in its cytoplasmic region, following CTLA-4 and PD-1. Although B7x had been proposed as a ligand for BTLA based on Ig fusion protein binding (Carreno and Collins 2003), this was later refuted. BTLA actually binds to the herpesvirus entry mediator (HVEM; TNFRSF14), which in turn binds to the B7 family in *cis* and *trans* situations (Gonzalez et al. 2005; Sedy et al. 2005). HVEM also binds three other distinct ligands, including lymphotoxin-like, inducible expression, which competes with herpes simplex virus glycoprotein D for HVEM; a receptor expressed by T lymphocytes (LIGHT), CD160; and lymphotoxin-alpha (LTα). The binding of LIGHT or LTα to HVEM delivers a co-stimulatory signal and counter-regulates the HVEM–BTLA-mediated inhibitory pathway (Cai and Freeman 2009; del Rio et al. 2010). CD160, which is a member of the Ig superfamily with one IgV-like domain in the extracellular region, competes with BTLA for binding to HVEM (Kojima et al. 2011). Details of the CD28 and B7 family molecules are provided in Chap. 2.

A considerable number of the tumor necrosis factor superfamily (TNFSF) and TNF receptor superfamily (TNFRSF) molecules also possess co-stimulatory activity in T cells and cooperate with the CD28-B7 family molecules (Ward-Kavanagh et al. 2016; Watts 2005). Most well-analyzed co-stimulatory pathways utilize the following three TNFSF–TNFRSF pathways, 4-1BB (TNFRSF9, CD137, ILA) and its ligand (4-1BBL, TNFSF9) (DeBenedette et al. 1995; Goodwin et al. 1993; Hurtado et al. 1995; Pollok et al. 1993), glucocorticoid-induced tumor necrosis factor (GITR, TNFRSF18, AITR, CD357) and its ligand (GITRL, TNFSF18) (Igarashi et al. 2008; Kanamaru et al. 2004; Tone et al. 2003), and OX40 (TNFRSF4, CD134) (Mallett et al. 1990) and its ligand (OX40L, TNFSF4) (Akiba et al. 1999; Ohshima et al. 1998). Although all three ligands are inducible on DCs, it seems that their major contribution lies in their interactions with naïve T cells. The receptors induced after TCR activation contribute to distinct phases and types of T-cell responses, by modulating T-cell proliferation, survival, and/or cytokine production (Ward-Kavanagh et al. 2016). Details of the TNFSF–TNFRSF family molecules are provided in Chap. 3.

The discovery of these co-stimulatory and co-inhibitory receptors and ligands necessitated further modification of the two-signal model of T-cell activation (Fig. 1.3). Signal 1 is delivered from the binding of an APC's MHC/antigen to the TCR. Multiple second signals (signal 2 + 2′) are delivered after the cell–cell interaction between a T cell and an APC. When co-inhibitory signals (signal 2′) outweigh the co-stimulatory signals (signal 2), a T cell does not induce a response and instead enters an antigen-specific unresponsive state known as anergy, or tolerance. When the co-stimulatory signals (signal 2) outweigh the co-inhibitory signals (signal 2′), a T cell proliferates and differentiates into an effector cell. Although the TCR signal (signal 1) is essential for a T-cell response, the co-stimulatory and co-inhibitory signals (signal 2 + 2′) determine the fate of the T-cell response. Details regarding signal transduction and molecular dynamics are provided in Chaps. 4 and 5.

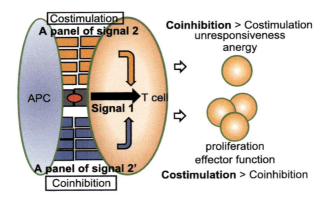

Fig. 1.3 Modified two-signal models of T-cell activation. Signal 1 is delivered from the binding of MHC/antigen on antigen-presenting cells (APCs) to the TCR. Multiple second signals (signal 2 + 2′) are delivered after the cell–cell interaction between a T cell and an APC. When co-inhibitory signals (signal 2′) outweigh the co-stimulatory signals (signal 2), a T cell does not induce a response and instead enters an antigen-specific unresponsive state. When the co-stimulatory signals (signal 2) outweigh the co-inhibitory signals (signal 2′), a T cell proliferates and differentiates into an effector cell. Although signal 1 is essential for a T-cell response, the co-stimulatory and co-inhibitory signals (signal 2 + 2′) determine the fate of the T-cell response

1.2 Perspective

1.2.1 Co-signals Required for CD8+ T-Cell Activation

Most early T-cell co-stimulation studies focused to CD4+ T-helper (Th) cells. Unlike CD4+ T cells, differentiation of naïve CD8+ T cells for full expansion and effector function requires additional inflammatory cytokine-mediated signals (signal 3) (Mescher et al. 2006) (Fig. 1.4). Because CD8+ T cells are initially unable to produce IL-2 by themselves, IL-12 and type I IFN (IFN-α and IFN-β) provided by the antigen-presenting DCs initiate CD8+ T-cell activation (Mescher et al. 2006; Valbon et al. 2016). During the priming and expansion phases in the lymphoid organs, the integration of signals 2 and 3 greatly influences the outcomes of CD8+ T-cell responses, which include full clonal expansion and acquisition of effector function (state 1), limited clonal expansion without effector function (state 2), or antigen-specific unresponsiveness/anergy (state 3). CD28 is also a critical co-stimulatory receptor during the priming and expansion phases of CD8+ T cells (Azuma et al. 1992a; Azuma and Lanier 1995; Harding and Allison 1993). In cooperation with CD28, the induction of 4-1BB after activation also contributes to the expansion phase of CD8+ T cells (Shuford et al. 1997; Tan et al. 1999). IL-2 secreted from CD4+ T cells and CD4+ T-cell-mediated DC activation through CD40 signals enables Ag-primed CD8+ T cells to achieve full clonal expansion and effector function (Bedoui et al. 2016). Clonally expanded CD8+ T cells with full effector function subsequently migrate to peripheral organs and then exert effector function.

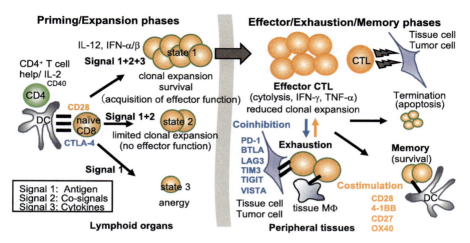

Fig. 1.4 Requirements of co-signals in CD8⁺ T cells at different phases. In addition to signals 1 and 2, full activation of naïve CD8⁺ T cells requires signal 3 during the priming and expansion phases. Signal 3 is provided by cytokines, such as IL-12 and type I IFNs. Lack of signal 3 induces limited clonal expansion without effector function. Fully differentiated CD8⁺ T cells recruit to the peripheral tissue sites to elicit effector function against infected tissue cells and tumor cells. Differential sets of co-stimulatory and co-inhibitory receptor–ligand interactions control the conversion of effector cytotoxic T lymphocytes (CTLs) into the exhausted or memory CD8⁺ T cells at peripheral tissue sites

Fully differentiated CD8⁺ T cells are able to directly interact with infected or noninfected inflammatory tissues cells, as well as tumor cells that express co-signal ligands and peptide-presenting class I MHC. It appears that the requirements for co-stimulation during the effector phase of cytolysis are much lower than during the expansion phase of CD8⁺ T-cell activation. Rather, recent reports indicate greater contributions of co-inhibitory signals, such as PD-1, which convert functional effector CD8⁺ T cells into exhausted CD8⁺ T cells (Okoye et al. 2017) and of co-stimulatory signals, such as CD28, 4-1BB, CD27, and OX40, to the survival and maintenance of memory CD8⁺ T cells (Duttagupta et al. 2009) (Fig. 1.4).

1.2.2 Co-inhibitory Receptors and CD8⁺ T-Cell Exhaustion

Exhausted CD8⁺ T cells arise at peripheral tissue sites during chronic infection and cancers. Exhausted T cells are a distinct cell lineage and are characterized by progressive loss of effector functions (e.g., production of cytokines, such as TNF-α and IFN-γ, and cytolytic function) and by sustained expression of multiple co-inhibitory receptors, such as PD-1(Okoye et al. 2017). These, co-inhibitory molecules were dubbed "immune checkpoints" by Allison, in reference to anti-CTLA-4 blockade in cancer immunotherapy (Korman et al. 2006). Ligands of co-inhibitory receptors, such as PD-L1, are abundantly induced on non-hematopoietic tissue cells, as well as on immune cells under chronic inflammatory conditions, where they bind to co-inhibitory receptors on tissue-infiltrating CD8[+] T cells (Ritprajak and Azuma 2015). Blockade of these pathways (immune checkpoint blockade) enables the conversion of exhausted CD8[+] T cells back into functional effector cells, to eliminate viral infected cells and tumor cells. CTLA-4 and/or PD-1 blockade in cancer immunotherapy demonstrates promise for tumor regression and improved patient survival (Pardoll 2012; Topalian et al. 2015). During chronic viral infections, such as human immunodeficiency virus (HIV), hepatitis C virus (HCV), cytomegalovirus (CMV), lymphocytic choriomeningitis virus (LCMV), and Epstein–Barr virus (EBV), PD-1 is also upregulated and contributes to T-cell exhaustion (Okoye et al. 2017; Rao et al. 2017).

Following CTLA-4 and PD-1, T-cell Ig and mucin-domain 3 (TIM 3) (Jones et al. 2008; Oikawa et al. 2006), lymphocyte activation gene-3 (LAG-3, CD223) (Nguyen and Ohashi 2015; Okazaki et al. 2011), V-domain Ig-containing suppressor of T-cell activation (VISTA) (Kondo et al. 2016; Wang et al. 2011), and T-cell immunoreceptor with Ig and ITIM domains (TIGIT) (Johnston et al. 2014; Yu et al. 2009) constitute the third generation of co-inhibitory receptors on exhausted CD8[+] T cells (Morris et al. 2018). These co-inhibitory pathways have also been targeted to restore the function of CD8[+] T cells in combination with PD-1 or CTLA-4 checkpoint blockade in cancer and viral infections. The mechanisms underlying sustained induction of these inhibitory receptors and how to control their expression and function will be discussed later.

1.2.3 Co-signals Required for Distinct Subsets of Helper and Regulatory T Cells

Distinct subsets of CD4[+] Th cells (Th1, Th2, Th17, and follicular helper T (T_{FH})) and regulatory T cells (Tregs) require both co-stimulatory and co-inhibitory signals for their differentiation, activation, and functional control (Gratz et al. 2013; Sun and Zhang 2014). Differential expression patterns of co-stimulatory ligands on antigen-presenting DCs, in cooperation with cytokines, polarizes Th subsets by affecting their differentiation and function. T-cell activation status via co-stimulatory signals, such as CD28, further induces additional co-signal receptors on T cells; furthermore, their activation status is fine-tuned during the differentiation process. Cytokines secreted by the polarized Th cell subsets induce various types of immune responses. Details of Th cells and their co-signal molecules are provided in Chap. 6.

Foxp3[+] Tregs are essential for maintaining self-tolerance and preventing autoimmunity. The two major types of Tregs are thymically derived Tregs and peripherally derived Tregs (Gratz et al. 2013). IL-2 is essential for their survival and function.

Despite the higher requirement for IL-2, Tregs themselves cannot produce IL-2 and instead deprive it from bystander conventional effector T cells. Otherwise, they need to receive activation signals via co-signal molecules (Zhang et al. 2015). Similar to conventional T cells, Tregs also differentiate from the resting stage to the activated functional and memory stages. Activated functional Tregs express high levels of Foxp3 and CTLA-4, which supports their suppressive function. Each stage of Tregs requires positive or negative co-signals for proliferation and functionality. The final outcomes in Tregs after receiving co-signals are very complicated and diverse (Bour-Jordan et al. 2011). For example, both GITR and OX40 are highly expressed on Tregs. GITR-mediated co-stimulation augments the suppressive activity of Tregs, whereas OX40-mediated co-stimulation inhibits the suppressive function of Tregs by downregulating Foxp3 expression (Igarashi et al. 2008; Kinnear et al. 2013; Valzasina et al. 2005; Vu et al. 2007). Details of Tregs and co-signal molecules are provided in Chap. 7.

1.2.4 Co-signals Beyond T Cells

T and B cells are not the only immune cells that require co-signals. Immune cells including NK, NKT cells, γδ T cells, monocytes, macrophages, DCs, and mast cells also require additional modification signals beyond primary triggering. For example, pattern recognition receptors (PRRs), such as Toll-like receptors (TLRs), trigger primary signals in macrophages and DCs, while activating NK receptors, such as NKG2D and NKp30/NKp44/NKp46, trigger primary signals in NK cells. Chen proposed the tide model of the control of immune responses (Zhu et al. 2011), in which co-signals, either co-stimulatory and co-inhibitory, are modulators that decide the direction and magnitude of the immune response. The primary signal is the initiator, but it is not sufficient to induce a biologically significant response. The balance between co-stimulatory and co-inhibitory molecules at each stage decides the cell's response. The ratio of primary triggering signals to co-signals for a given response is dependent on the state of the immune cell, which is tightly controlled by the different set of co-stimulatory and co-inhibitory molecules on the cell surface. Reverse or bidirectional signals have been demonstrated in many co-signal pathways. In addition to trans cell-cell interactions between a T cell and an APC, cis-interactions on a T cell or an APC further fine-tune the immune response. The interactions of co-signal molecules in immune responses are considerably more complicated than initially thought and help finely control immune responses across time and place.

References

Agata Y, Kawasaki A, Nishimura H, Ishida Y, Tsubata T, Yagita H, Honjo T (1996) Expression of the PD-1 antigen on the surface of stimulated mouse T and B lymphocytes. Int Immunol 8:765–772

Akiba H, Oshima H, Takeda K, Atsuta M, Nakano H, Nakajima A, Nohara C, Yagita H, Okumura K (1999) CD28-independent costimulation of T cells by OX40 ligand and CD70 on activated B cells. J Immunol 162:7058–7066

Ansari MJ, Salama AD, Chitnis T, Smith RN, Yagita H, Akiba H, Yamazaki T, Azuma M, Iwai H, Khoury SJ et al (2003) The programmed death-1 (PD-1) pathway regulates autoimmune diabetes in nonobese diabetic (NOD) mice. J Exp Med 198:63–69

Aruffo A, Seed B (1987) Molecular cloning of a CD28 cDNA by a high-efficiency COS cell expression system. Proc Natl Acad Sci U S A 84:8573–8577

Azuma M, Lanier LL (1995) The role of CD28 costimulation in the generation of cytotoxic T lymphocytes. Curr Top Microbiol Immunol 198:59–74

Azuma M, Cayabyab M, Buck D, Phillips JH, Lanier LL (1992a) CD28 interaction with B7 costimulates primary allogeneic proliferative responses and cytotoxicity mediated by small, resting T lymphocytes. J Exp Med 175:353–360

Azuma M, Cayabyab M, Buck D, Phillips JH, Lanier LL (1992b) Involvement of CD28 in MHC-unrestricted cytotoxicity mediated by a human natural killer leukemia cell line. J Immunol 149:1115–1123

Azuma M, Ito D, Yagita H, Okumura K, Phillips JH, Lanier LL, Somoza C (1993) B70 antigen is a second ligand for CTLA-4 and CD28. Nature 366:76–79

Baxter AG, Hodgkin PD (2002) Activation rules: the two-signal theories of immune activation. Nat Rev Immunol 2:439–446

Bedoui S, Heath WR, Mueller SN (2016) CD4(+) T-cell help amplifies innate signals for primary CD8(+) T-cell immunity. Immunol Rev 272:52–64

Bour-Jordan H, Esensten JH, Martinez-Llordella M, Penaranda C, Stumpf M, Bluestone JA (2011) Intrinsic and extrinsic control of peripheral T-cell tolerance by costimulatory molecules of the CD28/B7 family. Immunol Rev 241:180–205

Bradshaw JD, Lu P, Leytze G, Rodgers J, Schieven GL, Bennett KL, Linsley PS, Kurtz SE (1997) Interaction of the cytoplasmic tail of CTLA-4 (CD152) with a clathrin-associated protein is negatively regulated by tyrosine phosphorylation. Biochemistry 36:15975–15982

Bretscher P, Cohn M (1970) A theory of self-nonself discrimination. Science 169:1042–1049

Brunet JF, Denizot F, Luciani MF, Roux-Dosseto M, Suzan M, Mattei MG, Golstein P (1987) A new member of the immunoglobulin superfamily--CTLA-4. Nature 328:267–270

Cai G, Freeman GJ (2009) The CD160, BTLA, LIGHT/HVEM pathway: a bidirectional switch regulating T-cell activation. Immunol Rev 229:244–258

Carreno BM, Collins M (2002) The B7 family of ligands and its receptors: new pathways for costimulation and inhibition of immune responses. Annu Rev Immunol 20:29–53

Carreno BM, Collins M (2003) BTLA: a new inhibitory receptor with a B7-like ligand. Trends Immunol 24:524–527

Carter L, Fouser LA, Jussif J, Fitz L, Deng B, Wood CR, Collins M, Honjo T, Freeman GJ, Carreno BM (2002) PD-1:PD-L inhibitory pathway affects both CD4(+) and CD8(+) T cells and is overcome by IL-2. Eur J Immunol 32:634–643

Caux C, Vanbervliet B, Massacrier C, Azuma M, Okumura K, Lanier LL, Banchereau J (1994) B70/B7-2 is identical to CD86 and is the major functional ligand for CD28 expressed on human dendritic cells. J Exp Med 180:1841–1847

Chambers CA, Allison JP (1999) Costimulatory regulation of T cell function. Curr Opin Cell Biol 11:203–210

Chambers CA, Sullivan TJ, Allison JP (1997) Lymphoproliferation in CTLA-4-deficient mice is mediated by costimulation-dependent activation of CD4+ T cells. Immunity 7:885–895

1 Co-signal Molecules in T-Cell Activation

Chambers CA, Sullivan TJ, Truong T, Allison JP (1998) Secondary but not primary T cell responses are enhanced in CTLA-4-deficient CD8+ T cells. Eur J Immunol 28:3137–3143

Chambers CA, Kuhns MS, Allison JP (1999) Cytotoxic T lymphocyte antigen-4 (CTLA-4) regulates primary and secondary peptide-specific CD4(+) T cell responses. Proc Natl Acad Sci U S A 96:8603–8608

Chapoval AI, Ni J, Lau JS, Wilcox RA, Flies DB, Liu D, Dong H, Sica GL, Zhu G, Tamada K, Chen L (2001) B7-H3: a costimulatory molecule for T cell activation and IFN-gamma production. Nat Immunol 2:269–274

Chemnitz JM, Parry RV, Nichols KE, June CH, Riley JL (2004) SHP-1 and SHP-2 associate with immunoreceptor tyrosine-based switch motif of programmed death 1 upon primary human T cell stimulation, but only receptor ligation prevents T cell activation. J Immunol 173:945–954

Chen L (2004) Co-inhibitory molecules of the B7-CD28 family in the control of T-cell immunity. Nat Rev Immunol 4:336–347

Choi IH, Zhu G, Sica GL, Strome SE, Cheville JC, Lau JS, Zhu Y, Flies DB, Tamada K, Chen L (2003) Genomic organization and expression analysis of B7-H4, an immune inhibitory molecule of the B7 family. J Immunol 171:4650–4654

Cunningham AJ, Lafferty KJ (1977) A simple conservative explanation of the H-2 restriction of interactions between lymphocytes. Scand J Immunol 6:1–6

Damle NK, Hansen JA, Good RA, Gupta S (1981) Monoclonal antibody analysis of human T lymphocyte subpopulations exhibiting autologous mixed lymphocyte reaction. Proc Natl Acad Sci U S A 78:5096–5098

Dariavach P, Mattei MG, Golstein P, Lefranc MP (1988) Human Ig superfamily CTLA-4 gene: chromosomal localization and identity of protein sequence between murine and human CTLA-4 cytoplasmic domains. Eur J Immunol 18:1901–1905

DeBenedette MA, Chu NR, Pollok KE, Hurtado J, Wade WF, Kwon BS, Watts TH (1995) Role of 4-1BB ligand in costimulation of T lymphocyte growth and its upregulation on M12 B lymphomas by cAMP. J Exp Med 181:985–992

del Rio ML, Lucas CL, Buhler L, Rayat G, Rodriguez-Barbosa JI (2010) HVEM/LIGHT/BTLA/CD160 cosignaling pathways as targets for immune regulation. J Leukoc Biol 87:223–235

Dong H, Zhu G, Tamada K, Chen L (1999) B7-H1, a third member of the B7 family, co-stimulates T-cell proliferation and interleukin-10 secretion. Nat Med 5:1365–1369

Dong H, Zhu G, Tamada K, Flies DB, van Deursen JM, Chen L (2004) B7-H1 determines accumulation and deletion of intrahepatic CD8(+) T lymphocytes. Immunity 20:327–336

Duttagupta PA, Boesteanu AC, Katsikis PD (2009) Costimulation signals for memory CD8+ T cells during viral infections. Crit Rev Immunol 29:469–486

Fife BT, Guleria I, Gubbels Bupp M, Eagar TN, Tang Q, Bour-Jordan H, Yagita H, Azuma M, Sayegh MH, Bluestone JA (2006) Insulin-induced remission in new-onset NOD mice is maintained by the PD-1-PD-L1 pathway. J Exp Med 203:2737–2747

Fife BT, Pauken KE, Eagar TN, Obu T, Wu J, Tang Q, Azuma M, Krummel MF, Bluestone JA (2009) Interactions between PD-1 and PD-L1 promote tolerance by blocking the TCR-induced stop signal. Nat Immunol 10:1185–1192

Freeman GJ, Borriello F, Hodes RJ, Reiser H, Gribben JG, Ng JW, Kim J, Goldberg JM, Hathcock K, Laszlo G et al (1993a) Murine B7-2, an alternative CTLA4 counter-receptor that costimulates T cell proliferation and interleukin 2 production. J Exp Med 178:2185–2192

Freeman GJ, Borriello F, Hodes RJ, Reiser H, Hathcock KS, Laszlo G, McKnight AJ, Kim J, Du L, Lombard DB et al (1993b) Uncovering of functional alternative CTLA-4 counter-receptor in B7-deficient mice. Science 262:907–909

Freeman GJ, Gribben JG, Boussiotis VA, Ng JW, Restivo VA Jr, Lombard LA, Gray GS, Nadler LM (1993c) Cloning of B7-2: a CTLA-4 counter-receptor that costimulates human T cell proliferation. Science 262:909–911

Freeman GJ, Long AJ, Iwai Y, Bourque K, Chernova T, Nishimura H, Fitz LJ, Malenkovich N, Okazaki T, Byrne MC et al (2000) Engagement of the PD-1 immunoinhibitory receptor by a novel B7 family member leads to negative regulation of lymphocyte activation. J Exp Med 192:1027–1034

Gimmi CD, Freeman GJ, Gribben JG, Sugita K, Freedman AS, Morimoto C, Nadler LM (1991) B-cell surface antigen B7 provides a costimulatory signal that induces T cells to proliferate and secrete interleukin 2. Proc Natl Acad Sci U S A 88:6575–6579

Gimmi CD, Freeman GJ, Gribben JG, Gray G, Nadler LM (1993) Human T-cell clonal anergy is induced by antigen presentation in the absence of B7 costimulation. Proc Natl Acad Sci U S A 90:6586–6590

Goldberg MV, Maris CH, Hipkiss EL, Flies AS, Zhen L, Tuder RM, Grosso JF, Harris TJ, Getnet D, Whartenby KA et al (2007) Role of PD-1 and its ligand, B7-H1, in early fate decisions of CD8 T cells. Blood 110:186–192

Gonzalez LC, Loyet KM, Calemine-Fenaux J, Chauhan V, Wranik B, Ouyang W, Eaton DL (2005) A coreceptor interaction between the CD28 and TNF receptor family members B and T lymphocyte attenuator and herpesvirus entry mediator. Proc Natl Acad Sci U S A 102:1116–1121

Goodwin RG, Din WS, Davis-Smith T, Anderson DM, Gimpel SD, Sato TA, Maliszewski CR, Brannan CI, Copeland NG, Jenkins NA et al (1993) Molecular cloning of a ligand for the inducible T cell gene 4-1BB: a member of an emerging family of cytokines with homology to tumor necrosis factor. Eur J Immunol 23:2631–2641

Gratz IK, Rosenblum MD, Abbas AK (2013) The life of regulatory T cells. Ann N Y Acad Sci 1283:8–12

Greenwald RJ, Freeman GJ, Sharpe AH (2005) The B7 family revisited. Annu Rev Immunol 23:515–548

Grimbacher B, Hutloff A, Schlesier M, Glocker E, Warnatz K, Drager R, Eibel H, Fischer B, Schaffer AA, Mages HW et al (2003) Homozygous loss of ICOS is associated with adult-onset common variable immunodeficiency. Nat Immunol 4:261–268

Grohmann U, Orabona C, Fallarino F, Vacca C, Calcinaro F, Falorni A, Candeloro P, Belladonna ML, Bianchi R, Fioretti MC, Puccetti P (2002) CTLA-4-Ig regulates tryptophan catabolism in vivo. Nat Immunol 3:1097–1101

Habicht A, Dada S, Jurewicz M, Fife BT, Yagita H, Azuma M, Sayegh MH, Guleria I (2007) A link between PDL1 and T regulatory cells in fetomaternal tolerance. J Immunol 179:5211–5219

Hara T, Fu SM, Hansen JA (1985) Human T cell activation. II. A new activation pathway used by a major T cell population via a disulfide-bonded dimer of a 44 kilodalton polypeptide (9.3 antigen). J Exp Med 161:1513–1524

Harding FA, Allison JP (1993) CD28-B7 interactions allow the induction of CD8+ cytotoxic T lymphocytes in the absence of exogenous help. J Exp Med 177:1791–1796

Harding FA, McArthur JG, Gross JA, Raulet DH, Allison JP (1992) CD28-mediated signalling co-stimulates murine T cells and prevents induction of anergy in T-cell clones. Nature 356:607–609

Harper K, Balzano C, Rouvier E, Mattei MG, Luciani MF, Golstein P (1991) CTLA-4 and CD28 activated lymphocyte molecules are closely related in both mouse and human as to sequence, message expression, gene structure, and chromosomal location. J Immunol 147:1037–1044

Hashiguchi M, Kobori H, Ritprajak P, Kamimura Y, Kozono H, Azuma M (2008) Triggering receptor expressed on myeloid cell-like transcript 2 (TLT-2) is a counter-receptor for B7-H3 and enhances T cell responses. Proc Natl Acad Sci U S A 105:10495–10500

Hurtado JC, Kim SH, Pollok KE, Lee ZH, Kwon BS (1995) Potential role of 4-1BB in T cell activation. Comparison with the costimulatory molecule CD28. J Immunol 155:3360–3367

Hutloff A, Dittrich AM, Beier KC, Eljaschewitsch B, Kraft R, Anagnostopoulos I, Kroczek RA (1999) ICOS is an inducible T-cell co-stimulator structurally and functionally related to CD28. Nature 397:263–266

Igarashi H, Cao Y, Iwai H, Piao J, Kamimura Y, Hashiguchi M, Amagasa T, Azuma M (2008) GITR ligand-costimulation activates effector and regulatory functions of CD4+ T cells. Biochem Biophys Res Commun 369:1134–1138

Inaba K, Witmer-Pack M, Inaba M, Hathcock KS, Sakuta H, Azuma M, Yagita H, Okumura K, Linsley PS, Ikehara S et al (1994) The tissue distribution of the B7-2 costimulator in mice: abundant expression on dendritic cells in situ and during maturation in vitro. J Exp Med 180:1849–1860

Ishida Y, Agata Y, Shibahara K, Honjo T (1992) Induced expression of PD-1, a novel member of the immunoglobulin gene superfamily, upon programmed cell death. EMBO J 11:3887–3895

Iwai Y, Terawaki S, Ikegawa M, Okazaki T, Honjo T (2003) PD-1 inhibits antiviral immunity at the effector phase in the liver. J Exp Med 198:39–50

Jenkins MK, Schwartz RH (1987) Antigen presentation by chemically modified splenocytes induces antigen-specific T cell unresponsiveness in vitro and in vivo. J Exp Med 165:302–319

Jenkins MK, Pardoll DM, Mizuguchi J, Quill H, Schwartz RH (1987) T-cell unresponsiveness in vivo and in vitro: fine specificity of induction and molecular characterization of the unresponsive state. Immunol Rev 95:113–135

Johnston RJ, Comps-Agrar L, Hackney J, Yu X, Huseni M, Yang Y, Park S, Javinal V, Chiu H, Irving B et al (2014) The immunoreceptor TIGIT regulates antitumor and antiviral CD8(+) T cell effector function. Cancer Cell 26:923–937

Jones RB, Ndhlovu LC, Barbour JD, Sheth PM, Jha AR, Long BR, Wong JC, Satkunarajah M, Schweneker M, Chapman JM et al (2008) Tim-3 expression defines a novel population of dysfunctional T cells with highly elevated frequencies in progressive HIV-1 infection. J Exp Med 205:2763–2779

June CH, Ledbetter JA, Gillespie MM, Lindsten T, Thompson CB (1987) T-cell proliferation involving the CD28 pathway is associated with cyclosporine-resistant interleukin 2 gene expression. Mol Cell Biol 7:4472–4481

June CH, Ledbetter JA, Linsley PS, Thompson CB (1990) Role of the CD28 receptor in T-cell activation. Immunol Today 11:211–216

Jung G, Ledbetter JA, Muller-Eberhard HJ (1987) Induction of cytotoxicity in resting human T lymphocytes bound to tumor cells by antibody heteroconjugates. Proc Natl Acad Sci U S A 84:4611–4615

Kanamaru F, Youngnak P, Hashiguchi M, Nishioka T, Takahashi T, Sakaguchi S, Ishikawa I, Azuma M (2004) Costimulation via glucocorticoid-induced TNF receptor in both conventional and CD25+ regulatory CD4+ T cells. J Immunol 172:7306–7314

Kearney ER, Walunas TL, Karr RW, Morton PA, Loh DY, Bluestone JA, Jenkins MK (1995) Antigen-dependent clonal expansion of a trace population of antigen-specific CD4+ T cells in vivo is dependent on CD28 costimulation and inhibited by CTLA-4. J Immunol 155:1032–1036

Keir ME, Liang SC, Guleria I, Latchman YE, Qipo A, Albacker LA, Koulmanda M, Freeman GJ, Sayegh MH, Sharpe AH (2006) Tissue expression of PD-L1 mediates peripheral T cell tolerance. J Exp Med 203:883–895

Kinnear G, Wood KJ, Fallah-Arani F, Jones ND (2013) A diametric role for OX40 in the response of effector/memory CD4+ T cells and regulatory T cells to alloantigen. J Immunol 191:1465–1475

Kobori H, Hashiguchi M, Piao J, Kato M, Ritprajak P, Azuma M (2010) Enhancement of effector CD8+ T-cell function by tumour-associated B7-H3 and modulation of its counter-receptor triggering receptor expressed on myeloid cell-like transcript 2 at tumour sites. Immunology 130:363–373

Kojima R, Kajikawa M, Shiroishi M, Kuroki K, Maenaka K (2011) Molecular basis for herpesvirus entry mediator recognition by the human immune inhibitory receptor CD160 and its relationship to the cosignaling molecules BTLA and LIGHT. J Mol Biol 413:762–772

Kondo Y, Ohno T, Nishii N, Harada K, Yagita H, Azuma M (2016) Differential contribution of three immune checkpoint (VISTA, CTLA-4, PD-1) pathways to antitumor responses against squamous cell carcinoma. Oral Oncol 57:54–60

Korman AJ, Peggs KS, Allison JP (2006) Checkpoint blockade in cancer immunotherapy. Adv Immunol 90:297–339

Krummel MF, Sullivan TJ, Allison JP (1996) Superantigen responses and co-stimulation: CD28 and CTLA-4 have opposing effects on T cell expansion in vitro and in vivo. Int Immunol 8:519–523

Kuipers H, Muskens F, Willart M, Hijdra D, van Assema FB, Coyle AJ, Hoogsteden HC, Lambrecht BN (2006) Contribution of the PD-1 ligands/PD-1 signaling pathway to dendritic cell-mediated CD4+ T cell activation. Eur J Immunol 36:2472–2482

Lafage-Pochitaloff M, Costello R, Couez D, Simonetti J, Mannoni P, Mawas C, Olive D (1990) Human CD28 and CTLA-4 Ig superfamily genes are located on chromosome 2 at bands q33-q34. Immunogenetics 31:198–201

Lafferty KJ, Cunningham AJ (1975) A new analysis of allogeneic interactions. Aust J Exp Biol Med Sci 53:27–42

Lanier LL, O'Fallon S, Somoza C, Phillips JH, Linsley PS, Okumura K, Ito D, Azuma M (1995) CD80 (B7) and CD86 (B70) provide similar costimulatory signals for T cell proliferation, cytokine production, and generation of CTL. J Immunol 154:97–105

Latchman Y, Wood CR, Chernova T, Chaudhary D, Borde M, Chernova I, Iwai Y, Long AJ, Brown JA, Nunes R et al (2001) PD-L2 is a second ligand for PD-1 and inhibits T cell activation. Nat Immunol 2:261–268

Lee KM, Chuang E, Griffin M, Khattri R, Hong DK, Zhang W, Straus D, Samelson LE, Thompson CB, Bluestone JA (1998) Molecular basis of T cell inactivation by CTLA-4. Science 282:2263–2266

Lenschow DJ, Su GH, Zuckerman LA, Nabavi N, Jellis CL, Gray GS, Miller J, Bluestone JA (1993) Expression and functional significance of an additional ligand for CTLA-4. Proc Natl Acad Sci U S A 90:11054–11058

Lesslauer W, Koning F, Ottenhoff T, Giphart M, Goulmy E, van Rood JJ (1986) T90/44 (9.3 antigen). A cell surface molecule with a function in human T cell activation. Eur J Immunol 16:1289–1296

Lindstein T, June CH, Ledbetter JA, Stella G, Thompson CB (1989) Regulation of lymphokine messenger RNA stability by a surface-mediated T cell activation pathway. Science 244:339–343

Linsley PS, Brady W, Grosmaire L, Aruffo A, Damle NK, Ledbetter JA (1991a) Binding of the B cell activation antigen B7 to CD28 costimulates T cell proliferation and interleukin 2 mRNA accumulation. J Exp Med 173:721–730

Linsley PS, Brady W, Urnes M, Grosmaire LS, Damle NK, Ledbetter JA (1991b) CTLA-4 is a second receptor for the B cell activation antigen B7. J Exp Med 174:561–569

Linsley PS, Greene JL, Tan P, Bradshaw J, Ledbetter JA, Anasetti C, Damle NK (1992a) Coexpression and functional cooperation of CTLA-4 and CD28 on activated T lymphocytes. J Exp Med 176:1595–1604

Linsley PS, Wallace PM, Johnson J, Gibson MG, Greene JL, Ledbetter JA, Singh C, Tepper MA (1992b) Immunosuppression in vivo by a soluble form of the CTLA-4 T cell activation molecule. Science 257:792–795

Linsley PS, Bradshaw J, Greene J, Peach R, Bennett KL, Mittler RS (1996) Intracellular trafficking of CTLA-4 and focal localization towards sites of TCR engagement. Immunity 4:535–543

Mak TW, Shahinian A, Yoshinaga SK, Wakeham A, Boucher LM, Pintilie M, Duncan G, Gajewska BU, Gronski M, Eriksson U et al (2003) Costimulation through the inducible costimulator ligand is essential for both T helper and B cell functions in T cell-dependent B cell responses. Nat Immunol 4:765–772

Mallett S, Fossum S, Barclay AN (1990) Characterization of the MRC OX40 antigen of activated CD4 positive T lymphocytes--a molecule related to nerve growth factor receptor. EMBO J 9:1063–1068

Marengere LE, Waterhouse P, Duncan GS, Mittrucker HW, Feng GS, Mak TW (1996) Regulation of T cell receptor signaling by tyrosine phosphatase SYP association with CTLA-4. Science 272:1170–1173

Mescher MF, Curtsinger JM, Agarwal P, Casey KA, Gerner M, Hammerbeck CD, Popescu F, Xiao Z (2006) Signals required for programming effector and memory development by CD8+ T cells. Immunol Rev 211:81–92

Morris AB, Adams LE, Ford ML (2018) Influence of T cell Coinhibitory molecules on CD8(+) recall responses. Front Immunol 9:1810

Nakajima A, Azuma M, Kodera S, Nuriya S, Terashi A, Abe M, Hirose S, Shirai T, Yagita H, Okumura K (1995) Preferential dependence of autoantibody production in murine lupus on CD86 costimulatory molecule. Eur J Immunol 25:3060–3069

Nguyen LT, Ohashi PS (2015) Clinical blockade of PD1 and LAG3--potential mechanisms of action. Nat Rev Immunol 15:45–56

Nishimura H, Minato N, Nakano T, Honjo T (1998) Immunological studies on PD-1 deficient mice: implication of PD-1 as a negative regulator for B cell responses. Int Immunol 10:1563–1572

Nishimura H, Nose M, Hiai H, Minato N, Honjo T (1999) Development of lupus-like autoimmune diseases by disruption of the PD-1 gene encoding an ITIM motif-carrying immunoreceptor. Immunity 11:141–151

Nishimura H, Okazaki T, Tanaka Y, Nakatani K, Hara M, Matsumori A, Sasayama S, Mizoguchi A, Hiai H, Minato N, Honjo T (2001) Autoimmune dilated cardiomyopathy in PD-1 receptor-deficient mice. Science 291:319–322

Nuriya S, Yagita H, Okumura K, Azuma M (1996) The differential role of CD86 and CD80 co-stimulatory molecules in the induction and the effector phases of contact hypersensitivity. Int Immunol 8:917–926

Ohshima Y, Yang LP, Uchiyama T, Tanaka Y, Baum P, Sergerie M, Hermann P, Delespesse G (1998) OX40 costimulation enhances interleukin-4 (IL-4) expression at priming and promotes the differentiation of naive human CD4(+) T cells into high IL-4-producing effectors. Blood 92:3338–3345

Oikawa T, Kamimura Y, Akiba H, Yagita H, Okumura K, Takahashi H, Zeniya M, Tajiri H, Azuma M (2006) Preferential involvement of Tim-3 in the regulation of hepatic CD8+ T cells in murine acute graft-versus-host disease. J Immunol 177:4281–4287

Okazaki T, Maeda A, Nishimura H, Kurosaki T, Honjo T (2001) PD-1 immunoreceptor inhibits B cell receptor-mediated signaling by recruiting src homology 2-domain-containing tyrosine phosphatase 2 to phosphotyrosine. Proc Natl Acad Sci U S A 98:13866–13871

Okazaki T, Okazaki IM, Wang J, Sugiura D, Nakaki F, Yoshida T, Kato Y, Fagarasan S, Muramatsu M, Eto T et al (2011) PD-1 and LAG-3 inhibitory co-receptors act synergistically to prevent autoimmunity in mice. J Exp Med 208:395–407

Okoye IS, Houghton M, Tyrrell L, Barakat K, Elahi S (2017) Coinhibitory receptor expression and immune checkpoint blockade: maintaining a balance in CD8(+) T cell responses to chronic viral infections and Cancer. Front Immunol 8:1215

Pardoll DM (2012) The blockade of immune checkpoints in cancer immunotherapy. Nat Rev Cancer 12:252–264

Pentcheva-Hoang T, Egen JG, Wojnoonski K, Allison JP (2004) B7-1 and B7-2 selectively recruit CTLA-4 and CD28 to the immunological synapse. Immunity 21:401–413

Pollok KE, Kim YJ, Zhou Z, Hurtado J, Kim KK, Pickard RT, Kwon BS (1993) Inducible T cell antigen 4-1BB. Analysis of expression and function. J Immunol 150:771–781

Prasad DV, Richards S, Mai XM, Dong C (2003) B7S1, a novel B7 family member that negatively regulates T cell activation. Immunity 18:863–873

Rao M, Valentini D, Dodoo E, Zumla A, Maeurer M (2017) Anti-PD-1/PD-L1 therapy for infectious diseases: learning from the cancer paradigm. Int J Infect Dis 56:221–228

Ritprajak P, Azuma M (2015) Intrinsic and extrinsic control of expression of the immunoregulatory molecule PD-L1 in epithelial cells and squamous cell carcinoma. Oral Oncol 51:221–228

Ritprajak P, Hashiguchi M, Tsushima F, Chalermsarp N, Azuma M (2010) Keratinocyte-associated B7-H1 directly regulates cutaneous effector CD8+ T cell responses. J Immunol 184:4918–4925

Rudd CE (2008) The reverse stop-signal model for CTLA4 function. Nat Rev Immunol 8:153–160

Salama AD, Chitnis T, Imitola J, Ansari MJ, Akiba H, Tushima F, Azuma M, Yagita H, Sayegh MH, Khoury SJ (2003) Critical role of the programmed death-1 (PD-1) pathway in regulation of experimental autoimmune encephalomyelitis. J Exp Med 198:71–78

Schildberg FA, Klein SR, Freeman GJ, Sharpe AH (2016) Coinhibitory pathways in the B7-CD28 ligand-receptor family. Immunity 44:955–972

Schneider H, Downey J, Smith A, Zinselmeyer BH, Rush C, Brewer JM, Wei B, Hogg N, Garside P, Rudd CE (2006) Reversal of the TCR stop signal by CTLA-4. Science 313:1972–1975

Schwartz RH (1990) A cell culture model for T lymphocyte clonal anergy. Science 248:1349–1356

Schwartz RH (1992) Costimulation of T lymphocytes: the role of CD28, CTLA-4, and B7/BB1 in interleukin-2 production and immunotherapy. Cell 71:1065–1068

Sedy JR, Gavrieli M, Potter KG, Hurchla MA, Lindsley RC, Hildner K, Scheu S, Pfeffer K, Ware CF, Murphy TL, Murphy KM (2005) B and T lymphocyte attenuator regulates T cell activation through interaction with herpesvirus entry mediator. Nat Immunol 6:90–98

Sheppard KA, Fitz LJ, Lee JM, Benander C, George JA, Wooters J, Qiu Y, Jussif JM, Carter LL, Wood CR, Chaudhary D (2004) PD-1 inhibits T-cell receptor induced phosphorylation of the ZAP70/CD3zeta signalosome and downstream signaling to PKCtheta. FEBS Lett 574:37–41

Shiratori T, Miyatake S, Ohno H, Nakaseko C, Isono K, Bonifacino JS, Saito T (1997) Tyrosine phosphorylation controls internalization of CTLA-4 by regulating its interaction with clathrin-associated adaptor complex AP-2. Immunity 6:583–589

Shuford WW, Klussman K, Tritchler DD, Loo DT, Chalupny J, Siadak AW, Brown TJ, Emswiler J, Raecho H, Larsen CP et al (1997) 4-1BB costimulatory signals preferentially induce CD8+ T cell proliferation and lead to the amplification in vivo of cytotoxic T cell responses. J Exp Med 186:47–55

Sica GL, Choi IH, Zhu G, Tamada K, Wang SD, Tamura H, Chapoval AI, Flies DB, Bajorath J, Chen L (2003) B7-H4, a molecule of the B7 family, negatively regulates T cell immunity. Immunity 18:849–861

Smith KM, Brewer JM, Webb P, Coyle AJ, Gutierrez-Ramos C, Garside P (2003) Inducible costimulatory molecule-B7-related protein 1 interactions are important for the clonal expansion and B cell helper functions of naive, Th1, and Th2 cells. J Immunol 170:2310–2315

Suh WK, Gajewska BU, Okada H, Gronski MA, Bertram EM, Dawicki W, Duncan GS, Bukczynski J, Plyte S, Elia A et al (2003) The B7 family member B7-H3 preferentially down-regulates T helper type 1-mediated immune responses. Nat Immunol 4:899–906

Sun B, Zhang Y (2014) Overview of orchestration of CD4+ T cell subsets in immune responses. Adv Exp Med Biol 841:1–13

Sun M, Richards S, Prasad DV, Mai XM, Rudensky A, Dong C (2002) Characterization of mouse and human B7-H3 genes. J Immunol 168:6294–6297

Tan JT, Whitmire JK, Ahmed R, Pearson TC, Larsen CP (1999) 4-1BB ligand, a member of the TNF family, is important for the generation of antiviral CD8 T cell responses. J Immunol 163:4859–4868

Tanaka K, Albin MJ, Yuan X, Yamaura K, Habicht A, Murayama T, Grimm M, Waaga AM, Ueno T, Padera RF et al (2007) PDL1 is required for peripheral transplantation tolerance and protection from chronic allograft rejection. J Immunol 179:5204–5210

Thompson CB, Allison JP (1997) The emerging role of CTLA-4 as an immune attenuator. Immunity 7:445–450

Tivol EA, Borriello F, Schweitzer AN, Lynch WP, Bluestone JA, Sharpe AH (1995) Loss of CTLA-4 leads to massive lymphoproliferation and fatal multiorgan tissue destruction, revealing a critical negative regulatory role of CTLA-4. Immunity 3:541–547

Tone M, Tone Y, Adams E, Yates SF, Frewin MR, Cobbold SP, Waldmann H (2003) Mouse glucocorticoid-induced tumor necrosis factor receptor ligand is costimulatory for T cells. Proc Natl Acad Sci U S A 100:15059–15064

Topalian SL, Drake CG, Pardoll DM (2015) Immune checkpoint blockade: a common denominator approach to cancer therapy. Cancer Cell 27:450–461

Tseng SY, Otsuji M, Gorski K, Huang X, Slansky JE, Pai SI, Shalabi A, Shin T, Pardoll DM, Tsuchiya H (2001) B7-DC, a new dendritic cell molecule with potent costimulatory properties for T cells. J Exp Med 193:839–846

Valbon SF, Condotta SA, Richer MJ (2016) Regulation of effector and memory CD8(+) T cell function by inflammatory cytokines. Cytokine 82:16–23

Valzasina B, Guiducci C, Dislich H, Killeen N, Weinberg AD, Colombo MP (2005) Triggering of OX40 (CD134) on CD4(+)CD25+ T cells blocks their inhibitory activity: a novel regulatory role for OX40 and its comparison with GITR. Blood 105:2845–2851

Vu MD, Xiao X, Gao W, Degauque N, Chen M, Kroemer A, Killeen N, Ishii N, Li XC (2007) OX40 costimulation turns off Foxp3+ Tregs. Blood 110:2501–2510

Wang S, Zhu G, Chapoval AI, Dong H, Tamada K, Ni J, Chen L (2000) Costimulation of T cells by B7-H2, a B7-like molecule that binds ICOS. Blood 96:2808–2813

Wang L, Rubinstein R, Lines JL, Wasiuk A, Ahonen C, Guo Y, Lu LF, Gondek D, Wang Y, Fava RA et al (2011) VISTA, a novel mouse Ig superfamily ligand that negatively regulates T cell responses. J Exp Med 208:577–592

Ward-Kavanagh LK, Lin WW, Sedy JR, Ware CF (2016) The TNF receptor superfamily in co-stimulating and co-inhibitory responses. Immunity 44:1005–1019

Watanabe N, Gavrieli M, Sedy JR, Yang J, Fallarino F, Loftin SK, Hurchla MA, Zimmerman N, Sim J, Zang X et al (2003) BTLA is a lymphocyte inhibitory receptor with similarities to CTLA-4 and PD-1. Nat Immunol 4:670–679

Waterhouse P, Penninger JM, Timms E, Wakeham A, Shahinian A, Lee KP, Thompson CB, Griesser H, Mak TW (1995) Lymphoproliferative disorders with early lethality in mice deficient in Ctla-4. Science 270:985–988

Watts TH (2005) TNF/TNFR family members in costimulation of T cell responses. Annu Rev Immunol 23:23–68

Yamazaki T, Akiba H, Iwai H, Matsuda H, Aoki M, Tanno Y, Shin T, Tsuchiya H, Pardoll DM, Okumura K et al (2002) Expression of programmed death 1 ligands by murine T cells and APC. J Immunol 169:5538–5545

Yi KH, Chen L (2009) Fine tuning the immune response through B7-H3 and B7-H4. Immunol Rev 229:145–151

Yokosuka T, Takamatsu M, Kobayashi-Imanishi W, Hashimoto-Tane A, Azuma M, Saito T (2012) Programmed cell death 1 forms negative costimulatory microclusters that directly inhibit T cell receptor signaling by recruiting phosphatase SHP2. J Exp Med 209:1201–1217

Yu X, Harden K, Gonzalez LC, Francesco M, Chiang E, Irving B, Tom I, Ivelja S, Refino CJ, Clark H et al (2009) The surface protein TIGIT suppresses T cell activation by promoting the generation of mature immunoregulatory dendritic cells. Nat Immunol 10:48–57

Zang X, Loke P, Kim J, Murphy K, Waitz R, Allison JP (2003) B7x: a widely expressed B7 family member that inhibits T cell activation. Proc Natl Acad Sci U S A 100:10388–10392

Zhang R, Borges CM, Fan MY, Harris JE, Turka LA (2015) Requirement for CD28 in effector regulatory T cell differentiation, CCR6 induction, and skin homing. J Immunol 195:4154–4161

Zhu Y, Yao S, Chen L (2011) Cell surface signaling molecules in the control of immune responses: a tide model. Immunity 34:466–478

Chapter 2
The CD28–B7 Family of Co-signaling Molecules

Shigenori Nagai and Miyuki Azuma

Abstract Immune responses are controlled by the optimal balance between protective immunity and immune tolerance. T-cell receptor (TCR) signals are modulated by co-signaling molecules, which are divided into co-stimulatory and co-inhibitory molecules. By expression at the appropriate time and location, co-signaling molecules positively and negatively control T-cell differentiation and function. For example, ligation of the CD28 on T cells provides a critical secondary signal along with TCR ligation for naive T-cell activation. In contrast, co-inhibitory signaling by the CD28–B7 family is important to regulate immune homeostasis and host defense, as these signals limit the strength and duration of immune responses to prevent autoimmunity. At the same time, microorganisms or tumor cells can use these pathways to establish an immunosuppressive environment to inhibit the immune responses against themselves. Understanding these co-inhibitory pathways will support the development of new immunotherapy for the treatment of tumors and autoimmune and infectious diseases. Here, we introduce diverse molecules belonging to the members of the CD28–B7 family.

Keywords Co-stimulation · Co-inhibition · TCR signaling · Immunoglobulin superfamily · IgV · IgC

2.1 Introduction of B7/CD28 Members

Although T-cell receptors (TCRs) were initially discovered through their role in T cells' recognition of antigens, it soon became clear that TCRs alone do not completely control the activation of T cells because ligation of TCRs results in T-cell

---

S. Nagai (✉) · M. Azuma
Department of Molecular Immunology, Graduate School of Medical and Dental Sciences,
Tokyo Medical and Dental University, Tokyo, Japan
e-mail: nagai.mim@tmd.ac.jp; miyuki.mim@tmd.ac.jp

© Springer Nature Singapore Pte Ltd. 2019
M. Azuma, H. Yagita (eds.), *Co-signal Molecules in T Cell Activation*,
Advances in Experimental Medicine and Biology 1189,
https://doi.org/10.1007/978-981-32-9717-3_2

unresponsiveness (anergy). This finding drove researchers to discover the secondary signals called "co-stimulatory signals" in the 1980s. It was revealed that a monoclonal antibody against CD28 could provide a secondary signal which, in combination with the immobilization of TCR, induced T-cell activation (Weiss et al. 1986). CD28 itself induces several intracellular events, such as the production of cytokines and the transduction of signals triggering T cells to survive or to differentiate. Of note, treatment with a soluble antagonist of CD28 affected immune tolerance by preventing the development of autoimmune diseases as well as graft-versus-host reaction. In contrast, CD28 agonists have emerged as a new type of immunostimulator, especially in antitumor treatments. It has become clear that the CD28 molecule not only supports TCR signaling but engages in its own signaling to regulate intracellular events, such as phosphorylation or epigenetic changes in T cells. Furthermore, several surface molecules sharing homology with CD28 and its ligands have been identified, which makes the complete picture of the roles of receptor–ligand interaction much more complicated. For example, although CD80 (B7-1) and CD86 (B7-2) were initially identified as ligands by which CD28 could induce positive, that is, T-cell proliferative signals, they can also bind with CTLA-4 to suppress excessive T-cell proliferation. We introduce the function of CD28–B7-related co-signaling in this chapter.

CD28 is an originator of co-stimulatory molecules, each of which has an immunoglobulin-like domain in its extracellular region. Other members of this family include CTLA-4, ICOS, PD-1, TMIGD2, and VISTA. Although CD28 is constitutively expressed on T cells, ICOS and CTLA-4 are induced after stimulation of T cells. The ligands of CD28, CD80 and CD86 give diverse expression patterns, which have led to some confusion about the function of CD28 signaling. CD80 exists as a dimer on the cell surface, whereas CD86 exists as a monomer (Bhatia et al. 2005). Compared to CD80, CD86 expression is more rapidly upregulated on the surface of antigen-presenting cells (APCs) after stimulation, indicating that CD86 plays more important roles in the initial immune responses (Hathcock et al. 1994). For example, CD86-deficient mice immunized using antigens without adjuvant could not switch antibody isotypes or form germinal centers, though there were no such defects in CD80-deficient mice (Borriello et al. 1997).

CTLA-4 shares homology with CD28, and the two molecules compete with one another to bind their ligands, which are CD80 and CD86 (Linsley et al. 1991). The binding affinity of CTLA-4 for these ligands is stronger than its affinity for CD28, leading to the suppression of effector T-cell responses (Engelhardt et al. 2006). Yet although the binding affinity of CTLA-4 to CD80 and CD86 is stronger than that of CD28, when CTLA-4 and CD28 are in competition, CD86 prefers to CD28, which binds strongly to CTLA-4. In the context, the expression of CD86 followed by that of CD80 may act to increase the suppression by CTLA-4 when an immune response has initiated, given that the interaction between CTLA-4 and CD80 in the later phase is so strong (van der Merwe and Davis 2003).

In T-cell response, CD28 and CTLA-4 serve as activating or an inhibitory signals, respectively, and are regarded as prototypes for immune checkpoint molecules (Krummel and Allison 1995). In addition, ICOS, which is involved in T-cell activation, binds to ICOSL (B7-H2), which can also bind to human CD28 and CTLA-4 as a ligand (Chen et al. 2013). The existence of many possible combinations of these receptors and ligands increases the complexity of the immunological phenotype. Altogether, the opposing effects of these molecules regulate the immune responses via competition between activating and inhibitory signals. These complexities of these binding characteristics yield complex biological effects. However, these receptors are not able to substitute for each other in terms of their biological function. For example, although the *ICOS* gene emerged through the duplication of *CD28*, which is the adjacent and evolutionarily more ancient gene, the differences between these molecules is critical because, whereas ICOSL is ubiquitously and constitutively expressed, ligands for CD28 are inducible (Linterman et al. 2009). CD80 and CD86 may act as receptors for signal transduction because these molecules regulate tryptophan metabolism in APCs when these molecules are ligated with CTLA-4 Ig (Grohmann et al. 2002).

2.2 CD28

2.2.1 Structure and Ligand Binding of CD28

Human CD28 is composed of four exons encoding 220 amino acids. It is expressed on the cell surface, glycosylated, and homodimerized by disulfide bonds. Members of the CD28 family share a number of common features (Fig. 2.1). This molecule consists of

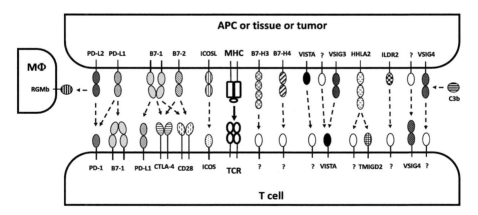

Fig. 2.1 Co-inhibitory pathways in the CD28-B7 family. T cells are activated by the recognition of antigen peptides presented by APCs. T-cell co-stimulatory signals are provided by CD28 interactions with CD80 and CD86. Upon T-cell activation, the expression levels of many co-inhibitory molecules are upregulated; these molecules attenuate TCR and its co-stimulatory signals to control T-cell responses in naive, effector, regulatory, memory, and exhausted T cells. These receptors are expressed on T cells and some are also expressed on other leukocytes. The ligands can be expressed on APCs, nonhematopoietic tissue cells, and tumor cells. In addition, some molecules are expressed on both APCs and T cells. The binding partners for some molecules have not yet been identified

a paired V-set of immunoglobulin (Ig) superfamily domains attached to single-transmembrane domains and cytoplasmic domains that contain signaling motifs (Carreno and Collins 2002). The ligands of CD28 are CD80 and CD86, each of which consists of a single V-set and C1-set Ig superfamily domains. The interaction is mediated through the MYPPPY motif of the V-set domains in the receptor (Metzler et al. 1997).

Analyses of the crystal structure have revealed that both CTLA-4 and CD28 share highly similar CDR3 analogous loops (Schwartz et al. 2002) (Zhang et al. 2003). Important insights into the different binding specificities and stoichiometric properties of CD28 have been gained through analyses of the crystal structure of the monomeric form of the ectodomain of CD28 complexed with the Fab of anti-CD28 antibody (Evans et al. 2005). Binding of CD80 onto the CD28 homodimer showed important differences in the orientations of CD28–CD80 versus CTLA-4 complexes. Since the two CD80 molecules come together in the CD28-CD80 complex, their membrane proximal domains clash three-dimensionally in spite of the accessibility of ligand-binding sites on CD28. In contrast, in the interface of the CTLA-dimer, a greater angle between the ligand-binding sites removes steric interference and allows for bivalent binding (Evans et al. 2005; Stamper et al. 2001). These results indicate that oligomeric interaction is more feasible between CTLA-4 and CD80 than between CD28 and CD80.

Oligomerization of protein is involved in a critical regulatory feature in the interaction of counter-receptor on T cells (Bhatia et al. 2005). CD86 exists as a monomer on the cell surface whereas CD80 predominantly exists as a dimer on the cell surface (Girard et al. 2014). IgC domains of these molecules prevent higher oligomer formation to maintain optimal binding to CD28 in T cells. Because CD28 prefers to bind with monomeric ligands whereas CTLA-4 prefers to bind with dimeric ligands, the ratio of CD80/CD86 in monomeric or oligomeric forms may play an important role regulating T-cell signaling by affecting the avidity of these interactions.

2.2.2 Regulation of T-Cell Activation by CD28 Pathway

It has been reported that CD28 augments the TCR signaling pathway as well as mediating unique signaling events (Boomer and Green 2010). However, it is difficult to clarify the mechanisms by which CD28 is involved in optimizing T-cell responses unless we study CD28-interacting proteins or mutate its cytoplasmic domain. CD28 co-stimulation has several effects on T cells, including biological events at the immunological synapse, downstream phosphorylation and post-translational modifications, transcriptional changes, and cytoskeletal remodeling. Basically, CD28 signals increase the glycolytic rate and thereby generate the energy for proliferation (Frauwirth et al. 2002).

2 The CD28–B7 Family of Co-signaling Molecules

2.2.2.1 CD28 and the Immunological Synapse

At the contact site between the APC and T cell, specific molecules must be organized and coordinated in a particular way for TCR signaling and co-signaling to occur. The immunological synapse (IS), a highly organized and spatially distinct structure, is composed of central, peripheral, and distal supramolecular activation complexes (SMACs). The CD28 molecule associates with these interactions and is enriched adjacent to the central supramolecular activation cluster (cSMAC) with TCR, CD4, Lck, and so on (Saito et al. 2010; Sanchez-Lockhart et al. 2008). Many molecules are known to localize onto and below the T-cell membrane for IS formation, including CD28, which regulates the spatial localization of PKCθ (Yokosuka et al. 2008).

2.2.2.2 CD28 and Actin Remodeling

The function of CD28 is highlighted in thymocytes, in which CD28-mediated actin cytoskeletal changes are required to fully activate TCR signaling (Tan et al. 2014). This remodeling of the actin cytoskeleton by CD28 is necessary for phosphorylated phospholipase Cγ1 (PLCγ1) to hydrolyze its substrate PIP2. Vav1, which can potentially link with CD28, can be recruited for the stimulation of CD28 via Grb2 binding (Ramos-Morales et al. 1995). The Vav1 GEF activates Rho GTPases, which are the regulators of the actin cytoskeleton in T cells (Fischer et al. 1998a). Additionally, the constitutive binding of Vav1 to talin and vinculin, anchoring the actin cytoskeleton to the cell membrane, is regulated in a GEF-independent manner (Fischer et al. 1998b). PIP5Kα is known to be essential for CD28-mediated actin polymerization because Vav1 associated with PIP5 kinase α (PIP5Kα) is recruited to the proline-rich motif of CD28, which promotes actin polymerization (Muscolini et al. 2015). Filamin-A, which binds to the PYAP motif of CD28, tethers CD28 to lipid rafts and recruits Rac and Rho GTPases to the vicinity of Vav1 in T cells (Tavano et al. 2006).

2.2.2.3 Transcriptional and Posttranscriptional Program

CD28 signals are important for IL-2 production and Bcl-xL upregulation, both of which serve as survival factors for T cells (Boise et al. 1995; Watts 2010). CD28 ligation stabilizes the mRNA of several cytokines (Lindstein et al. 1989) and generally amplifies the gene expression patterns initiated by T-cell receptor ligation (Diehn et al. 2002). CD28 ligation alone has little effect on transcription in the absence of TCR signals, but research with CD28-dependent naïve CD4[+] T-cell subsets has shown that CD28 co-stimulation has a qualitative effect on a large number of genes after TCR stimulation (Butte et al. 2012) and that this effect is amplified over the first 24 hours after stimulation (Martinez-Llordella et al. 2013). T cells that receive TCR signaling alone in the absence of CD28 signaling are more similar to cells that have never been activated by 24 hours than they are to cells that have received both first (TCR) signaling and second (CD28) signaling. IL-2 signals are not able to rescue the transcriptional phenotype of cells stimulated with TCR alone. CD28 signals affect alternative splicing in T cells dependent on the function of hnRNPLL because the hnRNPLL transcript itself is upregulated by CD28 ligation rather than by TCR stimulation alone (Butte et al. 2012). CD28 also regulates gene expression by epigenetic changes, for example, Ezh2 induced by CD28 signals is essential to maintain Treg fate after activation because Ezh2 contributes to Foxp3-induced transcriptional repression (DuPage et al. 2015). In addition, CD28 signals induce histone acetylation and loss of cytosine methylation at the IL-2 promoter, which leads to nucleosome repositioning and binding of transcription factors to the *Il2* locus (Attema et al. 2002; Thomas et al. 2005). c-Rel is known to be required for maximal expression of IL-2, one of the CD28-dependent genes. The mechanism of c-Rel activation is due to RE/AP, a c-Rel/AP-1 composite-binding site in the promoter region of *Il2* (Kontgen et al. 1995; Shapiro et al. 1997). The role of c-Rel is involved in chromatin remodeling of the *Il2* promoter (Rao et al. 2003). Furthermore, c-Rel appears to induce Foxp3 expression which contributes to the development of Tregs in the thymus (Isomura et al. 2009; Long et al. 2009). Interestingly, c-Rel is activated by O-glycosylation on Ser350, as evidenced by the finding that mutation of this amino acid residue results in loss of binding activity to a CD28 response element (Ramakrishnan et al. 2013).

In summary, the CD28 pathway has both quantitative effects, amplifying signals initiated by TCR signaling, and qualitative effects on a variety of processes.

2.3 CTLA-4 (Cytotoxic T Lymphocyte-Associated-4)

2.3.1 Structure of CTLA-4

The *Ctla4* gene consists of four exons: the signal peptide in exon 1, the IgV-like domain composing B7 binding domain in exon 2, the transmembrane domain in exon 3, and the cytoplasmic tail in exon 4 (Brunet et al. 1987). The overall homology between the human and mouse CTLA-4 homology is 76% (Dariavach et al. 1988). The CTLA-4 has four splicing variants. Full length of CTLA-4 has four exons and possesses an IgV-like domain containing the MYPPPY motif, which is involved in binding B7-1 or B7-2 molecules (Vijayakrishnan et al. 2004). Soluble CTLA-4 lacks the TM domain which is spliced out of exon 3 (Magistrelli et al. 1999) (Oaks et al. 2000) and has a transcript encoding only exons 1 and 4, which lacks both ligand binding and TM domains (Ueda et al. 2003). Although full-length CTLA-4 is induced immediately after activation of T cells (Perkins et al. 1996), soluble CTLA-4 is detected in resting T cells (Magistrelli et al. 1999).

2.3.2 Expression of CTLA-4

CTLA-4 is induced on Foxp3 conventional T cells after activation (Freeman et al. 1992; Linsley et al. 1992), but is constitutively expressed on Foxp3$^+$CD4$^+$ Treg cell (Takahashi et al. 2000). Furthermore, CTLA-4 is also expressed on other leukocytes, such as DCs, monocytes, B cells, granulocytes, and CD34$^+$ stem cells (Pistillo et al. 2003). CTLA-4 expression is controlled by transcriptional and posttranscriptional regulation in T cells. Two transcription factors Foxp3 and NFAT are able to regulate *Ctla4* (Gibson et al. 2007; Miller et al. 2002; Wu et al. 2006; Zheng et al. 2007). The stability of mRNA is regulated by the 3' UTR, and this affects the translation efficiency of CTLA-4 (Malquori et al. 2008). In addition, miR145 and miR-155 regulates CTLA-4 expression (de Jong et al. 2013; Sonkoly et al. 2010).

A small proportion of CTLA-4 is detected on the cell surface of resting T cells, and most of CTLA-4 molecules are localized in Golgi apparatus, endosomes, and lysosomes. CTLA-4 circulates to the cell surface, but is then internalized by unphosphorylated cytoplasmic domains and either recycled to the plasma membrane or subjected to lysosomal degradation (Qureshi et al. 2012). Intracellular trafficking of CTLA-4 is mediated by the association of the cytoplasmic domain of CTLA-4 with AP-1 and AP-2, clathrin-associated adaptor proteins involved in the recognition, and recruitment of proteins into coated pits (Schneider et al. 1999). The cytoplasmic region of unphosphorylated CTLA-4 binds to AP-2, thereby promoting rapid internalization, while at the same time the phosphorylation of the cytoplasmic domain retards internalization of CTLA-4. Association with AP-1 blocks access from the trans-Golgi network to lysosomal compartments for degradation of CTLA-4, regulating the amount of CTLA-4 in the trans-Golgi network. Endosomes containing CTLA-4 are recruited to the cell surface upon T-cell activation by the regulation of lipopolysaccharide-responsive and beige-like anchor protein (LRBA), which rescues CTLA-4 from entering the lysosomal pathway (Lo et al. 2015).

Upon TCR stimulation, CTLA-4 is released to the cell surface and localizes to the immune synapses in quantities relative to the strength of TCR stimulation (Linsley et al. 1996). These mechanisms might give feedback that inhibits T-cell activation. T-cell receptor-interacting molecule (TRIM) transports CTLA-4 to the cell surface in cooperation with phospholipase D (PLD) and ADP ribosylation factor-1 (ARF-1) (Mead et al. 2005; Valk et al. 2006). These findings demonstrate that CTLA-4 expression is regulated by both transcriptional and posttranscriptional machinery, such as vesicle transport, endocytosis, and recycling, which allow spatiotemporal inhibition of T-cell activation by the CTLA-4-mediated signaling pathway.

2.3.3 CTLA-4 Functions

The main function of CTLA-4 is to regulate T-cell activation and T-cell tolerance. CTLA-4 negatively regulates IL-2 production, IL-2R expression, and cell cycle progression of activated T cells (Walunas et al. 1996). CTLA-4 also affects helper T

(Th)-cell differentiation. CTLA-4 deficiency increases Th2 differentiation (Bour-Jordan et al. 2003), while CTLA-4 blockade enhances Th17 differentiation (Ying et al. 2010). It is particularly worth noting that Foxp3[+] Treg cells constitutively express CTLA-4, which is a target of Foxp3 (Wu et al. 2006; Zheng et al. 2007). Foxp3-specific CTLA-4 deletion results in autoimmune diseases due to the lymphoprolifera-tive effect, since these Tregs in this situation lose their suppressive activity and also increase in number (Wing et al. 2008). However, Tregs retain their suppressive activ-ity when CTLA-4 is deleted by tamoxifen treatment in adult mice (Paterson et al. 2015), suggesting that CTLA-4 has different roles in neonatal period and adulthood.

CTLA-4 can inhibit T-cell responses by several mechanisms. Intrinsically, CTLA-4 competes with CD28 for their shared ligands, B7-1 and B7-2 (van der Merwe et al. 1997); CTLA-4 also delivers inhibitory signals that induce cell cycle arrest and inhibit IL-2 production (Krummel and Allison 1996; Walunas et al. 1996) and limits T-cell staying time with APCs (Schneider et al. 2006). Within T cells, the phosphorylated cytoplasmic domain of CTLA-4 interacts with phosphatases, such as PP2A, inhibiting TCR/CD28 activation (Chuang et al. 2000). Especially in Tregs, interaction between CTLA-4 and phosphorylated PKC requires contact-dependent suppression of effector T-cell function (Kong et al. 2014). The extrinsic effects of CTLA-4 are thought to down-modulate B7-1 and B7-2 expression on APCs, reducing the availability of B7-CD28 co-stimulatory signals (Qureshi et al. 2012; Wing et al. 2008). Alternatively, CTLA-4 on T cells could occupy B7 molecules on APCs (Linsley et al. 1992). In addition, by the binding of CTLA-4 and B7s, DCs produce indoleamine 2,3-dioxygenase (IDO), which catalyzes oxidative catabolism of tryptophan, an important amino acid for regulating T-cell-mediated immune responses (Fallarino et al. 2003; Grohmann et al. 2002).

CTLA-4 is also expressed on DCs, B cells, and NK cells, but the roles of CTLA-4 in these cells are still not clear. CTLA-4[+] DCs have suppressive activity against T-cell responses through their expression of IL-10 and/or IDO, which define a regulatory DC subset (Han et al. 2014; Laurent et al. 2010). Heterozygous muta-tions of CTLA-4 lead to increased frequencies of autoreactive CD21 (lo) B cells (Kuehn et al. 2014). IL-2-activated NK cells express CTLA-4, which inhibits IFNγ production in response to B7-1 (Stojanovic et al. 2014).

2.4 PD-1

2.4.1 The Expression of PD-1

In T cells, PD-1 (programed cell death-1) is a 288-amino acid protein type I trans-membrane protein that consists of an immunoglobulin (Ig) domain, a short amino acid stalk, a transmembrane domain, and an intracellular domain including an immunoreceptor tyrosine-based inhibitory motif (ITIM) (Keir et al. 2008). PD-1 is induced by T-cell receptor (TCR) activation and cytokine signaling via interleukin receptors sharing the common gamma chain, such as IL-2, IL-7, IL-15, and IL-21

(Okazaki et al. 2013) (Kinter et al. 2008). The PD-1 molecule was originally identified as a preferential protein expressed in apoptotic cells by the subtractive hybridization technique (Ishida et al. 1992). Subsequently, however, its physiological role was discovered to be unrelated to cell death. Furthermore, PD-1 is also expressed on a variety of immune cells, such as B cells, monocytes, activated NK T cells, immature Langerhans cells, and others (Okazaki and Honjo 2007). NFATc is a critical factor in the transcription of *PDCD1*, enabling it to bind to the promoter region (Oestreich et al. 2008). IRF9 activated via IFNα (Terawaki et al. 2011), Notch signaling (Mathieu et al. 2013), and FoxO1 downstream of Akt (Staron et al. 2014) also enhance PDCD1 transcription in T cells, while T-bet represses its transcription (Kao et al. 2011). The kinetics of PD-1 expression indicates that PD-1 expression is upregulated as a natural consequence of activation and is required to terminate the immune responses. PD-1 expression is detected on the naïve T cells within 24 hours after activation, but its expression declines with clearance of the antigen. If T cells are constitutively stimulated with antigens, as in cases of chronic infection or tumor, PD-1 expression remains high, and T cells fall into dysfunctional "exhaustion" status (Barber et al. 2006). Posttranscriptional regulation changes PD-1 expression; metabolic status in T cells, such as aerobic glycolysis, reduces PD-1 expression on activated T cell (Chang et al. 2013). In B cells, BCR stimulation upregulates PD-1 expression, but this upregulation is suppressed by certain TLR ligands or cytokines, such as IFNγ and IL-4 (Zhong et al. 2004). In contrast, TLR ligands or inflammatory cytokines induce the expression of PD-1 on macrophages (Cho et al. 2008).

2.4.2 Ligands of PD-1: PD-L1 and PD-L2

Both PD-L1 (B7-H1) and PD-L2 (B7-DC) are the ligands for PD-1, but they have different patterns of expression. PD-L1 is constitutively expressed on immune cells, such as T cells, B cells, macrophages, and dendritic cells, and is upregulated by any inflammatory stimulation (Yamazaki et al. 2002). In addition, PD-L1 is also expressed on a variety of nonhematopoietic cells including vascular endothelium, pancreatic islets, and placental syncytiotrophoblasts (Keir et al. 2008). Particularly, PD-L1 is physiologically expressed on the dorsal surface of the tongue, gingiva, and hard palate but not on other squamous epithelia in the masticatory mucosa in the oral cavity (Kang et al. 2017). PD-L1 expression is induced by proinflammatory cytokines including interferons (IFNs), tumor necrosis factor alpha (TNFα), and vascular endothelial growth factor (VEGF). In contrast, PD-L2 expression is limited to dendritic cells, macrophages (MΦs), and 50–70% of resting B1 B cells and is not seen on conventional B2 B cells (Zhong et al. 2007). PD-L2 expression on DCs and MΦs is also upregulated after activation. The kinetics of PD-1 expression, the induction of PD-L1 or PD-L2 by proinflammatory stimuli, and the constitutive expression of PD-L1 on nonlymphoid tissues underscore the role of the PD-1 pathway in the suppression of effector T-cell activity, which preserves self-tolerance and accelerates the resolution of inflammation during immune responses. In addition to PD-1, PD-L1 also binds to B7-1 expressed on T cells and transduces inhibitory signals (Butte et al. 2007). In contrast, PD-L2 on lung DCs interacts with repulsive guidance molecule b (RGMb), a co-receptor for bone morphogenetic proteins expressed on resting lung interstitial MΦs and alveolar epithelial cells (Xiao et al. 2014). This interaction is thought to regulate respiratory tolerance.

2.4.3 Function of PD-1

Although "programed cell death-1" was cloned from T-cell hybridoma undergoing cell death, PD-1 is not able to activate caspases or other cell death pathways directly. Rather, PD-1 signals regulate the TCR signaling pathway in several ways. Ligation of PD-1 suppresses T-cell activation and cytokine production. By binding PD-1 to its ligands, tyrosines in the ITIM and ITSM motifs are phosphorylated, and phosphatases, such as SHP-1 or SHP-2, are recruited, resulting in the downregulation of TCR signaling by the dephosphorylation of CD3ζ, ZAP70, and PKCθ in T cells (Chemnitz et al. 2004) (Sheppard et al. 2004). The binding of tyrosine-phosphorylated ITSM to SHP-2 is required for the inhibitory effect of PD-1, as evidenced by the finding that this effect is lost due to the mutation of ITSM. Furthermore, research using live-cell imaging systems has revealed that SHP-2 forms central supramolecular activation clusters (c-SMACs) with ITSM of PD-1 (Yokosuka et al. 2012). The recruitment of PD-1 to c-SMACs is correlated with dephosphorylation of components of TCR microclusters, resulting in inhibition of T-cell activation.

PD-1 ligation inhibits the PI3K–Akt and MEK–ERK pathways. Although the activity of PTEN, a counter enzyme of PI3K, is suppressed during TCR/CD28 activation, PD-1 increases the phosphatase activity of PTEN, thereby inhibiting the PI3K–Akt signaling pathways (Patsoukis et al. 2013). PD-1 ligation also inhibits the MEK–ERK pathway via dephosphorylation of PLCγ1 by SHP-2 (Patsoukis et al. 2012). And eventually, PD-1 inhibits cell cycle by inhibiting cyclin-dependent kinase 2 (Cdk2). Furthermore, PD-1 reduces the cytokine expression and transcription factors in T cells in relation to effector function (Nurieva et al. 2006). PD-1 signaling also reduces the cytotoxic activity of T cells by inhibiting the production of cytotoxic effector molecules. PD-1 modulates T-cell motility and the length of interaction with DCs and target cells (Fife et al. 2009). PD-1/PD-L1 signaling also develops induced Tregs (iTregs) and sustains their function through antagonizing the Akt–mTOR pathway (Francisco et al. 2009), which negatively regulates iTreg differentiation (Sauer et al. 2008). Therefore, PD-1 signaling modifies T cells in several ways to inhibit immune responses.

PD-1 signaling is a key pathway involved in determining the threshold for the activation of T cells and suppressing T-cell responses. Expression of ligands of PD-1 in tissues weakens the local immune responses and maintains immune tolerance. PD-1 can bind to CD80, which inhibits T cells (Butte et al. 2007). Since tumors exploit the PD-1 pathway to inhibit their exclusion by T cells, antagonists against the PD-1 pathway are utilized in clinical therapy to restore effector T-cell function.

2.5 ICOS

ICOS (inducible co-stimulator) was firstly identified from activated T cells in humans (Hutloff et al. 1999); the mouse homolog was cloned thereafter (Mages et al. 2000). ICOS has significant homology with both CD28 and CTLA-4 and is composed of a single IgV in the extracellular domain and a YMFM motif for binding to PI3K in the cytoplasmic tail. The engagement of ICOS has been shown to induce PI3K signaling more stronger than CD28 co-stimulation does (Parry et al. 2003). ICOS expression has been detected in secondary lymphoid organs, such as the spleen, lymph nodes, and Peyer's patches (Mages et al. 2000). In contrast, the ligand of ICOS is ICOSL, another member of the B7 family that is expressed in APCs, such as B cells (Hu et al. 2011), MΦs, and DCs (Aicher et al. 2000; Yoshinaga et al. 2000). ICOSL can be induced by proinflammatory cytokines in nonlymphoid cells including endothelial cells (Khayyamian et al. 2002) and lung epithelial cells (Qian et al. 2006). Appropriately termed "inducible," ICOS is not constitutively expressed on resting T cells, but instead rapidly induced after TCR stimulation and/ or CD28 stimulation (Yoshinaga et al. 1999) (McAdam et al. 2000). During the initial priming of T cells, the contribution of ICOS seems minimum compared to that of CD28 because ICOS-deficient T cells proliferate comparably to control T cells (Dong et al. 2001a; Tafuri et al. 2001). Furthermore, the lymph nodes of ICOS-deficient mice were smaller than those from WT mice, indicating the defect of proliferation in vivo. Similarly, during parasite infections, CD4[+] T cells from ICOS-deficient mice exhibited some defects in proliferation and activation but not in differentiation (Wilson et al. 2006). In addition, when CD4[+] T cells from OVA-specific TCR transgenic mice, which were differentiated into Th1 or Th2 cells, were transferred into naïve mice, ICOS was found to be required for expansion of these subsets (Smith et al. 2003). However, when ICOS-deficient mice were immunized with KLH conjugated with complete Freund's adjuvant, there was no defect in T cell activation and proliferation (Dong et al. 2001a). These opposing results may be attributed to the fact that IL-2 production promotes T-cell clonal expansion, given that, in contrast to CD28 ligation, ICOS cross-linking in vitro induces not IL-2 (Arimura et al. 2002; Coyle et al. 2000; Dong et al. 2001a) but rather the anti-inflammatory cytokine IL-10 (Hutloff et al. 1999; Witsch et al. 2002). Therefore, the role of ICOS in T-cell proliferation seems to be independent of IL-2 signaling, and the molecular basis for the role of ICOS in T-cell proliferation remains unclear.

While a number of studies have examined the function of ICOS in T cells, the predominant phenotype that has emerged from the characterization of ICOS- and ICOSL-deficient mice indicates that ICOS is involved with class-switched antibodies against thymus-dependent antigens (Wong et al. 2003), a role that has been identified as responsible for the observed reduction in the number and size of germinal centers (GCs) in the absence of ICOS signaling (Dong et al. 2001b; McAdam et al. 2001). Within the GCs, follicular helper T (Tfh) cells play a critical role in promoting the selection and survival of B cells expressing high-affinity B-cell receptors (Victora and Nussenzweig 2012). A critical function of the Tfh phenotype is the expression of the chemokine receptor CXCR5, which can bind to CXCL13 produced by follicular DCs to enhance the migration of Tfh cells to the B-cell follicle. In addition, Tfh cells produce IL-21, a key cytokine in promoting the GC reaction, as well as reinforcing the Tfh phenotype itself in an autocrine manner (Crotty 2014). Treatment with anti-ICOS Abs abrogated expression of CXCR5 on CD4[+] T cells, suggesting that ICOS supports CXCR5 expression on Tfh cells during GC responses (Akiba et al. 2005).

2.6 B7–H3

B7–H3, also known as CD276, was discovered in the EST data base in 2001 and has since been identified as involved in both co-stimulatory and co-inhibitory functions in T-cell responses (Chapoval et al. 2001). The extracellular domain of B7–H3 is composed of a single pair of IgV and IgC domains of B7-family molecules (two IgB7–H3) in humans and mice, though human B7–H3 can also contain two pairs of IgV and IgC (four IgB7-H3) in the event of alternative splicing into two proteins (Ling et al. 2003). There are no signaling motifs in the cytoplasmic tail of B7–H3. The receptor of B7–H3 has not yet been identified (Leitner et al. 2009; Vigdorovich et al. 2013). The soluble form of B7–H3 (sB7–H3) is produced only from two IgB7–H3 shed by MMPs (Ling et al. 2003) (Zhang et al. 2008). B7–H3 mRNA is ubiquitously expressed on various tissues, such as the uterus, testis, thymus, lung, heart, and brain (Sun et al. 2002), and is evolutionarily conserved across various species (Sun et al. 2011). Although its mRNA expression is broad, its protein expression is restricted to low level in steady state, suggesting the presence of a posttranscriptional regulatory mechanism. B7–H3 protein is expressed on nonimmune resting cells, such as fibroblasts and epithelial cells (Picarda et al. 2016). Furthermore, its expression is induced on T cells, NK cells, and APCs, such as DCs and MΦs (Chapoval et al. 2001). In vitro, B7–H3 on bone marrow-derived DCs (BMDCs) is induced by IFNγ or LPS plus anti-CD40 Ab stimulation, but the addition of IL-4 abrogates its expression (Suh et al. 2003). Initially, it was reported that B7–H3 supports the proliferation of CD4[+] and CD8[+] T cells by TCR stimulation using immobilized Ig-fusion protein (Chapoval et al. 2001). In addition, it has been shown that ectopic expression of B7–H3 leads to activation of tumor-specific CTLs in mouse cancer models (Luo et al. 2004). These studies demonstrated that mouse B7–H3 acts as a co-stimulatory molecule. However, most data published to date have supported the notion that B7-H3 inhibits T-cell activation, that is, it causes T-cell co-inhibition. Both human and mouse B7–H3 inhibit CD4[+] T-cell activation and production of effector cytokines (Prasad et al. 2004; Suh et al. 2003). This inhibition may mediate transcription factors NF-AT, NF-κB, and AP-1, which regulate gene transcription via T-cell receptor (TCR) signaling. These opposing effects of B7–H3 may be due to the existence of multiple receptors, or the presence of other co-stimulatory or co-inhibitory molecules. B7–H3 also inhibits NK cell activity, such as cell lysis of neuroblastoma and glioma cell lines (Castriconi et al. 2004) (Lemke et al. 2012).

2.7 B7–H4

By searching the human EST data base for sequences containing the IgV and IgC domains of B7-family molecules, the B7–H4 nucleotide sequence encoding a putative protein of 282 amino acids was identified (V-set domain containing T-cell activation inhibitor 1; Vtcn1) (Sica et al. 2003). These transcripts are ubiquitously expressed, but protein expression is restricted, indicating that translation of B7-H4 is strictly regulated. In immune cells, B7–H4, also known as B7S1 and B7x, is expressed on T cells, B cells, monocytes, and DCs after the stimulation. It is known that B7–H4 suppresses cell-cycle progression, cell proliferation, and cytokine secretion from T cells (Zang et al. 2003). In B7–H4-deficient mice, although Th1 response was mildly upregulated and parasite burdens upon *Leishmania major* were slightly lower than that in WT mice, there was little effect on hypersensitive immune responses or the development of CTL reaction (Suh et al. 2006). These results collectively suggest that B7–H4 acts a fine-tuner for T-cell-mediated immunity. In addition, B7–H4 suppresses immune responses mediated by neutrophils in response to *Listeria* infection (Zhu et al. 2009). It is worth noting that, in spite of the restricted expression of B7–H4 in normal tissues, aberrant expression of B7–H4 was observed in human cancer cells (He et al. 2011). Because B7–H4-positive cancer has bad outcomes, B7–H4 can be a biomarker in cancer prognosis (Bignotti et al. 2006). These findings serve as a basis for targeting B7–H4 in cancer therapy. Furthermore, B7–H4 molecules elicit a cell-intrinsic effect in tumor cells. For example, overexpression of B7–H4 in a tumor avoided cell death and enhanced tumor formation in immunodeficient mice, while knockdown of B7–H4 markedly induced apoptosis by activating caspases (Qian et al. 2013).

2.8 HHLA2

Examination of the EST database led to the discovery of HHLA2 (human endogenous retrovirus (HERV)-H long terminal repeat-associating 2), which is polyadenylated within a long-term repeat (LTR) of the HERV-H endogenous retrovirus family (Mager et al. 1999). HHLA-2 is a type I transmembrane molecule with three extracellular Ig domains. It shares 10–18% amino acid identity and 23–33% similarity to other human B7 proteins (Table 2.1) and phylogenetically forms a subfamily with B7x and B7–H3 within the family (Zhao et al. 2013). Evolutionarily, the LTR of the HHLA2 locus has been integrated into the primate genome because it has been detected only in gorillas, chimpanzees, and humans, but not in mice. Protein expression in normal tissues is limited to epithelial cells in the intestine, kidney, gallbladder, and breast (Janakiram et al. 2015). HHLA is constitutively expressed on human monocytes and induced on B cells by stimulation with LPS and IFNγ (Zhao et al. 2013). HHLA2 Ig fusion protein binds to both resting and activated T cells and other

Table 2.1 Amino acid identities (%) of human B7 family receptors (A) and B7 family ligands (B) were calculated according to the Needleman–Wunsch algorithm

A

	Protein identities (%) among human B7 family receptors					
Protein	CTLA-4	PD-1	ICOS	TMIGD2	VISTA	VSIG4
CD28	28	17	24	19	14	14
CTLA-4		14	18	15	19	12
PD-1			12	15	14	15
ICOS				21	20	14
TMIGD2					18	15
VISTA						17

B

	Protein identities (%) among human B7 family ligands									
Protein	CD86	PD-L1	PD-L2	ICOSL	B7-H3	B7-H4	HHLA2	VISTA	VSIG4	ILDR2
CD80	21	21	20	21	14	21	17	16	16	11
CD86		19	20	20	15	19	16	16	18	14
PD-L1			36	21	16	21	16	18	16	12
PD-L2				22	16	21	18	18	14	11
ICOSL					18	21	19	18	17	13
B7-H3						16	18	16	17	17
B7-H4							19	17	14	11
HHLA2								18	18	14
VISTA									17	14
VSIG4										16

cells, suggesting that constitutive (but unknown) receptors are expressed on these cell surfaces. HHLA2 acts as a T-cell co-inhibitory molecule as evidenced by the finding that HHLA2-Ig can inhibit T-cell proliferation and the production of several cytokines including IFNγ, TNFα, IL-5, IL-10, IL-13, IL-17A, and IL-22. However, it has been reported that the interaction between HHLA2 and TMIGD2, which is expressed on MΦs or DCs, selectively co-stimulates human T-cell growth and cytokine production (Zhu et al. 2013). As well as in normal tissue, HHLA2 is expressed in various human tumor specimens, such as the breast, lung, thyroid, ovarian, and pancreatic cancer and melanoma (Janakiram et al. 2015). High expression levels in human cancers are associated with worse prognosis.

2.9 VISTA

V-domain immunoglobulin suppressor or T-cell activation (VISTA), also known as PD-1H and DD1 alpha, is a novel co-inhibitory checkpoint molecule that has some similarities with the IgV domain of PD-L1 in the extracellular region (Wang et al. 2011). No obvious signaling motif has been identified, but the existence of two potential PKC binding sites in the cytoplasmic region of VISTA (Ohno et al. 2018) suggests that VISTA works as a receptor (Flies et al. 2014). Furthermore, several experiments have suggested that VISTA also function as a ligand (Lines et al. 2014) (Wang et al. 2011). VISTA is involved in homophilic interactions between apoptotic cells and MΦs (Yoon et al. 2015), and VSIG-3 has been identified as a binding partner of VISTA (Wang et al. 2019). There are two isoforms of VISTA, one with a 60 amino acid deletion and the other with an alternative start site. VISTA is cleaved by MMP-14 to release a soluble extracellular region (Sakr et al. 2010). VISTA is constitutively expressed on immune cells including T cells, NK cells, DCs, and MΦ, but not B cells. VISTA expression in T cells or MΦs is downregulated after stimulation (Flies et al. 2014) (Wang et al. 2011).

VISTA regulates T-cell responses and induces T-cell tolerance. T-cell activation, proliferation, and cytokine expression in vitro are inhibited by VISTA Ig fusion protein or VISTA on APCs (Wang et al. 2011). VISTA-deficient mice have increased numbers of activated T cells and an age-related multiorgan proinflammatory phenotype but no signs of spontaneous autoimmunity (Flies et al. 2014). However, VISTA-deficient mice are more likely to develop severe experimental autoimmune encephalomyelitis (EAE) compared to WT mice, and VISTA on both APCs and T cells contributes to the worsening of EAE (Wang et al. 2011). Furthermore, anti-VISTA Ab treatment also exacerbates EAE.

VISTA has inhibitory functions that are non-redundant with the PD-1/PD-L1 pathway (Liu et al. 2015). PD-1 and VISTA double-deficient mice exhibited accelerated severity of EAE compared to mice that are single deficient for either PD-1 or VISTA. In addition, anti-PD-L1 and anti-VISTA Abs synergized to enhance antitumor immunity in the CT26 tumor model. In the SCC-VII tumor model, in contrast, in which Treg-mediated immune regulation is dominant, the combination of anti-CTLA-4 and anti-VISTA blockade is more efficacious than the combination of anti-PD-L1 and anti-VISTA blockade (Kondo et al. 2016).

2.10 VSIG4

V-set and Ig domain-containing 4 (VSIG4) were cloned in silico on a translated EST database using a hidden Markov model profile of the ectodomain of known B7 family members (Vogt et al. 2006). This molecule is also referred to as complement receptor of the immunoglobulin superfamily (CRIg) (Helmy et al. 2006), and the human ortholog of VSIG4 is Z39Ig (Langnaese et al. 2000). The protein sequence encoded by the cDNA displays about 15% identity and shared conserved amino acids with known B7 family members (Table 2.1). VSIG4 is a type I transmembrane Ig superfamily member and exists as two alternatively spliced forms. The longer form of human VSIG4 encodes both IgV and IgC domains, while shorter form encodes a single IgV domain. In contrast, murine VSIG4 encodes only one form with an IgV domain. The highest levels of human transcripts are detected in many organs, such as the placenta and lung, while the murine transcript is detected in the liver and heart (Helmy et al. 2006). In immune cells, VSIG4 is selectively expressed on MΦs and F4/80+ Kupffer cells, but absent in B cells, T cells, NK cells, and granulocytes (Helmy et al. 2006). VSIG4 expressed on resting peritoneal MΦs is downregulated upon activation with LPS or thioglycolate (Vogt et al. 2006). Since VSIG4 can bind to complement component C3b or inactivated C3b (iC3b), this molecule mediates clearance of C3b-opsonized pathogens, such as *Listeria monocytogenes* and *Staphylococcus aureus* (Helmy et al. 2006). VSIG4 functionally inhibits IL-2 production and T-cell proliferation and promotes Foxp3+ Treg differentiation by binding an unknown ligand or receptor on T cells (Vogt et al. 2006) (Yuan et al. 2017). A VSIG4-Ig can protect against development of arthritis (Katschke et al. 2007), autoimmune uveoretinitis (Chen et al. 2010), and immune-mediated liver injury (Jung et al. 2012), indicating that VSIG4 can restrain inflammatory responses. Studies using VSIG4-deficient mice have demonstrated that VSIG4 inhibits activation of M1 MΦ by pyruvate oxidation and reactive oxygen species (ROS) generation (Li et al. 2017) and suppresses NLRP3-associated inflammasome via A20-mediated NF-κB inactivation (Huang et al. 2019), suggesting that VSIG4 acts as a receptor inhibiting proinflammatory MΦ activation.

2.11 ILDR2

Ig-like domain-containing receptor 2 (ILDR2) and its two paralogs, ILDR1 and lipolysis-stimulated receptor (LSR, also named ILDR3), are designated as angulin family members, following their identification as protein components of tricellular tight junctions (tTJs) required for recruitment of tricellulin to tTJs (Higashi et al. 2013). ILDR2 mRNA encodes a type I membrane protein containing a large IgV domain and stalk region in the ectodomain, a transmembrane (TM) domain, a cysteine and proline (CCP)-rich domain located at the juxtamembrane, and a long intracellular domain. ILDR2 has several splicing variants; its longest transcript, comprising ten coding exons, encodes the membrane protein described above. Shorter isoforms lack an intracellular, stalk, TM, and/or CCP-rich domain (Hecht et al. 2018) (Higashi et al. 2013). Human ILDR2 mRNA is highly expressed in the testis and brain and less abundantly expressed in the kidney, heart, and colon. Murine Ildr2 mRNA is also highly expressed in the brain and eye and moderately expressed in the kidney but not in the testis. At the protein level, strong expression of ILDR2 is observed in inflamed tissues, such as ulcerative colitis and Crohn's

2 The CD28–B7 Family of Co-signaling Molecules

disease, compared with normal colon and small intestine (Hecht et al. 2018). With regard to immune cells, the highest human ILDR2 expression is observed in CD16[+] monocytes, while a weak expression is observed in CD56[+] (NK or NKT subsets) lymphocytes. ILDR2 expression is enhanced when monocytes are differentiated into MΦs by M-CSF. The *Ildr2* gene has been associated with type 2 diabetes because this gene is related to reduced β cell mass and replication rates, as well as persistent hyperglycemia (Dokmanovic-Chouinard et al. 2008). Although the receptor or ligand of ILDR2 remains unknown, ILDR2-Ig can bind to activated but not resting T cells to inhibit T-cell activation and cytokine/chemokine expression in vitro (Hecht et al. 2018). Upon differentiation of Th subsets, ILDR2-Ig downregulates Th1 and Th17 but enhances Th2 and Treg differentiation (Podojil et al. 2018). Therefore, ILDR2-Ig has therapeutic effects against autoimmune diseases, such as EAE, collagen-induced arthritis (CIA), and type 1 diabetes (T1D) (Hecht et al. 2018) (Podojil et al. 2018).

2.12 Concluding Remarks

The co-inhibition effects exerted by CD28-B7 family molecules are indispensable for immune homeostasis and tolerance as well as for protective immune responses. Progress in understanding these co-inhibitory pathways will enable us to develop new treatments for tumors and autoimmune diseases, just as the success of checkpoint blockade therapy opened the way for new cancer treatments. However, we still do not know the biological reasons why many co-inhibitory pathways are required to regulate host immunity. Furthermore, several receptors for B7 family members have not yet been identified. There are many orphan B7-family molecules whose receptors are critical for understanding their functions. Conventional approaches for discovering new binding partners have not been successful because some of these molecules are not proteins but rather lipids, carbohydrates, or possibly multimeric complexes. It is hoped that this review of findings from many researchers provides a full picture of what is currently known about the roles and effects of the B7-family members.

References

Aicher A, Hayden-Ledbetter M, Brady WA, Pezzutto A, Richter G, Magaletti D, Buckwalter S, Ledbetter JA, Clark EA (2000) Characterization of human inducible costimulator ligand expression and function. J Immunol 164:4689–4696

Akiba H, Takeda K, Kojima Y, Usui Y, Harada N, Yamazaki T, Ma J, Tezuka K, Yagita H, Okumura K (2005) The role of ICOS in the CXCR5+ follicular B helper T cell maintenance in vivo. J Immunol 175:2340–2348

Arimura Y, Kato H, Dianzani U, Okamoto T, Kamekura S, Buonfiglio D, Miyoshi-Akiyama T, Uchiyama T, Yagi J (2002) A co-stimulatory molecule on activated T cells, H4/ICOS, delivers specific signals in T(h) cells and regulates their responses. Int Immunol 14:555–566

Attema JL, Reeves R, Murray V, Levichkin I, Temple MD, Tremethick DJ, Shannon MF (2002) The human IL-2 gene promoter can assemble a positioned nucleosome that becomes remodeled upon T cell activation. J Immunol 169:2466–2476

Barber DL, Wherry EJ, Masopust D, Zhu B, Allison JP, Sharpe AH, Freeman GJ, Ahmed R (2006) Restoring function in exhausted CD8 T cells during chronic viral infection. Nature 439:682–687

Bhatia S, Edidin M, Almo SC, Nathenson SG (2005) Different cell surface oligomeric states of B7-1 and B7-2: implications for signaling. Proc Natl Acad Sci U S A 102:15569–15574

Bignotti E, Tassi RA, Calza S, Ravaggi A, Romani C, Rossi E, Falchetti M, Odicino FE, Pecorelli S, Santin AD (2006) Differential gene expression profiles between tumor biopsies and short-term primary cultures of ovarian serous carcinomas: identification of novel molecular biomarkers for early diagnosis and therapy. Gynecol Oncol 103:405–416

Boise LH, Minn AJ, Noel PJ, June CH, Accavitti MA, Lindsten T, Thompson CB (1995) CD28 costimulation can promote T cell survival by enhancing the expression of Bcl-XL. Immunity 3:87–98

Boomer JS, Green JM (2010) An enigmatic tail of CD28 signaling. Cold Spring Harb Perspect Biol 2:a002436

Borriello F, Lederer J, Scott S, Sharpe AH (1997) MRC OX-2 defines a novel T cell costimulatory pathway. J Immunol 158:4548–4554

Bour-Jordan H, Grogan JL, Tang Q, Auger JA, Locksley RM, Bluestone JA (2003) CTLA-4 regulates the requirement for cytokine-induced signals in T(H)2 lineage commitment. Nat Immunol 4:182–188

Brunet JF, Denizot F, Luciani MF, Roux-Dosseto M, Suzan M, Mattei MG, Golstein P (1987) A new member of the immunoglobulin superfamily--CTLA-4. Nature 328:267–270

Butte MJ, Keir ME, Phamduy TB, Sharpe AH, Freeman GJ (2007) Programmed death-1 ligand 1 interacts specifically with the B7-1 costimulatory molecule to inhibit T cell responses. Immunity 27:111–122

Butte MJ, Lee SJ, Jesneck J, Keir ME, Haining WN, Sharpe AH (2012) CD28 costimulation regulates genome-wide effects on alternative splicing. PLoS One 7:e40032

Carreno BM, Collins M (2002) The B7 family of ligands and its receptors: new pathways for costimulation and inhibition of immune responses. Annu Rev Immunol 20:29–53

Castriconi R, Dondero A, Augugliaro R, Cantoni C, Carnemolla B, Sementa AR, Negri F, Conte R, Corrias MV, Moretta L et al (2004) Identification of 4Ig-B7-H3 as a neuroblastoma-associated molecule that exerts a protective role from an NK cell-mediated lysis. Proc Natl Acad Sci U S A 101:12640–12645

Chang CH, Curtis JD, Maggi LB Jr, Faubert B, Villarino AV, O'Sullivan D, Huang SC, van der Windt GJ, Blagih J, Qiu J et al (2013) Posttranscriptional control of T cell effector function by aerobic glycolysis. Cell 153:1239–1251

Chapoval AI, Ni J, Lau JS, Wilcox RA, Flies DB, Liu D, Dong H, Sica GL, Zhu G, Tamada K et al (2001) B7-H3: a costimulatory molecule for T cell activation and IFN-gamma production. Nat Immunol 2:269–274

Chemnitz JM, Parry RV, Nichols KE, June CH, Riley JL (2004) SHP-1 and SHP-2 associate with immunoreceptor tyrosine-based switch motif of programmed death 1 upon primary human T cell stimulation, but only receptor ligation prevents T cell activation. J Immunol 173:945–954

Chen M, Muckersie E, Luo C, Forrester JV, Xu H (2010) Inhibition of the alternative pathway of complement activation reduces inflammation in experimental autoimmune uveoretinitis. Eur J Immunol 40:2870–2881

Chen J, Wang F, Cai Q, Shen S, Chen Y, Hao C, Sun J (2013) A novel anti-human ICOSL monoclonal antibody that enhances IgG production of B cells. Monoclon Antib Immunodiagn Immunother 32:125–131

Cho HY, Lee SW, Seo SK, Choi IW, Choi I, Lee SW (2008) Interferon-sensitive response element (ISRE) is mainly responsible for IFN-alpha-induced upregulation of programmed death-1 (PD-1) in macrophages. Biochim Biophys Acta 1779:811–819

Chuang E, Fisher TS, Morgan RW, Robbins MD, Duerr JM, Vander Heiden MG, Gardner JP, Hambor JE, Neveu MJ, Thompson CB (2000) The CD28 and CTLA-4 receptors associate with the serine/threonine phosphatase PP2A. Immunity 13:313–322

Coyle AJ, Lehar S, Lloyd C, Tian J, Delaney T, Manning S, Nguyen T, Burwell T, Schneider H, Gonzalo JA et al (2000) The CD28-related molecule ICOS is required for effective T cell-dependent immune responses. Immunity 13:95–105

Crotty S (2014) T follicular helper cell differentiation, function, and roles in disease. Immunity 41:529–542

Dariavach P, Mattei MG, Golstein P, Lefranc MP (1988) Human Ig superfamily CTLA-4 gene: chromosomal localization and identity of protein sequence between murine and human CTLA-4 cytoplasmic domains. Eur J Immunol 18:1901–1905

de Jong VM, Zaldumbide A, van der Slik AR, Persengiev SP, Roep BO, Koeleman BP (2013) Post-transcriptional control of candidate risk genes for type 1 diabetes by rare genetic variants. Genes Immun 14:58–61

Diehn M, Alizadeh AA, Rando OJ, Liu CL, Stankunas K, Botstein D, Crabtree GR, Brown PO (2002) Genomic expression programs and the integration of the CD28 costimulatory signal in T cell activation. Proc Natl Acad Sci U S A 99:11796–11801

Dokmanovic-Chouinard M, Chung WK, Chevre JC, Watson E, Yonan J, Wiegand B, Bromberg Y, Wakae N, Wright CV, Overton J et al (2008) Positional cloning of "Lisch-Like", a candidate modifier of susceptibility to type 2 diabetes in mice. PLoS Genet 4:e1000137

Dong C, Juedes AE, Temann UA, Shresta S, Allison JP, Ruddle NH, Flavell RA (2001a) ICOS co-stimulatory receptor is essential for T-cell activation and function. Nature 409:97–101

Dong C, Temann UA, Flavell RA (2001b) Cutting edge: critical role of inducible costimulator in germinal center reactions. J Immunol 166:3659–3662

DuPage M, Chopra G, Quiros J, Rosenthal WL, Morar MM, Holohan D, Zhang R, Turka L, Marson A, Bluestone JA (2015) The chromatin-modifying enzyme Ezh2 is critical for the maintenance of regulatory T cell identity after activation. Immunity 42:227–238

Engelhardt JJ, Sullivan TJ, Allison JP (2006) CTLA-4 overexpression inhibits T cell responses through a CD28-B7-dependent mechanism. J Immunol 177:1052–1061

Evans EJ, Esnouf RM, Manso-Sancho R, Gilbert RJ, James JR, Yu C, Fennelly JA, Vowles C, Hanke T, Walse B et al (2005) Crystal structure of a soluble CD28-Fab complex. Nat Immunol 6:271–279

Fallarino F, Grohmann U, Hwang KW, Orabona C, Vacca C, Bianchi R, Belladonna ML, Fioretti MC, Alegre ML, Puccetti P (2003) Modulation of tryptophan catabolism by regulatory T cells. Nat Immunol 4:1206–1212

Fife BT, Pauken KE, Eagar TN, Obu T, Wu J, Tang Q, Azuma M, Krummel MF, Bluestone JA (2009) Interactions between PD-1 and PD-L1 promote tolerance by blocking the TCR-induced stop signal. Nat Immunol 10:1185–1192

Fischer KD, Kong YY, Nishina H, Tedford K, Marengere LE, Kozieradzki I, Sasaki T, Starr M, Chan G, Gardener S et al (1998a) Vav is a regulator of cytoskeletal reorganization mediated by the T-cell receptor. Curr Biol 8:554–562

Fischer KD, Tedford K, Penninger JM (1998b) Vav links antigen-receptor signaling to the actin cytoskeleton. Semin Immunol 10:317–327

Flies DB, Han X, Higuchi T, Zheng L, Sun J, Ye JJ, Chen L (2014) Coinhibitory receptor PD-1H preferentially suppresses CD4(+) T cell-mediated immunity. J Clin Invest 124:1966–1975

Francisco LM, Salinas VH, Brown KE, Vanguri VK, Freeman GJ, Kuchroo VK, Sharpe AH (2009) PD-L1 regulates the development, maintenance, and function of induced regulatory T cells. J Exp Med 206:3015–3029

Frauwirth KA, Riley JL, Harris MH, Parry RV, Rathmell JC, Plas DR, Elstrom RL, June CH, Thompson CB (2002) The CD28 signaling pathway regulates glucose metabolism. Immunity 16:769–777

Freeman GJ, Lombard DB, Gimmi CD, Brod SA, Lee K, Laning JC, Hafler DA, Dorf ME, Gray GS, Reiser H et al (1992) CTLA-4 and CD28 mRNA are coexpressed in most T cells after activation. Expression of CTLA-4 and CD28 mRNA does not correlate with the pattern of lymphokine production. J Immunol 149:3795–3801

Gibson HM, Hedgcock CJ, Aufiero BM, Wilson AJ, Hafner MS, Tsokos GC, Wong HK (2007) Induction of the CTLA-4 gene in human lymphocytes is dependent on NFAT binding the proximal promoter. J Immunol 179:3831–3840

Girard T, Gaucher D, El-Far M, Breton G, Sekaly RP (2014) CD80 and CD86 IgC domains are important for quaternary structure, receptor binding and co-signaling function. Immunol Lett 161:65–75

Grohmann U, Orabona C, Fallarino F, Vacca C, Calcinaro F, Falorni A, Candeloro P, Belladonna ML, Bianchi R, Fioretti MC et al (2002) CTLA-4-Ig regulates tryptophan catabolism in vivo. Nat Immunol 3:1097–1101

Han Y, Chen Z, Yang Y, Jiang Z, Gu Y, Liu Y, Lin C, Pan Z, Yu Y, Jiang M et al (2014) Human CD14+ CTLA-4+ regulatory dendritic cells suppress T-cell response by cytotoxic T-lymphocyte antigen-4-dependent IL-10 and indoleamine-2,3-dioxygenase production in hepatocellular carcinoma. Hepatology 59:567–579

Hathcock KS, Laszlo G, Pucillo C, Linsley P, Hodes RJ (1994) Comparative analysis of B7-1 and B7-2 costimulatory ligands: expression and function. J Exp Med 180:631–640

He C, Qiao H, Jiang H, Sun X (2011) The inhibitory role of b7-h4 in antitumor immunity: association with cancer progression and survival. Clin Dev Immunol 2011:695834

Hecht I, Toporik A, Podojil JR, Vaknin I, Cojocaru G, Oren A, Aizman E, Liang SC, Leung L, Dicken Y et al (2018) ILDR2 is a novel B7-like protein that negatively regulates T cell responses. J Immunol 200:2025–2037

Helmy KY, Katschke KJ Jr, Gorgani NN, Kljavin NM, Elliott JM, Diehl L, Scales SJ, Ghilardi N, van Lookeren Campagne M (2006) CRIg: a macrophage complement receptor required for phagocytosis of circulating pathogens. Cell 124:915–927

Higashi T, Tokuda S, Kitajiri S, Masuda S, Nakamura H, Oda Y, Furuse M (2013) Analysis of the 'angulin' proteins LSR, ILDR1 and ILDR2--tricellulin recruitment, epithelial barrier function and implication in deafness pathogenesis. J Cell Sci 126:966–977

Hu H, Wu X, Jin W, Chang M, Cheng X, Sun SC (2011) Noncanonical NF-kappaB regulates inducible costimulator (ICOS) ligand expression and T follicular helper cell development. Proc Natl Acad Sci U S A 108:12827–12832

Huang X, Feng Z, Jiang Y, Li J, Xiang Q, Guo S, Yang C, Fei L, Guo G, Zheng L et al (2019) VSIG4 mediates transcriptional inhibition of Nlrp3 and Il-1beta in macrophages. Sci Adv 5:eaau7426

Hutloff A, Dittrich AM, Beier KC, Eljaschewitsch B, Kraft R, Anagnostopoulos I, Kroczek RA (1999) ICOS is an inducible T-cell co-stimulator structurally and functionally related to CD28. Nature 397:263–266

Ishida Y, Agata Y, Shibahara K, Honjo T (1992) Induced expression of PD-1, a novel member of the immunoglobulin gene superfamily, upon programmed cell death. EMBO J 11:3887–3895

Isomura I, Palmer S, Grumont RJ, Bunting K, Hoyne G, Wilkinson N, Banerjee A, Proietto A, Gugasyan R, Wu L et al (2009) c-Rel is required for the development of thymic Foxp3+ CD4 regulatory T cells. J Exp Med 206:3001–3014

Janakiram M, Chinai JM, Fineberg S, Fiser A, Montagna C, Medavarapu R, Castano E, Jeon H, Ohaegbulam KC, Zhao R et al (2015) Expression, Clinical Significance, and Receptor Identification of the Newest B7 Family Member HHLA2 Protein. Clin Cancer Res 21:2359–2366

Jung K, Kang M, Park C, Hyun Choi Y, Jeon Y, Park SH, Seo SK, Jin D, Choi I (2012) Protective role of V-set and immunoglobulin domain-containing 4 expressed on kupffer cells during immune-mediated liver injury by inducing tolerance of liver T- and natural killer T-cells. Hepatology 56:1838–1848

Kang S, Zhang C, Ohno T, Azuma M (2017) Unique B7-H1 expression on masticatory mucosae in the oral cavity and trans-coinhibition by B7-H1-expressing keratinocytes regulating CD4(+) T cell-mediated mucosal tissue inflammation. Mucosal Immunol 10:650–660

Kao C, Oestreich KJ, Paley MA, Crawford A, Angelosanto JM, Ali MA, Intlekofer AM, Boss JM, Reiner SL, Weinmann AS et al (2011) Transcription factor T-bet represses expression of

2 The CD28–B7 Family of Co-signaling Molecules

the inhibitory receptor PD-1 and sustains virus-specific CD8+ T cell responses during chronic infection. Nat Immunol 12:663–671

Katschke KJ Jr, Helmy KY, Steffek M, Xi H, Yin J, Lee WP, Gribling P, Barck KH, Carano RA, Taylor RE et al (2007) A novel inhibitor of the alternative pathway of complement reverses inflammation and bone destruction in experimental arthritis. J Exp Med 204:1319–1325

Keir ME, Butte MJ, Freeman GJ, Sharpe AH (2008) PD-1 and its ligands in tolerance and immunity. Annu Rev Immunol 26:677–704

Khayyamian S, Hutloff A, Buchner K, Grafe M, Henn V, Kroczek RA, Mages HW (2002) ICOS-ligand, expressed on human endothelial cells, costimulates Th1 and Th2 cytokine secretion by memory CD4+ T cells. Proc Natl Acad Sci U S A 99:6198–6203

Kinter AL, Godbout EJ, McNally JP, Sereti I, Roby GA, O'Shea MA, Fauci AS (2008) The common gamma-chain cytokines IL-2, IL-7, IL-15, and IL-21 induce the expression of programmed death-1 and its ligands. J Immunol 181:6738–6746

Kondo Y, Ohno T, Nishii N, Harada K, Yagita H, Azuma M (2016) Differential contribution of three immune checkpoint (VISTA, CTLA-4, PD-1) pathways to antitumor responses against squamous cell carcinoma. Oral Oncol 57:54–60

Kong KF, Fu G, Zhang Y, Yokosuka T, Casas J, Canonigo-Balancio AJ, Becart S, Kim G, Yates JR 3rd, Kronenberg M et al (2014) Protein kinase C-eta controls CTLA-4-mediated regulatory T cell function. Nat Immunol 15:465–472

Kontgen F, Grumont RJ, Strasser A, Metcalf D, Li R, Tarlinton D, Gerondakis S (1995) Mice lacking the c-rel proto-oncogene exhibit defects in lymphocyte proliferation, humoral immunity, and interleukin-2 expression. Genes Dev 9:1965–1977

Krummel MF, Allison JP (1995) CD28 and CTLA-4 have opposing effects on the response of T cells to stimulation. J Exp Med 182:459–465

Krummel MF, Allison JP (1996) CTLA-4 engagement inhibits IL-2 accumulation and cell cycle progression upon activation of resting T cells. J Exp Med 183:2533–2540

Kuehn HS, Ouyang W, Lo B, Deenick EK, Niemela JE, Avery DT, Schickel JN, Tran DQ, Stoddard J, Zhang Y et al (2014) Immune dysregulation in human subjects with heterozygous germline mutations in CTLA4. Science 345:1623–1627

Langnaese K, Colleaux L, Kloos DU, Fontes M, Wieacker P (2000) Cloning of Z39Ig, a novel gene with immunoglobulin-like domains located on human chromosome X. Biochim Biophys Acta 1492:522–525

Laurent S, Carrega P, Saverino D, Piccioli P, Camoriano M, Morabito A, Dozin B, Fontana V, Simone R, Mortara L et al (2010) CTLA-4 is expressed by human monocyte-derived dendritic cells and regulates their functions. Hum Immunol 71:934–941

Leitner J, Klauser C, Pickl WF, Stockl J, Majdic O, Bardet AF, Kreil DP, Dong C, Yamazaki T, Zlabinger G et al (2009) B7-H3 is a potent inhibitor of human T-cell activation: No evidence for B7-H3 and TREML2 interaction. Eur J Immunol 39:1754–1764

Lemke D, Pfenning PN, Sahm F, Klein AC, Kempf T, Warnken U, Schnolzer M, Tudoran R, Weller M, Platten M et al (2012) Costimulatory protein 4IgB7H3 drives the malignant phenotype of glioblastoma by mediating immune escape and invasiveness. Clin Cancer Res 18:105–117

Li J, Diao B, Guo S, Huang X, Yang C, Feng Z, Yan W, Ning Q, Zheng L, Chen Y et al (2017) VSIG4 inhibits proinflammatory macrophage activation by reprogramming mitochondrial pyruvate metabolism. Nat Commun 8:1322

Lindstein T, June CH, Ledbetter JA, Stella G, Thompson CB (1989) Regulation of lymphokine messenger RNA stability by a surface-mediated T cell activation pathway. Science 244:339–343

Lines JL, Pantazi E, Mak J, Sempere LF, Wang L, O'Connell S, Ceeraz S, Suriawinata AA, Yan S, Ernstoff MS et al (2014) VISTA is an immune checkpoint molecule for human T cells. Cancer Res 74:1924–1932

Ling V, Wu PW, Spaulding V, Kieleczawa J, Luxenberg D, Carreno BM, Collins M (2003) Duplication of primate and rodent B7-H3 immunoglobulin V- and C-like domains: divergent history of functional redundancy and exon loss. Genomics 82:365–377

Linsley PS, Brady W, Urnes M, Grosmaire LS, Damle NK, Ledbetter JA (1991) CTLA-4 is a second receptor for the B cell activation antigen B7. J Exp Med 174:561–569

Linsley PS, Greene JL, Tan P, Bradshaw J, Ledbetter JA, Anasetti C, Damle NK (1992) Coexpression and functional cooperation of CTLA-4 and CD28 on activated T lymphocytes. J Exp Med 176:1595–1604

Linsley PS, Bradshaw J, Greene J, Peach R, Bennett KL, Mittler RS (1996) Intracellular trafficking of CTLA-4 and focal localization towards sites of TCR engagement. Immunity 4:535–543

Linterman MA, Rigby RJ, Wong R, Silva D, Withers D, Anderson G, Verma NK, Brink R, Hutloff A, Goodnow CC et al (2009) Roquin differentiates the specialized functions of duplicated T cell costimulatory receptor genes CD28 and ICOS. Immunity 30:228–241

Liu J, Yuan Y, Chen W, Putra J, Suriawinata AA, Schenk AD, Miller HE, Guleria I, Barth RJ, Huang YH et al (2015) Immune-checkpoint proteins VISTA and PD-1 nonredundantly regulate murine T-cell responses. Proc Natl Acad Sci U S A 112:6682–6687

Lo B, Zhang K, Lu W, Zheng L, Zhang Q, Kanellopoulou C, Zhang Y, Liu Z, Fritz JM, Marsh R et al (2015) AUTOIMMUNE DISEASE. Patients with LRBA deficiency show CTLA4 loss and immune dysregulation responsive to abatacept therapy. Science 349:436–440

Long M, Park SG, Strickland I, Hayden MS, Ghosh S (2009) Nuclear factor-kappaB modulates regulatory T cell development by directly regulating expression of Foxp3 transcription factor. Immunity 31:921–931

Luo L, Chapoval AI, Flies DB, Zhu G, Hirano F, Wang S, Lau JS, Dong H, Tamada K, Flies AS et al (2004) B7-H3 enhances tumor immunity in vivo by costimulating rapid clonal expansion of antigen-specific CD8+ cytolytic T cells. J Immunol 173:5445–5450

Mager DL, Hunter DG, Schertzer M, Freeman JD (1999) Endogenous retroviruses provide the primary polyadenylation signal for two new human genes (HHLA2 and HHLA3). Genomics 59:255–263

Mages HW, Hutloff A, Heuck C, Buchner K, Himmelbauer H, Oliveri F, Kroczek RA (2000) Molecular cloning and characterization of murine ICOS and identification of B7h as ICOS ligand. Eur J Immunol 30:1040–1047

Magistrelli G, Jeannin P, Herbault N, Benoit De Coignac A, Gauchat JF, Bonnefoy JY, Delneste Y (1999) A soluble form of CTLA-4 generated by alternative splicing is expressed by nonstimulated human T cells. Eur J Immunol 29:3596–3602

Malquori L, Carsetti L, Ruberti G (2008) The 3' UTR of the human CTLA4 mRNA can regulate mRNA stability and translational efficiency. Biochim Biophys Acta 1779:60–65

Martinez-Llordella M, Esensten JH, Bailey-Bucktrout SL, Lipsky RH, Marini A, Chen J, Mughal M, Mattson MP, Taub DD, Bluestone JA (2013) CD28-inducible transcription factor DEC1 is required for efficient autoreactive CD4+ T cell response. J Exp Med 210:1603–1619

Mathieu M, Cotta-Grand N, Daudelin JF, Thebault P, Labrecque N (2013) Notch signaling regulates PD-1 expression during CD8(+) T-cell activation. Immunol Cell Biol 91:82–88

McAdam AJ, Chang TT, Lumelsky AE, Greenfield EA, Boussiotis VA, Duke-Cohan JS, Chernova T, Malenkovich N, Jabs C, Kuchroo VK et al (2000) Mouse inducible costimulatory molecule (ICOS) expression is enhanced by CD28 costimulation and regulates differentiation of CD4+ T cells. J Immunol 165:5035–5040

McAdam AJ, Greenwald RJ, Levin MA, Chernova T, Malenkovich N, Ling V, Freeman GJ, Sharpe AH (2001) ICOS is critical for CD40-mediated antibody class switching. Nature 409:102–105

Mead KI, Zheng Y, Manzotti CN, Perry LC, Liu MK, Burke F, Powner DJ, Wakelam MJ, Sansom DM (2005) Exocytosis of CTLA-4 is dependent on phospholipase D and ADP ribosylation factor-1 and stimulated during activation of regulatory T cells. J Immunol 174:4803–4811

Metzler WJ, Bajorath J, Fenderson W, Shaw SY, Constantine KL, Naemura J, Leytze G, Peach RJ, Lavoie TB, Mueller L et al (1997) Solution structure of human CTLA-4 and delineation of a CD80/CD86 binding site conserved in CD28. Nat Struct Biol 4:527–531

Miller RE, Fayen JD, Mohammad SF, Stein K, Kadereit S, Woods KD, Sramkoski RM, Jacobberger JW, Templeton D, Shurin SB et al (2002) Reduced CTLA-4 protein and messenger RNA expression in umbilical cord blood T lymphocytes. Exp Hematol 30:738–744

Muscolini M, Camperio C, Porciello N, Caristi S, Capuano C, Viola A, Galandrini R, Tuosto L (2015) Phosphatidylinositol 4-phosphate 5-kinase alpha and Vav1 mutual cooperation in CD28-mediated actin remodeling and signaling functions. J Immunol 194:1323–1333

Nurieva R, Thomas S, Nguyen T, Martin-Orozco N, Wang Y, Kaja MK, Yu XZ, Dong C (2006) T-cell tolerance or function is determined by combinatorial costimulatory signals. EMBO J 25:2623–2633

Oaks MK, Hallett KM, Penwell RT, Stauber EC, Warren SJ, Tector AJ (2000) A native soluble form of CTLA-4. Cell Immunol 201:144–153

Oestreich KJ, Yoon H, Ahmed R, Boss JM (2008) NFATc1 regulates PD-1 expression upon T cell activation. J Immunol 181:4832–4839

Ohno T, Zhang C, Kondo Y, Kang S, Furusawa E, Tsuchiya K, Miyazaki Y, Azuma M (2018) The immune checkpoint molecule VISTA regulates allergen-specific Th2-mediated immune responses. Int Immunol 30:3–11

Okazaki T, Honjo T (2007) PD-1 and PD-1 ligands: from discovery to clinical application. Int Immunol 19:813–824

Okazaki T, Chikuma S, Iwai Y, Fagarasan S, Honjo T (2013) A rheostat for immune responses: the unique properties of PD-1 and their advantages for clinical application. Nat Immunol 14:1212–1218

Parry RV, Rumbley CA, Vandenberghe LH, June CH, Riley JL (2003) CD28 and inducible costimulatory protein Src homology 2 binding domains show distinct regulation of phosphatidylinositol 3-kinase, Bcl-xL, and IL-2 expression in primary human CD4 T lymphocytes. J Immunol 171:166–174

Paterson AM, Lovitch SB, Sage PT, Juneja VR, Lee Y, Trombley JD, Arancibia-Carcamo CV, Sobel RA, Rudensky AY, Kuchroo VK et al (2015) Deletion of CTLA-4 on regulatory T cells during adulthood leads to resistance to autoimmunity. J Exp Med 212:1603–1621

Patsoukis N, Brown J, Petkova V, Liu F, Li L, Boussiotis VA (2012) Selective effects of PD-1 on Akt and Ras pathways regulate molecular components of the cell cycle and inhibit T cell proliferation. Sci Signal 5:ra46

Patsoukis N, Li L, Sari D, Petkova V, Boussiotis VA (2013) PD-1 increases PTEN phosphatase activity while decreasing PTEN protein stability by inhibiting casein kinase 2. Mol Cell Biol 33:3091–3098

Perkins D, Wang Z, Donovan C, He H, Mark D, Guan G, Wang Y, Walunas T, Bluestone J, Listman J et al (1996) Regulation of CTLA-4 expression during T cell activation. J Immunol 156:4154–4159

Picarda E, Ohaegbulam KC, Zang X (2016) Molecular Pathways: Targeting B7-H3 (CD276) for Human Cancer Immunotherapy. Clin Cancer Res 22:3425–3431

Pistillo MP, Tazzari PL, Palmisano GL, Pierri I, Bolognesi A, Ferlito F, Capanni P, Polito L, Ratta M, Pileri S et al (2003) CTLA-4 is not restricted to the lymphoid cell lineage and can function as a target molecule for apoptosis induction of leukemic cells. Blood 101:202–209

Podojil JR, Hecht I, Chiang MY, Vaknin I, Barbiro I, Novik A, Neria E, Rotman G, Miller SD (2018) ILDR2-Fc Is a Novel Regulator of Immune Homeostasis and Inducer of Antigen-Specific Immune Tolerance. J Immunol 200:2013–2024

Prasad DV, Nguyen T, Li Z, Yang Y, Duong J, Wang Y, Dong C (2004) Murine B7-H3 is a negative regulator of T cells. J Immunol 173:2500–2506

Qian X, Agematsu K, Freeman GJ, Tagawa Y, Sugane K, Hayashi T (2006) The ICOS-ligand B7-H2, expressed on human type II alveolar epithelial cells, plays a role in the pulmonary host defense system. Eur J Immunol 36:906–918

Qian Y, Hong B, Shen L, Wu Z, Yao H, Zhang L (2013) B7-H4 enhances oncogenicity and inhibits apoptosis in pancreatic cancer cells. Cell Tissue Res 353:139–151

Qureshi OS, Kaur S, Hou TZ, Jeffery LE, Poulter NS, Briggs Z, Kenefeck R, Willox AK, Royle SJ, Rappoport JZ et al (2012) Constitutive clathrin-mediated endocytosis of CTLA-4 persists during T cell activation. J Biol Chem 287:9429–9440

Ramakrishnan P, Clark PM, Mason DE, Peters EC, Hsieh-Wilson LC, Baltimore D (2013) Activation of the transcriptional function of the NF-kappaB protein c-Rel by O-GlcNAc glycosylation. Sci Signal 6:ra75

Ramos-Morales F, Romero F, Schweighoffer F, Bismuth G, Camonis J, Tortolero M, Fischer S (1995) The proline-rich region of Vav binds to Grb2 and Grb3-3. Oncogene 11:1665–1669

Rao S, Gerondakis S, Woltring D, Shannon MF (2003) c-Rel is required for chromatin remodeling across the IL-2 gene promoter. J Immunol 170:3724–3731

Saito T, Yokosuka T, Hashimoto-Tane A (2010) Dynamic regulation of T cell activation and costimulation through TCR-microclusters. FEBS Lett 584:4865–4871

Sakr MA, Takino T, Domoto T, Nakano H, Wong RW, Sasaki M, Nakanuma Y, Sato H (2010) GI24 enhances tumor invasiveness by regulating cell surface membrane-type 1 matrix metalloproteinase. Cancer Sci 101:2368–2374

Sanchez-Lockhart M, Graf B, Miller J (2008) Signals and sequences that control CD28 localization to the central region of the immunological synapse. J Immunol 181:7639–7648

Sauer S, Bruno L, Hertweck A, Finlay D, Leleu M, Spivakov M, Knight ZA, Cobb BS, Cantrell D, O'Connor E et al (2008) T cell receptor signaling controls Foxp3 expression via PI3K, Akt, and mTOR. Proc Natl Acad Sci U S A 105:7797–7802

Schneider H, Martin M, Agarraberes FA, Yin L, Rapoport I, Kirchhausen T, Rudd CE (1999) Cytolytic T lymphocyte-associated antigen-4 and the TCR zeta/CD3 complex, but not CD28, interact with clathrin adaptor complexes AP-1 and AP-2. J Immunol 163:1868–1879

Schneider H, Downey J, Smith A, Zinselmeyer BH, Rush C, Brewer JM, Wei B, Hogg N, Garside P, Rudd CE (2006) Reversal of the TCR stop signal by CTLA-4. Science 313:1972–1975

Schwartz JC, Zhang X, Nathenson SG, Almo SC (2002) Structural mechanisms of costimulation. Nat Immunol 3:427–434

Shapiro VS, Truitt KE, Imboden JB, Weiss A (1997) CD28 mediates transcriptional upregulation of the interleukin-2 (IL-2) promoter through a composite element containing the CD28RE and NF-IL-2B AP-1 sites. Mol Cell Biol 17:4051–4058

Sheppard KA, Fitz LJ, Lee JM, Benander C, George JA, Wooters J, Qiu Y, Jussif JM, Carter LL, Wood CR et al (2004) PD-1 inhibits T-cell receptor induced phosphorylation of the ZAP70/CD3zeta signalosome and downstream signaling to PKCtheta. FEBS Lett 574:37–41

Sica GL, Choi IH, Zhu G, Tamada K, Wang SD, Tamura H, Chapoval AI, Flies DB, Bajorath J, Chen L (2003) B7-H4, a molecule of the B7 family, negatively regulates T cell immunity. Immunity 18:849–861

Smith KM, Brewer JM, Webb P, Coyle AJ, Gutierrez-Ramos C, Garside P (2003) Inducible costimulatory molecule-B7-related protein 1 interactions are important for the clonal expansion and B cell helper functions of naive, Th1, and Th2 T cells. J Immunol 170:2310–2315

Sonkoly E, Janson P, Majuri ML, Savinko T, Fyhrquist N, Eidsmo L, Xu N, Meisgen F, Wei T, Bradley M et al (2010) MiR-155 is overexpressed in patients with atopic dermatitis and modulates T-cell proliferative responses by targeting cytotoxic T lymphocyte-associated antigen 4. J Allergy Clin Immunol 126(581–589):e581–e520

Stamper CC, Zhang Y, Tobin JF, Erbe DV, Ikemizu S, Davis SJ, Stahl ML, Seehra J, Somers WS, Mosyak L (2001) Crystal structure of the B7-1/CTLA-4 complex that inhibits human immune responses. Nature 410:608–611

Staron MM, Gray SM, Marshall HD, Parish IA, Chen JH, Perry CJ, Cui G, Li MO, Kaech SM (2014) The transcription factor FoxO1 sustains expression of the inhibitory receptor PD-1 and survival of antiviral CD8(+) T cells during chronic infection. Immunity 41:802–814

Stojanovic A, Fiegler N, Brunner-Weinzierl M, Cerwenka A (2014) CTLA-4 is expressed by activated mouse NK cells and inhibits NK Cell IFN-gamma production in response to mature dendritic cells. J Immunol 192:4184–4191

Suh WK, Gajewska BU, Okada H, Gronski MA, Bertram EM, Dawicki W, Duncan GS, Bukczynski J, Plyte S, Elia A et al (2003) The B7 family member B7-H3 preferentially down-regulates T helper type 1-mediated immune responses. Nat Immunol 4:899–906

Suh WK, Wang S, Duncan GS, Miyazaki Y, Cates E, Walker T, Gajewska BU, Deenick E, Dawicki W, Okada H et al (2006) Generation and characterization of B7-H4/B7S1/B7x-deficient mice. Mol Cell Biol 26:6403–6411

Sun MY, Richards S, Prasad DVR, Mai XM, Rudensky A, Dong C (2002) Characterization of mouse and human B7-H3 genes. J Immunol 168:6294–6297

Sun J, Fu F, Gu W, Yan R, Zhang G, Shen Z, Zhou Y, Wang H, Shen B, Zhang X (2011) Origination of new immunological functions in the costimulatory molecule B7-H3: the role of exon duplication in evolution of the immune system. PLoS One 6:e24751

Tafuri A, Shahinian A, Bladt F, Yoshinaga SK, Jordana M, Wakeham A, Boucher LM, Bouchard D, Chan VS, Duncan G et al (2001) ICOS is essential for effective T-helper-cell responses. Nature 409:105–109

Takahashi T, Tagami T, Yamazaki S, Uede T, Shimizu J, Sakaguchi N, Mak TW, Sakaguchi S (2000) Immunologic self-tolerance maintained by CD25(+)CD4(+) regulatory T cells constitutively expressing cytotoxic T lymphocyte-associated antigen 4. J Exp Med 192:303–310

Tan C, Wei L, Vistica BP, Shi G, Wawrousek EF, Gery I (2014) Phenotypes of Th lineages generated by the commonly used activation with anti-CD3/CD28 antibodies differ from those generated by the physiological activation with the specific antigen. Cell Mol Immunol 11:305–313

Tavano R, Contento RL, Baranda SJ, Soligo M, Tuosto L, Manes S, Viola A (2006) CD28 interaction with filamin-A controls lipid raft accumulation at the T-cell immunological synapse. Nat Cell Biol 8:1270–1276

Terawaki S, Chikuma S, Shibayama S, Hayashi T, Yoshida T, Okazaki T, Honjo T (2011) IFN-alpha directly promotes programmed cell death-1 transcription and limits the duration of T cell-mediated immunity. J Immunol 186:2772–2779

Thomas RM, Gao L, Wells AD (2005) Signals from CD28 induce stable epigenetic modification of the IL-2 promoter. J Immunol 174:4639–4646

Ueda H, Howson JM, Esposito L, Heward J, Snook H, Chamberlain G, Rainbow DB, Hunter KM, Smith AN, Di Genova G et al (2003) Association of the T-cell regulatory gene CTLA4 with susceptibility to autoimmune disease. Nature 423:506–511

Valk E, Leung R, Kang H, Kaneko K, Rudd CE, Schneider H (2006) T cell receptor-interacting molecule acts as a chaperone to modulate surface expression of the CTLA-4 coreceptor. Immunity 25:807–821

van der Merwe PA, Davis SJ (2003) Molecular interactions mediating T cell antigen recognition. Annu Rev Immunol 21:659–684

van der Merwe PA, Bodian DL, Daenke S, Linsley P, Davis SJ (1997) CD80 (B7-1) binds both CD28 and CTLA-4 with a low affinity and very fast kinetics. J Exp Med 185:393–403

Victora GD, Nussenzweig MC (2012) Germinal centers. Annu Rev Immunol 30:429–457

Vigdorovich V, Ramagopal UA, Lazar-Molnar E, Sylvestre E, Lee JS, Hofmeyer KA, Zang X, Nathenson SG, Almo SC (2013) Structure and T cell inhibition properties of B7 family member, B7-H3. Structure 21:707–717

Vijayakrishnan L, Slavik JM, Illes Z, Greenwald RJ, Rainbow D, Greve B, Peterson LB, Hafler DA, Freeman GJ, Sharpe AH et al (2004) An autoimmune disease-associated CTLA-4 splice variant lacking the B7 binding domain signals negatively in T cells. Immunity 20:563–575

Vogt L, Schmitz N, Kurrer MO, Bauer M, Hinton HI, Behnke S, Gatto D, Sebbel P, Beerli RR, Sonderegger I et al (2006) VSIG4, a B7 family-related protein, is a negative regulator of T cell activation. J Clin Invest 116:2817–2826

Walunas TL, Bakker CY, Bluestone JA (1996) CTLA-4 ligation blocks CD28-dependent T cell activation. J Exp Med 183:2541–2550

Wang L, Rubinstein R, Lines JL, Wasiuk A, Ahonen C, Guo Y, Lu LF, Gondek D, Wang Y, Fava RA et al (2011) VISTA, a novel mouse Ig superfamily ligand that negatively regulates T cell responses. J Exp Med 208:577–592

Wang J, Wu G, Manick B, Hernandez V, Renelt M, Erickson C, Guan J, Singh R, Rollins S, Solorz A et al (2019) VSIG-3 as a ligand of VISTA inhibits human T-cell function. Immunology 156:74–85

Watts TH (2010) Staying alive: T cell costimulation, CD28, and Bcl-xL. J Immunol 185:3785–3787

Weiss A, Manger B, Imboden J (1986) Synergy between the T3/antigen receptor complex and Tp44 in the activation of human T cells. J Immunol 137:819–825

Wilson EH, Zaph C, Mohrs M, Welcher A, Siu J, Artis D, Hunter CA (2006) B7RP-1-ICOS interactions are required for optimal infection-induced expansion of CD4+ Th1 and Th2 responses. J Immunol 177:2365–2372

Wing K, Onishi Y, Prieto-Martin P, Yamaguchi T, Miyara M, Fehervari Z, Nomura T, Sakaguchi S (2008) CTLA-4 control over Foxp3+ regulatory T cell function. Science 322:271–275

Witsch EJ, Peiser M, Hutloff A, Buchner K, Dorner BG, Jonuleit H, Mages HW, Kroczek RA (2002) ICOS and CD28 reversely regulate IL-10 on re-activation of human effector T cells with mature dendritic cells. Eur J Immunol 32:2680–2686

Wong SC, Oh E, Ng CH, Lam KP (2003) Impaired germinal center formation and recall T-cell-dependent immune responses in mice lacking the costimulatory ligand B7-H2. Blood 102:1381–1388

Wu YQ, Borde M, Heissmeyer V, Feuerer M, Lapan AD, Stroud JC, Bates DL, Guo L, Han AD, Ziegler SF et al (2006) FOXP3 controls regulatory T cell function through cooperation with NFAT. Cell 126:375–387

Xiao Y, Yu S, Zhu B, Bedoret D, Bu X, Francisco LM, Hua P, Duke-Cohan JS, Umetsu DT, Sharpe AH et al (2014) RGMb is a novel binding partner for PD-L2 and its engagement with PD-L2 promotes respiratory tolerance. J Exp Med 211:943–959

Yamazaki T, Akiba H, Iwai H, Matsuda H, Aoki M, Tanno Y, Shin T, Tsuchiya H, Pardoll DM, Okumura K et al (2002) Expression of programmed death 1 ligands by murine T cells and APC. J Immunol 169:5538–5545

Ying H, Yang L, Qiao G, Li Z, Zhang L, Yin F, Xie D, Zhang J (2010) Cutting edge: CTLA-4--B7 interaction suppresses Th17 cell differentiation. J Immunol 185:1375–1378

Yokosuka T, Kobayashi W, Sakata-Sogawa K, Takamatsu M, Hashimoto-Tane A, Dustin ML, Tokunaga M, Saito T (2008) Spatiotemporal regulation of T cell costimulation by TCR-CD28 microclusters and protein kinase C theta translocation. Immunity 29:589–601

Yokosuka T, Takamatsu M, Kobayashi-Imanishi W, Hashimoto-Tane A, Azuma M, Saito T (2012) Programmed cell death 1 forms negative costimulatory microclusters that directly inhibit T cell receptor signaling by recruiting phosphatase SHP2. J Exp Med 209:1201–1217

Yoon KW, Byun S, Kwon E, Hwang SY, Chu K, Hiraki M, Jo SH, Weins A, Hakroush S, Cebulla A et al (2015) Control of signaling-mediated clearance of apoptotic cells by the tumor suppressor p53. Science 349:1261669

Yoshinaga SK, Whoriskey JS, Khare SD, Sarmiento U, Guo J, Horan T, Shih G, Zhang M, Coccia MA, Kohno T et al (1999) T-cell co-stimulation through B7RP-1 and ICOS. Nature 402:827–832

Yoshinaga SK, Zhang M, Pistillo J, Horan T, Khare SD, Miner K, Sonnenberg M, Boone T, Brankow D, Dai T et al (2000) Characterization of a new human B7-related protein: B7RP-1 is the ligand to the co-stimulatory protein ICOS. Int Immunol 12:1439–1447

Yuan X, Yang BH, Dong Y, Yamamura A, Fu W (2017) CRIg, a tissue-resident macrophage specific immune checkpoint molecule, promotes immunological tolerance in NOD mice, via a dual role in effector and regulatory T cells. elife 6:e29540

Zang X, Loke P, Kim J, Murphy K, Waitz R, Allison JP (2003) B7x: a widely expressed B7 family member that inhibits T cell activation. Proc Natl Acad Sci U S A 100:10388–10392

Zhang X, Schwartz JC, Almo SC, Nathenson SG (2003) Crystal structure of the receptor-binding domain of human B7-2: insights into organization and signaling. Proc Natl Acad Sci U S A 100:2586–2591

Zhang G, Hou J, Shi J, Yu G, Lu B, Zhang X (2008) Soluble CD276 (B7-H3) is released from monocytes, dendritic cells and activated T cells and is detectable in normal human serum. Immunology 123:538–546

Zhao R, Chinai JM, Buhl S, Scandiuzzi L, Ray A, Jeon H, Ohaegbulam KC, Ghosh K, Zhao A, Scharff MD et al (2013) HHLA2 is a member of the B7 family and inhibits human CD4 and CD8 T-cell function. Proc Natl Acad Sci U S A 110:9879–9884

Zheng Y, Josefowicz SZ, Kas A, Chu TT, Gavin MA, Rudensky AY (2007) Genome-wide analysis of Foxp3 target genes in developing and mature regulatory T cells. Nature 445:936–940

Zhong X, Bai C, Gao W, Strom TB, Rothstein TL (2004) Suppression of expression and function of negative immune regulator PD-1 by certain pattern recognition and cytokine receptor signals associated with immune system danger. Int Immunol 16:1181–1188

Zhong X, Tumang JR, Gao W, Bai C, Rothstein TL (2007) PD-L2 expression extends beyond dendritic cells/macrophages to B1 cells enriched for V(H)11/V(H)12 and phosphatidylcholine binding. Eur J Immunol 37:2405–2410

Zhu G, Augustine MM, Azuma T, Luo L, Yao S, Anand S, Rietz AC, Huang J, Xu H, Flies AS et al (2009) B7-H4-deficient mice display augmented neutrophil-mediated innate immunity. Blood 113:1759–1767

Zhu Y, Yao S, Iliopoulou BP, Han X, Augustine MM, Xu H, Phennicie RT, Flies SJ, Broadwater M, Ruff W et al (2013) B7-H5 costimulates human T cells via CD28H. Nat Commun 4:2043

Chapter 3
The TNF–TNFR Family of Co-signal Molecules

Takanori So and Naoto Ishii

Abstract Costimulatory signals initiated by the interaction between the tumor necrosis factor (TNF) ligand and cognate TNF receptor (TNFR) superfamilies promote clonal expansion, differentiation, and survival of antigen-primed CD4$^+$ and CD8$^+$ T cells and have a pivotal role in T-cell-mediated adaptive immunity and diseases. Accumulating evidence in recent years indicates that costimulatory signals via the subset of the TNFR superfamily molecules, OX40 (TNFRSF4), 4-1BB (TNFRSF9), CD27, DR3 (TNFRSF25), CD30 (TNFRSF8), GITR (TNFRSF18), TNFR2 (TNFRSF1B), and HVEM (TNFRSF14), which are constitutive or inducible on T cells, play important roles in protective immunity, inflammatory and autoimmune diseases, and tumor immunotherapy. In this chapter, we will summarize the findings of recent studies on these TNFR family of co-signaling molecules regarding their function at various stages of the T-cell response in the context of infection, inflammation, and cancer. We will also discuss how these TNFR co-signals are critical for immune regulation and have therapeutic potential for the treatment of T-cell-mediated diseases.

Keywords 4-1BB · CD27 · CD30 · DR3 · HVEM · GITR · OX40 · TNFR2 · TNFSF · TNFRSF

T. So (✉)
Department of Microbiology and Immunology, Tohoku University Graduate
School of Medicine, Sendai, Japan

Laboratory of Molecular Cell Biology, Graduate School of Medicine
and Pharmaceutical Sciences, University of Toyama, Toyama, Japan
e-mail: tso@pha.u-toyama.ac.jp

N. Ishii
Department of Microbiology and Immunology, Tohoku University Graduate
School of Medicine, Sendai, Japan
e-mail: ishiin@med.tohoku.ac.jp

© Springer Nature Singapore Pte Ltd. 2019
M. Azuma, H. Yagita (eds.), *Co-signal Molecules in T Cell Activation*,
Advances in Experimental Medicine and Biology 1189,
https://doi.org/10.1007/978-981-32-9717-3_3

Abbreviations

APC	antigen-presenting cell;
CAR	chimeric antigen receptor
CMV	cytomegalovirus
CTL	cytotoxic T lymphocyte
CTLA-4	cytotoxic T-lymphocyte-associated protein-4
DC	dendritic cell
DcR3	decoy receptor 3
DR3	death receptor 3
EAE	experimental autoimmune encephalomyelitis
EBV	Epstein–Barr virus
GC	germinal center
GITR	glucocorticoid-induced TNFR family-related protein
GVHD	graft-versus-host disease
HPV	human papillomavirus
HVEM	herpesvirus entry mediator
ICOS	inducible T-cell costimulator
LCMV	lymphocytic choriomeningitis virus
LIGHT	homologous to *l*ymphotoxins (LTs), *i*nducible expression, which competes with herpes simplex virus *g*lycoprotein D (HSV gD) for *H*VEM, a receptor expressed on *T* lymphocytes
mAb	monoclonal antibody
MAPK	mitogen-activated protein kinase
NF-κB	nuclear factor-kappa B
PD-1	programmed cell death-1
SLE	systemic lupus erythematosus
TCR	T-cell receptor
Tfh	T follicular helper
Th1	T-helper-1
Th17	T-helper-17
Th2	T-helper-2
Th9	T-helper-9
TL1A	TNF-like ligand 1A
TLR	Toll-like receptor
TNF	tumor necrosis factor
TNFR2	tumor necrosis factor receptor 2
TNFRSF	TNF receptor superfamily
TNFSF	TNF superfamily
TRAF	TNF receptor-associated factor
Treg cells	Foxp3$^+$ CD25$^+$ CD4$^+$ regulatory T cells

3.1 Introduction

The tumor necrosis factor (TNF) superfamily (TNFSF) of cytokines engages specific cognate cell surface receptors, the TNF receptor superfamily (TNFRSF). The TNFSF–TNFRSF interactions activate signaling pathways for cell survival, death, and differentiation that control immune function and disease, and several receptor–ligand pairs within TNF family molecules expressed by immune cells play key roles in T-cell immunity (Locksley et al. 2001; Aggarwal 2003; So et al. 2006; Croft 2009; Watts 2005; Ward-Kavanagh et al. 2016). The subset of TNFRSF molecules, 4-1BB, CD27, CD30, DR3 (death receptor 3), GITR (glucocorticoid-induced TNFR family-related protein), HVEM (herpesvirus entry mediator), OX40, and TNFR2 (tumor necrosis factor receptor 2), expressed by T cells, deliver activating signals, which are largely dependent on antigen recognition and participate in activation, clonal expansion, and differentiation of T cells. TNFRSF and TNFSF molecules that contribute to these additional signals in T cells function as a costimulatory receptor and a costimulatory ligand, respectively (Croft 2009; Watts 2005; So and Croft 2013) (Table 3.1, Fig. 3.1).

A dialogue between a naïve T cell and a dendritic cell (DC) plays an essential role for priming of naïve T cells in secondary lymph organs. The expression levels of 4-1BB, CD27, CD30, DR3, GITR, HVEM, OX40, and TNFR2 on T cells are positively or negatively controlled by activating signals through the T-cell receptor (TCR) and the costimulatory receptor CD28. At the same time, after recognition of microbes, immature DCs are activated via pattern recognition receptors and upregulate not only major histocompatibility complex (MHC) and B7 proteins but also TNFSF molecules including 4-1BBL, CD70, CD30L, TL1A (TNF-like ligand 1A), GITRL, LIGHT, OX40L, and TNF-α. The T cell-DC dialogue via each individual TNFSF–TNFRSF interaction provides additional costimulatory signals to antigen-primed naïve T cells, promotes the differentiation of naïve T cells into effector and memory T-cell populations, and supports the survival of these antigen-primed T cells in the periphery (Fig. 3.2).

In this chapter, we focus on the TNFRSF of costimulatory receptors, 4-1BB, CD27, CD30, DR3, GITR, HVEM, OX40, and TNFR2, and summarize the significance of costimulatory signals mediated by these receptors in terms of protective immunity, autoimmunity and inflammation, and cancer, in which these TNFRSF molecules play critical roles. Administration of agonistic or antagonistic agents (biologics) that can modulate the co-signaling activity of TNFRSF molecules can regulate T-cell functions in vivo, and thus these TNFSF–TNFRSF interactions have been considered as therapeutic targets for intervention in human diseases including autoimmunity and cancer.

3.2 Structure

3.2.1 Ligand

The costimulatory ligands of the TNFSF described in this chapter are type II (intracellular N terminus and extracellular C terminus) transmembrane proteins and have a C-terminal TNF homology domain (THD) that is responsible for receptor binding (Bodmer et al. 2002) (Table 3.1, Fig. 3.1). One TNFSF molecule assembles into a trimer on the surface of antigen-presenting cells (APCs), and its cognate monomer TNFRSF molecule on T cells is trimerized through binding to the trimeric configuration of the ligand THDs, resulting in formation of a quaternary organized hexamer complex at the T cell–APC interface (Fig. 3.2). TNFSF molecules can be produced as membrane-bound trimers or be released as soluble trimers from the cell surface after proteolytic processing in the stalk region. The membrane-bound TNFSF molecules that are engaged by their cognate receptors have been defined as inducers of signal transduction. This "reverse" signaling mediated by membrane-bound TNFSF molecules can regulate some cellular functions, such as pro-inflammatory cytokine production and cell maturation (Eissner et al. 2004; Sun and Fink 2007).

3.2.2 Receptor

The costimulatory receptors of the TNFRSF described in this chapter are type I (extracellular N terminus and intracellular C terminus) transmembrane proteins and have three to six cysteine-rich domains (CRDs) in their extracellular regions (Bodmer et al. 2002) (Table 3.1, Fig. 3.1). After binding to TNFSF timers via CRDs, TNFRSF molecules cluster on the T-cell membrane, which in turn initiates co-signaling cascades in antigen-recognized T cells. The cytoplasmic amino acid sequences divide TNFRSF molecules into three major groups: (1) TNF receptor-associated factor (TRAF) binding TNFRSF molecule, such as 4-1BB, CD27, CD30, DR3, GITR, HVEM, OX40, and TNFR2; (2) death domain (DD) containing TNFRSF molecule, such as DR3; and (3) decoy TNFRSF molecule lacking a functional cytoplasmic domain, such as DcR3 (decoy receptor 3). Upon binding of cognate TNFSF molecules, the TNFRSF of co-signaling molecules on T cells initiate "forward" signaling mediated by the TRAF family molecules, and this TRAF-mediated signaling contributes to activation of co-signaling cascades in antigen-primed T cells (Figs. 3.1 and 3.2). The extracellular domains of membrane-bound TNFRSF molecules can be cleaved to release soluble TNFRSF forms in some contexts.

Table 3.1 The receptor and ligand system responsible for TNFR co-signaling

Receptor	Symbol	Synonyms	Ligand	Symbol	Synonyms
OX40	TNFRSF4	CD134, ACT35, TXGP1L	**OX40L**	TNFSF4	CD134L, CD252, gp34, OX-40L, TXGP1
4-1BB	TNFRSF9	CD137, ILA	**4-1BBL**	TNFSF9	CD137L
CD27	CD27	S152, Tp55	**CD70**	CD70	CD27L, CD27LG, TNFSF7
DR3	TNFRSF25	APO-3, DDR3, LARD, TNFRSF12, TR3, TRAMP, WSL-1, WSL-LR	**TL1A**	TNFSF15	MGC129934, MGC129935, TL1, VEGI, VEGI192A
CD30	TNFRSF8	D1S166E, KI-1	**CD30L**	TNFSF8	CD30LG, CD153
GITR	TNFRSF18	AITR, CD357	**GITRL**	TNFSF18	AITRL, TL6
TNFR2	TNFRSF1B	CD120b, p75, TNF-R-II, TNF-R75, TNFBR, TNFR80	**TNF-α**	TNF	DIF, TNFA, TNF-alpha, TNFSF2
			LT-α	LTA	LT, $LT\alpha_3$, TNFB, TNFSF1
HVEM	TNFRSF14	ATAR, CD270, HVEA, LIGHTR, TR2	**LIGHT**	TNFSF14	CD258, HVEM-L, LTg
			LT-α	LTA	LT, $LT\alpha_3$, TNFB, TNFSF1
			BTLA	BTLA	BTLA1, CD272
			CD160	CD160	BY55, NK1, NK28
DcR3	TNFRSF6B	DCR3, M68, TR6	**TL1A**	TNFSF15	MGC129934, MGC129935, TL1, VEGI, VEGI192A
			LIGHT	TNFSF14	CD258, HVEM-L, LTg
			FASL	FASLG	APT1LG1, CD178, TNFSF6

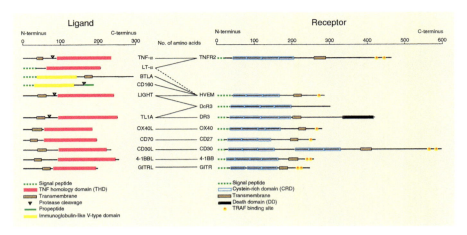

Fig. 3.1 Protein domain organization in the TNF–TNFR family of co-signaling molecules. Data are based on UniProt (www.uniprot.org). TNF-α, P01375; LT-α, P01374; BTLA, Q7Z6A9; CD160, O95971; LIGHT, O43557; TL1A, O95150; OX40L, P23510; CD70, P32970; CD30L, P32971; 4-1BBL, P41273; GITRL, Q9UNG2; TNFR2, P20333; HVEM, Q92956; DcR3, O95407; DR3, Q93038; OX40, P43489; CD27, P26842; CD30, P28908; 4-1BB, Q07011; GITR, Q9Y5U5. LT-α shows low affinity for HVEM (dashed line)

3.2.3 TRAF

After binding to cognate ligands of the TNFSF family molecules, the TNFRSF of co-signaling molecules recruits various intracellular TRAF molecules to their cytoplasmic tails, leading to activation of canonical and noncanonical nuclear factor-kappa B (NF-κB), mitogen-activated protein kinase (MAPK), and serine/threonine-protein kinase Akt (protein kinase B) cascades (Brenner et al. 2015; So and Croft 2013; Hayden and Ghosh 2014; Karin and Gallagher 2009) (Fig. 3.2). Thus, TRAFs mediate the link between receptor-proximal and cytosolic signaling events. Six TRAFs, TRAF1 to TRAF6, which share a conserved C-terminal TRAF-C domain, function both as ubiquitin E3 ligases and as adaptor molecules to potentiate signal transduction. Except for TRAF1, the N-terminal of TRAF contains a really interesting new gene (RING) and zinc-finger domains that are responsible for ubiquitin E3 ligase activity to promote the activation of downstream signaling cascades. The C-terminal of TRAF contains a coiled-coil (TRAF-N) domain and a TRAF-C domain that contributes to intermolecular interactions and sequence-specific interactions with receptor cytoplasmic tails, respectively (Ha et al. 2009; So et al. 2015).

3 The TNF–TNFR Family of Co-signal Molecules

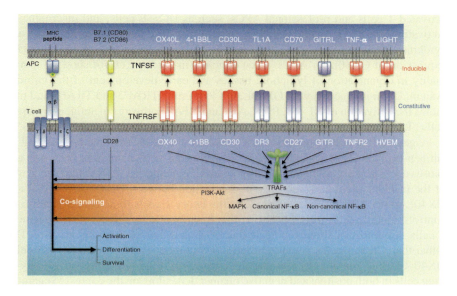

Fig. 3.2 T-cell signaling regulated by the TNF–TNFR family of co-signaling molecules. T cells are activated firstly by recognition of antigen by the T-cell receptor (TCR)/CD3 complex when antigenic peptides are presented by class I or class II molecules of the major histocompatibility complex (MHC) on antigen-presenting cell (APCs), such as dendritic cells, B cells, and macrophages. The second costimulatory signal is delivered via CD28 by interacting its ligands B7.1 (CD80) and/or B7.2 (CD86). After recognition of trimeric TNF ligand superfamily (TNFSF) molecules on APCs, TNF receptor superfamily (TNFRSF) molecules on T cells are trimerized and recruit TNF receptor-associated factors (TRAFs) to their cytoplasmic regions, which results in activation of canonical and noncanonical nuclear factor kappa B (NF-κB) and mitogen-activated protein kinase (MAPK) pathways. The TNFSF–TNFRSF interaction promotes costimulatory signaling pathways, which include phosphoinositide 3-kinase (PI3K)-Akt (protein kinase B), NF-κB, and MAPK pathways, initiated by the TCR and CD28, and plays important roles for T-cell activation, differentiation, and survival, at both early and later stages of the T-cell response. TNFSF and TNFRSF molecules constitutively and inducibly expressed by cells are indicated in blue and red, respectively

3.3 TNFR Co-signaling

3.3.1 OX40L-OX40

3.3.1.1 Expression and Function

Naïve CD4+ and CD8+ T cells do not express OX40. OX40 is induced on activated T cells upon antigen recognition and is downregulated after antigen clearance. Resting and memory T cells rapidly reexpress OX40 after antigen reencounter. CD28 co-signaling and pro-inflammatory cytokines including IL-1, IL-2, IL-4, and TNF-α can promote the expression of OX40. Foxp3+ CD25+ CD4+ regulatory T cells (Treg cells) constitutively express OX40 in mice. OX40L is induced on activated T cells and professional APCs, such as DCs, B cells, and macrophages. Activating signals via CD40, B-cell receptor (BCR), Toll-like receptors (TLRs), and cytokines, such as TSLP, type I IFN, and IL-18, and prostaglandin E2 promote the expression of OX40L on APCs. Mice deficient in *Ox40* or *Ox40l* show no abnormality in organization of lymphoid tissues and early development of the immune system. Upon interaction with OX40L, OX40 recruits TRAF2 and TRAF3 and promotes the activation of NF-κB, PI3K-Akt, and NFAT pathways in antigen-primed T cells (Table 3.1, Figs. 3.1 and 3.2).

A genetic deficiency of *Ox40* or *Ox40l* in mice leads to defective survival of antigen-primed CD4[+] and CD8[+] T cells during an active immune response and causes decreased accumulation of antigen-specific memory T cells in the later stages of the primary immune response. The interaction between OX40 on a T cell and OX40L on an APC provides critical costimulatory signals to activated T cells and controls not only cell survival but also other functional activities of effector/memory T cells. A number of studies indicate that OX40 has a more dominant role in CD4[+] rather than CD8[+] T-cell immunity because of its higher expression on CD4[+] T cells. OX40–OX40L interactions regulate the expansion, differentiation, and activity of Treg cells in both positive and negative manner depending on the context (Sugamura et al. 2004; Croft et al. 2009; Ishii et al. 2010; Croft 2010) (see Sect. 3.9).

3.3.1.2 Protective Immunity

Pathogen invasion results in activation of antigen-specific CD4[+] and CD8[+] T cells, and the OX40 co-signaling in primed T cells plays a key role in establishing protective immunity against infections by promoting the accumulation of antigen-specific effector/memory T cells. The OX40–OX40L interaction enhances pathogen-specific T-cell immunity in various models of infection including lymphocytic choriomeningitis virus (LCMV), influenza virus, vaccinia virus, human immunodeficiency virus, Epstein–Barr virus (EBV), cytomegalovirus (CMV), *Listeria monocytogenes*, and malaria. Although excessive stimulation of activated T cells with an agonistic monoclonal antibody (mAb) to OX40 induces adverse responses in some contexts, OX40 co-signaling generally augments both primary and memory T-cell responses to bacteria, virus, and parasite infections (Mousavi et al. 2008; Humphreys et al. 2007; Salek-Ardakani et al. 2008; Zander et al. 2015).

The cross talk and counterbalance between OX40 costimulatory and PD-1 (programmed cell death 1, CD279) co-inhibitory pathways play important roles for generation of protective CD4[+] T-cell immunity against malaria. OX40 is expressed by malaria-specific CD4[+] T cells but not CD8[+] T cells, and the expression is sustained after malaria infection. OX40L blockade and OX40 agonism exhibit enhanced and reduced parasite burdens, respectively. OX40 signaling supports the expansion of IFN-γ[+] T-bet[+] T-helper-1 (Th1) cells and Bcl-6[+] T follicular helper (Tfh) cells. OX40 signaling also enhances extra-follicular IgM[+] plasmablast formation, sustained Tfh responses, germinal center (GC) reactions, and T-dependent malaria-specific antibody class switching to IgG1. Both OX40 and PD-1 are expressed by malaria-specific CD4[+] T cells, and simultaneous PD-1 blockade and OX40 stimulation induce overproduction of IFN-γ, which limits Tfh cell-dependent humoral immunity that requires parasite control. This shows that OX40 co-signaling augments malaria-specific CD4[+] T-cell immunity and that PD-1 co-inhibitory signaling counterbalances the OX40 signaling to inhibit Th1 effector responses, which in turn facilitates the generation of optimal Tfh response required for humoral immunity to parasite (Zander et al. 2015).

In vaccinia virus infection in mice, the OX40–OX40L interaction promotes the development of Tfh cells, which is critical for GC development, plasma cell generation, and virus-specific antibody responses. OX40 is expressed by differentiating Tfh cells, and OX40L is expressed by CD11c[+] DCs in the periarteriolar lymphoid sheaths and the marginal zone bridging channels and by B220[+] B cells in the follicles. OX40L[+] DCs and OX40L[+] B cells are in contact with OX40[+] CD4[+] T cells at the T/B borders in the white pulp of the spleen. OX40 and ICOS (inducible T-cell costimulatory, CD278) are co-expressed by CXCR5[+] Bcl-6[+] Tfh cells in GC, and deficiency in *OX40* or OX40L blockade or ICOS blockade significantly inhibits the development of both Tfh cells and GC B cells. This demonstrates that OX40 co-signaling in synergy with ICOS co-signaling maximizes Tfh responses and GC reactions, which are important for humoral immunity against vaccinia virus (Tahiliani et al. 2017).

A case study that reports a nonfunctional *OX40* mutant in a patient strongly suggests that OX40 co-signaling plays a critical role in establishing a long-term T-cell immunity to pathogens in humans. The homozygous Arg65Cys missense/loss-of-function mutation in the first of four CRDs of extracellular region in OX40 causes a low level of OX40 expression on the T-cell surface, and this residual OX40 mutant protein does not show any binding activity to OX40L. The peripheral blood from this patient contains a decreased frequency of memory CD4[+] T cells. Consistent with this, in vitro recall T-cell responses to encountered antigens, including tuberculin purified protein derivatives (PPD), tetanus toxoid, EBV, CMV, and herpes simplex virus type 1, are severely impaired in this patient (Byun et al. 2013).

3.3.1.3 Autoimmunity and Inflammation

The OX40–OX40L interaction drives the development of autoimmunity and inflammation in many different animal models of asthma, colitis, graft-versus-host disease (GVHD), diabetes, multiple sclerosis, rheumatoid arthritis, atherosclerosis, and transplantation. Polymorphisms of the *OX40L* and *OX40* genes have been identified as risk factors in human diseases including systemic lupus erythematosus (SLE), rheumatoid arthritis, Sjögren syndrome, systemic sclerosis, cardiovascular disease, and narcolepsy (Table 3.2). Antigen-primed pathogenic T cells, but not naïve T cells, express OX40 or rapidly reexpress OX40 upon antigen reencounter, and thus the blockade of OX40L-OX40 interaction with a mAb or the depletion of OX40[+] T cells with a mAb to OX40 has been suggested to be effective for treatment of these T-cell-mediated diseases (Sugamura et al. 2004; Croft et al. 2009; Ishii et al. 2010; Croft 2010).

Table 3.2 Human disease linkage in the TNF-TNFR family of co-signaling molecules

Gene (Symbol)	Chromosomal location	OMIM No.	Disease phenotypes, symptoms, and molecular features	References, PubMed unique identifier (PMID) No.
OX40 (TNFRSF4)	1p36.33	600315	A homozygous loss-of-function mutation in the OX40 gene. Immunodeficiency. Childhood-onset classic Kaposi sarcoma.	23897980
OX40L (TNFSF4)	1q25.1	603594	A single risk haplotype for systemic lupus erythematosus in the OX40L gene that correlates with increased cell surface OX40L expression.	18059267
			Systemic lupus erythematosus, GWAS.	18204446, 19838195, 23273568, 26502338, 26663301, 27399966, 28714469
			Rheumatoid arthritis, GWAS.	23143596, 24532676
			Asthma, GWAS.	27182965, 31036433
4-1BB (TNFRSF9)	1p36.23	602250	A homozygous loss-of-function mutation in the 4-1BB gene. Immunodeficiency. Defective immunity against EBV.	30872117
			Rheumatoid arthritis, GWAS.	24390342, 30423114
			Breast carcinoma, GWAS.	29059683
CD27 (CD27)	12p13.31	186711	Homozygous, heterozygous, and compound heterozygous mutations in the CD27 gene. Immunodeficiency. Defective immunity against EBV.	22197273, 22801960, 25843314
CD70 (CD70)	19p13.3	602840	Homozygous loss-of-function mutations in the CD70 gene. Immunodeficiency. Defective immunity against EBV.	28011863, 28011864
TL1A (TNFSF15)	9q32	604052	Crohn's disease, GWAS.	18587394, 21102463, 23266558, 26192919, 26891255, 30500874
			Inflammatory bowel disease, GWAS.	18758464, 23128233, 26192919
			Ulcerative colitis, GWAS.	20848476, 21297633, 26192919
			Leprosy, GWAS.	20018961, 25642632
			Primary biliary cirrhosis, GWAS.	23000144, 28062665
			Chronic inflammatory diseases (ankylosing spondylitis, Crohn's disease, psoriasis, primary sclerosig cholangitis, ulcerative colitis), GWAS.	26974007

3 The TNF–TNFR Family of Co-signal Molecules

63

Gene	Location	OMIM	Disease/association	PubMed ID
TNF-α (TNF)	6p21.33	191160	Crohn's disease, GWAS.	21102463
			Oral cavity cancer, GWAS.	27749845
HVEM (TNFRSF14)	1p36.32	602746	Chronic inflammatory diseases (ankylosing spondylitis, Crohn's disease, psoriasis, primary sclerosig cholangitis, ulcerative colitis), GWAS.	26974007
LIGHT (TNFSF14)	19p13.3	604520	Multiple sclerosis, GWAS.	21833088, 24076602
LT-α (LTA)	6p21.33	153440	Cervical carcinoma, GWAS.	28806749
			Crohn's disease, GWAS.	21102463
DcR3 (TNFRSF6B)	20q13.33	603361	Glioma, GWAS.	19578366, 21531791, 22886559, 24908248, 26424050, 28346443, 29743610
			Allergic diseases (atopic dermatitis, asthma, hay fever, eczema), GWAS.	25574825, 26482879, 29083406, 29785011, 30929738
			Ulcerative colitis, GWAS.	21297633, 28067908
			Inflammatory bowel disease, GWAS.	26192919, 28067908
			Crohn's disease, GWAS.	28067908
			Colorectal cancer, GWAS.	30510241, 31089142
			Chronic inflammatory diseases (ankylosing spondylitis, Crohn's disease, psoriasis, primary sclerosig cholangitis, ulcerative colitis), GWAS.	26974007
TRAF1 (TRAF1)	9q33.2	601711	Rheumatoid arthritis, GWAS.	17804836, 20453842, 23143596, 24532676, 30891314
TRAF3 (TRAF3)	14q32.32	601896	A heterozygous dominant-negative mutation in the TRAF3 gene. A history of herpes simplex virus-1 encephalitis.	20832341
			Multiple sclerosis, GWAS.	24076602
			Asthma, GWAS.	30929738
			Systemic lupus erythematosus, GWAS.	28714469
TRAF6 (TRAF6)	11p12	602355	Rheumatoid arthritis, GWAS.	24390342, 30423114
			Myositis, GWAS.	26362759

Genome-wide association study (GWAS) data are based on the GWAS Catalog (www.ebi.ac.uk/gwas/home). EBV, Epstein-Barr virus

One human lupus study shows the correlation between the frequency of circulating OX40L[+] myeloid APCs in blood and the disease activity of SLE. OX40L is highly expressed in inflamed tissues including the tonsils, kidney, and skin from SLE patients. Sera from SLE patients contain immune complexes with RNA that can promote OX40L expression through TLR7 in APCs, and this OX40L activates human CD4[+] T cells to become Tfh-like cells possessing B-cell-helper activity. This proposes a hypothesis that excessive OX40 co-signaling through OX40L overproduction on APCs causes aberrant Tfh responses that lead to SLE (Jacquemin et al. 2015).

OX40L blockade in conjunction with traditional costimulation blockade is effective in preventing alloreactive T-cell responses that hinder long-term graft function and survival. In a murine allogeneic skin graft model, a blocking mAb to OX40L, but not to ICOSL (ICOS ligand, CD275), CD70, RANKL (receptor activator of NF-κB ligand, TNFSF11, CD254), or 4-1BBL, significantly improves allograft survival when combined with traditional blockade with anti-CD40L and CTLA-4 (cytotoxic T-lymphocyte-associated protein-4, CD152)-immunoglobulin (CTLA-4-Ig). This combined blockade effectively suppresses not only primary but also memory allogeneic T-cell responses. In a nonhuman primate renal transplantation model, treatment with combined humanized anti-OX40L mAb and belatacept (CTLA-4-Ig) exhibits a synergistic suppressive effect in prolonging allograft survival. This demonstrates that successful acceptance of allografts can be achieved by the simultaneous blockade of multiple costimulatory pathways and suggests that in this setting blockade of OX40 co-signaling is effective for dampening memory T-cell responses against allografts (Kitchens et al. 2017).

3.3.1.4 Cancer

Agonistic agents against OX40, such as anti-OX40 mAb and OX40L-Ig, provide potent costimulatory signals that can augment the expansion and proliferation of CD4[+] and CD8[+] T cells that recognize tumor antigens. In addition, the transduction of tumor cells or DCs with a vector that expresses OX40L can effectively boost antitumor T-cell responses. Although augmenting OX40 co-signaling can induce tumor regression and delay tumor growth, combination therapies of OX40 agonists with additional immune modulations, such as other mAbs to costimulatory/coinhibitory receptors, cytokines, vaccination, chemotherapy, and radiotherapy, have been suggested to be more effective in comparison to OX40 monotherapies (Moran et al. 2013; Linch et al. 2015).

OX40 agonism can effectively eradicate tumor cells in the presence of an immune checkpoint inhibitor and vaccination. Combination of mAb treatment of mice with anti-OX40 agonist and anti-CTLA-4 antagonist promotes the expansion and differentiation of tumor antigen-specific effector/memory CD8[+] T cells. In murine models of mammary carcinoma and spontaneous prostate adenocarcinoma, additional vaccination targeting to cross-presenting DCs using an anti-DEC205 (CD205) mAb conjugated with HER2, a tumor-associated antigen that is overexpressed in a subset of breast cancers, promotes the induction of IFN-γ-producing CD4+ and CD8+ T cells that infiltrate into the tumor, which leads to extensive tumor destruction and improved mice survival. This demonstrates that OX40 agonism in synergy with checkpoint inhibitor blockade and tumor antigen vaccination augments durable T-cell immunity that is effective for tumor eradication (Linch et al. 2016).

3.3.2 4-1BBL-4-1BB

3.3.2.1 Expression and Function

As with OX40, 4-1BB is not expressed by naïve or resting CD4+ and CD8+ T cells but is transiently upregulated on activated T cells upon TCR triggering. 4-1BBL is transiently induced on activated professional APCs by signals from CD40 and TLRs. A genetic deficiency of *4-1bb* or *4-1 bbl* in mice displays no abnormality in the development of lymphocytes and lymphoid organs. Co-signaling via 4-1BB promotes T-cell proliferation, cytokine production, and cell survival. 4-1BB plays more predominant effects on CD8+ T-cell responses because of its higher expression on CD8+ T cells in comparison with CD4+ T cells. Upon binding with 4-1BBL, 4-1BB recruits TRAF1 and TRAF2, which leads to activation of NF-κB, Akt, and MAPK pathways (Snell et al. 2011; Wortzman et al. 2013a; Croft 2009) (Table 3.1, Figs. 3.1 and 3.2).

4-1BB is expressed on Treg cells. Divergent expression of 4-1BB and CD40L can distinguish antigen-specific human Treg cells from conventional activated CD4+ T cells. In the course of short-term activation of human peripheral blood mononuclear cells (PBMCs) with antigens in vitro, Treg cells and conventional CD4+ T cells upregulate 4-1BB and CD40L, respectively. Purified 4-1BB+ Treg cells express Treg marker genes including *FOXP3*, *CD25*, *HELIOS*, and *CTLA4*. 4-1BB+ Treg cells display a complete demethylation of the Treg-specific demethylated region (TSDR) at the *FOXP3* gene locus and exhibit a potent antigen-specific suppressive activity. This indicates that the extremely low frequency of antigen-specific Treg cells can be isolated from human PBMCs based on the surface expression of 4-1BB (Bacher et al. 2016).

3.3.2.2 Protective Immunity

The predominant role for 4-1BB co-signaling in CD8+ T-cell immunity has been demonstrated in various murine infection models including LCMV, influenza virus, CMV, murine gammaherpesvirus 68, vesicular stomatitis virus, and *Listeria monocytogenes*. The requirement of 4-1BB co-signaling for both CD4+ and CD8+ T-cell responses depends on the antigen load, the persistence of the infection, and the nature of pathogens. The levels of 4-1BB on T cells can be sustained under conditions where the infection persists. In general, mice lacking *4-1bb* or *4-1 bbl* show defective pathogen clearance and impaired antigen-specific CD8+ T-cell memory formation, especially in chronic or highly infectious disease context with the higher antigenic load. On the other hand, in a situation where antigens are rapidly cleared or the infection induces minimal inflammation, the deficiency in *4-1bb* or *4-1 bbl* does not display defective antigen-specific T-cell responses (Snell et al. 2011; Wortzman et al. 2013a).

3.3.2.3 Cancer

Ligation of 4-1BB with agonistic antibodies or engineered 4-1BBL on the surface of tumor cells or DCs promotes 4-1BB co-signaling that leads to expansion of tumor antigen-specific effector CD4+ and CD8+ T cells. Anti-4-1BB agonists can induce significant tumor regressions in various established tumor models, although the associated immunopathology has been reported. The use of anti-4-1BB agonists in combination with other cancer therapeutics, such as checkpoint inhibitors, vaccination, anticancer drugs, radiation, cytokines, and adoptive T-cell therapy, has been shown to exert synergistic antitumor activity (Sanchez-Paulete et al. 2016; Bartkowiak and Curran 2015; Vinay and Kwon 2014).

4-1BB agonism combination with vaccination can induce durable antitumor T-cell immunity against vaginally implanted tumor cells. In a mouse model of human papillomavirus (HPV) syngeneic tumor, mice administered with anti-4-1BB agonistic mAb combination with a peptide vaccine, which is composed of peptides from HPV-16 E6/E7 oncoproteins and α-galactosylceramide, display stronger tumor regression, which is accompanied with expansion of HPV-specific cytotoxic CD4+ and CD8+ T cells and with robust infiltration of these cytotoxic T lymphocytes (CTLs) into the tumor microenvironment. Neither checkpoint inhibitors (anti-CTLA-4 or -PD-1) nor anti-TNFR agonists (anti-OX40, -CD40, or -GITR) cannot recapitulate the therapeutic effect of the 4-1BB agonism. This indicates that 4-1BB co-signaling plays a predominant role for induction of robust antitumor T-cell immunity against cervical neoplasia (Bartkowiak et al. 2015).

The cytoplasmic tail of 4-1BB has been utilized for a critical component of the chimeric antigen receptors (CARs) for adoptive T-cell therapy against B-cell leukemia, lymphoma, and myeloma. A T cell transduced to express a CAR that comprises of an extracellular tumor antigen-binding single-chain antibody fragment and intracellular 4-1BB and TCR CD3ζ signaling domains exhibits a potent cytotoxic activity after recognition of target antigens on the surface of tumor cells. This 4-1BB-CAR, but not CD28-CAR, ameliorates T-cell exhaustion or anergy that is induced by persistent activation of the CD3ζ domain (Long et al. 2015). After recognizing target antigens, human CD8+ T cells expressing 4-1BB-CAR display a phenotype with CD45RO+ CCR7+ central memory T cells that have an enhanced respiratory capacity, increased fatty acid oxidation, and increased mitochondrial biogenesis. In contrast, CD28-CAR promotes the induction of CD45RO+ CCR7− effector memory T cells with an enhanced aerobic glycolysis (Kawalekar et al. 2016). These studies demonstrate that the 4-1BB signaling domain is superior over the CD28 signaling domain in terms of inducing beneficial T-cell signaling activity and suggest that 4-1BB-CAR promotes a better T-cell response that is required for tumor regression.

3.3.3 CD70–CD27

3.3.3.1 Expression and Function

Unlike OX40 and 4-1BB, CD27 is constitutively expressed on naïve CD4+ and CD8+ T cells and Treg cells. CD70, the ligand for CD27, is induced on activated DCs and B cells, and signals from TLRs, CD40, and BCR enhance the expression of CD70. Activated T cells also express CD70. Mice deficient in *Cd27* or *Cd70* show normal development of lymphoid organs and lymphocytes. The CD27–CD70 interaction promotes the expansion of antigen-specific effector/memory CD4+ and CD8+ T cells, which contributes to the establishment of T-cell immunity. Upon binding with CD70, CD27 recruits TRAF2 and TRAF5 to activate NF-κB and MAPK pathways (Nolte et al. 2009; Bullock 2017) (Table 3.1, Figs. 3.1 and 3.2).

3.3.3.2 Protective Immunity

A population of APCs exclusively localized in the gut lamina propria expresses higher levels of CD70. This CD70+ APC population provides a critical CD27 co-signaling into T cells, which supports proliferation and differentiation of gut mucosal T cells after oral *Listeria monocytogenes* infection (Laouar et al. 2005).

Optimal CD27 co-signaling plays an important role for protective T-cell immunity against infections. Critical roles for CD27 co-signaling in pathogen clearance have been shown in murine infection models including influenza virus, LCMV, and CMV. *Cd27*−/− mice display impaired primary CD4+ and CD8+ T-cell responses to influenza virus, and a memory T-cell response to a secondary challenge with influenza is also greatly attenuated (Hendriks et al. 2000). Mice deficient in *Cd70* or injected with an anti-CD70 blocking mAb display diminished primary effector CD8+ T-cell responses to acute LCMV infection and delayed virus clearance (Penaloza-MacMaster et al. 2011; Munitic et al. 2013). By contrast, the prolonged and excessive CD27–CD70 interactions with higher antigenic load during chronic virus infection induce pathological cytokine responses and immunopathology, which promotes activation-induced T-cell death and limits viral clearance. Blockade of this adverse signaling can restore protective CD8+ T-cell responses (Penaloza-MacMaster et al. 2011; Wensveen et al. 2012; Clouthier and Watts 2015). These studies suggest that an optimal level of CD27 co-signaling is required for the differentiation of effector/memory T cells that are important for pathogen clearance.

Loss of function of *CD27* or *CD70* in humans is associated with higher susceptibility to EBV infection and EBV-related diseases. Homozygous mutations in

CD70 in patients abolish surface expression of CD70 on B cells or binding to its cognate receptor CD27 on T cells, which results in impaired T-cell proliferation, cytotoxic responses, and IFN-γ production toward CD70-negative EBV-infected B cells (Izawa et al. 2017; Abolhassani et al. 2017). These studies suggest that CD70–CD27 interactions are important for generating stable T-cell immunity against EBV.

3.3.3.3 Autoimmunity and Inflammation

CD27 co-signaling promotes intestinal inflammation mediated by CD4[+] T cells. Adoptive transfer of CD45RB[high] CD4[+] T cells into lymphocyte-deficient *Rag*[−/−] recipient mice leads to weight loss, diarrhea, and severe colitis. In this T-cell-dependent murine colitis model, either deficiency of *Cd27* in donor CD4[+] T cells or administration of a blocking mAb to CD70 into recipient mice prevents the development of colitis and suppresses the differentiation of effector CD4[+] T cells producing pro-inflammatory cytokines. CD70 blockade also suppresses Th1 cell-driven trinitrobenzene sulfonic acid (TNBS)-induced colitis, indicating that CD27–CD70 interactions enhance the accumulation of pathogenic T cells in the gut mucosa and play an important role for development of T-cell-driven colitis (Manocha et al. 2009).

CD27–CD70 interactions facilitate allograft rejection mediated by CD8[+] T cells. In a murine fully mismatched cardiac allograft model, CD70 blockade inhibits the expansion of alloreactive effector/memory CD8[+] T cells and prevents CD8[+] T cell-driven allograft rejection. Cardiac allografts can survive longer in *Cd28*[−/−] recipient mice, and this allograft survival is further prolonged in the presence of CD70 blockade, indicating that CD27 co-signaling plays a dominant role for the development of alloimmune responses even in the absence of CD28. Adoptive transfer of allograft-specific memory CD8[+] T cells into syngeneic recipient mice lacking secondary lymphoid organs induces rapid rejection of cardiac allografts, and CD70 blockade inhibits this memory recall response. This demonstrates that the CD27–CD70 pathway promotes the development of acute and chronic allograft rejection mediated by alloreactive effector/memory CD8[+] T cells (Yamada et al. 2005).

3.3.3.4 Cancer

Enhancing CD27 signaling via administration of CD27 agonists, transgenic expression of CD70 on APCs, or enforced expression of CD70 on tumor cells is effective for evoking and augmenting antitumor immunity (Bullock 2017).

Ligation of CD27 in combination with PD-1 blockade is effective at eradicating tumor cells expressing HPV antigens. CD4[+] T-cell-mediated help is critical for inducing optimal CD8[+] T-cell responses against HPV antigens, and CD70 blockade abrogates this helper activity and abolishes the therapeutic effect of tumor vaccination. Contrary to this, CD27 agonism mimics this help and enhances antitumor responses. Although in the absence of help from CD4[+] T cells, PD-1 blockade alone cannot improve tumor control, a combination of PD-1 blockade and CD27 agonism augments the therapeutic efficacy of vaccination. Thus, CD27 agonism provides a potent help to the endogenous T-cell immunity against tumor and enhances antitumor immunity either alone or in combination with PD-1 blockade (Ahrends et al. 2016).

Human T cells expressing a tumor antigen-specific CAR, which contains an intracellular TCR CD3ζ and a CD27 signaling domain, produce higher amounts of IFN-γ and exhibit increased cytotoxicity against tumors in vitro. Cognate recognition of tumor antigens supports the expansion of CD27–CAR-expressing T cells in vivo, and adoptive transfer of CD27–CAR T cells into highly immunodeficient mice that have been inoculated with human ovarian cancer cells expressing a specific antigen leads to increased regression of established tumors in recipient mice. This indicates that human T cells bearing CD27 costimulatory module in a CAR can exert enhanced antigen-specific CTL activity toward tumor cells (Song et al. 2012).

3.3.4 TL1A-DR3

3.3.4.1 Expression and Function

DR3 is constitutively expressed by naïve or resting CD4$^+$ and CD8$^+$ T cells, and its expression is upregulated following T-cell activation. DR3 is also expressed by Treg cells. TL1A, the ligand for DR3, is expressed on activated T cells and transiently induced on DCs and macrophages by pro-inflammatory stimuli, such as TLR and FcγR signaling. In humans, DcR3 binds to TL1A and inhibits the interaction between DR3 and TL1A. Upon binding to TL1A, DR3 provides costimulatory signals to T cells in concert with TCR signaling, which enhances pro-inflammatory cytokine production and promotes the clonal expansion and differentiation of effector T cells. Although $Dr3^{-/-}$ mice show a partial impairment in the negative selection of thymocytes, mice deficient in $Dr3$ or $Tl1a$ show normal development of lymphoid organs and lymphocytes. After interaction with TL1A, DR3 directly binds to TRADD. TRADD then recruits TRAF2 and RIP1 to the DR3 signaling complex and activates NF-κB and MAPK signaling pathways (Meylan et al. 2011; Pobezinskaya et al. 2011) (Table 3.1, Figs. 3.1 and 3.2).

3.3.4.2 Protective Immunity

DR3 co-signaling is critical for optimal expansion of IFN-γ producing CD4$^+$ T cells that facilitate killing of intracellular bacteria. Infection of mice with *Salmonella enterica* Typhimurium induces sustained expression of TL1A on F4/80$^+$ macrophages, and TL1A–DR3 interactions expand IFN-γ-producing Th1 cells, which leads to efficient clearance of *S. enterica* Typhimurium. Clonal expansion of $Dr3^{-/-}$ CD4$^+$ T cells is significantly impaired, and this reduced T-cell response results in compromised control of the bacterial burden in the spleens of $Dr3^{-/-}$ mice (Buchan et al. 2012).

DR3 co-signaling is critical for inducing antiviral immunity against murine CMV and vaccinia virus. $Dr3^{-/-}$ mice cannot mount effective antiviral CD4[+] and CD8[+] T-cell immunity during acute virus infection, which is associated with impaired control of virus replication and increased morbidity and mortality. The impaired T-cell response in $Dr3^{-/-}$ mice is caused by defects in the capacity of CD4[+] and CD8[+] T cells to divide and produce IFN-γ in response to cognate viral antigens (Twohig et al. 2012).

3.3.4.3 Autoimmunity and Inflammation

TL1A–DR3 interactions enhance immunopathology in a number of T-cell-dependent animal models of multiple sclerosis, rheumatoid arthritis, inflammatory bowel disease, and allergic lung diseases (Richard et al. 2015a; Meylan et al. 2011). Indeed, increased expression of both TL1A and DR3 is observed in patients with ulcerative colitis and Crohn's disease, and TL1A is one of the definitive susceptible genes to Crohn's disease in humans (Strober and Fuss 2011) (Table 3.2).

DR3 co-signaling in CD4[+] T cells exacerbates inflammatory responses in the target organs of autoimmune and inflammatory diseases. Although CD4[+] T cells from the spleen and lymph nodes of antigen-immunized $Dr3^{-/-}$ mice proliferate normally in response to recall antigen stimulation in vitro, $Dr3^{-/-}$ mice display reduced inflammation in experimental autoimmune encephalomyelitis (EAE) and allergic airway inflammation with decreased effector CD4[+] T-cell accumulation in the local tissues (Meylan et al. 2008).

TL1A expression in DCs supports the expansion and differentiation of inflammatory IL-17-producing helper T cells (Th17 cells), and thus $Tl1a^{-/-}$ mice show reduced clinical severity in EAE that is dependent on autoimmune Th17 cells (Pappu et al. 2008).

TL1A promotes the differentiation of IL-9-producing helper T cells (Th9 cells) by augmenting signals through DR3 on CD4[+] T cells, and endogenous TL1A enhances allergic pathology mediated by Th9 cells in murine models of experimental eye inflammation and allergic airway disease (Richard et al. 2015b).

3.3.4.4 Cancer

DR3 co-signaling augments antitumor CD8[+] T-cell immunity. Engagement of DR3 with soluble TL1A enhances both primary and secondary expansion of antigen-specific CD8[+] T cells in vivo. Mice inoculated with TL1A-expressing tumor cells generate protective antitumor CD8[+] CTL responses and effectively eradicate the tumor cells in a CD8[+] T-cell-dependent manner (Slebioda et al. 2011).

3.3.5 CD30L–CD30

3.3.5.1 Expression and Function

CD30 is expressed by activated CD4+ and CD8+ T cells and Treg cells. CD30 is also well recognized as a marker for malignant tumors including Hodgkin's lymphoma and anaplastic large cell lymphoma. CD30L is induced on activated T cells and professional APCs. CD30–CD30L interactions promote the expansion and survival of effector and memory T cells. *Cd30*$^{-/-}$ mice have no obvious defects in peripheral T-cell or B-cell lineages. The phenotype of immune homeostasis of *Cd30l*$^{-/-}$ mice has not been described so far. CD30 utilizes TRAF2 and TRAF3 to activate NF-κB and MAPK pathways (Watts 2005; Ward-Kavanagh et al. 2016) (Table 3.1, Figs. 3.1 and 3.2).

3.3.5.2 Protective Immunity

CD30–CD30L interactions establish optimal T-cell immunity against *Mycobacterium avium*. During infection with *M. avium*, CD30L blockade leads to increased mycobacterial burdens. *Cd30*$^{-/-}$ mice display higher susceptibility to *M. avium* infection, and the defective antibacterial response is associated with a decreased expansion of IFN-γ-producing CD4+ T cells specific for bacterial antigens (Florido et al. 2004). *Cd30l*$^{-/-}$ mice are susceptible to *Mycobacterium bovis* Bacillus Calmette–Guérin (BCG) infection and exhibit higher bacterial burden. The numbers of antigen-specific IFN-γ-producing CD4+ T cells in the spleen, lung, and peritoneal cavity of *Cd30l*$^{-/-}$ mice are greatly diminished after BCG infection (Tang et al. 2008).

CD30 signaling promotes the differentiation of memory CD8+ T cells and is required for protective immunity against *Listeria monocytogenes*. Following *L. monocytogenes* infection, *Cd30l*$^{-/-}$ mice can generate a normal antigen-specific effector CD8+ T-cell response at an early stage of infection but display a defective recall memory CD8+ T-cell response against reinfection (Nishimura et al. 2005).

Double knockout mice deficient in both *Cd30* and *Ox40* exhibit defective Th1 immunity against *Salmonella typhimurium*. Antigen-specific *Cd30*$^{-/-}$*Ox40*$^{-/-}$ donor CD4+ T cells fail to persist after transfer into infected *Rag*$^{-/-}$ recipient mice, and these recipient mice exhibit an impaired capacity to control *S. typhimurium* infection, indicating that both CD30 and OX40 signals promote Th1 immunity against *Salmonella* (Gaspal et al. 2008).

3.3.5.3 Autoimmunity and Inflammation

The CD30–CD30L interaction augments allergic airway inflammation mediated by T-helper-2 (Th2) cells. *Cd30*$^{-/-}$ or *Cd30l*$^{-/-}$ mice primed with ovalbumin (OVA) antigen and challenged with OVA display diminished eosinophilic infiltration into the airway and pulmonary inflammation. In these mice, the levels of pro-inflammatory cytokines IL-5 and IL-13 in bronchoalveolar lavage fluids (BALF) are reduced, and lung-draining lymph node CD4[+] T cells produce lesser amount of IL-5 and IL-13 in response to OVA in vitro. Thus, CD30 signaling contributes to allergic lung inflammation through accumulation of pathogenic effector/memory Th2 cells during the course of airway inflammation (Polte et al. 2006; Nam et al. 2008; Fuchiwaki et al. 2011).

CD30 signaling in CD4[+] T cells enhances the development of pathogenic IL-17- and/or IFN-γ-producing CD4[+] T cells in autoimmune neuroinflammation. EAE disease is ameliorated in $Cd30^{-/-}$ and $Cd30l^{-/-}$ mice. CD4[+] T cells from draining lymph node of $Cd30^{-/-}$ or $Cd30l^{-/-}$ mice exhibit reduced proliferative and cytokine responses to recall antigen in vitro. Infiltration of inflammatory cells including CD4[+] T cell, macrophage/microglia, and granulocyte in the spinal cords is significantly attenuated in these knockout mice. CD30 blockade in the course of disease development ameliorates EAE in wild-type mice. Accordingly, adoptive transfer of antigen-specific wild-type CD4[+] T cells into $Cd30l^{-/-}$ mice induces significantly attenuated EAE (Shinoda et al. 2015).

Signals through both CD30 and OX40 promote autoimmune tissue damage mediated by effector CD4[+] T cells in the context of $Foxp3$ deficiency. Although $Foxp3^{-/-}$ mice develop lethal autoimmune disease, mice with combined deficiency in $Foxp3$, $Cd30$, and $Ox40$ develop and grow normally. Pathogenic CD62L^{low}CD44^{high}CD4[+] effector/memory T cells, which reside in $Foxp3^{-/-}$ mice and secrete higher amounts of IL-4 and IFN-γ, are substantially decreased in $Foxp3^{-/-}$ $Cd30^{-/-}Ox40^{-/-}$ mice. Accordingly, blockade of both CD30 and OX40 signaling can prevent the development of lethal autoimmune responses that are mediated by auto-reactive T cells existing in $Foxp3^{-/-}$ mice (Gaspal et al. 2011).

3.3.6 GITRL–GITR

3.3.6.1 Expression and Function

GITR is expressed on naïve or resting CD4[+] and CD8[+] T cells at basal levels and is upregulated after T-cell activation. GITR is highly expressed by Treg cells. GITRL is expressed at low levels on APCs and is transiently upregulated after cell activation. GITR provides costimulatory signals to CD4[+] and CD8[+] T cells to enhance proliferation, effector function, and cell survival. $Gitr^{-/-}$ mice show normal development of lymphoid organs and homeostasis of T cells. A study regarding $Gitrl^{-/-}$ mice has not been reported so far. GITR interacts with TRAF2 and TRAF5 and activates NF-κB and MAPK pathways (Snell et al. 2011; Clouthier and Watts 2014) (Table 3.1, Figs. 3.1 and 3.2).

GITR co-signaling plays critical roles in both conventional CD4[+] and CD8[+] T cells and Treg cells, and the effect of GITR co-signaling on conventional T cells versus Treg cells depends on the context of the immune response (see Sect. 3.9).

3.3.6.2 Protective Immunity

GITR co-signaling plays a critical role in control of virus infection. GITR is required for primary and recall CD8[+] T-cell responses and for survival of antigen-specific CD8[+] T cells during viral infection, and GITR signaling protects mice from death during severe respiratory influenza infection (Snell et al. 2010).

T-cell-intrinsic GITR co-signaling increases the frequency and number of LCMV-specific CD8[+] T cells, which results in decreased viral load. GITRL is transiently induced on APCs at early time points of LCMV infection and is downregulated to below baseline levels thereafter. GITR is also transiently upregulated on CD8[+] T cells but is sustained at low but above baseline levels at chronic stages of LCMV infection. Thus, GITR on T cells is not efficiently engaged by endogenously expressed GITRL on APCs at the chronic stage of infection. However, an agonistic mAb to GITR can overcome the insufficiency of GITRL and activates LCMV-specific CD8[+] T cells, which leads to lower viral load without causing overt immune pathology (Clouthier et al. 2014).

GITR signaling in CD4[+] T cells is required for antiviral CD8[+] T-cell responses and humoral immunity that are important for control of chronic LCMV infection. $Gitr^{-/-}$ mice display impaired accumulation of IL-2[+] IFN-γ[+] Th1 cells as well as Tfh cells and have decreased IgG responses to LCMV. CD8[+] T cells from $Gitr^{-/-}$ mice express higher levels of exhaustion markers PD-1 and Tim-3. GITR-mediated priming of Th1 cells promotes cell-mediated immunity as well as humoral immunity to optimally regulate chronic LCMV infection (Clouthier et al. 2015).

3.3.6.3 Autoimmunity and Inflammation

GITR agonism exacerbates CD4[+] T-cell-dependent murine models of autoimmune/ inflammatory diseases, such as asthma, collagen-induced arthritis (CIA), diabetes, and EAE. Treatment of mice with an agonistic mAb to GITR promotes migration, proliferation, and activation of diabetogenic T cells within the pancreatic islets and exacerbates T-cell-driven destructive insulitis in nonobese diabetic (NOD) mice (You et al. 2009).

$Gitr^{-/-}$ mice develop significantly attenuated CIA. Draining lymph node CD4[+] T cells from type II collagen (CII)-immunized $Gitr^{-/-}$ mice secrete lower amounts of IFN-γ in response to CII *in vitro*. Donor splenic T cells from CII-immunized $Gitr^{-/-}$ mice fail to induce sufficient disease symptoms of CIA in severe combined immunodeficient (SCID) recipient mice, suggesting that GITR signaling is required for CD4[+] T cells to attain full pathogenic potential to promote CIA (Cuzzocrea et al. 2005).

3.3.6.4 Cancer

GITR signaling boosts antitumor immunity by enhancing effector function of tumor antigen-specific T cells (Schaer et al. 2012).

Although either GITR agonism or PD-1 blockade alone exhibits little antitumor effect, a combination of GITR agonism and PD-1 blockade enhances a potent antitumor immunity against ovarian cancer. Anti-GITR/PD-1 mAbs increase the frequency of IFN-γ-producing CD4$^+$ and CD8$^+$ T cells with cytotoxic activity against tumors. Combined treatment of anti-GITR/PD-1 mAbs and chemotherapeutic drugs further enhances the antitumor responses (Lu et al. 2014). Treatment of mice bearing B16 melanoma with anti-GITR/PD-1 mAbs in combination with tumor antigen vaccination leads to markedly better inhibition of tumor growth and prolonged mice survival. The tumor regression correlates with the induction of tumor-infiltrating antigen-specific effector/memory CD8$^+$ T cells producing IFN-γ and TNF-α, and depletion of these CD8$^+$ T cells abrogates the beneficial effects provided by the therapy (Villarreal et al. 2017).

Anti-GITR agonist facilitates antitumor immunity by promoting the differentiation of IL-9-producing Th9 cells. Administration of anti-GITR mAb into CT26 colon tumor- or B16F10 melanoma-bearing mice inhibits growth of tumors, which is mediated by GITR signal-driven differentiation of Th9 cells. Neutralization of IL-9 prevents the tumor regression, and IL-9 from Th9 cells promotes the development of tumor antigen-specific cytotoxic CD8$^+$ T cells through activation of tumor-associated DCs (Kim et al. 2015).

3.3.7 TNFα-TNFR2

3.3.7.1 Expression and Function

A low level of TNFR2 is expressed by resting or naïve CD4$^+$ and CD8$^+$ T cells, and its expression is further upregulated after T-cell activation. TNFR2 binds to cognate ligands TNF-α and LT-α (lymphotoxin-α). TNF-α is produced by activated macrophages, T cells, and many other cell types during inflammation and exists as a transmembrane trimer whose proteolysis by TNF-converting enzyme (TACE or ADAM17) leads to a soluble form. LT-α is produced as a soluble form. TNFR2 is more efficiently engaged by transmembrane TNF-α than by soluble TNF-α. Interaction of TNF-α with TNFR2 is costimulatory to TCR-mediated T-cell activation and promotes the activation, differentiation, and survival of T cells. $Tnfr2^{-/-}$ mice show normal development of peripheral lymphoid organs and lymphocytes. Unlike TNFR1, TNFR2 lacks an intracellular DD and directly recruits TRAF1, TRAF2, and TRAF3 to activate NF-κB and MAPK pathways (Kim et al. 2006; Calzascia et al. 2007; Faustman and Davis 2010; Mehta et al. 2016) (Table 3.1, Figs. 3.1 and 3.2).

Mutations in *TNFR2* that lead to enhanced NF-κB signaling have been found in patients with T-cell lymphoma (Ungewickell et al. 2015).

TNFR2 is expressed on Treg cells. Similar to other TNFRSF molecules, such as GITR and OX40, the effect of TNF-α on conventional CD4$^+$ and CD8$^+$ T cells versus Treg cells depends on the context of inflammatory environments (see Sect. 3.9).

Although the TNF-α-TNFR2 interaction provides costimulatory signals into T cells, signals from TNFR2 limit activity of effector CD8$^+$ T cells in some contexts (Wortzman et al. 2013b; Punit et al. 2015).

3.3.7.2 Protective Immunity

TNF-α-TNFR2 interactions are critical for generating cytotoxic CD8$^+$ T-cell responses against adenovirus in the liver. Intrahepatic lymphocytes isolated from adenovirus-infected *Tnfa$^{-/-}$* or *Tnfr2$^{-/-}$* mice display decreased CTL responses against antigen-expressing target hepatocytes (Kafrouni et al. 2003).

TNFR2 signaling plays an important role for T-cell-mediated immunity against *Listeria monocytogenes*. After *L. monocytogenes* infection, *Tnfr2$^{-/-}$* mice display reduced expansion and survival of antigen-specific CD4$^+$ and CD8$^+$ T cells producing IFN-γ and delayed bacterial clearance upon challenge with higher dose of bacteria. Antigen-specific donor *Tnfr2$^{-/-}$* CD8$^+$ T cells display a marked reduction in clonal expansion and survival in infected recipient mice (Kim et al. 2006).

3.3.7.3 Autoimmunity and Inflammation

In a model of murine GVHD, TNFR2 signaling in both donor CD4$^+$ and CD8$^+$ T cells is required for induction of acute GVHD responses mediated by alloantigen-specific CD8$^+$ CTL. Recipient mice transferred with donor *Tnfr2$^{-/-}$*T cells exhibit a reduced cytotoxic phenotype and a decreased elimination of host spleen cell populations mediated by allo-specific donor CD8$^+$ T cells. Whereas TNFR2 signaling in donor CD4$^+$ T cells is critical for their gaining of optimal helper activity for donor CD8$^+$ T cells, TNFR2 signaling in donor CD8$^+$ T cells promotes the maturation of fully competent KLRG1$^+$ CCR7$^-$ CD8$^+$ T cells, termed short-lived effector cells (SLECs). This indicates that induction of optimal donor CD8$^+$ CTL activity requires TNFR2 signaling in both donor CD4$^+$ and CD8$^+$ T-cell populations (Soloviova et al. 2013).

TNF-α blockers are well established for treatment of human inflammatory diseases, such as rheumatoid arthritis and Crohn's disease. Although T cells might not be the main target cells in the therapy, blockade of TNF-α-TNFR2 interactions promotes apoptosis of mucosal CD4$^+$ T cells from patients with inflammatory bowel disease (IBD). CD14$^+$ macrophages and CD4$^+$ T cells isolated from the lamina propria of IBD patients express higher levels of membrane-bound TNF-α (mTNF-α) and TNFR2, respectively. Clinically effective anti-TNF-α mAbs in IBD induce apoptosis of TNFR2[+] CD4[+] T cells when these T cells are cocultured with mTNF-α[+] CD14[+] macrophages, suggesting that disruption of mTNF-α-TNFR2 interactions with anti-TNF-α leads to suppression of gut inflammation in IBD through inducing apoptosis of pathogenic CD4[+] T cells in the intestine (Atreya et al. 2011).

TNFR2 signaling in CD4[+] T cells expands pathogenic effector T cells that promote colitis in mice. Adoptive transfer of donor naïve CD4[+] T cells from *Tnfr2[-/-]* mice fails to induce severe colitis in lymphopenic *Rag1[-/-]* mice. *Tnfr2[-/-]* CD4[+] T cells are defective in clonal expansion and differentiation into IFN-γ-producing colitogenic effector T cells in the lymphopenic environment (Chen et al. 2016).

3.3.8 LIGHT–HVEM

3.3.8.1 Expression and Function

HVEM, a member of the TNFRSF, binds to four different molecules, TNFSF molecules LIGHT and LT-α and immunoglobulin superfamily molecules BTLA and CD160, in distinct configurations, and these molecular networks activate both inflammatory and anti-inflammatory signaling pathways. Ligation of HVEM on T cells by the canonical TNF-related ligand LIGHT provides costimulatory signals to T cells. HVEM is expressed on naïve or resting CD4[+] and CD8[+] T cells and Treg cells. LIGHT is expressed on activated lymphoid cells including APC populations and T cells either as a membrane-bound or a soluble form. In human, DcR3 binds to LIGHT and inhibits the interaction between HVEM and LIGHT. HVEM co-signaling promotes the activation, differentiation, and survival of T cells. *Hvem[-/-]* and *Light[-/-]* mice have no significant abnormalities in the development of lymphoid organs and lymphocytes. HVEM recruits TRAF2 and TRAF3 to activate NF-κB pathway (Ward-Kavanagh et al. 2016) (Table 3.1, Figs. 3.1 and 3.2).

Although ligation of HVEM by BTLA activates pro-survival HVEM signaling pathways in effector and memory T cells after antigen recognition (Steinberg et al. 2013; Flynn et al. 2013; Sakoda et al. 2011), we mainly focus on the canonical HVEM–LIGHT interaction that controls HVEM co-signaling in T cells.

3.3.8.2 Autoimmunity and Inflammation

HVEM co-signaling promotes the differentiation of pathogenic effector CD4[+] T cells that exacerbate experimental autoimmune uveitis (EAU). Pathogenic responses and clinical scores of EAU are significantly decreased in *Hvem[-/-]* mice and draining lymph node T cells from *Hvem[-/-]* mice display reduced cell proliferation and production of Th1- and Th17-related cytokines in response to antigen restimulation in vitro. *Light[-/-]*, *Btla[-/-]*, and *Light[-/-]Btla[-/-]* mice also display attenuated EAU disease phenotypes and decreased Th1-/Th17-type responses. A blocking mAb to

HVEM that can inhibit both HVEM–LIGHT and HVEM–BTLA interactions ameliorates pathogenic Th1/Th17 responses in EAU (Sakoda et al. 2016).

In a T-cell-dependent allergic lung inflammation model, the HVEM–LIGHT interaction plays a dominant role in the survival of pathogenic memory Th2 cells. After antigen recall challenges, adoptively transferred donor OVA-specific *Hvem*$^{-/-}$ Th2 cells display reduced accumulation in the airways, lungs, and draining mediastinal lymph nodes of recipient mice and induce decreased airway eosinophilia and Th2 cytokine responses. Interruption of HVEM–LIGHT interactions also inhibits the accumulation of inflammatory memory Th2 cells in the lung. Although *Light*$^{-/-}$ donor CD4$^+$ T cells cannot sustain after antigen exposure in vivo, cotransfer of wild-type and *Light*$^{-/-}$ donor T cells rescues the survival defect of *Light*$^{-/-}$ donor T cells, suggesting that HVEM induces cell survival signals into T cells through interacting with LIGHT expressing on neighboring antigen-specific T cells. This demonstrates that HVEM expressed by CD4$^+$ T cells induces cell survival signals and controls T-cell-driven allergic lung inflammation (Soroosh et al. 2011).

In a T-cell-dependent murine colitis model, HVEM signaling in donor CD4$^+$ T cells promotes intestinal inflammation and contributes to the immunopathology mediated by differentiated colitogenic T cells. *Rag*$^{-/-}$ recipient mice with donor CD45RB^{high} CD4$^+$ T cells from *Hvem*$^{-/-}$ or *Light*$^{-/-}$ mice display reduced intestinal inflammation, indicating that both HVEM and LIGHT on CD4$^+$ T cells are required for the development of inflammatory T cells within the intestine during colitis development. *Rag*$^{-/-}$ recipient mice receiving *Hvem*$^{-/-}$ CD4$^+$ T cells express lesser amounts of IL-6, TNF-α, and IL-12 mRNAs in the colon and have a decreased number of donor T cells producing IFN-γ or IL-17. In the absence of HVEM signaling, donor CD4$^+$ T cells expand normally at early time points but cannot persist at later time points in lymphopenic hosts. These results suggest that T-cell-expressing LIGHT interacting with HVEM expressed by an adjacent T cell plays a critical role for the expansion, differentiation, and survival of gut-homing pathogenic T cells driving colitis (Schaer et al. 2011; Steinberg et al. 2008).

HVEM–LIGHT interactions contribute to GVHD pathogenesis. Adoptive transfer of allogeneic T cells from *Hvem*$^{-/-}$ or *Light*$^{-/-}$ mice into recipient mice induces attenuated anti-host CTL responses, which results in prolonged survival of recipient mice. *Hvem*$^{-/-}$ and *Light*$^{-/-}$ donor T cells undergo apoptosis after transfer into recipient mice. Accordingly, administration of an anti-HVEM mAb, which interferes with HVEM–LIGHT interactions, ameliorates GVHD responses and prolongs the survival of recipient mice (Xu et al. 2007).

3.3.8.3 Cancer

HVEM co-signaling via LIGHT plays an important role for establishing robust T-cell immunity against tumors. Mice inoculated with tumor cells expressing an agonistic mAb to HVEM on the cell surface generate protective antitumor immunity in a manner dependent on both CD4$^+$ and CD8$^+$ T cells. The potent antitumor CTL activity is associated with increased IFN-γ production, and mice which have rejected this tumor are resistant to rechallenge of parental tumors, indicating that HVEM signaling facilitates tumor-reactive T-cell responses, induction of long-term antitumor immunity, and tumor regression (Park et al. 2012).

LIGHT expression in the tumor environment elicits potent antitumor immunity leading to tumor regression (Yu and Fu 2008). Combined immunotherapy with LIGHT expression on tumors and antigen-specific vaccination is effective for generating tumor-infiltrating CD8+ T-cell responses that are important for tumor eradication. Adenovirus-mediated forced expression of LIGHT in HPV16-induced tumors results in upregulation of IFN-γ and chemoattractant cytokines in the tumor, which results in induction of antigen-specific CD8+ T cells in the peripheral lymphoid organs and within the tumor. However, antigen-specific T cells induced by LIGHT cannot induce complete tumor regression. More importantly, additional vaccination with HPV16 antigen boosts the frequency of antigen-specific T cells and prevents the outgrowth of tumors. This suggests that LIGHT expressed by tumors expands incoming T cells via HVEM signaling and that these LIGHT–HVEM interactions in the presence of antigenic signals play an important role for generating robust antitumor immunity that can eradicate tumors (Kanodia et al. 2010).

3.3.9 The Role of TNFRSF Molecules in Immune Regulation Mediated by Treg Cells

Treg cells play important roles for regulation of conventional CD4+ and CD8+ T-cell responses. TNFRSF molecules described in this chapter are all expressed by both Treg cells and conventional T-cell populations, and the cognate TNFSF–TNFRSF interaction regulates the balance between Treg cells and conventional T cells, which is critical for determining all aspects of the immune response. Although the cell-intrinsic effects of the TNFRSF signaling in Treg cells are still unclear (Shevach and Stephens 2006; So et al. 2008; Croft 2014; Mbanwi and Watts 2014), it has been demonstrated that signals from TNFRSF molecules influence the Treg and conventional T-cell balance through (1) promoting the development of natural or thymus-derived Treg cells, (2) antagonizing the development of induced or periphery-derived Treg cells, (3) promoting the expansion and survival of Treg cells, (4) downregulating Treg cell suppressive functions, and (5) enhancing resistance of naïve/effector/memory responder CD4+ and CD8+ T cells to the Treg cell-mediated suppression.

3.4 Conclusion

Five out of eight TNFRSF molecules, CD27, DR3, HVEM, GITR, and TNFR2, discussed in this chapter are constitutively expressed on most CD4+ and CD8+ T cells, whereas other three TNFRSF molecules, 4-1BB, CD30, and OX40, are upregulated on activated T cells after antigen recognition. Most of the cognate ligands for these TNFRSF molecules are not highly expressed by APC populations or other cell types and are induced by antigen recognition or innate stimuli or inflammation. The co-signaling activated by the cognate TNFSF–TNFRSF interaction quantitatively and/or qualitatively augments signals that are initiated by the TCR and CD28 and controls not only in early phases of T-cell responses to enhance cell proliferation, differentiation, and survival but also in later phases of memory T-cell responses (Fig. 3.2). Thus, TNFRSF molecules expressed by T cells have central roles in infection, immune-mediated diseases, and cancer that are critically regulated by various populations of antigen-primed T cells. Understanding of co-signaling functions of TNFRSF molecules in health and disease has progressed over the past few decades, and biologics or gene engineering technologies that inhibit or stimulate co-signaling functions of TNFRSF molecules have proven to be clinically efficacious for autoimmune and inflammatory diseases and cancer (Sugamura et al. 2004; Croft et al. 2013; Moran et al. 2013; Ward-Kavanagh et al. 2016). However, there are still fundamental questions regarding signaling mechanisms of the TNF–TNFR family of co-signal molecules: (1) qualitative and/or quantitative contribution of the TNFR co-signaling to the TCR, (2) cross talk between TNFR and co-inhibitory molecules, (3) intrinsic TNFR signaling functions in Treg cells, (4) utilization patterns of individual TRAF molecules in each individual TNFR signaling complex that might explain the qualitative difference in co-signaling activity, (5) cross talk of costimulatory signals among TNFRSF molecules, (6) roles of reverse signaling mediated by membrane-bound TNFSF ligands expressed by T cells, and (7) adverse (death) signaling effects of co-stimulatory TNFRSF molecules expressed by T cells. Further research will uncover these unresolved issues and may provide novel information regarding the potential usefulness of blockade or agonism of the TNFR co-signaling pathways in human diseases (Table 3.2).

Acknowledgments This work was supported by JSPS KAKENHI Grant Numbers 24590571 (to T.S.), 15H04640 (to T.S.), 18H02572 (to T.S.), 24390118 (to N.I.), 15H04742 (to N.I.), and 16K15508 (to N.I.), as well as by grants from the Takeda Science Foundation (to T.S.), the Suzuken Memorial Foundation (to T.S.), the SENSHIN Medical Research Foundation (to T.S.), the Astellas Foundation for Research on Metabolic Disorders (to T.S.), the Yamaguchi Educational and Scholarship Foundation (to T.S.), and the Daiichi-Sankyo Foundation of Life Science (to N.I. and T.S.).

References

Abolhassani H, Edwards ES, Ikinciogullari A et al (2017) Combined immunodeficiency and Epstein-Barr virus-induced B cell malignancy in humans with inherited CD70 deficiency. J Exp Med 214:91–106

Aggarwal BB (2003) Signalling pathways of the TNF superfamily: a double-edged sword. Nat Rev Immunol 3:745–756

Ahrends T, Babala N, Xiao Y et al (2016) CD27 Agonism plus PD-1 blockade recapitulates CD4+ T-cell help in therapeutic anticancer vaccination. Cancer Res 76:2921–2931

Atreya R, Zimmer M, Bartsch B et al (2011) Antibodies against tumor necrosis factor (TNF) induce T-cell apoptosis in patients with inflammatory bowel diseases via TNF receptor 2 and intestinal CD14(+) macrophages. Gastroenterology 141:2026–2038

Bacher P, Heinrich F, Stervbo U et al (2016) Regulatory T cell specificity directs tolerance versus allergy against Aeroantigens in humans. Cell 167:1067–1078

Bartkowiak T, Curran MA (2015) 4-1BB agonists: multi-potent Potentiators of tumor immunity. Front Oncol 5:117

Bartkowiak T, Singh S, Yang G et al (2015) Unique potential of 4-1BB agonist antibody to promote durable regression of HPV+ tumors when combined with an E6/E7 peptide vaccine. Proc Natl Acad Sci U S A 112:E5290–E5299

Bodmer JL, Schneider P, Tschopp J (2002) The molecular architecture of the TNF superfamily. Trends Biochem Sci 27:19–26

Brenner D, Blaser H, Mak TW (2015) Regulation of tumour necrosis factor signalling: live or let die. Nat Rev Immunol 15:362–374

Brown GR, Thiele DL (2000) Enhancement of MHC class I-stimulated alloresponses by TNF/TNF receptor (TNFR)1 interactions and of MHC class II-stimulated alloresponses by TNF/TNFR2 interactions. Eur J Immunol 30:2900–2907

Buchan SL, Taraban VY, Slebioda TJ et al (2012) Death receptor 3 is essential for generating optimal protective CD4(+) T-cell immunity against Salmonella. Eur J Immunol 42:580–588

Bullock TN (2017) Stimulating CD27 to quantitatively and qualitatively shape adaptive immunity to cancer. Curr Opin Immunol 45:82–88

Byun M, Ma CS, Akcay A et al (2013) Inherited human OX40 deficiency underlying classic Kaposi sarcoma of childhood. J Exp Med 210:1743–1759

Calzascia T, Pellegrini M, Hall H et al (2007) TNF-alpha is critical for antitumor but not antiviral T cell immunity in mice. J Clin Invest 117:3833–3845

Chen X, Nie Y, Xiao H et al (2016) TNFR2 expression by CD4 effector T cells is required to induce full-fledged experimental colitis. Sci Rep 6:32834

Clouthier DL, Watts TH (2014) Cell-specific and context-dependent effects of GITR in cancer, autoimmunity, and infection. Cytokine Growth Factor Rev 25:91–106

Clouthier DL, Watts TH (2015) TNFRs and control of chronic LCMV infection: implications for therapy. Trends Immunol 36:697–708

Clouthier DL, Zhou AC, Watts TH (2014) Anti-GITR agonist therapy intrinsically enhances CD8 T cell responses to chronic lymphocytic choriomeningitis virus (LCMV), thereby circumventing LCMV-induced downregulation of costimulatory GITR ligand on APC. J Immunol 193:5033–5043

Clouthier DL, Zhou AC, Wortzman ME et al (2015) GITR intrinsically sustains early type 1 and late follicular helper CD4 T cell accumulation to control a chronic viral infection. PLoS Pathog 11:e1004517

Croft M (2009) The role of TNF superfamily members in T-cell function and diseases. Nat Rev Immunol 9:271–285

Croft M (2010) Control of immunity by the TNFR-related molecule OX40 (CD134). Annu Rev Immunol 28:57–78

Croft M (2014) The TNF family in T cell differentiation and function-unanswered questions and future directions. Semin Immunol 26:183–190

Croft M, So T, Duan W et al (2009) The significance of OX40 and OX40L to T-cell biology and immune disease. Immunol Rev 229:173–191

Croft M, Benedict CA, Ware CF (2013) Clinical targeting of the TNF and TNFR superfamilies. Nat Rev Drug Discov 12:147–168

Cuzzocrea S, Ayroldi E, Di Paola R et al (2005) Role of glucocorticoid-induced TNF receptor family gene (GITR) in collagen-induced arthritis. FASEB J 19:1253–1265

Eissner G, Kolch W, Scheurich P (2004) Ligands working as receptors: reverse signaling by members of the TNF superfamily enhance the plasticity of the immune system. Cytokine Growth Factor Rev 15:353–366

Faustman D, Davis M (2010) TNF receptor 2 pathway: drug target for autoimmune diseases. Nat Rev Drug Discov 9:482–493

Florido M, Borges M, Yagita H et al (2004) Contribution of CD30/CD153 but not of CD27/CD70, CD134/OX40L, or CD137/4-1BBL to the optimal induction of protective immunity to Mycobacterium avium. J Leukoc Biol 76:1039–1046

Flynn R, Hutchinson T, Murphy KM et al (2013) CD8 T cell memory to a viral pathogen requires trans Cosignaling between HVEM and BTLA. PLoS One 8:e77991

Fuchiwaki T, Sun X, Fujimura K et al (2011) The central role of CD30L/CD30 interactions in allergic rhinitis pathogenesis in mice. Eur J Immunol 41:2947–2954

Gaspal F, Bekiaris V, Kim MY et al (2008) Critical synergy of CD30 and OX40 signals in CD4 T cell homeostasis and Th1 immunity to Salmonella. J Immunol 180:2824–2829

Gaspal F, Withers D, Saini M et al (2011) Abrogation of CD30 and OX40 signals prevents autoimmune disease in FoxP3-deficient mice. J Exp Med 208:1579–1584

Ha H, Han D, Choi Y (2009) TRAF-mediated TNFR-family signaling. Curr Protoc Immunol Suppl.87:Unit11.9D.1–Unit 11.9D.19

Hayden MS, Ghosh S (2014) Regulation of NF-kappaB by TNF family cytokines. Semin Immunol 26:253–266

Hendriks J, Gravestein LA, Tesselaar K et al (2000) CD27 is required for generation and long-term maintenance of T cell immunity. Nat Immunol 1:433–440

Humphreys IR, de Trez C, Kinkade A et al (2007) Cytomegalovirus exploits IL-10-mediated immune regulation in the salivary glands. J Exp Med 204:1217–1225

Ishii N, Takahashi T, Soroosh P et al (2010) OX40-OX40 ligand interaction in T-cell-mediated immunity and immunopathology. Adv Immunol 105:63–98

Izawa K, Martin E, Soudais C et al (2017) Inherited CD70 deficiency in humans reveals a critical role for the CD70-CD27 pathway in immunity to Epstein-Barr virus infection. J Exp Med 214:73–89

Jacquemin C, Schmitt N, Contin-Bordes C et al (2015) OX40 ligand contributes to human lupus pathogenesis by promoting T follicular helper response. Immunity 42:1159–1170

Kafrouni MI, Brown GR, Thiele DL (2003) The role of TNF-TNFR2 interactions in generation of CTL responses and clearance of hepatic adenovirus infection. J Leukoc Biol 74:564–571

Kanodia S, Da Silva DM, Karamanukyan T et al (2010) Expression of LIGHT/TNFSF14 combined with vaccination against human papillomavirus type 16 E7 induces significant tumor regression. Cancer Res 70:3955–3964

Karin M, Gallagher E (2009) TNFR signaling: ubiquitin-conjugated TRAFfic signals control stop-and-go for MAPK signaling complexes. Immunol Rev 228:225–240

Kawalekar OU, O'Connor RS, Fraietta JA et al (2016) Distinct signaling of coreceptors regulates specific metabolism pathways and impacts memory development in CAR T cells. Immunity 44:380–390

Kim EY, Priatel JJ, Teh SJ et al (2006) TNF receptor type 2 (p75) functions as a costimulator for antigen-driven T cell responses in vivo. J Immunol 176:1026–1035

Kim IK, Kim BS, Koh CH et al (2015) Glucocorticoid-induced tumor necrosis factor receptor-related protein co-stimulation facilitates tumor regression by inducing IL-9-producing helper T cells. Nat Med 21:1010–1017

Kitchens WH, Dong Y, Mathews DV et al (2017) Interruption of OX40L signaling prevents costimulation blockade-resistant allograft rejection. JCI Insight 2:e90317

Laouar A, Haridas V, Vargas D et al (2005) CD70+ antigen-presenting cells control the proliferation and differentiation of T cells in the intestinal mucosa. Nat Immunol 6:698–706

Linch SN, McNamara MJ, Redmond WL (2015) OX40 agonists and combination immunotherapy: putting the pedal to the metal. Front Oncol 5:34

Linch SN, Kasiewicz MJ, McNamara MJ et al (2016) Combination OX40 agonism/CTLA-4 blockade with HER2 vaccination reverses T-cell anergy and promotes survival in tumor-bearing mice. Proc Natl Acad Sci U S A 113:E319–E327

Locksley RM, Killeen N, Lenardo MJ (2001) The TNF and TNF receptor superfamilies: integrating mammalian biology. Cell 104:487–501

Long AH, Haso WM, Shern JF et al (2015) 4-1BB costimulation ameliorates T cell exhaustion induced by tonic signaling of chimeric antigen receptors. Nat Med 21:581–590

Lu L, Xu X, Zhang B et al (2014) Combined PD-1 blockade and GITR triggering induce a potent antitumor immunity in murine cancer models and synergizes with chemotherapeutic drugs. J Transl Med 12:36

Manocha M, Rietdijk S, Laouar A et al (2009) Blocking CD27-CD70 costimulatory pathway suppresses experimental colitis. J Immunol 183:270–276

Mbanwi AN, Watts TH (2014) Costimulatory TNFR family members in control of viral infection: outstanding questions. Semin Immunol 26:210–219

Mehta AK, Gracias DT, Croft M (2016) TNF activity and T cells. Cytokine 101:14–18

Meylan F, Davidson TS, Kahle E et al (2008) The TNF-family receptor DR3 is essential for diverse T cell-mediated inflammatory diseases. Immunity 29:79–89

Meylan F, Richard AC, Siegel RM (2011) TL1A and DR3, a TNF family ligand-receptor pair that promotes lymphocyte costimulation, mucosal hyperplasia, and autoimmune inflammation. Immunol Rev 244:188–196

Moran AE, Kovacsovics-Bankowski M, Weinberg AD (2013) The TNFRs OX40, 4-1BB, and CD40 as targets for cancer immunotherapy. Curr Opin Immunol 25:230–237

Mousavi SF, Soroosh P, Takahashi T et al (2008) OX40 costimulatory signals potentiate the memory commitment of effector CD8+ T cells. J Immunol 181:5990–6001

Munitic I, Kuka M, Allam A et al (2013) CD70 deficiency impairs effector CD8 T cell generation and viral clearance but is dispensable for the recall response to lymphocytic choriomeningitis virus. J Immunol 190:1169–1179

Nam SY, Kim YH, Do JS et al (2008) CD30 supports lung inflammation. Int Immunol 20:177–184

Nishimura H, Yajima T, Muta H et al (2005) A novel role of CD30/CD30 ligand signaling in the generation of long-lived memory CD8+ T cells. J Immunol 175:4627–4634

Nolte MA, van Olffen RW, van Gisbergen KP et al (2009) Timing and tuning of CD27-CD70 interactions: the impact of signal strength in setting the balance between adaptive responses and immunopathology. Immunol Rev 229:216–231

Pappu BP, Borodovsky A, Zheng TS et al (2008) TL1A-DR3 interaction regulates Th17 cell function and Th17-mediated autoimmune disease. J Exp Med 205:1049–1062

Park JJ, Anand S, Zhao Y et al (2012) Expression of anti-HVEM single-chain antibody on tumor cells induces tumor-specific immunity with long-term memory. Cancer Immunol Immunother 61:203–214

Penaloza-MacMaster P, Ur Rasheed A, Iyer SS et al (2011) Opposing effects of CD70 costimulation during acute and chronic lymphocytic choriomeningitis virus infection of mice. J Virol 85:6168–6174

Pobezinskaya YL, Choksi S, Morgan MJ et al (2011) The adaptor protein TRADD is essential for TNF-like ligand 1A/death receptor 3 signaling. J Immunol 186:5212–5216

Polte T, Behrendt AK, Hansen G (2006) Direct evidence for a critical role of CD30 in the development of allergic asthma. J Allergy Clin Immunol 118:942–948

Punit S, Dube PE, Liu CY et al (2015) Tumor necrosis factor receptor 2 restricts the pathogenicity of CD8(+) T cells in mice with colitis. Gastroenterology 149:993–1005

Richard AC, Ferdinand JR, Meylan F et al (2015a) The TNF-family cytokine TL1A: from lymphocyte costimulator to disease co-conspirator. J Leukoc Biol 98:333–345

Richard AC, Tan C, Hawley ET et al (2015b) The TNF-family ligand TL1A and its receptor DR3 promote T cell-mediated allergic immunopathology by enhancing differentiation and pathogenicity of IL-9-producing T cells. J Immunol 194:3567–3582

Sakoda Y, Park JJ, Zhao Y et al (2011) Dichotomous regulation of GVHD through bidirectional functions of the BTLA-HVEM pathway. Blood 117:2506–2514

Sakoda Y, Nagai T, Murata S et al (2016) Pathogenic function of herpesvirus entry mediator in experimental autoimmune uveitis by induction of Th1-and Th17-type T cell responses. J Immunol 196:2947–2954

Salek-Ardakani S, Moutaftsi M, Crotty S et al (2008) OX40 drives protective vaccinia virus-specific CD8 T cells. J Immunol 181:7969–7976

Sanchez-Paulete AR, Labiano S, Rodriguez-Ruiz ME et al (2016) Deciphering CD137 (4-1BB) signaling in T-cell costimulation for translation into successful cancer immunotherapy. Eur J Immunol 46:513–522

Schaer C, Hiltbrunner S, Ernst B et al (2011) HVEM signalling promotes colitis. PLoS One 6:e18495

Schaer DA, Murphy JT, Wolchok JD (2012) Modulation of GITR for cancer immunotherapy. Curr Opin Immunol 24:217–224

Shevach EM, Stephens GL (2006) The GITR-GITRL interaction: co-stimulation or contrasuppression of regulatory activity? Nat Rev Immunol 6:613–618

Shinoda K, Sun X, Oyamada A et al (2015) CD30 ligand is a new therapeutic target for central nervous system autoimmunity. J Autoimmun 57:14–23

Slebioda TJ, Rowley TF, Ferdinand JR et al (2011) Triggering of TNFRSF25 promotes CD8(+) T-cell responses and anti-tumor immunity. Eur J Immunol 41:2606–2611

Snell LM, McPherson AJ, Lin GH et al (2010) CD8 T cell-intrinsic GITR is required for T cell clonal expansion and mouse survival following severe influenza infection. J Immunol 185:7223–7234

Snell LM, Lin GH, McPherson AJ et al (2011) T-cell intrinsic effects of GITR and 4-1BB during viral infection and cancer immunotherapy. Immunol Rev 244:197–217

So T, Croft M (2013) Regulation of PI-3-kinase and Akt signaling in T lymphocytes and other cells by TNFR family molecules. Front Immunol 4:139

So T, Lee SW, Croft M (2006) Tumor necrosis factor/tumor necrosis factor receptor family members that positively regulate immunity. Int J Hematol 83:1–11

So T, Lee SW, Croft M (2008) Immune regulation and control of regulatory T cells by OX40 and 4-1BB. Cytokine Growth Factor Rev 19:253–262

So T, Nagashima H, Ishii N (2015) TNF receptor-associated factor (TRAF) signaling network in CD4(+) T-lymphocytes. Tohoku J Exp Med 236:139–154

Soloviova K, Puliaiev M, Haas M et al (2013) In vivo maturation of Allo-specific CD8 CTL and prevention of lupus-like graft-versus-host disease is critically dependent on T cell signaling through the TNF p75 receptor but not the TNF p55 receptor. J Immunol 190:4562–4572

Song DG, Ye Q, Poussin M et al (2012) CD27 costimulation augments the survival and antitumor activity of redirected human T cells in vivo. Blood 119:696–706

Soroosh P, Doherty TA, So T et al (2011) Herpesvirus entry mediator (TNFRSF14) regulates the persistence of T helper memory cell populations. J Exp Med 208:797–809

Steinberg MW, Turovskaya O, Shaikh RB et al (2008) A crucial role for HVEM and BTLA in preventing intestinal inflammation. J Exp Med 205:1463–1476

Steinberg MW, Huang YJ, Wang-Zhu Y et al (2013) BTLA interaction with HVEM expressed on CD8(+) T cells promotes survival and memory generation in response to a bacterial infection. PLoS One 8:e77992

Strober W, Fuss IJ (2011) Proinflammatory cytokines in the pathogenesis of inflammatory bowel diseases. Gastroenterology 140:1756–1767

Sugamura K, Ishii N, Weinberg AD (2004) Therapeutic targeting of the effector T-cell co-stimulatory molecule OX40. Nat Rev Immunol 4:420–431

Sun M, Fink PJ (2007) A new class of reverse signaling costimulators belongs to the TNF family. J Immunol 179:4307–4312

Tahiliani V, Hutchinson TE, Abboud G et al (2017) OX40 cooperates with ICOS to amplify follicular Th cell development and germinal center reactions during infection. J Immunol 198:218–228

Tang C, Yamada H, Shibata K et al (2008) A novel role of CD30L/CD30 signaling by T-T cell interaction in Th1 response against mycobacterial infection. J Immunol 181:6316–6327

Twohig JP, Marsden M, Cuff SM et al (2012) The death receptor 3/TL1A pathway is essential for efficient development of antiviral CD4(+) and CD8(+) T-cell immunity. FASEB J 26:3575–3586

Ungewickell A, Bhaduri A, Rios E et al (2015) Genomic analysis of mycosis fungoides and Sezary syndrome identifies recurrent alterations in TNFR2. Nat Genet 47:1056–1060

Villarreal DO, Chin D, Smith MA et al (2017) Combination GITR targeting/PD-1 blockade with vaccination drives robust antigen-specific antitumor immunity. Oncotarget 8:39117–39130

Vinay DS, Kwon BS (2014) 4-1BB (CD137), an inducible costimulatory receptor, as a specific target for cancer therapy. BMB Rep 47:122–129

Ward-Kavanagh LK, Lin WW, Sedy JR et al (2016) The TNF receptor superfamily in co-stimulating and co-inhibitory responses. Immunity 44:1005–1019

Watts TH (2005) TNF/TNFR family members in costimulation of T cell responses. Annu Rev Immunol 23:23–68

Wensveen FM, Unger PP, Kragten NA et al (2012) CD70-driven costimulation induces survival or Fas-mediated apoptosis of T cells depending on antigenic load. J Immunol 188:4256–4267

Wortzman ME, Clouthier DL, McPherson AJ et al (2013a) The contextual role of TNFR family members in CD8(+) T-cell control of viral infections. Immunol Rev 255:125–148

Wortzman ME, Lin GH, Watts TH (2013b) Intrinsic TNF/TNFR2 interactions fine-tune the CD8 T cell response to respiratory influenza virus infection in mice. PLoS One 8:e68911

Xu Y, Flies AS, Flies DB et al (2007) Selective targeting of the LIGHT-HVEM costimulatory system for the treatment of graft-versus-host disease. Blood 109:4097–4104

Yamada A, Salama AD, Sho M et al (2005) CD70 signaling is critical for CD28-independent CD8+ T cell-mediated alloimmune responses in vivo. J Immunol 174:1357–1364

You S, Poulton L, Cobbold S et al (2009) Key role of the GITR/GITRLigand pathway in the development of murine autoimmune diabetes: a potential therapeutic target. PLoS One 4:e7848

Yu P, Fu YX (2008) Targeting tumors with LIGHT to generate metastasis-clearing immunity. Cytokine Growth Factor Rev 19:285–294

Zander RA, Obeng-Adjei N, Guthmiller JJ et al (2015) PD-1 co-inhibitory and OX40 co-stimulatory crosstalk regulates helper T cell differentiation and anti-plasmodium humoral immunity. Cell Host Microbe 17:628–641

Chapter 4
Signal Transduction Via Co-stimulatory and Co-inhibitory Receptors

Shuhei Ogawa and Ryo Abe

Abstract T-cell receptor (TCR)-mediated antigen-specific stimulation is essential for initiating T-cell activation. However, signaling through the TCR alone is not sufficient for inducing an effective response. In addition to TCR-mediated signaling, signaling through antigen-independent co-stimulatory or co-inhibitory receptors is critically important not only for the full activation and functional differentiation of T cells but also for the termination and suppression of T-cell responses. Many studies have investigated the signaling pathways underlying the function of each molecular component. Co-stimulatory and co-inhibitory receptors have no kinase activity, but their cytoplasmic region contains unique functional motifs and potential phosphorylation sites. Engagement of co-stimulatory receptors leads to recruitment of specific binding partners, such as adaptor molecules, kinases, and phosphatases, via recognition of a specific motif. Consequently, each co-stimulatory receptor transduces a unique pattern of signaling pathways. This review focuses on our current understanding of the intracellular signaling pathways provided by co-stimulatory and co-inhibitory molecules, including B7:CD28 family members, immunoglobulin, and members of the tumor necrosis factor receptor superfamily.

Keywords Co-stimulatory receptor · Co-inhibitory receptor · Signal transduction · B7:CD28 family members · Ig superfamily members · TNFR superfamily members

---

S. Ogawa (✉)
Division of Experimental Animal Immunology, Research Institute for Biomedical Sciences, Tokyo University of Science, Chiba, Japan
e-mail: shugyaba@rs.noda.tus.ac.jp

R. Abe
Strategic Innovation and Research Center, Teikyo University, Tokyo, Japan

Division of Immunobiology, Research Institute for Biomedical Sciences, Tokyo University of Science, Chiba, Japan

© Springer Nature Singapore Pte Ltd. 2019
M. Azuma, H. Yagita (eds.), *Co-signal Molecules in T Cell Activation*,
Advances in Experimental Medicine and Biology 1189,
https://doi.org/10.1007/978-981-32-9717-3_4

4.1 Introduction

TCR-mediated antigen-specific signaling is essential for T-cell responses. Upon TCR stimulation, the immunoreceptor tyrosine-based activation motif (ITAM, consensus sequence [D/E]x_{0-2}Yxx[L/I]x_{6-9}Yxx[L/I], where x is any amino acid) in the cytoplasmic tail of CD3 is phosphorylated by src family kinases, mainly Lck and Fyn. This event recruits tandem Src homology 2 (SH2) domain-containing tyrosine kinase ZAP70 initiating a cascade of events involving the assembly of intracellular components and the activation of downstream signaling pathways (Au-Yeung et al. 2009). Numerous co-stimulatory and co-inhibitory receptors have been identified, and each co-stimulatory and co-inhibitory molecule has unique functions determined by various factors, including expression on a specific cell type, the kinetics of its expression, its binding to a ligand partner, and the activation of intracellular signaling. The utilization of the signaling molecules recruited and activated by receptor ligation is the most determinant of the receptor function. In general, positive co-stimulatory receptors support T-cell activation and differentiation not only by augmenting TCR-mediated signaling but also by activating unique signaling pathways (Fig. 4.1). Co-inhibitory receptors diminish the activity of the TCR and co-stimulatory receptor signaling by recruiting phosphatase and/or by competing with the co-stimulatory receptor–ligand interaction. Engagement of a co-stimulatory receptor with a specific ligand triggers the protein tyrosine kinase-induced phosphorylation of tyrosine residues within the intracellular region. Tyrosine phosphorylation of receptors is critical for interactions with SH2 domain-containing proteins, such as Lck, Itk, Vav, PI3K, Grb2, and Gads, in T cells. The SH2 domain of each intracellular molecule recognizes the phosphorylated tyrosine and surrounding amino acids. For example, the SH2 domain of the p85 PI3K regulatory subunit binds to pYxxM, whereas the SH2 domain of Grb2 recognizes pYxNx. The proline-rich region is a potential binding site for SH3-containing molecules, such as Lck, Fyn, Itk, Tec, Grb2, and Gads.

Several co-inhibitory receptors possess an immunoreceptor tyrosine-based inhibitory motif (ITIM, consensus sequence [V/I]xYxx[L/V]) and an immunoreceptor tyrosine-based switch motif (ITSM, consensus sequence TxYxx[V/I]). When the tyrosine residue is phosphorylated within the ITIM or ITSM, SH2-contianing phosphatase (SHP) and SH2-containing inositol phosphatase (SHIP) associate with these consensus sequences and dephosphorylate the target molecules.

The tumor necrosis factor (TNF) receptor superfamily (TNFRSF) is critically involved in T-cell survival, cell death, cell cycle progression, and effector and memory formation. TNFRSF members are classified into two primary types: one group has co-stimulatory functions that induce the activation of NF-κB, PI3K, and MAPK, and the other group induces cell death. The latter group contains a death domain (DD) in the cytoplasmic region, which mediates apoptotic signals through interactions with components of the death machinery. This review focuses on the signal transduction through TNFRSF members, which transmit co-stimulatory signals to T cells. In general, engagement of the TNF receptor on T cells by its trimeric ligand

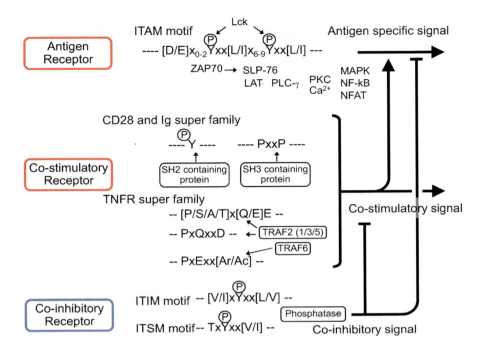

Fig. 4.1 General concepts of antigen-specific, co-stimulatory, and co-inhibitory signaling
Upon TCR stimulation, ITAM motifs in the CD3 cytoplasmic tail are phosphorylated by Lck, and this event initiates activation of the signaling cascade downstream of the TCR. Co-stimulatory receptor signals not only amplify the TCR-mediated signals but also deliver unique signals. In general, tyrosine phosphorylation induced by tyrosine kinase is critical for interaction with SH2-containing protein, such as Lck, Itk, Vav, PI3K, Grb2, and Gads. A proline-rich region comprises the binding site for SH3-containing proteins, such as Lck, Fyn, Itk, Tec, Grb2, and Gads. TNF receptor superfamily members have TRAF binding sequences that recruit different combinations of TRAFs. Several co-inhibitory receptors diminish TCR and co-stimulatory receptor signaling by recruiting phosphatase through ITIM motif and/or ITSM motif

recruits TNF receptor-associated factor (TRAF) adaptor proteins (Aggarwal 2003; Arch and Thompson 1998). TRAF2, TRAF1, TRAF3, and TRAF5 bind to a major motif, [P/S/A/T]x[Q/E], and a minor motif, PxQxxD (Ye et al. 1999; Park et al. 1999). TRAF6 binds to the PxExx[aromatic (Ar)/acidic (Ac)] motif (Ye et al. 2002). The TRAF4-binding motif has not been identified. TRAFs function as E3 ubiquitin ligases and are important for the activation of NF-κB, PI3K, and MAPK through the K63-linked polyubiquitination of target proteins (Deng et al. 2000; Shi and Kehrl 2003). One of the important features of TNFRSF is that several TNFRSF can activate noncanonical NF-κB signaling pathways. TRAF3 binds to NF-κB inducing kinase (NIK), and the TRAF2-TRAF3 dimer recruits the cellular inhibitor of apoptosis (cIAP)1 and cIAP2, which are ubiquitin E3 ligases. These complexes limit the NIK activity by K48 ubiquitination-induced degradation of NIK under unstimulated conditions. After TNFRS ligation, cIAP degrades TRAF3, and NIK is consequently released from TRAF3. Cellular accumulation of NIK activates noncanonical NF-κB by IKKα activation. Although each of TNFR utilizes different sets of TRAFs, several TNFRs have overlapping combinations for recruiting TRAFs. The mechanisms underlying the unique and diverse functions of each TNFR have not been fully elucidated; however, differences in expression patterns, TNFR–TRAF binding affinities, and recruitment of other adaptor proteins in addition to TRAFs probably contribute to the specific features of each TNFR (Chung et al. 2002).

Because co-stimulatory or co-inhibitory receptor-mediated signaling has a strong impact on T-cell responses, many of these receptors are potential therapeutic targets for autoimmune disease, graft survival, and cancer immune therapy. In this review, we summarize the recruiting molecules associated with the functional motifs in the intracellular region of several co-stimulatory and co-inhibitory receptors, including B7:CD28, immunoglobulin (Ig), and TNFR superfamily members.

4.2 CD28

CD28-mediated co-stimulatory signals not only amplify the TCR-mediated signals but also deliver unique signals that control T-cell activation, growth, survival, and differentiation by changing the activation of signaling molecules that regulate the formation of the following: immunological synapses (Viola et al. 1999), transcription (Fraser et al. 1991; Shapiro et al. 1997; June et al. 1987; Thompson et al. 1989), epigenetic modification of promoter regions (Thomas et al. 2005), alternative splicing of mRNA (Butte et al. 2012), mRNA stabilization (Lindstein et al. 1989), post-translational modification (Blanchet et al. 2006; Blanchet et al. 2005), and metabolic reprogramming (Frauwirth et al. 2002; Chang et al. 2013; Michalek et al. 2011; Klein Geltink et al. 2017).

Like other CD28 receptor members, CD28 has no enzymatic activity in the intracellular domain but contains four tyrosine residues and several functional motifs, such as Y^{170}MNM motif, which recruits SH2 domain-containing proteins and two PxxP motifs, which interact with SH3 domain-containing molecules (Fig. 4.2). CD28 ligation induces the activation of several protein tyrosine kinases, such as Lck, Fyn, and Itk, and results in the phosphorylation of CD28 tyrosine residues (Hutchcroft and Bierer 1994; August et al. 1994; King et al. 1997; Sadra et al. 1999; Raab et al. 1995; Holdorf et al. 1999). Several studies have shown the importance of the C-terminal PYAP motif of CD28 in Lck kinase activity (Holdorf et al. 1999, 2002). However, we found that tyrosine phosphorylation of CD28 could be induced by CD28 crosslinking in the CD28 mutant bearing substitutions the proline residues (PYAP to AYAA), whereas the Y^{170}F CD28 mutant abrogated tyrosine phosphorylation of CD28 (Ogawa et al. 2013). The N-terminal PRRP motif in CD28 is thought to be an Itk/Tec binding site. Therefore, it is possible that Itk-induced tyrosine phosphorylation of CD28 triggers full activation of Lck. A recent study showed that the cytoplasmic domain of CD28 binds to the plasma membrane (Dobbins et al. 2016)

4 Signal Transduction Via Co-stimulatory and Co-inhibitory Receptors

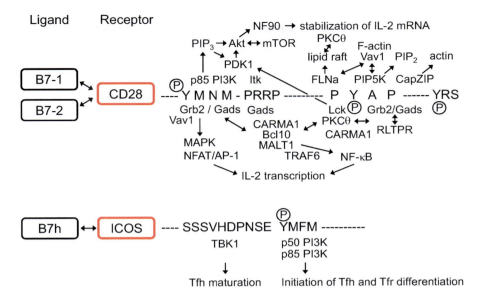

Fig. 4.2 Cytoplasmic motifs and interacting molecules of CD28 and ICOS
Upon CD28 ligation, tyrosine residues are phosphorylated by the Src family tyrosine kinase, Lck, and Itk, leading to recruitment of intracellular signaling molecules. The YMNM motif recruits p85 PI3K, Grb2, and Gads; the PRRP motif binds to Itk and Grb2. The PYAP motif binds to Lck, FLNa, and Gads and is also important for recruitment of CapZIP, RLTPR, and PIP5K. Recruitment of these molecules contributes to the interaction of PKCθ with CD28. These events are critical for effective CD28-mediated co-stimulation leading to activation of T cells and cytokine production Engagement of ICOS recruits p50 and p85 PI3K via the YMFM motif, and the IProx motif binds to TBK1. The Y to F mutant in the ICOS YMFM motif causes a defect in the early stages of Tfh and Tfr differentiation. The ICOS IProx motif is required for the development of fully mature Tfh cells

and CD28 ligation releases the cytoplasmic region from the plasma membrane. Yang et al. demonstrated concentration of Ca^{2+} around CD28 induced by TCR ligation disrupted the CD28-lipid interaction, leading to an open conformation of the CD28 cytoplasmic domain (Yang et al. 2017). Consequently, these events may allow Lck to access CD28 and phosphorylate the tyrosine residues of CD28. Regarding phosphorylation of other tyrosine residues in CD28, the recent global analysis of protein phosphorylation revealed that the most C-terminal tyrosine residue in CD28 is also phosphorylated (Tian et al. 2015); however, the role of this phosphorylation in CD28-mediated co-stimulation needs further analysis.

CD28 recruits several adaptor proteins, including the p85 regulatory subunit of PI3K (August and Dupont 1994; Pages et al. 1994; Prasad et al. 1994), Grb2, and Gads (Cai et al. 1995; Kim et al. 1998; Okkenhaug et al. 2001; Okkenhaug and Rottapel 1998; Raab et al. 1995; Stein et al. 1994), to its YMNM motif in a phosphorylation-dependent manner. Although each SH2 domain of PI3K, Grb2, and Gads binds to the CD28 YMNM motif, these three molecules interact with CD28 in strikingly different ways that depend on the binding sequence, conformation, and affinity (Higo et al. 2013, 2014; Inaba et al. 2017). In turn, these interactions activate MAPK, Akt, NFAT, and NF-κB, which lead to T-cell activation. We demonstrated that CD28 stimulation induces translocation of the CARMA1, Bcl10, and MALT1 (CBM) complex to the plasma membrane and the protein kinase C (PKC) θ kinase activity and association of the CD28 YMNM motif with the SH2 domain of Grb2/Gads have a greater impact on interleukin (IL)-2 transcription than does that with p85 PI3K (Takeda et al. 2008; Harada et al. 2001a). Other studies revealed that both TCR and CD28 activate NF-κB, but each signaling uses distinct adaptor signaling complexes. TCR and CD28 activate NF-κB via LAT/ADAP and Grb2/Vav1 pathways, respectively (Thaker et al. 2015). Schneider et al. demonstrated that Grb2 is required for recruitment of Vav1 to CD28 and NFAT/AP-1 activity (Schneider and Rudd 2008).

In addition to the role of CD28 in elevating IL-2 transcription, CD28-mediated co-stimulation stabilizes IL-2 mRNA (Lindstein et al. 1989). Two elements of IL-2 mRNA have been related to stabilization of IL-2 mRNA: one element located within its 5′ UTR is regulated by JNK (Chen et al. 1998) and another element, located within the 3′ UTR of IL-2 mRNA, is an AU-rich element regulated by the Akt/NF90 axis. Recruitment of Grb2/Gads and PI3K to the CD28 YMNM motif contributes to the stabilization of IL-2 mRNA (Sanchez-Lockhart et al. 2004; Sanchez-Lockhart and Miller 2006; Pei et al. 2008; Zhu et al. 2010).

It has been reported that CD28 PRRP and PYAP motifs recruit several intracellular molecules including the Itk/Tec family kinase, Lck, Grb2/Gads, PKCθ, filamin A (FLNa), and RLTPR (also known as CARMIL2). The Itk/Tec family kinase binds to the CD28 PRRP motif. It is possible that this interaction triggers tyrosine phosphorylation of CD28 and augments TCR signaling by inducing PLC-γ phosphorylation. However, the functional importance of Itk downstream of CD28 is uncertain (Tai et al. 2005, 2007; Li and Berg 2005; Jain et al. 2013).

Since several studies in the 2000s demonstrated that PKCθ downstream of CD28 is critically important for activation of NF-κB, AP-1, and NFAT (Coudronniere et al. 2000; Lin et al. 2000), the regulation of PKCθ localization and its activity have been studied intensively. A recent imaging study showed that stimulation of CD28 with TCR induces co-localization of CD28 with PKCθ at the T cell-antigen-presenting cell (APC) interface (Yokosuka et al. 2008). Although the CD28 PYAP motif-PKCθ association appears to be more involved in the CD28-mediated co-stimulatory function, both tyrosine residues within the YMNM and PYAP motifs are involved in the recruitment of PKCθ. Kong et al. demonstrated that Lck plays a role in the association between CD28 and PKCθ (Kong et al. 2011). In this context, the SH2 domain of Lck binds to the CD28 PYAP motif, and the SH3 domain of Lck binds to the proline-rich region within the V3 domain of PKCθ. These results are consistent with the finding that the SH2 domain of Lck has a much higher affinity than the SH3 domain for the phosphorylated PYAP motif of CD28 (Hofinger and Sticht 2005). Mutations of tyrosine residues at 185 and 188 around the C-terminal proline-rich motif strongly reduced CD28-mediated NF-κB activation (Muscolini et al. 2011). Another report showed that interaction of Lck with the PYAP motif of CD28 is required for tyrosine phosphorylation of PDK1 on Y^9. Subsequently, PDK1 phosphorylates Akt T^{308} and PKCθ Y^{538} (Dodson et al. 2009). Wang et al. revealed that TCR-induced sumoylation of PKCθ does not affect its kinase activity but is involved in the interaction of PKCθ with CD28 and FLNa. Mutation in the sumoylation site of PKCθ decreases the interaction with CD28 and impairs the formation of a mature immunological synapse (Wang et al. 2015). The SH3 domain of Grb2/Gads, but not that of p85 PI3K, also binds to CD28 PxxP motifs (Okkenhaug and Rottapel 1998; Higo et al. 2014; Watanabe et al. 2006), and these interactions might contribute to the elevation of IL-2 production through the recruitment of the CBM complex and PKCθ activation. Therefore, PKCθ is important for CD28-mediated co-stimulation, and its localization and kinase activity are regulated in multiple steps.

CD28-induced cytoskeletal remodeling is also important for efficient TCR and CD28 signaling pathways through the polarization of T cells toward the APC, which is based on the localization of surface and intracellular molecules. Association of the actin-binding protein FLNa with CD28 is involved in lipid-raft accumulation at the immunological synapse. Mutation in the CD28 PYAP motif resulted in impaired association with FLNa (Tavano et al. 2006). FLNa knockdown decreased the CD3/CD28 stimulation-induced membrane translocation of PKCθ and the activation of PKCθ-dependent transcription factors, including NF-κB, NFAT, and AP-1 (Hayashi and Altman 2006). Among the phosphoinositides, the amounts and localization of phosphatidylinositol 3,4,5-triphosphate (PIP₃) and phosphatidylinositol 4,5-biphosphate (PIP₂) affect actin cytoskeleton reorganization. The optimal activation of PI3K requires the replenishment of PIP₂ pools to ensure the direct regulation of actin cytoskeleton rearrangements. CD28 also recruits phosphatidylinositol 4-phosphate 5-kinases (PIP5K)-α and PIP5K-β as well as PI3K, which ensures the PIP₂ pool necessary for the CD28 signaling function (Muscolini et al. 2015; Kallikourdis et al. 2016). Overexpression of the PIP5K kinase-dead mutant impaired recruitment of Vav1 and accumulation of F-actin. Consequently, the CD28-mediated activation of NF-κB and NFAT was significantly inhibited by kinase-dead PIP5K expression. A mutant CD28, containing changes from proline to alanine at the PYAP motif, decreased its functional ability to recruit Vav1 and PIP5K. Kallikourdis et al. also found that Vav1 is required for CD28-induced recruitment of FLNa and PIP5K to the membrane (Kallikourdis et al. 2016). Furthermore, Tian et al. found that CapZ-interacting protein, which regulates actin cytoskeleton, is phosphorylated by CD28 stimulation and plays a critical role in CD28-mediated IL-2 production (Tian et al. 2015). Recently, RLPTR, a lymphoid lineage-specific actin-uncapping protein, was found to be critically important for CD28-mediated co-stimulation. Liang et al. showed that the functional ability of CD28 to recruit CARMA1 and PKCθ is dependent on RLPTR (Liang et al. 2013). It has been reported that humans with homozygous RLTPR mutations have immunodeficiency syndromes (Schober et al. 2017; Wang et al. 2016; Sorte et al. 2016; Roncagalli et al. 2016). The RLTPR acts as a scaffold protein in CD28-mediated co-stimulation, and RLTPR is pivotal for recruitment of CARMA1 and PKCθ to CD28 (Roncagalli et al. 2016). They discussed that the proline-rich region of RLTPR binds to Grb2/Gads and RLTPR is coupled to the CD28 PYAP motif via Grb2/Gads.

CD28 co-stimulation regulates the thymic development of Foxp3[+] regulatory T cells (Tregs) in a cell-intrinsic manner (Tai et al. 2005), although IL-2 is also a key factor for maintaining Treg homeostasis (Tang et al. 2003; Hombach et al. 2007; Long et al. 2010; Cheng et al. 2013). The contribution of CD28-mediated co-stimulation to the development and homeostasis of peripheral Tregs remains an open issue (Guo et al. 2008; Semple et al. 2011). Mice with a Foxp3[+] Treg-specific deletion of CD28, CD28$^{fl/fl}$ Foxp3^{Cre} mice, develop severe autoimmune-like disease, although Treg development is unchanged (Zhang et al. 2013b; Gogishvili et al. 2013). This finding indicates that CD28-mediated co-stimulation is also critical for the homeostasis and suppressive functions of Tregs. Analysis of mutant CD28 knock-in mice with Y^{170}F and AYAA revealed that the PYAP motif of CD28 is responsible for the development of Tregs (Lio et al. 2010). The *Foxp3* locus contains three conserved non-coding DNA sequences (CNSs) (Zheng et al. 2010b). These CNSs contribute to the stability of Foxp3 expression by interacting with NFAT, AP-1, Smad3, and PAR-RXR in CNS1; CREB-ATF, STAT5, Foxo1/2, Runx, Cbfb, and Foxp3 in CNS2 (known as the Treg-specific demethylation region, TSDR); and c-Rel in CNS3 (Zheng et al. 2010b; Cobbold and Waldmann 2013). Furthermore, c-Rel also binds to the Foxp3 promoter. Several studies demonstrated that c-Rel is a key regulator of Foxp3 expression and the development of thymic Tregs (Ruan et al. 2009; Long et al. 2009; Isomura et al. 2009). Vang et al. demonstrated that activation of c-Rel downstream of CD28 is involved in the development of Tregs (Vang et al. 2010). RelA, another NF-κB protein, is related to the development of peripheral Tregs (Soligo et al. 2011). True Tregs show demethylation of the TSDR; the methylation level of TSDR – which is regulated by DNA (cytosine-5)-methyltransferases (DNMTs), tet methylcytosine dioxygenase (TET), and/or enhancer of zeste homolog 2 (Ezh2) – affects Treg stabilization (Wang et al. 2013; Yang et al. 2015; Sarmento et al. 2017). Further analysis is required to determine how CD28-mediated co-stimulation contributes to Foxp3 expression and its stability.

Overall, the relevance of YMNM and PYAP motifs in CD28-mediated co-stimulation requires further investigation. Analyses using mutant CD28 knock-in mice demonstrated that the PYAP motif is more critical for CD28-mediated co-stimulatory function than is the YMNM motif with regard to immune responses involving antibody formation, allergic airways, and induction of experimental allergic encephalomyelitis (EAE) (Dodson et al. 2009; Friend et al. 2006). However, a subsequent study demonstrated that YMNM and PYAP double-mutant knock-in mice showed more severe impairment of CD28-mediated co-stimulation compared to either single mutant, although they maintain residual CD28-dependent responses (Boomer et al. 2014). Therefore, the YMNM motif also plays important roles in CD28-mediated co-stimulation. Our study consistently showed that CD28 Y^{170}F transgenic T cells failed to induce an acute graft-versus-host reaction (Harada et al. 2001b). Furthermore, under highly immunogenic conditions, such as during bacterial or viral infection, the YMNM and PYAP double-mutant knock-in mice develop

4 Signal Transduction Via Co-stimulatory and Co-inhibitory Receptors 93

T-cell responses against the microorganism, even though CD28-deficient mice show decreasing clonal expansion of T cells under the same conditions (Pagan et al. 2012; Boomer et al. 2014). These data imply that unknown functional motifs or amino acids recruit these intracellular molecules. Further studies are needed to explore the unknown functional domains and clarify the entire picture of CD28-mediated co-stimulation.

4.3 Inducible Co-stimulator (ICOS, Known as AILIM, H4, and CD278)

ICOS is a CD28 family co-stimulatory receptor. Whereas ICOS expression levels are low on naive T cells, increased levels are induced on recently activated or antigen-experienced T cells. Upon ICOS engagement by binding of the ICOS ligand (B7h, also known as B7RP-1 or CD275) or by crosslinking with anti-ICOS monoclonal antibody (mAb), ICOS derives positive co-stimulatory signals that augment the proliferation of T cells and promote the secretion of cytokines, including IL-4, IL-5, IL-10, and IL-21 but not IL-2. Analysis of ICOS-deficient mice showed that the production of basal and antigen-specific IgG1 and IgG2 antibodies was significantly reduced. Spontaneous systemic autoimmune animal model in MRL/*lpr* mice or fatal lymphoproliferating disease arise form CTLA-4 deficiency was prevented or reduced by ICOS deficiency or blockade of the ICOS–ICOS ligand interaction (Odegard et al. 2008; van Berkel et al. 2005). Therefore, ICOS-mediated co-stimulation is thought to be critical for the effector and regulatory functions of CD4+ T cells and particularly for the development of follicular helper T cells (Tfh) and follicular regulatory T cells (Tfr) (Choi et al. 2011; Akiba et al. 2005; Leavenworth et al. 2015).

ICOS possesses a YMFM motif in the cytoplasmic region corresponding to the CD28 YMNM motif (Fig. 4.2). However, unlike CD28, ICOS lacks a proline-rich region, which is a binding motif of SH3-containing molecules, such as Lck, Itk, Grb2, and Gads. Engagement of ICOS recruits the PI3K regulatory subunit via the YMFM–SH2 domain interaction. To examine the in vivo function of the ICOS–PI3K interaction, Gigoux and Shang et al. generated ICOS YF knock-in mice, in which Y was changed to F mutant in the YMFM motif. The authors showed that ICOS-mediated PI3K signaling is critical for Tfh generation (Gigoux et al. 2009). Germinal center formation, antibody class switching, and affinity maturation are significantly diminished in the ICOS YF knock-in mice. Although both CD28 and ICOS promote PI3K activity, the importance of PI3K driven by ICOS in Tfh development might be related to evidence that ICOS can induce high PIP_3 production and Akt phosphorylation compared to CD28 stimulation (Parry et al. 2003; Fos et al. 2008).

Recently, Pedros et al. found that ICOS has an evolutionarily conserved proximal membrane motif, named IProx (SSSVHDPNGE at positions 170–179), and a distal motif (AVNTAKK at positions 185–191) in addition to the PI3K YMFM-binding motif (Pedros et al. 2016). The IProx motif shares homology with TRAF2 and

TRAF3. An ICOS mutant, with replacement of all residues in the IProx motif with a string of 10 alanine residues, abolished the association of the serine-threonine kinase TBK1 with ICOS but still bound to p85 PI3K. On the other hand, the ICOS YF mutant retained the interaction with TBK1 but lacked the binding ability to p85 PI3K. In the early stages after antigen priming, ICOS-deficient CD4[+] T cells reconstituted with the ICOS IProx mutant differentiated into CXCR5[+]Bcl6[+] nascent Tfh cells comparable to those with wild-type (WT) ICOS. However, the ICOS IProx mutant-reconstituted CD4[+] T cells did not develop fully mature Tfh cells. The ICOS YF mutant exhibited a defect in early-stage Tfh differentiation. The antigen-specific antibody secretion and plasma cell differentiation of B cells were significantly impaired in both IProx and YF mutants. Furthermore, they also revealed a critical role for TBK1 in Tfh differentiation and antibody production. Therefore, both ICOS-PI3K and IProx-dependent ICOS-TBK1 pathways are non-redundant and required for Tfh development and humoral immune responses. Further analysis is needed to explore the role of TBK1 in the differentiation of nascent Tfh cells into fully mature Tfh cells.

4.4 Cytotoxic T-Lymphocyte-Associated Antigen-4 (CTLA-4, Known as CD152)

CTLA-4 is the most characterized CD28 family co-inhibitory receptor (Fig. 4.3). CTLA-4 shares the B7-1 and B7-2 ligands with CD28, using a MYPPPY extracellular binding motif. The binding affinity of CTLA-4 to B7s is quite higher than that of CD28. CTLA-4 expression is very low on resting T cells but is induced after T-cell activation; Foxp3[+] Tregs constitutively express CTLA-4. Surface expression of CTLA-4 after translation is dynamically regulated by endocytosis, lysosomal degradation, and recycling to the cell surface. Binding of clathrin adaptor protein-2 (AP-2) to the cytoplasmic YVKM motif of CTLA-4 promotes the internalization of CTLA-4 to endosomes and lysosomes. AP-2 can bind to unphosphorylated but not phosphorylated CTLA-4. Therefore, upon tyrosine phosphorylation of the YVKM motif within the intracellular domain of CTLA-4 initiated by TCR and/or CD28/CTLA-4 ligation, CTLA-4 dissociates from AP-2, and consequently cell surface expression of CTLA-4 is sustained. Recently, several groups reported that lipopolysaccharide-responsive beige-like anchor (LRBA) and CTLA-4 colocalized within recycling endosomes and the trans-Golgi network (Lo et al. 2015). LRBA protects CTLA-4 from being degraded within lysosomes. Mutations in the LRBA gene or LRBA knockdown increased CTLA-4 degradation and consequently reduced the expression and protein level of CTLA-4 in Foxp3[+] Tregs, augmenting T-cell activation. These data are consistent with the clinical observation that humans bearing a mutation in LRBR develop a syndrome of immune deficiency and autoimmunity (Lopez-Herrera et al. 2012; Bratanic et al. 2017; Hou et al. 2017). Furthermore, tyrosine phosphorylation within the YVKM motif is critical for the interaction with LRBA. Therefore, the clathrin-associated adaptor protein complex

4 Signal Transduction Via Co-stimulatory and Co-inhibitory Receptors

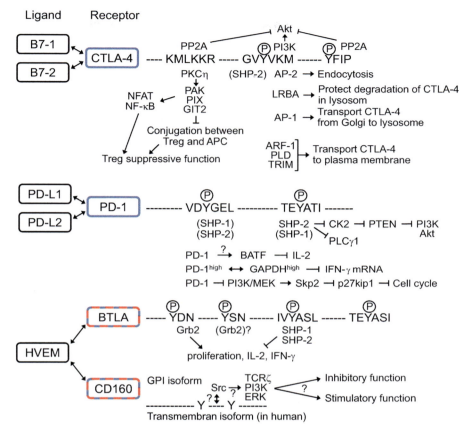

Fig. 4.3 Cytoplasmic motifs of CTLA-4, PD-1, BTLA, and CD160 and interacting molecules Clathrin adaptor protein (AP)-1, AP-2, and LRBA bind to the CTLA-4 YVKM motif to regulate the localization and degradation of CTLA-4. The CTLA-4–PP2A interaction may inhibit Akt activation. The Y to F mutant in the CTLA-4 YVKM motif increases CTLA-4 surface expression and impairs Treg-suppressive activity but has no effect on the conventional T-cell phenotype. PKCη interacts with a conserved three-lysine (KMLKKR) motif in the juxtamembrane of CTLA-4

PD-1 contains ITIM (VDYGEL) and ITSM (TEYATI) motifs. The interaction of SHP-2 with the ITSM motif is essential for the PD-1-mediated suppressive function. PD-1 increases PTEN phosphatase activity by inhibition of CK2 activity. PD-1-mediated signal induces expression of BATF, which inhibits IL-2 production. PD-1 expression correlated with GAPDH. Under glucose-restricted conditions, GAPDH binds to the 3' UTR of cytokine mRNA and suppresses cytokine production. PD-1 ligation suppresses ubiquitin ligase Skp2 transcription. The expression of p27^{kip1}, the target of Skp2, is sustained, which thereby inhibits the cell cycle

BTLA contains ITIM (IVYASL), ITSM (TEYASI), and Grb2-binding motifs. BTLA recruits SHP-1 and SHP-2 via ITIM and ITSM, resulting in suppression of T-cell function. The Grb2-binding motif of BTLA has a positive function in IL-2 production and the proliferation of T cells

CD160 is mainly GPI-anchored protein and has an alternative TM isoform. In T cells, CD160 co-precipitates with Lck and the phosphorylated TCRζ chain. The function of CD160-mediated signaling in T cells is unclear. It is possible that CD160 has differing functions in various cell types and conditions

and LRBA might mutually inhibit CTLA-4 binding in a YVKM-phosphorylation-dependent manner. AP-1 also binds to the CTLA-4 YVKM motif at the Golgi apparatus, and the CTLA-4–AP-1 complex appears to play a role in shuttling excess CTLA-4 from the Golgi to the lysosome for degradation (Schneider et al. 1999). GTPase ADP ribosylation factor-1 (ARF-1), phospholipase D (PLD), and T-cell receptor-interacting molecule (TRIM) function to transport CTLA-4 from the trans-Golgi network toward the plasma membrane but do not inhibit the endocytosis of CTLA-4 (Mead et al. 2005; Valk et al. 2006). TRIM binds to the cytoplasmic portion of CTLA-4 cytoplasm in a region other than the YVKM motif; direct interactions involving CTLA-4, ARF, or PLD have not been examined.

The mechanisms of inhibitory function of CTLA-4 have been investigated intensively and discussed by many researchers. CTLA-4 negatively regulates immune responses by both cell-intrinsic and cell-extrinsic mechanisms. The cell-extrinsic mechanisms include secretion of soluble CTLA-4 (sCTLA-4) (Oaks et al. 2000), reducing B7-1/B7-2 expression on APCs by downregulation and transendocytosis (Oderup et al. 2006; Cederbom et al. 2000; Qureshi et al. 2011), production of indoleamine 2,3-dioxygenase (IDO) from the APC through a CTLA-4–B7 reverse signal, and functional involvement of Treg cells (Grohmann et al. 2002). Cell-intrinsic factors include competition of interactions of CD28 with B7-1/B7-2, CTLA-4-mediated inhibitory signaling, modulation of TCR and CD28 signaling, inhibition of ZAP-70 microcluster formation, and altered immunological synapses (IS). CTLA-4 lacks ITIM and ITSM motifs but has a YVKM motif in the cytoplasmic region (Fig. 4.3). CTLA-4 recruits SH2 domain-containing phosphatase-2 (SHP-2) (Marengere et al. 1996; Lee et al. 1998), protein phosphatase 2A (PP2A) (Parry et al. 2005; Chuang et al. 2000), and PI3K (Hu et al. 2001). SHP-2 is associated with CTLA-4 in a manner dependent on tyrosine phosphorylation within the YVKM motif (Marengere et al. 1996). However, it remains unclear whether the CTLA-4 YVKM motif is required in the association with SHP-2 (Lee et al. 1998). Furthermore, a recent imaging study failed to show accumulation of SHP-2 at the T-APC interaction site and colocalization of CTLA-4 with SHP-2 (Yokosuka et al. 2010). Therefore, the role of SHP-2–CTLA-4 interactions in the CTLA-4-mediated inhibitory function is controversial. Regarding the negative function of CTLA-4 YVKM motif, a CTLA-4 $Y^{201}V$ mutant knock-in mice showed increased expression levels of CTLA-4 on T cells and impaired suppressive activity of Treg cells; however, CTLA-4 $Y^{201}V$ had little effect on the conventional T-cell homeostasis and activation (Stumpf et al. 2014).

PP2A is thought to be important for CTLA-4-mediated inhibitory functions. Several studies investigated the binding mode of PP2A and the cytoplasmic tail of CTAL-4. The PP2A scaffolding A subunit interacts with a conserved three-lysine motif in the juxtamembrane of the CTLA-4 cytoplasmic region and Y^{218} within the YFIP motif (Teft et al. 2009). Whereas TCR ligation induces tyrosine phosphorylation of PP2AA, TCR/CTLA-4 co-ligation dissociates PP2AA from CTLA-4. The PP2AA/C core dimer released from CTLA-4 interacts with the PP2A B subunit, providing the cellular localization, and dephosphorylates target molecule. CTLA-4-mediated suppression of Akt phosphorylation and IL-2 transcription are inhibited by treatment with okadaic acid, which is a PP2A inhibitor. Okadaic acid enhances CD28-dependent IL-2 transcription. Furthermore, PP2A also binds to the cytoplasmic tail of CD28, and the interaction of PP2A with CD28 inhibits Lck-dependent CD28 tyrosine phosphorylation (Chuang et al. 2000). Therefore, it is possible that CD28 may be the target of PP2A downstream of CTLA-4. CTLA-4 associates with PI3K and increases Akt activity (Schneider et al. 2008; Hu et al. 2001). Activation of the PI3K/Akt pathway downstream of CTLA-4 may be related to the function of CTLA-4 in anergy induction without cell death (Da Rocha Dias and Rudd 2001).

Recently, Kong et al. revealed that the positively charged KMLKKR motif in the membrane-proximal region of CTLA-4 could interact with PKCη (Kong et al. 2014). Phosphorylated PKCη bound predominantly to CTLA-4; mutagenesis showed that Ser^{28} and Ser^{32} in the C2 domain or Ser^{317} in the V3 domain of PKCη are critical for the association with CTLA-4. Tregs in PKCη-deficient mice developed normally. However, Tregs from PKCη-deficient mice exhibited impaired contact-dependent suppressive activity. Furthermore, focal adhesion complexes composed of p21-activated kinase (PAK), PAK-interacting exchange factor (PIX), and G protein-coupled receptor kinase-interacting protein 2 (GIT2) were physically associated with CTLA-4 and PKCη. The association of CTLA-4 with the PAK–PIX–GIT2 complex and the activity of this complex was reduced in Tregs in PKCη-deficient mice. PKCη-deficient Tregs displayed impaired dissociation from engaged APCs and diminished NFAT and NF-κB activities. Therefore, a CTLA-4–PKCη signaling axis is required for the suppressive function of Tregs.

As mentioned above, although it is unclear whether the cytoplasmic tail of CTLA-4 directly inhibits the signaling pathways related to T-cell activation, the cytoplasmic region of CTLA-4 clearly contributes to the regulation of immune responses through multistep regulation of CTLA-4 localization within T cells.

4.5 Programmed Death 1 (PD-1, Known as CD279)

PD-1 has two ligands, PD-L1 (known as CD274 and B7-H1) (Freeman et al. 2000; Dong et al. 1999) and PD-L2 (known as CD273 and B7-DC) (Tseng et al. 2001; Latchman et al. 2001). PD-1-mediated signaling engaged in by PD-L1 and PD-L2 regulates the threshold of T-cell activation and affects effector T-cell responses, differentiation of T cells, T-cell tolerance, T-cell exhaustion, and inflammation in the periphery. PD-1 is inducibly expressed on $CD4^+$ and $CD8^+$ T cells, NK, NKT, B cells, macrophages, and several dendritic cells (DCs) subsets during immune responses, chronic inflammation, and exhaustion (Moll et al. 2009; Keir et al. 2006; Yamazaki et al. 2002; Agata et al. 1996). Exhausted T cells such as those involved in chronic viral infections (e.g., HIV) have increased amounts of inhibitory receptors, including PD-1. In exhausted T cells, basic leucine transcription factor, ATF-like (BATF), which binds to c-Jun and competitively inhibits AP-1 transcriptional activity, undergoes PD-1-mediated upregulation by an unknown mechanism. PD-1-mediated upregulation of BATF impairs T-cell proliferation and cytokine production, whereas BATF silencing causes an increase in IL-2 secretion (Quigley et al. 2010). PD-1 signaling can decrease the production of cytotoxic effector molecules and effector function – such as proliferation and production of IL-2, TNF-α, IFN-γ, and MIP-1β – in a PD-1-signaling dose-dependent manner (Wei et al. 2013). Aerobic glycolysis is required for T cells to acquire full effector function, which is regulated by bifunctional enzyme GAPDH. Under glucose-sufficient conditions, GAPDH engages in its enzymatic function; however, under glucose-restricted conditions, GAPDH suppresses effector cytokine production by binding to the 3' UTR of cytokine mRNA. In exhausted T cells, high GAPDH expression correlates with PD-1 expression but inversely correlates with effector cytokine production (Chang et al. 2013). Furthermore, anti-PD-1 immune checkpoint therapy restores glucose in the tumor microenvironment. Therefore, PD-1 signaling affects the metabolic reprogramming of T cells by inhibiting aerobic glycolysis and promoting fatty acid oxidation. This PD-1-mediated metabolic reprogramming influences effector T-cell and Tregs differentiation (Chang et al. 2013; Patsoukis et al. 2015; Chang et al. 2015; Michalek et al. 2011). PD-1 signals also modulate T-cell motility and the duration of interaction with DCs and target cells. PD-1 suppressed TCR-driven stop signals, and inversed blockade of PD-1 inhibited T-cell migration, prolonged T cell–DC engagement, enhanced T-cell cytokine production, boosted TCR signaling, and abrogated peripheral tolerance (Fife et al. 2009).

PD-1 consists of several domains, including IgV-like, stalk, transmembrane (TM), and cytoplasmic domains. Although many CD28 family members share a cysteine residue in the stalk region that mediates homodimerization and a ligand-binding site, PD-1 lacks the cysteine residues; therefor, PD-1 cannot form a covalent homodimer (Zhang et al. 2004). The cytoplasmic region of PD-1 contains an ITIM motif and an ITSM motif (Okazaki et al. 2001; Shinohara et al. 1994; Ishida et al. 1992) (Fig. 4.3). Upon PD-1 stimulation by interaction with PD-L1 or PD-L2, two tyrosine residues of PD-1 are phosphorylated within the ITIM (Y^{223}) and ITSM (Y^{248}) motifs (Chemnitz et al. 2004), triggering the recruitment of SH2 domain-containing molecules and decreasing the activation of membrane-proximal T-cell signaling events through the dephosphorylation of signaling molecules, such as CD3ζ, ZAP70, and PKCθ, in T cells (Sheppard et al. 2004; Chemnitz et al. 2004; Okazaki et al. 2001). Engagement of PD-1 recruits SHP-1 and SHP-2 (Chemnitz et al. 2004). Binding of SHP-2 to the ITSM motif of PD-1 is more critical for the PD-1-mediated inhibitory function (Parry et al. 2005; Chemnitz et al. 2004). A molecular imaging and mutagenesis approach clarified the importance of the localization of PD-1 on effector T cells in the co-inhibitory function of PD-1 and revealed the role of tyrosine residues within ITIM and ITSM motifs (Yokosuka et al. 2012). Ligand-dependent localization of PD-1 to the TCR microcluster and the central supramolecular activation cluster (c-SMAC) is critical for the inhibitory function of PD-1. Imaging analysis revealed that the association of SHP-2 with PD-1 via the ITSM motif is required for the PD-1-mediated suppression of T-cell activation by the dephosphorylation of TCR proximal signaling molecules. However, the ITIM motif plays only a partial role in the PD-1-mediated inhibitory function. PD-1-mediated signaling predominantly dephosphorylates tyrosine residues in CD28. Hui et al. demonstrated that tyrosine phosphorylation of CD28 is the most sensitive target of the PD-1–SHP-2 signal compared to phosphorylation of the proximal molecules of TCR, such as CD3ζ, ZAP70, LAT, SLP76, and another co-stimulatory molecule, ICOS (Hui et al. 2017). Kamphorst et al. reported that CD28-mediated co-stimulatory signaling is essential for effective anti-PD-1 immune checkpoint therapy (Kamphorst et al. 2017).

PD-1-mediated signaling affects the activation of many intracellular signaling pathways downstream of TCR and CD28. Many studies have reported that PD-1 inhibits PI3K activation (Yang et al. 2016; Ding et al. 2016; Patsoukis et al. 2013; Saunders et al. 2005). In a collagen-induced arthritis (CIA) murine RA model, the severity was significantly higher in PD-1-deficient mice than in WT mice. This severe CIA in PD-1-deficient mice was attenuated by administration of the PI3K inhibitor, LY294002 (Yang et al. 2016). Parry et al. showed that PD-1-mediated PI3K inhibition is dependent on the ITSM motif of PD-1 (Parry et al. 2005). Recently, Patsoukis et al. demonstrated that PD-1 inhibits activity of casein kinase 2 (CK2), which phosphorylates serine-threonine cluster within the C-terminal domain of PTEN (Patsoukis et al. 2013). Phosphorylation of this cluster by CK2 leads to the stabilization of PTEN and inversely decreases the phosphatase activity of PTEN. Therefore, PD-1 signaling inhibits phosphorylation of the serine-threonine cluster of PTEN but increases PTEN phosphatase activity, thereby inhibiting the PI3K–Akt signaling axis. In contrast, CTLA-4 preserves PI3K activity and expression of certain genes, such as Bcl-xL, and directly inhibits Akt via the PP2A phosphatase (Parry et al. 2005).

PD-1 ligation inhibits the MEK–ERK signaling pathway (Patsoukis et al. 2012). Activation of both PI3K–Akt and MEK–ERK signaling pathways is required for the induction of ubiquitin ligase SCF[Skp2], which degrades cyclin-dependent kinase inhibitor p27[kip1]. Therefore, PD-1-mediated inhibition of the PI3K–Akt and MEK–ERK pathways suppresses SKP2 expression and inhibits cell cycle progression via the inhibition of cyclin-dependent kinase-2 (Cdk2) activation (Patsoukis et al. 2012).

Further downstream, PD-1 modulates T-cell effector function and T-cell tolerance by reducing expression of cytokines and key transcription factors (e.g., GATA-3, T-bet, and Eomes) and increasing expression of Grail, Itch, and Cbl-b (Tang et al. 2016; Nurieva et al. 2006). Furthermore, as PD-1-mediated signaling downregulates activation of PI3K–Akt, mTOR, and ERK and upregulates PTEN phosphatase activity – which are key signaling molecules for inducible Treg (iTreg) development – PD-1 can promote the development and maintenance of iTreg cells (Francisco et al. 2009).

4.6 B- and T-Lymphocyte Attenuator (BTLA, Known as CD272)

BTLA is expressed on B cells, $\alpha\beta$ and $\gamma\delta$ T cells, mature DCs, and macrophages (Watanabe et al. 2003; Loyet et al. 2005; Otsuki et al. 2006). Upon TCR engagement, naive T cells express transiently upregulated BTLA, which is downregulated in fully activated T cells (Hurchla et al. 2005; Otsuki et al. 2006). BTLA is highly expressed on anergic and exhausted T cells. BTLA has the ability to provide both stimulatory and inhibitory signals to T cells. The cytoplasmic region of BTLA contains ITIM, ITSM, and Grb2-binding motifs (Watanabe et al. 2003; Gavrieli and Murphy 2006) (Fig. 4.3). Engagement of BTLA by its herpes virus entry mediator (HVEM)-containing ligands recruits SHP-1 and SHP-2 to ITIM and ITSM, resulting in suppression of T-cell proliferation and production of cytokines, including IFN-γ, IL-2, and IL-10 (Watanabe et al. 2003; Sedy et al. 2005; Otsuki et al. 2006). BTLA possesses four tyrosine residues; mutation of all four tyrosine residues is required to abolish the BTLA-mediated inhibitory function (Chemnitz et al. 2006). Ritthipichai et al. showed that a Y to F mutation in the Grb2-binding motif of BTLA abrogates the BTLA-dependent proliferation and IL-2 production in T cells (Ritthipichai et al. 2017). Therefore, the Grb2-binding motif functions to provide a positive co-stimulatory signal to T cells. The balance between the positive and negative aspects of BTLA functions is not well understood. As HVEM interacts with at least five ligands – including lymphotoxin alpha (LTα) and LIGHT (Mauri et al. 1998; Granger et al. 2001), which transmits a positive signal, and CD160 (Cai et al. 2008) and glycoprotein D (gD) of the herpes simplex virus (Whitbeck et al. 1997), which have an inhibitory function, as well as BTLA – it appears that the expression and localization of the BTLAs or other receptors influence whether the signal is positive or negative signals to T cells.

4.7 CD160 (Known as BY55)

CD160 is expressed on NK, NKT, and $\gamma\delta$T cells, CD8$^+$ T cells, and a small subset of CD4$^+$ T cells, but not on B or myeloid cells (DEL Rio et al. 2017; Tsujimura et al. 2006; Maeda et al. 2005). The expression level of CD160 is downregulated in CD3/CD28 stimulated cells (Vigano et al. 2014) and upregulated under exhaustive conditions, such as HIV infection. CD160 protein mainly forms a single IgV-like domain – a stalk domain to glycosylphosphatidylinositol (GPI)-anchor (CD160-GPI). In addition to this form, human isoforms originating from alternative splicing encode a TM and intracellular domain (CD160-TM), sharing the same extracellular domain as the original GPI-anchored CD160 (Giustiniani et al. 2009) (Fig. 4.3). An alternative isoform of murine CD160 with a short cytoplasmic domain lacks a tyrosine residue. CD160 interacts with HVEM and weakly binds to classical and non-classical MHCs. In NK cells, CD160-mediated signaling appears to have a co-stimulatory function. The soluble form of CD160 blocks the CD160–MHC class I interaction and inhibits specific cytotoxicities of NK cells (Giustiniani et al. 2007). Furthermore, CD160 promotes survival and production of effector cytokines (IFN-γ, TNF-α, and IL-6) by activating Syk, PI3K, and ERK pathways in NK cells and chronic lymphocytic leukemia (CLL) (Liu et al. 2010; Rabot et al. 2007; Sedy et al. 2013; Tu et al. 2015). The function of CD160-mediated signaling in T cells remains unclear. Cai et al. demonstrated that crosslinking CD160 with anti-CD160 mAb inhibits anti-CD3/anti-CD28-induced activation and proliferation of human CD4$^+$ T cells (Cai et al. 2008). Blockade of CD160 restored the proliferative capacity in exhausted CD8[+] T cells (Vigano et al. 2014). However, Nikolova et al. reported that upon TCR-CD3 activation, CD160 co-precipitates with Lck and phosphorylated ζ chains and anti-CD160 mAb enhances CD3-induced proliferation of a CD28-negative T-cell subset (Nikolova et al. 2002). Blocking CD160 using CD160-Ig prolonged graft survival in CD28-deficient hosts (D'addio et al. 2013). Therefore, the function of CD160 may differ in various cell types and under different conditions. A number of mAbs against CD160 (clone names: BY55, CL1-R2, 5D.10A11, and 5D.8E10) (Maiza et al. 1993; Agrawal et al. 1999; Cai et al. 2008) and anti-murine CD160 mAbs (clone names: 7H1 and CNX46-3) (Tsujimura et al. 2006, Maeda et al. 2005) or CD160-Fc fusion proteins show promise as tools with which to investigate the function of CD160. Therefore, we need to recognize the properties of these reagents, and further analysis concerning intracellular mechanisms downstream of CD160 is expected.

4.8 DNAM-1/TIGIT/CD96

DNAX accessory protein-1 (DNAM-1, known as CD226) is a co-stimulatory and adhesion molecule expressed mainly on NK and CD8[+] T cells (Shibuya et al. 1996). T-cell immunoreceptor with Ig and ITIM domains (TIGIT, known as Vstms3, WUCAM, and VSIG9), a member of the Ig superfamily, is expressed on activated and memory T cells and on Treg, NK, and NKT cells (Yu et al. 2009; Boles et al. 2009). CD96 (known as tactile), another member of the Ig superfamily, is expressed on αβ and γδ T cells, NK cells, and NKT cells (Wang et al. 1992). Activation of T cells increases CD96 expression with a slow kinetics. DNAM-1 is a positive co-stimulatory receptor. On the other hand, TIGIT and CD96 have inhibitory functions.

DNAM-1 and TIGIT bind to the same two ligands, which are CD112 (known as PVRL2) and CD155 (known as Necl-5 or Tage4), which are expressed on APCs, tumor cells, and infected cells (Bottino et al. 2003; Yu et al. 2009). CD96 also binds to CD155 and uniquely binds to CD111 (Meyer et al. 2009; Seth et al. 2007) (Fig. 4.4).

DNAM-1 is important for the NK cell-mediated killing of tumor cells (Lakshmikanth et al. 2009; Verhoeven et al. 2008; Gilfillan et al. 2008; Iguchi-Manaka et al. 2008) and the elimination of virus-infected cells (Magri et al. 2011; Nabekura et al. 2014) and is critical for the development of acute graft-vs.-host disease (Nabekura et al. 2010). Zhang et al. examined the intrinsic biochemical signals downstream of DNAM-1 in detail (Zhang et al. 2015). DNAM-1 contains a conserved YVN motif, which recruits Grb2 in a tyrosine phosphorylation-dependent manner. Tyrosine phosphorylation of Y^{319} within the YVN motif was induced by Src family kinases in NK cells. Fyn dominantly induces phosphorylation of DNAM-1; however, Lyn Src and Lck could also induce it (Shibuya et al. 1999; Zhang et al. 2015). Engagement of DNAM-1 leads to activation of Vav1, PI3K, and PLCγ.

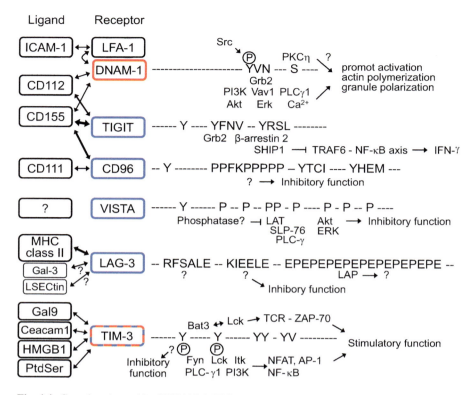

Fig. 4.4 Cytoplasmic motifs of DNAM-1, TIGIT, CD96, VIST, LAG-3, and TIM-3
DNAM-1 contains an YVN Grb2-binding motif. Engagement of DNAM-1 leads to activation of Vav1, PI3K, and PLCγ, thereby promoting Erk, Akt, and Ca^{2+} flux. The interaction of DNAM-1 with Grb2 is important for the activity of these signaling molecules. The DNAM-1–Grb2 association also contributes to actin polymerization and granule polarization

TIGIT contains an Ig tail-tyrosine (ITT)-like motif and an ITIM motif. Both ITT-like and ITIM motifs contribute to the inhibitory function of TIGIT. The ITT-like motif associates with adaptor protein β-arrestin 2, Grb2, and SHIP1, dampening the activity of PI3K and MAPK

CD96 contains a proline-rich motif and an ITIM-like domain, indicating the potential inhibitory function. However, intracellular signaling downstream of CD96 has not been well characterized

VISTA lacks typical ITIMs and ITSMs but possesses several tyrosine residues and proline-rich regions; however, the intracellular binding partners have yet to be identified

LAG-3 contains the KIEELE motif and glutamic acid–proline (EP) repetitive sequence. The KIEELE motif is indispensable to the inhibitory function of LAG-3, but the molecular mechanism remains unclear. LAP binds to the EP repetitive sequence (EP motif), but deletion of the EP motif has no effect on LAG-3 function

TIM-3 has no ITIM or ITSM in its cytoplasmic region, and obvious interactions between TIM-3 and inhibitory phosphatase have not been reported. TIM-3 contains five conserved tyrosine residues; two membrane-proximal tyrosine residues are important for coupling to the downstream signaling molecules. In the absence of TIM-3 ligands, Bat3 binds to unphosphorylated TIM-3 and bridges Lck to the TCR complex. Upon TIM-3 ligation by ligands, tyrosine residues are phosphorylated, recruiting several molecules, such as Fyn, Lck, PI3-kinase p85, PLC-γ1, and Itk. However, Bat3 does not bind to phosphorylated TIM-3. Therefore, Lck-dependent TCR signaling and TIM-3 phosphorylation are diminished in the presence of TIM-3 ligands. It is unclear whether TIM-3 directly transmits co-inhibitory signaling

Consequently, these kinases promote activation of Erk, Akt, and Ca^{2+} flux. The DNAM-1 $Y^{319}F$ mutant abrogated the binding ability to Grb2, causing reduced activity of these signaling molecules. DNAM-1 functions to induce cell–cell conjugation, actin polymerization, and granule polarization. A DNAM-1 mutant lacking the ability to interact with Grb2 diminished actin polymerization and granule polarization; however, cell–cell conjugation was normal (Zhang et al. 2015). In humans and mice, but not all other species, DNAM-1 contains a serine residue at 326, which is phosphorylated by the crosslinking of DNAM-1 or PMA stimulation (Shibuya et al. 1998). Serine phosphorylation of DNAM-1 induces the association of DNAM-1 with LFA-1, which drives DNAM-1 into lipid raft compartments (Shirakawa et al. 2006). The requirement of S^{326} in the DNAM-1-mediated costimulatory function is controversial. Nabekura et al. demonstrated that the DNAM-1 $S^{326}F$ mutant has a lower capacity to induce NK responses and NK cell responses are impaired by PKCη deficiency (Nabekura et al. 2014). However, a later study revealed that S^{326} appears to be dispensable for the DNAM-1-mediated costimulatory function, as the DNAM-1 mutant carrying $S^{326}A$ did not show a defect in DNAM-1 function (Zhang et al. 2015). Further analysis is needed to explore the molecular mechanisms of DNAM-1 in T cells.

As TIGIT has higher affinity for CD155 than DNAM-1, the expression of TIGIT cell-intrinsically interferes with DNAM-1-CD155 interaction (Yu et al. 2009). The cytoplasmic region of TIGIT contains an immunoreceptor tyrosine-based inhibitory motif (ITIM) and an Ig tail-tyrosine (ITT)-like motif (Yu et al. 2009). Although both ITT-like and ITIM motifs contribute to the inhibitory function of TIGIT, it is unclear which of these motifs is critical for TIGIT function. In mouse NK cells, phosphorylation of the tyrosine residues in either the ITT-like motif or the ITIM motif is sufficient for the TIGIT inhibitory function (Stanietsky et al. 2013). Li et al. demonstrated that TIGIT associates with adaptor protein β-arrestin 2 through the phosphorylated ITT-like motif (Y^{225}) and recruits SHIP1 (Li et al. 2014). SHIP1 inhibits activation of the TRAF6-NF-κB axis, leading to suppression of IFN-γ production. Liu et al. also showed that tyrosine phosphorylation within the ITT-like motif induces the interaction with Grb2 and recruits SHIP1, dampening the activity of PI3-kinase and MAPK (Liu et al. 2013). Recent studies demonstrated the role of TIGIT-mediated co-inhibitory signaling in Treg cells. Joller et al. showed that ligation of TIGIT on Treg cells induced IL-10 and fibrinogen-like protein 2 (Fgl2), which promote the suppressive activity of Treg cells (Joller et al. 2014). TIGIT + TIM-3 double-positive Treg cells are abundant in tumor-infiltrating lymphocytes (TIL), and TIM-3 and TIGIT act synergistically to suppress antitumor immune responses (Kurtulus et al. 2015).

Expression of CD96 competes in the interaction between DNAM-1 and CD155, resulting in decreased IFN-γ production in NK cells (Chan et al. 2014). The cytoplasmic region of CD96 contains a short basic/proline-rich motif and an ITIM-like domain, indicating a potential inhibitory function (Meyer et al. 2009). The CD96 cytoplasmic region in humans, but not other species, contains an YxxM motif, which is a potential binding site of the SH2 domain of p85 PI3K. However, intracellular signaling downstream of CD96 has not been well characterized. CD96 is expressed on cancer stem cells in acute myeloid leukemia, T-cell acute lymphoblastic leukemia, and myelodysplastic syndromes. Therefore, CD96 is potential target for cancer immunotherapy. Further analysis is needed to clarify the molecular mechanisms of CD96.

4.9 V-Domain Ig Suppressor of T-Cell Activation (VISTA, Known as PD-1 Homolog (PD-1H), Death Domain 1 α (DD1α), and Gi24)

VISTA is highly expressed on many hematopoietic cell types including $CD4^+$, $CD8^+$ T cells, and Tregs, but its expression of B cells is low (Wang et al. 2011; Flies et al. 2011). VISTA consists of a single IgV domain, a stalk domain, a TM domain, and a 95 amino acid cytoplasmic region. The entire VISTA shares similarities with PD-1, CD28, and CTLA-4, but the IgV domain of VISTA shares homology with PD-L1. Although a specific ligand for VISTA has not been identified, treatment with anti-VISTA neutralizing antibody augments T-cell responses. The phenotype in VISTA-deficient mice indicates that VISTA serves as both a ligand and a receptor, with both having inhibitory functions (Wang et al. 2011; Yoon et al. 2015; Wang et al. 2014; Flies et al. 2014; Ceeraz et al. 2017). Anti-CD3-induced T-cell proliferation is suppressed by immobilized VISTA-Ig, and this stimulation promotes conversion of naive $CD4^+$ T cells to $Foxp3^+$ T cells (Lines et al. 2014). Although the cytoplasmic domain of VISTA does not contain the typical ITIM and ITSM motifs, it possesses two or three tyrosine residues, which are potential SH2 binding sites, and several proline-rich regions, which are potential SH3-containing protein binding sites (Flies et al. 2011) (Fig. 4.4). Liu et al. showed that immobilized VISTA-Ig impairs the anti-CD3-induced phosphorylation of LAT, SLP-76, PLCγ1, Akt, and ERK (Liu et al. 2015). However, the actual binding of intracellular molecules with VISTA has yet to be identified. VISTA is a promising candidate therapeutic target for promoting anti-cancer immune responses. To elucidate the molecular mechanisms of VISTA-mediated co-inhibitory signaling, further studies are needed to identify the binding partners.

4.10 Lymphocyte-Activated Gene-3 (LAG-3, Known as CD223)

LAG-3 is an Ig superfamily member and expressed on activated CD4, CD8, Treg, NK, and B cells and plasmacytoid DCs. The structure of LAG-3 is highly homologous to that of CD4, with more than 20% homology at the amino acid level. The affinity of LAG-3 to MHC class II molecules is higher than that of CD4 (Huard et al. 1997). LAG-3 is heavily glycosylated, and it has been reported that galectin-3 and liver sinusoidal endothelial cell lection (LSECtin) bind to LAG-3 as alternative ligands (Kouo et al. 2015; Xu et al. 2014). Recently, α-synuclein (α-syn) was identified as an additional another ligand for LAG-3 (Mao et al. 2016). Misfolded preformed fibrils (PFF) of α-syn bound to LAG-3 on neurons initiate α-syn PFF endocytosis, transmission, and toxicity. The LAG-3-mediated spreading of α-syn from neuron to neuron is a pathogenic mechanism in Parkinson's disease. The function of α-syn-LAG-3 in T-cell responses has not been examined.

In resting T cells, localized LAG-3 is degraded within lysosomal compartments. After TCR stimulation, LAG-3 is rapidly translocated to the cell surface (Bae et al. 2014). LAG-3 expression is inhibited by TCR-induced metalloproteases, such as ADAM10 and ADAM17 (Li et al. 2007). TCR engagement triggers the association of LAG-3 with the TCR/CD3 complex, and LAG-3 negatively regulates TCR signaling. Although LAG-3-associated protein (LAP) binds to glutamic acid–proline (EP) repetitive sequences in the cytoplasmic tail of LAG-3 (Iouzalen et al. 2001), an EP motif deletion mutant had no effect on LAG-3 function (Workman et al. 2002) (Fig. 4.4). LAG-3 has a potential serine phosphorylation site (S454); however, the $S^{454}A$ mutant retains the LAG-3-mediated co-inhibitory function. Additionally, LAG-3 has a conserved KIEELE motif in the cytoplasmic region, and this motif plays an important role in the LAG-3-mediated inhibitory function. In particular, a lysine residue (Lys^{468} in mice) in this motif is indispensable for the inhibitory function of LAG-3 (Workman and Vignali 2003; Workman et al. 2002). Future identification of LAG-3-associated proteins will be important for elucidating the molecular mechanisms of LAG-3-mediated inhibitory signaling.

4.11 T-Cell Immunoglobulin and Mucin-Containing Protein 3 (TIM-3)

TIM-3 is expressed on Th1, Tc1, Treg, monocyte, and DC. Galectin-9 (Zhu et al. 2005), Ceacam1 (Huang et al. 2015, 2016; Bonsor et al. 2015; Cao et al. 2007; Zhu et al. 2005), HMGB1(Chiba et al. 2012), and PtdSer (Dekruyff et al. 2010; Nakayama et al. 2009) are the ligands of TIM-3. TIM-3 lacks ITIMs or ITSMs in its cytoplasmic region, and no obvious interaction between TIM-3 and inhibitory phosphatase has been reported (Fig. 4.4). Blocking the interaction of TIM-3 with its ligands suggests that TIM-3 has an inhibitory function in T-cell responses (Sabatos et al. 2003; Sanchez-Fueyo et al. 2003). However, TIM-3 promotes not only negative but also stimulatory signals, depending on the situation of the T cells and/or the binding partner of the intracellular signaling molecules (Anderson et al. 2007). The cytoplasmic region of TIM-3 contains five conserved tyrosine residues, with two of five the tyrosine residues being important for TIM-3-mediated co-stimulatory signaling. Engagement of TIM-3 induces phosphorylation of Y^{256} and Y^{263} in mice (Y^{265} and Y^{272} in human) and recruits several molecules, including Fyn, Lck, p85 PI3K, PLC-γ1, and Itk (Anderson et al. 2007). Lee et al. showed that expression of TIM-3 on

Jurkat cells and ligation of TIM-3 by antibodies augments NFAT/AP-1- and NF-κB-dependent transcription, leading to IL-2 production. Conversely, another agonistic antibody to TIM-3 inhibited T-cell activation (Lee et al. 2011). van de Weyer et al. indicated that Y^{256} is phosphorylated by Itk and stimulation of TIM-3 by its ligand, galectin-9, results in phosphorylation of Y^{256} (van de Weyer et al. 2006). The authors proposed that galectin-9-induced TIM-3 Y^{256} phosphorylation might recruit SH2-containing proteins, including negative regulators. It is possible that the conformation or aggregation of TIM-3 alters the function of TIM-3-mediated signaling. Recently, Rangachari et al. reported that expression of HLA-B associated transcript 3 (Bat3), which binds to the C-terminal region of TIM-3, affects the positive and negative functions of TIM-3 (Rangachari et al. 2012). Bat3 is preferentially expressed on Th1 cells compared to Th0 and Th17 cells. Under unstimulated conditions, Bat3 binds to residues 252–270 on TIM-3, which contain two tyrosine residues (Y^{256} and Y^{263} in mice, Y^{265} and Y^{272} in humans). Overexpression of Bat3 in $CD4^+$ T cells enhances IFN-γ and IL-2 production and prevents galectin-9-mediated cell death. In contrast, disruption of Bat3 expression increases the exhaustion-associated molecules (e.g., TIM-3, LAG3, Prdm1, and Pbx3) and markedly decreases the production of IFN-γ and IL-2. Furthermore, this report showed that Bat3 binds and recruits catalytically active Lck to the TIM-3 and engagement of TIM-3 induces dissociation of the TIM-3–Bat3–active Lck complex. Therefore, expression levels of Bat3 might affect the balance of TIM-3-mediated signaling. A high Bat3 expression level blocks the inhibitory signaling of the TIM-3 by the formation of the TIM-3–Bat3–active Lck axis; however, under low Bat3 conditions, TIM-3 transduces inhibitory signals mediated by the recruitment of SH2 domain-containing proteins.

4.12 4-1BB (Known as TNFRSF9 and CD137)

4-1BB is an inducible molecule expressed on activated T cells. 4-1BBL (known as TNFSF9) is the ligand for 4-1BB, which is expressed on activated APCs. 4-1BB has two TRAF-binding motifs (QEED and EEEE) in the cytoplasmic region that recruits TRAF1, TRAF2, and TRAF3 (Saoulli et al. 1998; Jang et al. 1998; Arch and Thompson 1998) (Fig. 4.5). 4-1BB induces ERK activation through the recruitment of TRAF1 and leukocyte-specific protein 1 (LSP1) (Sabbagh et al. 2013). 4-1BB-mediated ERK activation contributes to the upregulation of Bcl-xL and the downregulation of Bim, promoting $CD8^+$ T-cell survival (Sabbagh et al. 2008). 4-1BB-mediated recruitment of TRAF2 is important for the activation of canonical NF-κB and apoptosis signal-regulating kinase 1 (ASK1) in $CD8^+$ T cells, which leads to the upregulation of Bcl-xL and Bfl-1 and the activation of JNK and p38 (Lee et al. 2002; Nam et al. 2005; Cannons et al. 2000; Cannons et al. 1999). TRAF2 trimer and TRAF1:(TRAF2)2 heterotrimer interact with the cellular inhibitor of apoptosis (cIAP) 1 and cIAP2 of the ubiquitin E3 ligase (Zheng et al. 2010a).

Giardino Torchia et al. demonstrated that the E3 ligase activity of cIAP is required for 4-1BB-mediated signaling and maintenance of memory CD8$^+$ T cells (Giardino Torchia et al. 2015). These data indicate that 4-1BB-mediated co-stimulation plays an important role in CD8$^+$ T-cell-dependent immune responses.

4.13 OX40 (Known as TNFRSF4, CD134, and ACT35)

OX40 is induced on T cells after activation and promotes the growth, survival, expansion, and longevity of effector and memory T cells (Rogers et al. 2001; Mousavi et al. 2008; Soroosh et al. 2007; Humphreys et al. 2007; Pakala et al. 2004; Bansal-Pakala et al. 2004; Murata et al. 2000; Gramaglia et al. 2000). OX40L (known as TNFSF4) is expressed on professional APCs. OX40 possesses a PIQEE motif in the cytoplasmic domain, which recruits TRAF1, TRAF2, TRAF3, and TRAF5 (Arch and Thompson 1998; Kawamata et al. 1998) (Fig. 4.5). Upon OX40 stimulation, OX40 translocates to detergent-insoluble membrane lipid microdomains and assembles a signaling complex composed of TRAF2, PKCθ, p85 PI3K, RIP1, cIAP1, cIAP2, and IKKα/β/γ complex, leading to effective canonical NF-κB and Akt activation (Song et al. 2004, 2008; So et al. 2011a, b). Knockdown of TRAF2 results in impaired recruitment of PKCθ, IKK complex, and PI3K. Therefore, TRAF2 is a key factor for OX40-mediated function. TRAF3 inhibits TRAF2-dependent OX40-mediated NF-κB activation (Kawamata et al. 1998; Arch and Thompson 1998). OX40-mediated co-stimulation upregulates NIK and contributes to the activation of noncanonical NF-κB. OX40 does not directly bind TRAF6, but TRAF6 deficiency critically reduces OX40-mediated noncanonical NF-κB activation (Xiao et al. 2012). Therefore, TRAF6 is also important for OX40-mediated co-stimulation.

4.14 CD27 (Known as TNFRSF7)

CD27, which is expressed on mature T cells, is upregulated upon T-cell activation (Hintzen et al. 1994a). The CD27 ligand, CD70 (known as TNFSF7), is transiently expressed on T and B cells and professional APCs (Tesselaar et al. 2003; Lens et al. 1997; Hintzen et al. 1994b). Analysis of CD27-deficient mice demonstrated that CD27 is dispensable for primary T-cell responses but critically important for the memory T-cell formation (Hendriks et al. 2000). CD27 has a PIQED motif in the cytoplasmic region and recruits TRAF2, TRAF3, and TRAF5 (Fig. 4.5). Ligation of CD27 induces activation of NF-κB and JNK through interaction with TRAF2 and TRAF5 (Nakano et al. 1999; Yamamoto et al. 1998; Gravestein et al. 1998; Akiba et al. 1998). TRAF3 downstream of CD27 appears to function as an inhibitor for CD27-mediated co-stimulation (Yamamoto et al. 1998). CD27 is also expressed on B cells. In B cells, co-crosslinking of BCR along with CD27 ligation augments

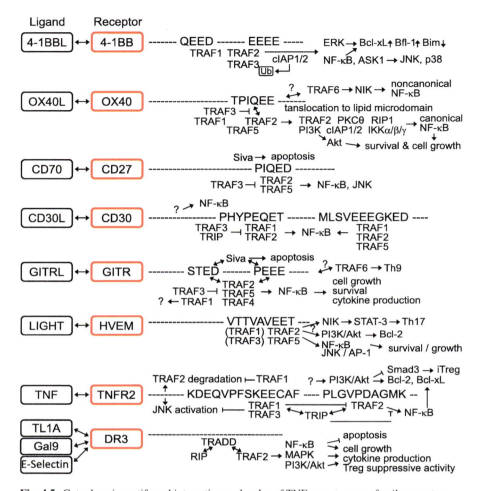

Fig. 4.5 Cytoplasmic motifs and interacting molecules of TNF receptor superfamily receptors
4-1BB contains QEED and EEEE motifs. TRAF1 binds to the QEED motif, and TRAF2 and TRAF3 bind to both motifs. The 4-1BB–TRAF1 interaction induces activation of ERK. The 4-1BB–TRAF2 interaction is important for the activation of canonical NF-κB and ASK1

OX40 contains the TPIQEE motif; TRAF1, TRAF2, TRAF3, and TRAF5 bind to this motif. The OX40–TRAF2 interaction is indispensable to the OX40 co-stimulatory function. TRAF6 contributes to OX40 co-stimulation, although TRAF6 does not bind directly to OX40

CD27 contains the PIQED motif; TRAF2, TRAF3, and TRAF5 bind to this motif. TRAF2 and TRAF5 induce NF-κB and JNK activation, leading to T-cell activation. TRAF3 inhibits this activation. Siva also binds to CD27, inducing apoptosis

CD30 contains the PHYPEQET and MLSVEEEGKED motifs. PHYPEQET recruits TRAF1, TRAF2, TRAF3, and TRIP. The MLSVEEEGKED motif recruits TRAF1, TRAF2, and TRAF5. TRAF1, TRAF2, and TRAF5 activate NF-κB. TRAF3 and TRIP negatively regulate this activation

4 Signal Transduction Via Co-stimulatory and Co-inhibitory Receptors 109

CD27-mediated apoptosis. The interaction of Siva – which has a death domain (DD) homology region, a box-B-like ring finger, and a zinc finger-like domain – with the cytoplasmic tail of CD27 is related to CD27-induced apoptosis (Prasad et al. 1997). Py et al. found that the Siva N- and C-terminal regions, which do not contain DDs, could induce CD27-mediated apoptosis in T cells (Py et al. 2004).

4.15 CD30 (Known as TNFRSF8 and KI-1)

CD30 is expressed on activated and memory T cells (Ellis et al. 1993; del Prete et al. 1995). CD30L (known as CD153) is expressed on APCs (Bowen et al. 1996; Smith et al. 1993; Kim et al. 2003b). CD30 has two TRAF-binding motifs (PHYPEQET and MLSVEEEGKED) in the cytoplasmic region that recruit TRAF1, TRAF2, TRAF3, and TRAF5 (Duckett et al. 1997; Gedrich et al. 1996; Aizawa et al. 1996, 1997; Boucher et al. 1997; Lee et al. 1996) (Fig. 4.5). The PEQER motif binds to TRAF1, TRAF2, and TRAF3, whereas the EEEGKE motif binds to TRAF1, TRAF2, and TRAF5 (Gedrich et al. 1996; Aizawa et al. 1997). The interaction of CD30 with TRAF1, TRAF2, and TRAF5 induces NF-κB activation (Duckett et al. 1997; Aizawa et al. 1997). In contrast, TRAF3 and TRAF-interacting protein (TRIP) downstream of CD30 inhibits TRAF1- and TRAF2-dependent NF-κB activation (Duckett et al. 1997; Lee et al. 1997). The membrane-proximal region also contributes to NF-κB activation, without direct interaction of TRAF2 or TRAF5 (Horie et al. 1998). CD30 also functions to induce apoptosis, and this function is inversely related to the expression level of TRAF2 (Duckett and Thompson 1997).

Abnormal expression of CD30 has been observed on anaplastic large cell lymphoma (ALCL) and Hodgkin lymphoma (HL) cells (Mir et al. 2000). In these cells, CD30 activates both canonical and noncanonical NF-κB activation independent of CD30 ligand and induces IκBζ expression (Wright et al. 2007; Ishikawa et al. 2015). Wright et al. determined that the cytoplasmic region of CD30 interacts with aryl

---

Fig. 4.5 (continued) GITR contains STED and PEEE motifs; TRAF1 and TRAF3 bind to the STED motif. TRAF2, TRAF4, and TRAF5 bind to both motifs and induce NF-κB activation, leading to T-cell activation. TRAF3 inhibits this activation. Siva also binds to STED and PEEE motifs and promotes apoptosis

HVEM contains the VTTVAVEET motif; TRAF2 and TRAF5 bind to this motif and trigger the activation of canonical and noncanonical NF-κB and JNK/AP-1 and PI3K/Akt pathways

TNFR2 contains KDEQVPFSKEECAF and PLGVPDAGMK motifs. TRAF1 and TRAF3 bind to SKEE, and TRAF2 binds to the PLGVPDAGMK region; TRIP binds to both regions. TRAF2 activates the NF-κB pathway, and overexpression of TRAF1 and TRAF3 inhibits TRAF2 activity. TNFR2 stimulation induces degradation of TRAF2, and TRAF1 inhibits this event. TNFR2 has the capacity to induce JNK activation

DR3 lacks TRAF-binding motif. DR3 ligation recruits TRADD, and this DR3–TRADD interaction is important for recruitment of TRAF2 and RIP. TRAF2 downstream of DR3 activates NF-κB, MAPK, and PI3K signaling pathways

hydrocarbon receptor nuclear translocator (ARNT) (Wright and Duckett 2009). CD30-mediated hyperactivation of NF-κB suppresses the cell cycle and induces apoptosis. ARNT and IκBζ negatively modulate NF-κB hyperactivation, thereby allowing these transforming cells to survive (Ishikawa et al. 2015; Wright and Duckett 2009; Wright et al. 2007). Further analysis is required to determine whether these mechanisms apply to a range of CD30 co-stimulation in T cells.

4.16 Glucocorticoid-Induced TNFR (GITR, Known as TNFRSF18, CD357, and AITR)

GITR is expressed at high levels on Tregs but at low levels on naive T cells; GITR expression is upregulated on activated T cells (Shimizu et al. 2002; Mchugh et al. 2002). GITR is also expressed on NK cells, eosinophils, basophils, macrophages, and B cells at low levels (Nocentini et al. 1997; Kwon et al. 1999; Gurney et al. 1999; Zhan et al. 2004). GITR ligand (GITRL) is expressed on APCs, such as DC, macrophages, and resting-state B cells, and it is upregulated after activation (Kwon et al. 1999; Kim et al. 2003a; Gurney et al. 1999; Tone et al. 2003). GITRL is also expressed on activated T cells and endothelial cells (Stephens et al. 2004; Ronchetti et al. 2007). GITR-mediated stimulation promotes proliferation, survival, and cytokine production. GITR-induced signaling is also important for Treg to suppress effector T-cell activity and prevent autoimmune diseases. GITR has two TRAF-binding motifs (STED and PEEE) in the cytoplasmic region that recruit TRAF1, TRAF2, TRAF3, TRAF4, and TRAF5 (Kwon et al. 1999; Esparza and Arch 2005; Esparza and Arch 2004; Snell et al. 2010; Esparza et al. 2006) (Fig. 4.5). GITR activates several signaling pathways such as canonical and noncanonical NF-κB and MAPK. Both TRAF2 and TRAF5 are required for efficient canonical NF-κB activation. TRAF1 seems to be dispensable for the GITR-mediated co-stimulation. TRAF3 appears to negatively regulate NF-κB signaling downstream of GITR. Although the physiological function of TRAF4 in T-cell responses is unclear, overexpression of TRAF4 promotes GITR-dependent NF-κB activation. GITR also binds to Siva, an intracellular molecule possessing a DD (Spinicelli et al. 2002). Siva binds near the TRAF2-binding site of GITR. Therefore, it is possible that the interaction of Siva with GITR regulates GITR-mediated NF-κB activation by mutually inhibiting the GITR–TRAF2 interaction. Recently, Kim et al. demonstrated that an agonistic antibody to GITR (also known as DTA-1) enhances the differentiation of IL-9-producing CD4$^+$ T cells (Th9) in a TRAF6- and NF-κB-dependent manner (Kim et al. 2015). Further study is required to determine the molecular mechanisms of the GITR–TRAF6 pathway in Th9 differentiation.

GITR and GITRL are structurally different in species. For example, murine GITRL (mGITRL) does not interact with human GITR receptor and vice versa. Furthermore, crystallographic studies of the mGITRL crystal structure revealed a dimeric assembly, with a likely stoichiometry of receptor to ligand of 2:2 (Chattopadhyay et al. 2008; Zhou et al. 2008b). On the other hand, hGITRL assembles into an atypical loose homotrimer (Chattopadhyay et al. 2007; Zhou et al. 2008a). Therefore, it is possible that GITRs of differing species may activate different signal transductions.

4.17 HVEM (Known as TNFRSF14 or CD270 or ATAR)

HVEM is widely expressed on many cell types, including naive and activated T cells (Kwon et al. 1997). HVEM serves not only as a receptor but also as a ligand binding to LIGHT (also known as TNFSF14), glycoprotein D (gD) of herpes simplex virus origin, LTα, BTLA, and CD160 (Mauri et al. 1998; Montgomery et al. 1996; Gonzalez et al. 2005; Sedy et al. 2005; Cai et al. 2008). The extracellular region of HVEM has three full cysteine-rich domains (CRD), with the fourth CRD being only two of three disulfide bonds that form a CRD. CD160 and BTLA bind to the CRD1/CRD2 region of HVEM, whereas LIGHT binds to the CRD2/CRD3 region on the opposite side from CD160 and BTLA (Cai and Freeman 2009). A HVEM deletion mutant lacking CRD1 has no co-inhibitory function and functions solely as a co-stimulatory receptor (Cai et al. 2008). Expression of LIGHT is induced on T cells, DC, and B cells upon activation (Ware and Sedy 2011; Steinberg et al. 2011). Engagement of HVEM by LIGHT provides co-stimulatory signals to T cells, promoting activation, differentiation, and survival. HVEM has a TRAF-binding motif (VTTVAVEET) in the cytoplasmic region and recruits TRAF1, TRAF2, TRAF3, and TRAF5 (Hsu et al. 1997; Marsters et al. 1997; Cheung et al. 2009) (Fig. 4.5). Signaling through HVEM activates NF-κB and JNK/AP-1. HVEM-mediated canonical NF-κB activation is dependent on TRAF2, providing a survival signal for T cells (Cheung et al. 2009). It is possible that TRAF5 also contributes to NF-κB activation, as co-expression of HVEM and TRAF5 strongly induces NF-κB activation in 293 cells (Hsu et al. 1997). HVEM also activates the PI3K–Akt axis supporting T-cell survival via sustaining Bcl-2 expression at the later phase of T-cell responses (Soroosh et al. 2011). HVEM also activates the signal transducer and activator of transcription 3 (STAT3) through noncanonical NF-κB activation, possibly facilitating Th17 differentiation (Shui et al. 2012; Jin et al. 2009).

4.18 TNFR2 (Known as TNFRSF1B, CD120b, and p75)

TNFR2, which is expressed on naive T cells, is upregulated after activation. TNFα (known as TNFSF2) and LTα (known as TNFSF1) are the ligands, which are expressed on many cell types, including macrophages and T cells. TNF forms as a TM trimer or a soluble form (Grell et al. 1995; Faustman and Davis 2010). TNFR2-mediated co-stimulation contributes to activation and effector T-cell differentiation (Kim and Teh 2001, 2004; Aspalter et al. 2003; Kim et al. 2006). TNFR2 has two TRAF-binding motifs (KDEQVPFSKEECAF and KPLPLGVPDAGMK) in the cytoplasmic region that recruit TRAF1, TRAF2, and TRAF3 (Rothe et al. 1995; Cabal-Hierro et al. 2014) (Fig. 4.5). TRAF2 preferentially binds to the C-terminal KPLPLGVPDAGMK motif, whereas TRAF1 and TRAF3 recognize the SKEE motif. Co-expression of TNFR2 and TRAF2 augments NF-κB activation, and this TNFR2-dependent NF-κB activation is inhibited by TRAF1 and TRAF3 overexpression (Cabal-Hierro et al. 2014). However, a separate report showed that TRAF1 inhibits TNFR2-induced degradation of TRAF2 and the physiological expression levels of TRAF1 enhance the NF-κB activation induced by TNFR2 (Wicovsky et al. 2009). It is possible that the expression levels of TRAF1 and TRAF2 affect the TNFR2-mediated co-stimulatory function. TRIP associates with TNFR2 through TRAF1 and TRAF2, and TRIP inhibits TNFR2-mediated NF-κB activation (Lee et al. 1997). TNFR2 induces JNK activation. JNK activation downstream of TNFR2 is related to a region different from the TRAF-binding sequences, and this region is responsible for inducing TRAF2 degradation (Cabal-Hierro et al. 2014; Cabal-Hierro and Lazo 2012; Rodriguez et al. 2011). TNFR2 also functions to sustain Akt activity after engagement of the TCR and CD28 (Kim and Teh 2004). TNFR2-mediated co-stimulation upregulates the expression of survivin, Bcl-2, and Bcl-xL (Kim and Teh 2004; Kim et al. 2006). TNFR2-mediated NF-κB and PI3K/Akt activation support TCR/CD28-mediated IL-2 induction, clonal expansion, and survival of T cells. Furthermore, ligation of TNFR2 inhibits TGF-β-induced iTreg differentiation through the induction of Akt–Smad3 interaction, resulting in suppression of Smad3-dependent Foxp3 transcription (Zhang et al. 2013a).

4.19 DR3 (Known as TNFRSF25 and TRAMP)

DR3, expressed at low levels on T cells, is upregulated after activation and highly expressed on Tregs (Schreiber et al. 2010). TNF-like ligand 1A (TL1A; known as TNFSF15) is a ligand for DR3, which is induced by pro-inflammatory stimuli on APCs (Migone et al. 2002). DR3 lacks a TRAF-binding sequence but possesses a DD (Chinnaiyan et al. 1996) (Fig. 4.5). However, DR3 functions to promote T-cell activation and expansion rather than induce apoptosis (Wen et al. 2003). DR3 associates with TRADD and RIP but not with FADD, and a truncated DD mutant of DR3 lacks the ability to bind to TRADD. This DR3–TRADD interaction is important for recruitment of TRAF2 and RIP. Formation of these complexes, especially DR3–TRADD–TRAF2, likely induces DR3-mediated activation of NF-κB, MAPK, and PI3K (Pobezinskaya et al. 2011; Schreiber et al. 2010). Wen et al. demonstrated that engagement of DR3 activates NF-κB and MAPK; activation of NF-κB, but not of MAPK, is responsible for resistance to apoptosis (Wen et al. 2003). Galectin-9 binds to the extracellular domain of DR3. The DR3–galectin-9 interaction is important for DR3 ligation-induced IL-2 and IFN-γ production from CD4[+] T cells and for the expansion and suppressive activity of Tregs (Madireddi et al. 2017). E-Selectin is an alternate ligand for DR3, and E-Selectin triggers DR3-dependent PI3K–NF-κB and MAPK activation in colon cancer cells (Porquet et al. 2011; Gout et al. 2006).

Further analysis is required to explore whether this mechanism utilizes DR3-mediated signaling in T cells.

4.20 Concluding Remarks

The two-signal model for T-cell activation was proposed more than four decades ago (Bretscher and Cohn 1970). T cells are central players in the regulation of immune response and tolerance. Because co-stimulatory and co-inhibitory signals critically affect the fate of T cells, we must characterize each molecule to add to our understanding of the immune response and to develop effective therapeutics for autoimmune diseases, organ transplantation, and anticancer immune responses. Several agents targeting CD28, CTLA-4, and PD-1 have been approved for the treatment of rheumatoid arthritis, renal transplantation, and cancer immunotherapy. Furthermore, chimeric antigen receptor (CAR) T-cell therapy is highlighted in cancer immunotherapy (Gill and June 2015). CAR is composed of an antibody-derived single chain variable fragment (scFv), TM domain (CD8 or CD28), and TCRζ chain. Second-generation CAR constructs contain one co-stimulatory receptor (e.g., CD28, ICOS, 4-1BB, OX40, and CD27) linked to a TCRζ chain; a third-generation of CAR is engineered with more than one additional co-stimulatory molecule, such as CD28–4-1BB–TCRζ. A recent study revealed that CD28–TCRζ CAR promotes effector CD8$^+$ T cells with enhanced glycolysis; on the other hand, 4-1BB–TCRζ CAR enhances respiratory capacity and mitochondria biogenesis leading to enhanced development of central memory CD8$^+$ T cells (Kawalekar et al. 2016). Therefore, it is important to understand precise molecular mechanisms and integrated functions of the CD28 family members and TNFRSF members when developing new therapeutic agents.

Successful anti-CTLA-4 and anti-PD-1 immune checkpoint therapies and the potential of CAR-T cell therapy show promise in the field of co-stimulation. Numerous studies have investigated the therapeutic potential of antagonistic/agonistic antibodies to co-stimulatory and co-inhibitory molecules used alone or in combination with other therapies. However, the molecular mechanisms of regulating T-cell responses require further elucidation. For example, the intracellular binding partners with VISTA have yet to be identified. Additionally, the in vivo role of the cytoplasmic functional motif, TNFRSF, is relatively unknown compared with those of CD28 family members. Furthermore, recent data suggests that the cytoplasmic motif and signaling pathways downstream of CTLA-4, the best characterized co-inhibitory molecule, might not play the primary role in the suppressive mechanisms in conventional T cells. Recent studies reported the presence of unknown functional motifs (i.e., other than the YMNM and PYAP motifs) in the cytoplasmic region of CD28 and identified a new functional IProx motif in the cytoplasmic region of ICOS. Global proteomic and imaging analyses in combination with conventional mutagenesis and biochemical approaches using T cells from physiological conditions are necessary for the identification of novel mechanisms underlying the function of each molecule. Understanding the detailed molecular mechanisms of co-stimulatory or co-inhibitory receptors will lead to the development of selective inhibitors and therapeutics with potential relevance to autoimmune diseases, direct cancer immunotherapies, effective vaccines, and predictors of drug efficacy or side effects.

References

Agata Y, Kawasaki A, Nishimura H, Ishida Y, Tsubata T, Yagita H, Honjo T (1996) Expression of the PD-1 antigen on the surface of stimulated mouse T and B lymphocytes. Int Immunol 8:765–772

Aggarwal BB (2003) Signalling pathways of the TNF superfamily: a double-edged sword. Nat Rev Immunol 3:745–756

Agrawal S, Marquet J, Freeman GJ, Tawab A, Bouteiller PL, Roth P, Bolton W, Ogg G, Boumsell L, Bensussan A (1999) Cutting edge: MHC class I triggering by a novel cell surface ligand costimulates proliferation of activated human T cells. J Immunol 162:1223–1226

Aizawa S, Satoh H, Horie R, Ito K, Choi SH, Takeuchi H, Watanabe T (1996) Cloning and characterization of a cDNA for rat CD30 homolog and chromosomal assignment of the genomic gene. Gene 182:155–162

Aizawa S, Nakano H, Ishida T, Horie R, Nagai M, Ito K, Yagita H, Okumura K, Inoue J, Watanabe T (1997) Tumor necrosis factor receptor-associated factor (TRAF) 5 and TRAF2 are involved in CD30-mediated NFkappaB activation. J Biol Chem 272:2042–2045

Akiba H, Nakano H, Nishinaka S, Shindo M, Kobata T, Atsuta M, Morimoto C, Ware CF, Malinin NL, Wallach D, Yagita H, Okumura K (1998) CD27, a member of the tumor necrosis factor receptor superfamily, activates NF-kappaB and stress-activated protein kinase/c-Jun N-terminal kinase via TRAF2, TRAF5, and NF-kappaB-inducing kinase. J Biol Chem 273:13353–13358

Akiba H, Takeda K, Kojima Y, Usui Y, Harada N, Yamazaki T, Ma J, Tezuka K, Yagita H, Okumura K (2005) The role of ICOS in the CXCR5+ follicular B helper T cell maintenance in vivo. J Immunol 175:2340–2348

Anderson AC, Anderson DE, Bregoli L, Hastings WD, Kassam N, Lei C, Chandwaskar R, Karman J, Su EW, Hirashima M, Bruce JN, Kane LP, Kuchroo VK, Hafler DA (2007) Promotion of tissue inflammation by the immune receptor Tim-3 expressed on innate immune cells. Science 318:1141–1143

Arch RH, Thompson CB (1998) 4-1BB and Ox40 are members of a tumor necrosis factor (TNF)-nerve growth factor receptor subfamily that bind TNF receptor-associated factors and activate nuclear factor kappaB. Mol Cell Biol 18:558–565

Aspalter RM, Eibl MM, Wolf HM (2003) Regulation of TCR-mediated T cell activation by TNF-RII. J Leukoc Biol 74:572–582

August A, Dupont B (1994) CD28 of T lymphocytes associates with phosphatidylinositol 3-kinase. Int Immunol 6:769–774

August A, Gibson S, Kawakami Y, Kawakami T, Mills GB, Dupont B (1994) CD28 is associated with and induces the immediate tyrosine phosphorylation and activation of the Tec family kinase ITK/EMT in the human Jurkat leukemic T-cell line. Proc Natl Acad Sci U S A 91:9347–9351

Au-Yeung BB, Deindl S, Hsu LY, Palacios EH, Levin SE, Kuriyan J, Weiss A (2009) The structure, regulation, and function of ZAP-70. Immunol Rev 228:41–57

Bae J, Lee SJ, Park CG, Lee YS, Chun T (2014) Trafficking of LAG-3 to the surface on activated T cells via its cytoplasmic domain and protein kinase C signaling. J Immunol 193:3101–3112

Bansal-Pakala P, Halteman BS, Cheng MH, Croft M (2004) Costimulation of CD8 T cell responses by OX40. J Immunol 172:4821–4825

4 Signal Transduction Via Co-stimulatory and Co-inhibitory Receptors

van Berkel ME, Schrijver EH, Hofhuis FM, Sharpe AH, Coyle AJ, Broeren CP, Tesselaar K, Oosterwegel MA (2005) ICOS contributes to T cell expansion in CTLA-4 deficient mice. J Immunol 175:182–188

Blanchet F, Cardona A, Letimier FA, Hershfield MS, Acuto O (2005) CD28 costimulatory signal induces protein arginine methylation in T cells. J Exp Med 202:371–377

Blanchet F, Schurter BT, Acuto O (2006) Protein arginine methylation in lymphocyte signaling. Curr Opin Immunol 18:321–328

Boles KS, Vermi W, Facchetti F, Fuchs A, Wilson TJ, Diacovo TG, Cella M, Colonna M (2009) A novel molecular interaction for the adhesion of follicular CD4 T cells to follicular DC. Eur J Immunol 39:695–703

Bonsor DA, Gunther S, Beadenkopf R, Beckett D, Sundberg EJ (2015) Diverse oligomeric states of CEACAM IgV domains. Proc Natl Acad Sci U S A 112:13561–13566

Boomer JS, Deppong CM, Shah DD, Bricker TL, Green JM (2014) Cutting edge: A double-mutant knockin of the CD28 YMNM and PYAP motifs reveals a critical role for the YMNM motif in regulation of T cell proliferation and Bcl-xL expression. J Immunol 192:3465–3469

Bottino C, Castriconi R, Pende D, Rivera P, Nanni M, Carnemolla B, Cantoni C, Grassi J, Marcenaro S, Reymond N, Vitale M, Moretta L, Lopez M, Moretta A (2003) Identification of PVR (CD155) and Nectin-2 (CD112) as cell surface ligands for the human DNAM-1 (CD226) activating molecule. J Exp Med 198:557–567

Boucher LM, Marengere LE, Lu Y, Thukral S, Mak TW (1997) Binding sites of cytoplasmic effectors TRAF1, 2, and 3 on CD30 and other members of the TNF receptor superfamily. Biochem Biophys Res Commun 233:592–600

Bowen MA, Lee RK, Miragliotta G, Nam SY, Podack ER (1996) Structure and expression of murine CD30 and its role in cytokine production. J Immunol 156:442–449

Bratanic N, Kovac J, Pohar K, Trebusak Podkrajsek K, Ihan A, Battelino T, Avbelj Stefanija M (2017) Multifocal gastric adenocarcinoma in a patient with LRBA deficiency. Orphanet J Rare Dis 12:131

Bretscher P, Cohn M (1970) A theory of self-nonself discrimination. Science 169:1042–1049

Butte MJ, Lee SJ, Jesneck J, Keir ME, Haining WN, Sharpe AH (2012) CD28 costimulation regulates genome-wide effects on alternative splicing. PLoS One 7:e40032

Cabal-Hierro L, Lazo PS (2012) Signal transduction by tumor necrosis factor receptors. Cell Signal 24:1297–1305

Cabal-Hierro L, Rodriguez M, Artime N, Iglesias J, Ugarte L, Prado MA, Lazo PS (2014) TRAF-mediated modulation of NF-κB AND JNK activation by TNFR2. Cell Signal 26:2658–2666

Cai G, Freeman GJ (2009) The CD160, BTLA, LIGHT/HVEM pathway: a bidirectional switch regulating T-cell activation. Immunol Rev 229:244–258

Cai YC, Cefai D, Schneider H, Raab M, Nabavi N, Rudd CE (1995) Selective CD28pYMNM mutations implicate phosphatidylinositol 3-kinase in CD86-CD28-mediated costimulation. Immunity 3:417–426

Cai G, Anumanthan A, Brown JA, Greenfield EA, Zhu B, Freeman GJ (2008) CD160 inhibits activation of human CD4+ T cells through interaction with herpesvirus entry mediator. Nat Immunol 9:176–185

Cannons JL, Hoeflich KP, Woodgett JR, Watts TH (1999) Role of the stress kinase pathway in signaling via the T cell costimulatory receptor 4-1BB. J Immunol 163:2990–2998

Cannons JL, Choi Y, Watts TH (2000) Role of TNF receptor-associated factor 2 and p38 mitogen-activated protein kinase activation during 4-1BB-dependent immune response. J Immunol 165:6193–6204

Cao E, Zang X, Ramagopal UA, Mukhopadhaya A, Fedorov A, Fedorov E, Zencheck WD, Lary JW, Cole JL, Deng H, Xiao H, Dilorenzo TP, Allison JP, Nathenson SG, Almo SC (2007) T cell immunoglobulin mucin-3 crystal structure reveals a galectin-9-independent ligand-binding surface. Immunity 26:311–321

Cederbom L, Hall H, Ivars F (2000) CD4+CD25+ regulatory T cells down-regulate co-stimulatory molecules on antigen-presenting cells. Eur J Immunol 30:1538–1543

Ceeraz S, Sergent PA, Plummer SF, Schned AR, Pechenick D, Burns CM, Noelle RJ (2017) VISTA deficiency accelerates the development of fatal murine lupus nephritis. Arthritis Rheumatol 69:814–825

Chan CJ, Martinet L, Gilfillan S, Souza-Fonseca-Guimaraes F, Chow MT, Town L, Ritchie DS, Colonna M, Andrews DM, Smyth MJ (2014) The receptors CD96 and CD226 oppose each other in the regulation of natural killer cell functions. Nat Immunol 15:431–438

Chang CH, Curtis JD, Maggi LB Jr, Faubert B, Villarino AV, O'sullivan D, Huang SC, van der Windt GJ, Blagih J, Qiu J, Weber JD, Pearce EJ, Jones RG, Pearce EL (2013) Posttranscriptional control of T cell effector function by aerobic glycolysis. Cell 153:1239–1251

Chang CH, Qiu J, O'sullivan D, Buck MD, Noguchi T, Curtis JD, Chen Q, Gindin M, Gubin MM, van der Windt GJ, Tonc E, Schreiber RD, Pearce EJ, Pearce EL (2015) Metabolic competition in the tumor microenvironment is a driver of Cancer progression. Cell 162:1229–1241

Chattopadhyay K, Ramagopal UA, Mukhopadhaya A, Malashkevich VN, Dilorenzo TP, Brenowitz M, Nathenson SG, Almo SC (2007) Assembly and structural properties of glucocorticoid-induced TNF receptor ligand: implications for function. Proc Natl Acad Sci U S A 104:19452–19457

Chattopadhyay K, Ramagopal UA, Brenowitz M, Nathenson SG, Almo SC (2008) Evolution of GITRL immune function: murine GITRL exhibits unique structural and biochemical properties within the TNF superfamily. Proc Natl Acad Sci U S A 105:635–640

Chemnitz JM, Parry RV, Nichols KE, June CH, Riley JL (2004) SHP-1 and SHP-2 associate with immunoreceptor tyrosine-based switch motif of programmed death 1 upon primary human T cell stimulation, but only receptor ligation prevents T cell activation. J Immunol 173:945–954

Chemnitz JM, Lanfranco AR, Braunstein I, Riley JL (2006) B and T lymphocyte attenuator-mediated signal transduction provides a potent inhibitory signal to primary human CD4 T cells that can be initiated by multiple phosphotyrosine motifs. J Immunol 176:6603–6614

Chen CY, Del Gatto-Konczak F, Wu Z, Karin M (1998) Stabilization of interleukin-2 mRNA by the c-Jun NH2-terminal kinase pathway. Science 280:1945–1949

Cheng G, Yu A, Dee MJ, Malek TR (2013) IL-2R signaling is essential for functional maturation of regulatory T cells during thymic development. J Immunol 190:1567–1575

Cheung TC, Steinberg MW, Oborne LM, Macauley MG, Fukuyama S, Sanjo H, D'souza C, Norris PS, Pfeffer K, Murphy KM, Kronenberg M, Spear PG, Ware CF (2009) Unconventional ligand activation of herpesvirus entry mediator signals cell survival. Proc Natl Acad Sci U S A 106:6244–6249

Chiba S, Baghdadi M, Akiba H, Yoshiyama H, Kinoshita I, Dosaka-Akita H, Fujioka Y, Ohba Y, Gorman JV, Colgan JD, Hirashima M, Uede T, Takaoka A, Yagita H, Jinushi M (2012) Tumor-infiltrating DCs suppress nucleic acid-mediated innate immune responses through interactions between the receptor TIM-3 and the alarmin HMGB1. Nat Immunol 13:832–842

Chinnaiyan AM, O'rourke K, Yu GL, Lyons RH, Garg M, Duan DR, Xing L, Gentz R, Ni J, Dixit VM (1996) Signal transduction by DR3, a death domain-containing receptor related to TNFR-1 and CD95. Science 274:990–992

Choi YS, Kageyama R, Eto D, Escobar TC, Johnston RJ, Monticelli L, Lao C, Crotty S (2011) ICOS receptor instructs T follicular helper cell versus effector cell differentiation via induction of the transcriptional repressor Bcl6. Immunity 34:932–946

Chuang E, Fisher TS, Morgan RW, Robbins MD, Duerr JM, Vander Heiden MG, Gardner JP, Hambor JE, Neveu MJ, Thompson CB (2000) The CD28 and CTLA-4 receptors associate with the serine/threonine phosphatase PP2A. Immunity 13:313–322

Chung JY, Park YC, Ye H, Wu H (2002) All TRAFs are not created equal: common and distinct molecular mechanisms of TRAF-mediated signal transduction. J Cell Sci 115:679–688

Cobbold SP, Waldmann H (2013) Regulatory cells and transplantation tolerance. Cold Spring Harb Perspect Med 3

Coudronniere N, Villalba M, Englund N, Altman A (2000) NF-kappa B activation induced by T cell receptor/CD28 costimulation is mediated by protein kinase C-theta. Proc Natl Acad Sci U S A 97:3394–3399

4 Signal Transduction Via Co-stimulatory and Co-inhibitory Receptors

Da Rocha Dias S, Rudd CE (2001) CTLA-4 blockade of antigen-induced cell death. Blood 97:1134–1137

D'addio F, Ueno T, Clarkson M, Zhu B, Vergani A, Freeman GJ, Sayegh MH, Ansari MJ, Fiorina P, Habicht A (2013) CD160Ig fusion protein targets a novel costimulatory pathway and prolongs allograft survival. PLoS One 8:e60391

Dekruyff RH, Bu X, Ballesteros A, Santiago C, Chim YL, Lee HH, Karisola P, Pichavant M, Kaplan GG, Umetsu DT, Freeman GJ, Casasnovas JM (2010) T cell/transmembrane, Ig, and mucin-3 allelic variants differentially recognize phosphatidylserine and mediate phagocytosis of apoptotic cells. J Immunol 184:1918–1930

DEL Rio ML, Bravo Moral AM, Fernandez-Renedo C, Buhler L, Perez-Simon JA, Chaloin O, Alvarez Nogal R, Fernandez-Caso M, Rodriguez-Barbosa JI (2017) Modulation of cytotoxic responses by targeting CD160 prolongs skin graft survival across major histocompatibility class I barrier. Transl Res 181(83–95):e3

Deng L, Wang C, Spencer E, Yang L, Braun A, You J, Slaughter C, Pickart C, Chen ZJ (2000) Activation of the IkappaB kinase complex by TRAF6 requires a dimeric ubiquitin-conjugating enzyme complex and a unique polyubiquitin chain. Cell 103:351–361

Ding Y, Han R, Jiang W, Xiao J, Liu H, Chen X, Li X, Hao J (2016) Programmed death ligand 1 plays a Neuroprotective role in experimental autoimmune neuritis by controlling peripheral nervous system inflammation of rats. J Immunol 197:3831–3840

Dobbins J, Gagnon E, Godec J, Pyrdol J, Vignali DA, Sharpe AH, Wucherpfennig KW (2016) Binding of the cytoplasmic domain of CD28 to the plasma membrane inhibits Lck recruitment and signaling. Sci Signal 9:ra75

Dodson LF, Boomer JS, Deppong CM, Shah DD, Sim J, Bricker TL, Russell JH, Green JM (2009) Targeted knock-in mice expressing mutations of CD28 reveal an essential pathway for costimulation. Mol Cell Biol 29:3710–3721

Dong H, Zhu G, Tamada K, Chen L (1999) B7-H1, a third member of the B7 family, co-stimulates T-cell proliferation and interleukin-10 secretion. Nat Med 5:1365–1369

Duckett CS, Thompson CB (1997) CD30-dependent degradation of TRAF2: implications for negative regulation of TRAF signaling and the control of cell survival. Genes Dev 11:2810–2821

Duckett CS, Gedrich RW, Gilfillan MC, Thompson CB (1997) Induction of nuclear factor kappaB by the CD30 receptor is mediated by TRAF1 and TRAF2. Mol Cell Biol 17:1535–1542

Ellis TM, Simms PE, Slivnick DJ, Jack HM, Fisher RI (1993) CD30 is a signal-transducing molecule that defines a subset of human activated CD45RO+ T cells. J Immunol 151:2380–2389

Esparza EM, Arch RH (2004) TRAF4 functions as an intermediate of GITR-induced NF-kappaB activation. Cell Mol Life Sci 61:3087–3092

Esparza EM, Arch RH (2005) Glucocorticoid-induced TNF receptor, a costimulatory receptor on naive and activated T cells, uses TNF receptor-associated factor 2 in a novel fashion as an inhibitor of NF-kappa B activation. J Immunol 174:7875–7882

Esparza EM, Lindsten T, Stockhausen JM, Arch RH (2006) Tumor necrosis factor receptor (TNFR)-associated factor 5 is a critical intermediate of costimulatory signaling pathways triggered by glucocorticoid-induced TNFR in T cells. J Biol Chem 281:8559–8564

Faustman D, Davis M (2010) TNF receptor 2 pathway: drug target for autoimmune diseases. Nat Rev Drug Discov 9:482–493

Fife BT, Pauken KE, Eagar TN, Obu T, Wu J, Tang Q, Azuma M, Krummel MF, Bluestone JA (2009) Interactions between PD-1 and PD-L1 promote tolerance by blocking the TCR-induced stop signal. Nat Immunol 10:1185–1192

Flies DB, Wang S, Xu H, Chen L (2011) Cutting edge: A monoclonal antibody specific for the programmed death-1 homolog prevents graft-versus-host disease in mouse models. J Immunol 187:1537–1541

Flies DB, Han X, Higuchi T, Zheng L, Sun J, Ye JJ, Chen L (2014) Coinhibitory receptor PD-1H preferentially suppresses CD4(+) T cell-mediated immunity. J Clin Invest 124:1966–1975

Fos C, Salles A, Lang V, Carrette F, Audebert S, Pastor S, Ghiotto M, Olive D, Bismuth G, Nunes JA (2008) ICOS ligation recruits the p50alpha PI3K regulatory subunit to the immunological synapse. J Immunol 181:1969–1977

Francisco LM, Salinas VH, Brown KE, Vanguri VK, Freeman GJ, Kuchroo VK, Sharpe AH (2009) PD-L1 regulates the development, maintenance, and function of induced regulatory T cells. J Exp Med 206:3015–3029

Fraser JD, Irving BA, Crabtree GR, Weiss A (1991) Regulation of interleukin-2 gene enhancer activity by the T cell accessory molecule CD28. Science 251:313–316

Frauwirth KA, Riley JL, Harris MH, Parry RV, Rathmell JC, Plas DR, Elstrom RL, June CH, Thompson CB (2002) The CD28 signaling pathway regulates glucose metabolism. Immunity 16:769–777

Freeman GJ, Long AJ, Iwai Y, Bourque K, Chernova T, Nishimura H, Fitz LJ, Malenkovich N, Okazaki T, Byrne MC, Horton HF, Fouser L, Carter L, Ling V, Bowman MR, Carreno BM, Collins M, Wood CR, Honjo T (2000) Engagement of the PD-1 immunoinhibitory receptor by a novel B7 family member leads to negative regulation of lymphocyte activation. J Exp Med 192:1027–1034

Friend LD, Shah DD, Deppong C, Lin J, Bricker TL, Juehne TI, Rose CM, Green JM (2006) A dose-dependent requirement for the proline motif of CD28 in cellular and humoral immunity revealed by a targeted knockin mutant. J Exp Med 203:2121–2133

Gavrieli M, Murphy KM (2006) Association of Grb-2 and PI3K p85 with phosphotyrosile peptides derived from BTLA. Biochem Biophys Res Commun 345:1440–1445

Gedrich RW, Gilfillan MC, Duckett CS, van Dongen JL, Thompson CB (1996) CD30 contains two binding sites with different specificities for members of the tumor necrosis factor receptor-associated factor family of signal transducing proteins. J Biol Chem 271:12852–12858

Giardino Torchia ML, Munitic I, Castro E, Herz J, Mcgavern DB, Ashwell JD (2015) -IAP ubiquitin protein ligase activity is required for 4-1BB signaling and CD8(+) memory T-cell survival. Eur J Immunol 45:2672–2682

Gigoux M, Shang J, Pak Y, Xu M, Choe J, Mak TW, Suh WK (2009) Inducible costimulator promotes helper T-cell differentiation through phosphoinositide 3-kinase. Proc Natl Acad Sci U S A 106:20371–20376

Gilfillan S, Chan CJ, Cella M, Haynes NM, Rapaport AS, Boles KS, Andrews DM, Smyth MJ, Colonna M (2008) DNAM-1 promotes activation of cytotoxic lymphocytes by nonprofessional antigen-presenting cells and tumors. J Exp Med 205:2965–2973

Gill S, June CH (2015) Going viral: chimeric antigen receptor T-cell therapy for hematological malignancies. Immunol Rev 263:68–89

Giustiniani J, Marie-Cardine A, Bensussan A (2007) A soluble form of the MHC class I-specific CD160 receptor is released from human activated NK lymphocytes and inhibits cell-mediated cytotoxicity. J Immunol 178:1293–1300

Giustiniani J, Bensussan A, Marie-Cardine A (2009) Identification and characterization of a transmembrane isoform of CD160 (CD160-TM), a unique activating receptor selectively expressed upon human NK cell activation. J Immunol 182:63–71

Gogishvili T, Luhder F, Goebbels S, Beer-Hammer S, Pfeffer K, Hunig T (2013) Cell-intrinsic and -extrinsic control of Treg-cell homeostasis and function revealed by induced CD28 deletion. Eur J Immunol 43:188–193

Gonzalez LC, Loyet KM, Calemine-Fenaux J, Chauhan V, Wranik B, Ouyang W, Eaton DL (2005) A coreceptor interaction between the CD28 and TNF receptor family members B and T lymphocyte attenuator and herpesvirus entry mediator. Proc Natl Acad Sci U S A 102:1116–1121

Gout S, Morin C, Houle F, Huot J (2006) Death receptor-3, a new E-Selectin counter-receptor that confers migration and survival advantages to colon carcinoma cells by triggering p38 and ERK MAPK activation. Cancer Res 66:9117–9124

Gramaglia I, Jember A, Pippig SD, Weinberg AD, Killeen N, Croft M (2000) The OX40 costimulatory receptor determines the development of CD4 memory by regulating primary clonal expansion. J Immunol 165:3043–3050

4 Signal Transduction Via Co-stimulatory and Co-inhibitory Receptors

Granger SW, Butrovich KD, Houshmand P, Edwards WR, Ware CF (2001) Genomic characterization of LIGHT reveals linkage to an immune response locus on chromosome 19p13.3 and distinct isoforms generated by alternate splicing or proteolysis. J Immunol 167:5122–5128

Gravestein LA, Amsen D, Boes M, Calvo CR, Kruisbeek AM, Borst J (1998) The TNF receptor family member CD27 signals to Jun N-terminal kinase via Traf-2. Eur J Immunol 28:2208–2216

Grell M, Douni E, Wajant H, Lohden M, Clauss M, Maxeiner B, Georgopoulos S, Lesslauer W, Kollias G, Pfizenmaier K, Scheurich P (1995) The transmembrane form of tumor necrosis factor is the prime activating ligand of the 80 kDa tumor necrosis factor receptor. Cell 83:793–802

Grohmann U, Orabona C, Fallarino F, Vacca C, Calcinaro F, Falorni A, Candeloro P, Belladonna ML, Bianchi R, Fioretti MC, Puccetti P (2002) CTLA-4-Ig regulates tryptophan catabolism in vivo. Nat Immunol 3:1097–1101

Guo F, Iclozan C, Suh WK, Anasetti C, Yu XZ (2008) CD28 controls differentiation of regulatory T cells from naive CD4 T cells. J Immunol 181:2285–2291

Gurney AL, Marsters SA, Huang RM, Pitti RM, Mark DT, Baldwin DT, Gray AM, Dowd AD, Brush AD, Heldens AD, Schow AD, Goddard AD, Wood WI, Baker KP, Godowski PJ, Ashkenazi A (1999) Identification of a new member of the tumor necrosis factor family and its receptor, a human ortholog of mouse GITR. Curr Biol 9:215–218

Harada Y, Tanabe E, Watanabe R, Weiss BD, Matsumoto A, Ariga H, Koiwai O, Fukui Y, Kubo M, June CH, Abe R (2001a) Novel role of phosphatidylinositol 3-kinase in CD28-mediated costimulation. J Biol Chem 276:9003–9008

Harada Y, Tokushima M, Matsumoto Y, Ogawa S, Otsuka M, Hayashi K, Weiss BD, June CH, Abe R (2001b) Critical requirement for the membrane-proximal cytosolic tyrosine residue for CD28-mediated costimulation in vivo. J Immunol 166:3797–3803

Hayashi K, Altman A (2006) Filamin A is required for T cell activation mediated by protein kinase C-theta. J Immunol 177:1721–1728

Hendriks J, Gravestein LA, Tesselaar K, van Lier RA, Schumacher TN, Borst J (2000) CD27 is required for generation and long-term maintenance of T cell immunity. Nat Immunol 1:433–440

Higo K, Ikura T, Oda M, Morii H, Takahashi J, Abe R, Ito N (2013) High resolution crystal structure of the Grb2 SH2 domain with a phosphopeptide derived from CD28. PLoS One 8:e74482

Higo K, Oda M, Morii H, Takahashi J, Harada Y, Ogawa S, Abe R (2014) Quantitative analysis by surface plasmon resonance of CD28 interaction with cytoplasmic adaptor molecules Grb2, gads and p85 PI3K. Immunol Investig 43:278–291

Hintzen RQ, de Jong R, Lens SM, van Lier RA (1994a) CD27: marker and mediator of T-cell activation? Immunol Today 15:307–311

Hintzen RQ, Lens SM, Koopman G, Pals ST, Spits H, van Lier RA (1994b) CD70 represents the human ligand for CD27. Int Immunol 6:477–480

Hofinger E, Sticht H (2005) Multiple modes of interaction between Lck and CD28. J Immunol 174:3839–3840

Holdorf AD, Green JM, Levin SD, Denny MF, Straus DB, Link V, Changelian PS, Allen PM, Shaw AS (1999) Proline residues in CD28 and the Src homology (SH)3 domain of Lck are required for T cell costimulation. J Exp Med 190:375–384

Holdorf AD, Lee KH, Burack WR, Allen PM, Shaw AS (2002) Regulation of Lck activity by CD4 and CD28 in the immunological synapse. Nat Immunol 3:259–264

Hombach AA, Kofler D, Hombach A, Rappl G, Abken H (2007) Effective proliferation of human regulatory T cells requires a strong costimulatory CD28 signal that cannot be substituted by IL-2. J Immunol 179:7924–7931

Horie R, Aizawa S, Nagai M, Ito K, Higashihara M, Ishida T, Inoue J, Watanabe T (1998) A novel domain in the CD30 cytoplasmic tail mediates NFkappaB activation. Int Immunol 10:203–210

Hou TZ, Verma N, Wanders J, Kennedy A, Soskic B, Janman D, Halliday N, Rowshanravan B, Worth A, Qasim W, Baxendale H, Stauss H, Seneviratne S, Neth O, Olbrich P, Hambleton S, Arkwright PD, Burns SO, Walker LS, Sansom DM (2017) Identifying functional defects in patients with immune dysregulation due to LRBA and CTLA-4 mutations. Blood 129:1458–1468

Hsu H, Solovyev I, Colombero A, Elliott R, Kelley M, Boyle WJ (1997) ATAR, a novel tumor necrosis factor receptor family member, signals through TRAF2 and TRAF5. J Biol Chem 272:13471–13474

Hu H, Rudd CE, Schneider H (2001) Src kinases Fyn and Lck facilitate the accumulation of phosphorylated CTLA-4 and its association with PI-3 kinase in intracellular compartments of T-cells. Biochem Biophys Res Commun 288:573–578

Huang YH, Zhu C, Kondo Y, Anderson AC, Gandhi A, Russell A, Dougan SK, Petersen BS, Melum E, Pertel T, Clayton KL, Raab M, Chen Q, Beauchemin N, Yazaki PJ, Pyzik M, Ostrowski MA, Glickman JN, Rudd CE, Ploegh HL, Franke A, Petsko GA, Kuchroo VK, Blumberg RS (2015) CEACAM1 regulates TIM-3-mediated tolerance and exhaustion. Nature 517:386–390

Huang YH, Zhu C, Kondo Y, Anderson AC, Gandhi A, Russell A, Dougan SK, Petersen BS, Melum E, Pertel T, Clayton KL, Raab M, Chen Q, Beauchemin N, Yazaki PJ, Pyzik M, Ostrowski MA, Glickman JN, Rudd CE, Ploegh HL, Franke A, Petsko GA, Kuchroo VK, Blumberg RS (2016) Corrigendum: CEACAM1 regulates TIM-3-mediated tolerance and exhaustion. Nature 536:359

Huard B, Mastrangeli R, Prigent P, Bruniquel D, Donini S, El-Tayar N, Maigret B, Dreano M, Triebel F (1997) Characterization of the major histocompatibility complex class II binding site on LAG-3 protein. Proc Natl Acad Sci U S A 94:5744–5749

Hui E, Cheung J, Zhu J, Su X, Taylor MJ, Wallweber HA, Sasmal DK, Huang J, Kim JM, Mellman I, Vale RD (2017) T cell costimulatory receptor CD28 is a primary target for PD-1-mediated inhibition. Science 355:1428–1433

Humphreys IR, Loewendorf A, de Trez C, Schneider K, Benedict CA, Munks MW, Ware CF, Croft M (2007) OX40 costimulation promotes persistence of cytomegalovirus-specific CD8 T cells: A CD4-dependent mechanism. J Immunol 179:2195–2202

Hurchla MA, Sedy JR, Gavrieli M, Drake CG, Murphy TL, Murphy KM (2005) B and T lymphocyte attenuator exhibits structural and expression polymorphisms and is highly induced in anergic CD4+ T cells. J Immunol 174:3377–3385

Hutchcroft JE, Bierer BE (1994) Activation-dependent phosphorylation of the T-lymphocyte surface receptor CD28 and associated proteins. Proc Natl Acad Sci U S A 91:3260–3264

Iguchi-Manaka A, Kai H, Yamashita Y, Shibata K, Tahara-Hanaoka S, Honda S, Yasui T, Kikutani H, Shibuya K, Shibuya A (2008) Accelerated tumor growth in mice deficient in DNAM-1 receptor. J Exp Med 205:2959–2964

Inaba S, Numoto N, Ogawa S, Morii H, Ikura T, Abe R, Ito N, Oda M (2017) Crystal structures and thermodynamic analysis reveal distinct mechanisms of CD28 Phosphopeptide binding to the Src homology 2 (SH2) domains of three adaptor proteins. J Biol Chem 292:1052–1060

Iouzalen N, Andreae S, Hannier S, Triebel F (2001) LAP, a lymphocyte activation gene-3 (LAG-3)-associated protein that binds to a repeated EP motif in the intracellular region of LAG-3, may participate in the down-regulation of the CD3/TCR activation pathway. Eur J Immunol 31:2885–2891

Ishida Y, Agata Y, Shibahara K, Honjo T (1992) Induced expression of PD-1, a novel member of the immunoglobulin gene superfamily, upon programmed cell death. EMBO J 11:3887–3895

Ishikawa C, Senba M, Mori N (2015) Induction of IkappaB-zeta by Epstein-Barr virus latent membrane protein-1 and CD30. Int J Oncol 47:2197–2207

Isomura I, Palmer S, Grumont RJ, Bunting K, Hoyne G, Wilkinson N, Banerjee A, Proietto A, Gugasyan R, Wu L, Mcnally A, Steptoe RJ, Thomas R, Shannon MF, Gerondakis S (2009) -Rel is required for the development of thymic Foxp3+ CD4 regulatory T cells. J Exp Med 206:3001–3014

Jain N, Miu B, Jiang JK, Mckinstry KK, Prince A, Swain SL, Greiner DL, Thomas CJ, Sanderson MJ, Berg LJ, Kang J (2013) CD28 and ITK signals regulate autoreactive T cell trafficking. Nat Med 19:1632–1637

Jang IK, Lee ZH, Kim YJ, Kim SH, Kwon BS (1998) Human 4-1BB (CD137) signals are mediated by TRAF2 and activate nuclear factor-kappa B. Biochem Biophys Res Commun 242:613–620

Jin W, Zhou XF, Yu J, Cheng X, Sun SC (2009) Regulation of Th17 cell differentiation and EAE induction by MAP3K NIK. Blood 113:6603–6610

Joller N, Lozano E, Burkett PR, Patel B, Xiao S, Zhu C, Xia J, Tan TG, Sefik E, Yajnik V, Sharpe AH, Quintana FJ, Mathis D, Benoist C, Hafler DA, Kuchroo VK (2014) Treg cells expressing the coinhibitory molecule TIGIT selectively inhibit proinflammatory Th1 and Th17 cell responses. Immunity 40:569–581

June CH, Ledbetter JA, Gillespie MM, Lindsten T, Thompson CB (1987) T-cell proliferation involving the CD28 pathway is associated with cyclosporine-resistant interleukin 2 gene expression. Mol Cell Biol 7:4472–4481

Kallikourdis M, Trovato AE, Roselli G, Muscolini M, Porciello N, Tuosto L, Viola A (2016) Phosphatidylinositol 4-phosphate 5-kinase beta controls recruitment of lipid rafts into the immunological synapse. J Immunol 196:1955–1963

Kamphorst AO, Wieland A, Nasti T, Yang S, Zhang R, Barber DL, Konieczny BT, Daugherty CZ, Koenig L, Yu K, Sica GL, Sharpe AH, Freeman GJ, Blazar BR, Turka LA, Owonikoko TK, Pillai RN, Ramalingam SS, Araki K, Ahmed R (2017) Rescue of exhausted CD8 T cells by PD-1-targeted therapies is CD28-dependent. Science 355:1423–1427

Kawalekar OU, O'connor RS, Fraietta JA, Guo L, Mcgettigan SE, Posey AD Jr, Patel PR, Guedan S, Scholler J, Keith B, Snyder NW, Blair IA, Milone MC, June CH (2016) Distinct signaling of Coreceptors regulates specific metabolism pathways and impacts memory development in CAR T cells. Immunity 44:380–390

Kawamata S, Hori T, Imura A, Takaori-Kondo A, Uchiyama T (1998) Activation of OX40 signal transduction pathways leads to tumor necrosis factor receptor-associated factor (TRAF) 2- and TRAF5-mediated NF-kappaB activation. J Biol Chem 273:5808–5814

Keir ME, Liang SC, Guleria I, Latchman YE, Qipo A, Albacker LA, Koulmanda M, Freeman GJ, Sayegh MH, Sharpe AH (2006) Tissue expression of PD-L1 mediates peripheral T cell tolerance. J Exp Med 203:883–895

Kim EY, Teh HS (2001) TNF type 2 receptor (p75) lowers the threshold of T cell activation. J Immunol 167:6812–6820

Kim EY, Teh HS (2004) Critical role of TNF receptor type-2 (p75) as a costimulator for IL-2 induction and T cell survival: a functional link to CD28. J Immunol 173:4500–4509

Kim HH, Tharayil M, Rudd CE (1998) Growth factor receptor-bound protein 2 SH2/SH3 domain binding to CD28 and its role in co-signaling. J Biol Chem 273:296–301

Kim JD, Choi BK, Bae JS, Lee UH, Han IS, Lee HW, Youn BS, Vinay DS, Kwon BS (2003a) Cloning and characterization of GITR ligand. Genes Immun 4:564–569

Kim MY, Gaspal FM, Wiggett HE, Mcconnell FM, Gulbranson-Judge A, Raykundalia C, Walker LS, Goodall MD, Lane PJ (2003b) CD4(+)CD3(−) accessory cells costimulate primed CD4 T cells through OX40 and CD30 at sites where T cells collaborate with B cells. Immunity 18:643–654

Kim EY, Priatel JJ, Teh SJ, Teh HS (2006) TNF receptor type 2 (p75) functions as a costimulator for antigen-driven T cell responses in vivo. J Immunol 176:1026–1035

Kim IK, Kim BS, Koh CH, Seok JW, Park JS, Shin KS, Bae EA, Lee GE, Jeon H, Cho J, Jung Y, Han D, Kwon BS, Lee HY, Chung Y, Kang CY (2015) Glucocorticoid-induced tumor necrosis factor receptor-related protein co-stimulation facilitates tumor regression by inducing IL-9-producing helper T cells. Nat Med 21:1010–1017

King PD, Sadra A, Teng JM, Xiao-Rong L, Han A, Selvakumar A, August A, Dupont B (1997) Analysis of CD28 cytoplasmic tail tyrosine residues as regulators and substrates for the protein tyrosine kinases, EMT and LCK. J Immunol 158:580–590

Klein Geltink RI, O'sullivan D, Corrado M, Bremser A, Buck MD, Buescher JM, Firat E, Zhu X, Niedermann G, Caputa G, Kelly B, Warthorst U, Rensing-Ehl A, Kyle RL, Vandersarren L, Curtis JD, Patterson AE, Lawless S, Grzes K, Qiu J, Sanin DE, Kretz O, Huber TB, Janssens S, Lambrecht BN, Rambold AS, Pearce EJ, Pearce EL (2017) Mitochondrial priming by CD28. Cell

Kong KF, Yokosuka T, Canonigo-Balancio AJ, Isakov N, Saito T, Altman A (2011) A motif in the V3 domain of the kinase PKC-theta determines its localization in the immunological synapse and functions in T cells via association with CD28. Nat Immunol 12:1105–1112

Kong KF, Fu G, Zhang Y, Yokosuka T, Casas J, Canonigo-Balancio AJ, Becart S, Kim G, Yates JR 3rd, Kronenberg M, Saito T, Gascoigne NR, Altman A (2014) Protein kinase C-eta controls CTLA-4-mediated regulatory T cell function. Nat Immunol 15:465–472

Kouo T, Huang L, Pucsek AB, Cao M, Solt S, Armstrong T, Jaffee E (2015) Galectin-3 shapes antitumor immune responses by suppressing CD8+ T cells via LAG-3 and inhibiting expansion of Plasmacytoid dendritic cells. Cancer Immunol Res 3:412–423

Kurtulus S, Sakuishi K, Ngiow SF, Joller N, Tan DJ, Teng MW, Smyth MJ, Kuchroo VK, Anderson AC (2015) TIGIT predominantly regulates the immune response via regulatory T cells. J Clin Invest 125:4053–4062

Kwon BS, Tan KB, Ni J, Oh KO, Lee ZH, Kim KK, Kim YJ, Wang S, Gentz R, Yu GL, Harrop J, Lyn SD, Silverman C, Porter TG, Truneh A, Young PR (1997) A newly identified member of the tumor necrosis factor receptor superfamily with a wide tissue distribution and involvement in lymphocyte activation. J Biol Chem 272:14272–14276

Kwon B, Yu KY, Ni J, Yu GL, Jang IK, Kim YJ, Xing L, Liu D, Wang SX, Kwon BS (1999) Identification of a novel activation-inducible protein of the tumor necrosis factor receptor superfamily and its ligand. J Biol Chem 274:6056–6061

Lakshmikanth T, Burke S, Ali TH, Kimpfler S, Ursini F, Ruggeri L, Capanni M, Umansky V, Paschen A, Sucker A, Pende D, Groh V, Biassoni R, Hoglund P, Kato M, Shibuya K, Schadendorf D, Anichini A, Ferrone S, Velardi A, Karre K, Shibuya A, Carbone E, Colucci F (2009) NCRs and DNAM-1 mediate NK cell recognition and lysis of human and mouse melanoma cell lines in vitro and in vivo. J Clin Invest 119:1251–1263

Latchman Y, Wood CR, Chernova T, Chaudhary D, Borde M, Chernova I, Iwai Y, Long AJ, Brown JA, Nunes R, Greenfield EA, Bourque K, Boussiotis VA, Carter LL, Carreno BM, Malenkovich N, Nishimura H, Okazaki T, Honjo T, Sharpe AH, Freeman GJ (2001) PD-L2 is a second ligand for PD-1 and inhibits T cell activation. Nat Immunol 2:261–268

Leavenworth JW, Verbinnen B, Yin J, Huang H, Cantor H (2015) A p85alpha-osteopontin axis couples the receptor ICOS to sustained Bcl-6 expression by follicular helper and regulatory T cells. Nat Immunol 16:96–106

Lee SY, Lee SY, Kandala G, Liou ML, Liou HC, Choi Y (1996) CD30/TNF receptor-associated factor interaction: NF-kappa B activation and binding specificity. Proc Natl Acad Sci U S A 93:9699–9703

Lee SY, Lee SY, Choi Y (1997) TRAF-interacting protein (TRIP): a novel component of the tumor necrosis factor receptor (TNFR)- and CD30-TRAF signaling complexes that inhibits TRAF2-mediated NF-kappaB activation. J Exp Med 185:1275–1285

Lee KM, Chuang E, Griffin M, Khattri R, Hong DK, Zhang W, Straus D, Samelson LE, Thompson CB, Bluestone JA (1998) Molecular basis of T cell inactivation by CTLA-4. Science 282:2263–2266

Lee HW, Park SJ, Choi BK, Kim HH, Nam KO, Kwon BS (2002) 4-1BB promotes the survival of CD8+ T lymphocytes by increasing expression of Bcl-xL and Bfl-1. J Immunol 169:4882–4888

Lee J, Su EW, Zhu C, Hainline S, Phuah J, Moroco JA, Smithgall TE, Kuchroo VK, Kane LP (2011) Phosphotyrosine-dependent coupling of Tim-3 to T-cell receptor signaling pathways. Mol Cell Biol 31:3963–3974

Lens SM, Baars PA, Hooibrink B, van Oers MH, van Lier RA (1997) Antigen-presenting cell-derived signals determine expression levels of CD70 on primed T cells. Immunology 90:38–45

Li CR, Berg LJ (2005) Itk is not essential for CD28 signaling in naive T cells. J Immunol 174:4475–4479

Li N, Wang Y, Forbes K, Vignali KM, Heale BS, Saftig P, Hartmann D, Black RA, Rossi JJ, Blobel CP, Dempsey PJ, Workman CJ, Vignali DA (2007) Metalloproteases regulate T-cell proliferation and effector function via LAG-3. EMBO J 26:494–504

4 Signal Transduction Via Co-stimulatory and Co-inhibitory Receptors

Li M, Xia P, Du Y, Liu S, Huang G, Chen J, Zhang H, Hou N, Cheng X, Zhou L, Li P, Yang X, Fan Z (2014) T-cell immunoglobulin and ITIM domain (TIGIT) receptor/poliovirus receptor (PVR) ligand engagement suppresses interferon-gamma production of natural killer cells via beta-arrestin 2-mediated negative signaling. J Biol Chem 289:17647–17657

Liang Y, Cucchetti M, Roncagalli R, Yokosuka T, Malzac A, Bertosio E, Imbert J, Nijman IJ, Suchanek M, Saito T, Wulfing C, Malissen B, Malissen M (2013) The lymphoid lineage-specific actin-uncapping protein Rltpr is essential for costimulation via CD28 and the development of regulatory T cells. Nat Immunol 14:858–866

Lin X, O'mahony A, Mu Y, Geleziunas R, Greene WC (2000) Protein kinase C-theta participates in NF-kappaB activation induced by CD3-CD28 costimulation through selective activation of IkappaB kinase beta. Mol Cell Biol 20:2933–2940

Lindstein T, June CH, Ledbetter JA, Stella G, Thompson CB (1989) Regulation of lymphokine messenger RNA stability by a surface-mediated T cell activation pathway. Science 244:339–343

Lines JL, Pantazi E, Mak J, Sempere LF, Wang L, O'connell S, Ceeraz S, Suriawinata AA, Yan S, Ernstoff MS, Noelle R (2014) VISTA is an immune checkpoint molecule for human T cells. Cancer Res 74:1924–1932

Lio CW, Dodson LF, Deppong CM, Hsieh CS, Green JM (2010) CD28 facilitates the generation of Foxp3(−) cytokine responsive regulatory T cell precursors. J Immunol 184:6007–6013

Liu FT, Giustiniani J, Farren T, Jia L, Bensussan A, Gribben JG, Agrawal SG (2010) CD160 signaling mediates PI3K-dependent survival and growth signals in chronic lymphocytic leukemia. Blood 115:3079–3088

Liu S, Zhang H, Li M, Hu D, Li C, Ge B, Jin B, Fan Z (2013) Recruitment of Grb2 and SHIP1 by the ITT-like motif of TIGIT suppresses granule polarization and cytotoxicity of NK cells. Cell Death Differ 20:456–464

Liu J, Yuan Y, Chen W, Putra J, Suriawinata AA, Schenk AD, Miller HE, Guleria I, Barth RJ, Huang YH, Wang L (2015) Immune-checkpoint proteins VISTA and PD-1 nonredundantly regulate murine T-cell responses. Proc Natl Acad Sci U S A 112:6682–6687

Lo B, Zhang K, Lu W, Zheng L, Zhang Q, Kanellopoulou C, Zhang Y, Liu Z, Fritz JM, Marsh R, Husami A, Kissell D, Nortman S, Chaturvedi V, Haines H, Young LR, Mo J, Filipovich AH, Bleesing JJ, Mustillo P, Stephens M, Rueda CM, Chougnet CA, Hoebe K, Mcelwee J, Hughes JD, Karakoc-Aydiner E, Matthews HF, Price S, Su HC, Rao VK, Lenardo MJ, Jordan MB (2015) AUTOIMMUNE DISEASE. Patients with LRBA deficiency show CTLA4 loss and immune dysregulation responsive to abatacept therapy. Science 349:436–440

Long M, Park SG, Strickland I, Hayden MS, Ghosh S (2009) Nuclear factor-kappaB modulates regulatory T cell development by directly regulating expression of Foxp3 transcription factor. Immunity 31:921–931

Long SA, Cerosaletti K, Bollyky PL, Tatum M, Shilling H, Zhang S, Zhang ZY, Pihoker C, Sanda S, Greenbaum C, Buckner JH (2010) Defects in IL-2R signaling contribute to diminished maintenance of FOXP3 expression in CD4(+)CD25(+) regulatory T-cells of type 1 diabetic subjects. Diabetes 59:407–415

Lopez-Herrera G, Tampella G, Pan-Hammarstrom Q, Herholz P, Trujillo-Vargas CM, Phadwal K, Simon AK, Moutschen M, Etzioni A, Mory A, Srugo I, Melamed D, Hultenby K, Liu C, Baronio M, Vitali M, Philippet P, Dideberg V, Aghamohammadi A, Rezaei N, Enright V, Du L, Salzer U, Eibel H, Pfeifer D, Veelken H, Stauss H, Lougaris V, Plebani A, Gertz EM, Schaffer AA, Hammarstrom L, Grimbacher B (2012) Deleterious mutations in LRBA are associated with a syndrome of immune deficiency and autoimmunity. Am J Hum Genet 90:986–1001

Loyet KM, Ouyang W, Eaton DL, Stults JT (2005) Proteomic profiling of surface proteins on Th1 and Th2 cells. J Proteome Res 4:400–409

Madireddi S, Eun SY, Mehta AK, Birta A, Zajonc DM, Niki T, Hirashima M, Podack ER, Schreiber TH, Croft M (2017) Regulatory T cell-mediated suppression of inflammation induced by DR3 signaling is dependent on Galectin-9. J Immunol 199:2721–2728

Maeda M, Carpenito C, Russell RC, Dasanjh J, Veinotte LL, Ohta H, Yamamura T, Tan R, Takei F (2005) Murine CD160, Ig-like receptor on NK cells and NKT cells, recognizes classical and nonclassical MHC class I and regulates NK cell activation. J Immunol 175:4426–4432

Magri G, Muntasell A, Romo N, Saez-Borderias A, Pende D, Geraghty DE, Hengel H, Angulo A, Moretta A, Lopez-Botet M (2011) NKp46 and DNAM-1 NK-cell receptors drive the response to human cytomegalovirus-infected myeloid dendritic cells overcoming viral immune evasion strategies. Blood 117:848–856

Maiza H, Leca G, Mansur IG, Schiavon V, Boumsell L, Bensussan A (1993) A novel 80-kD cell surface structure identifies human circulating lymphocytes with natural killer activity. J Exp Med 178:1121–1126

Mao X, Ou MT, Karuppagounder SS, Kam TI, Yin X, Xiong Y, Ge P, Umanah GE, Brahmachari S, Shin JH, Kang HC, Zhang J, Xu J, Chen R, Park H, Andrabi SA, Kang SU, Goncalves RA, Liang Y, Zhang S, Qi C, Lam S, Keiler JA, Tyson J, Kim D, Panicker N, Yun SP, Workman CJ, Vignali DA, Dawson VL, Ko HS, Dawson TM (2016) Pathological alpha-synuclein transmission initiated by binding lymphocyte-activation gene 3. Science 353

Marengere LE, Waterhouse P, Duncan GS, Mittrucker HW, Feng GS, Mak TW (1996) Regulation of T cell receptor signaling by tyrosine phosphatase SYP association with CTLA-4. Science 272:1170–1173

Marsters SA, Ayres TM, Skubatch M, Gray CL, Rothe M, Ashkenazi A (1997) Herpesvirus entry mediator, a member of the tumor necrosis factor receptor (TNFR) family, interacts with members of the TNFR-associated factor family and activates the transcription factors NF-kappaB and AP-1. J Biol Chem 272:14029–14032

Mauri DN, Ebner R, Montgomery RI, Kochel KD, Cheung TC, YU GL, Ruben S, Murphy M, Eisenberg RJ, Cohen GH, Spear PG, Ware CF (1998) LIGHT, a new member of the TNF superfamily, and lymphotoxin alpha are ligands for herpesvirus entry mediator. Immunity 8:21–30

Mchugh RS, Whitters MJ, Piccirillo CA, Young DA, Shevach EM, Collins M, Byrne MC (2002) CD4(+)CD25(+) immunoregulatory T cells: gene expression analysis reveals a functional role for the glucocorticoid-induced TNF receptor. Immunity 16:311–323

Mead KI, Zheng Y, Manzotti CN, Perry LC, Liu MK, Burke F, Powner DJ, Wakelam MJ, Sansom DM (2005) Exocytosis of CTLA-4 is dependent on phospholipase D and ADP ribosylation factor-1 and stimulated during activation of regulatory T cells. J Immunol 174:4803–4811

Meyer D, Seth S, Albrecht J, Maier MK, DU Pasquier L, Ravens I, Dreyer L, Burger R, Gramatzki M, Schwinzer R, Kremmer E, Foerster R, Bernhardt G (2009) CD96 interaction with CD155 via its first Ig-like domain is modulated by alternative splicing or mutations in distal Ig-like domains. J Biol Chem 284:2235–2244

Michalek RD, Gerriets VA, Jacobs SR, Macintyre AN, Maciver NJ, Mason EF, Sullivan SA, Nichols AG, Rathmell JC (2011) Cutting edge: distinct glycolytic and lipid oxidative metabolic programs are essential for effector and regulatory CD4+ T cell subsets. J Immunol 186:3299–3303

Migone TS, Zhang J, Luo X, Zhuang L, Chen C, Hu B, Hong JS, Perry JW, Chen SF, Zhou JX, Cho YH, Ullrich S, Kanakaraj P, Carrell J, Boyd E, Olsen HS, Hu G, Pukac L, Liu D, Ni J, Kim S, Gentz R, Feng P, Moore PA, Ruben SM, Wei P (2002) TL1A is a TNF-like ligand for DR3 and TR6/DcR3 and functions as a T cell costimulator. Immunity 16:479–492

Mir SS, Richter BW, Duckett CS (2000) Differential effects of CD30 activation in anaplastic large cell lymphoma and Hodgkin disease cells. Blood 96:4307–4312

Moll M, Kuylenstierna C, Gonzalez VD, Andersson SK, Bosnjak L, Sonnerborg A, Quigley MF, Sandberg JK (2009) Severe functional impairment and elevated PD-1 expression in CD1d-restricted NKT cells retained during chronic HIV-1 infection. Eur J Immunol 39:902–911

Montgomery RI, Warner MS, Lum BJ, Spear PG (1996) Herpes simplex virus-1 entry into cells mediated by a novel member of the TNF/NGF receptor family. Cell 87:427–436

Mousavi SF, Soroosh P, Takahashi T, Yoshikai Y, Shen H, Lefrancois L, Borst J, Sugamura K, Ishii N (2008) OX40 costimulatory signals potentiate the memory commitment of effector CD8+ T cells. J Immunol 181:5990–6001

Murata K, Ishii N, Takano H, Miura S, Ndhlovu LC, Nose M, Noda T, Sugamura K (2000) Impairment of antigen-presenting cell function in mice lacking expression of OX40 ligand. J Exp Med 191:365–374

Muscolini M, Sajeva A, Caristi S, Tuosto L (2011) A novel association between filamin A and NF-kappaB inducing kinase couples CD28 to inhibitor of NF-kappaB kinase alpha and NF-kappaB activation. Immunol Lett 136:203–212

Muscolini M, Camperio C, Porciello N, Caristi S, Capuano C, Viola A, Galandrini R, Tuosto L (2015) Phosphatidylinositol 4-phosphate 5-kinase alpha and Vav1 mutual cooperation in CD28-mediated actin remodeling and signaling functions. J Immunol 194:1323–1333

Nabekura T, Shibuya K, Takenaka E, Kai H, Shibata K, Yamashita Y, Harada K, Tahara-Hanaoka S, Honda S, Shibuya A (2010) Critical role of DNAX accessory molecule-1 (DNAM-1) in the development of acute graft-versus-host disease in mice. Proc Natl Acad Sci U S A 107:18593–18598

Nabekura T, Kanaya M, Shibuya A, Fu G, Gascoigne NR, Lanier LL (2014) Costimulatory molecule DNAM-1 is essential for optimal differentiation of memory natural killer cells during mouse cytomegalovirus infection. Immunity 40:225–234

Nakano H, Sakon S, Koseki H, Takemori T, Tada K, Matsumoto M, Munechika E, Sakai T, Shirasawa T, Akiba H, Kobata T, Santee SM, Ware CF, Rennert PD, Taniguchi M, Yagita H, Okumura K (1999) Targeted disruption of Traf5 gene causes defects in CD40- and CD27-mediated lymphocyte activation. Proc Natl Acad Sci U S A 96:9803–9808

Nakayama M, Akiba H, Takeda K, Kojima Y, Hashiguchi M, Azuma M, Yagita H, Okumura K (2009) Tim-3 mediates phagocytosis of apoptotic cells and cross-presentation. Blood 113:3821–3830

Nam KO, Kang H, Shin SM, Cho KH, Kwon B, Kwon BS, Kim SJ, Lee HW (2005) Cross-linking of 4-1BB activates TCR-signaling pathways in CD8+ T lymphocytes. J Immunol 174:1898–1905

Nikolova M, Marie-Cardine A, Boumsell L, Bensussan A (2002) BY55/CD160 acts as a co-receptor in TCR signal transduction of a human circulating cytotoxic effector T lymphocyte subset lacking CD28 expression. Int Immunol 14:445–451

Nocentini G, Giunchi L, Ronchetti S, Krausz LT, Bartoli A, Moraca R, Migliorati G, Riccardi C (1997) A new member of the tumor necrosis factor/nerve growth factor receptor family inhibits T cell receptor-induced apoptosis. Proc Natl Acad Sci U S A 94:6216–6221

Nurieva R, Thomas S, Nguyen T, Martin-Orozco N, Wang Y, Kaja MK, Yu XZ, Dong C (2006) T-cell tolerance or function is determined by combinatorial costimulatory signals. EMBO J 25:2623–2633

Oaks MK, Hallett KM, Penwell RT, Stauber EC, Warren SJ, Tector AJ (2000) A native soluble form of CTLA-4. Cell Immunol 201:144–153

Odegard JM, Marks BR, Diplacido LD, Poholek AC, Kono DH, Dong C, Flavell RA, Craft J (2008) ICOS-dependent extrafollicular helper T cells elicit IgG production via IL-21 in systemic autoimmunity. J Exp Med 205:2873–2886

Oderup C, Cederbom L, Makowska A, Cilio CM, Ivars F (2006) Cytotoxic T lymphocyte antigen-4-dependent down-modulation of costimulatory molecules on dendritic cells in CD4+ CD25+ regulatory T-cell-mediated suppression. Immunology 118:240–249

Ogawa S, Watanabe M, Sakurai Y, Inutake Y, Watanabe S, Tai X, Abe R (2013) CD28 signaling in primary CD4(+) T cells: identification of both tyrosine phosphorylation-dependent and phosphorylation-independent pathways. Int Immunol 25:671–681

Okazaki T, Maeda A, Nishimura H, Kurosaki T, Honjo T (2001) PD-1 immunoreceptor inhibits B cell receptor-mediated signaling by recruiting src homology 2-domain-containing tyrosine phosphatase 2 to phosphotyrosine. Proc Natl Acad Sci U S A 98:13866–13871

Okkenhaug K, Rottapel R (1998) Grb2 forms an inducible protein complex with CD28 through a Src homology 3 domain-proline interaction. J Biol Chem 273:21194–21202

Okkenhaug K, Wu L, Garza KM, La Rose J, Khoo W, Odermatt B, Mak TW, Ohashi PS, Rottapel R (2001) A point mutation in CD28 distinguishes proliferative signals from survival signals. Nat Immunol 2:325–332

Otsuki N, Kamimura Y, Hashiguchi M, Azuma M (2006) Expression and function of the B and T lymphocyte attenuator (BTLA/CD272) on human T cells. Biochem Biophys Res Commun 344:1121–1127

Pagan AJ, Pepper M, Chu HH, Green JM, Jenkins MK (2012) CD28 promotes CD4+ T cell clonal expansion during infection independently of its YMNM and PYAP motifs. J Immunol 189:2909–2917

Pages F, Ragueneau M, Rottapel R, Truneh A, Nunes J, Imbert J, Olive D (1994) Binding of phosphatidylinositol-3-OH kinase to CD28 is required for T-cell signalling. Nature 369:327–329

Pakala SV, Bansal-Pakala P, Halteman BS, Croft M (2004) Prevention of diabetes in NOD mice at a late stage by targeting OX40/OX40 ligand interactions. Eur J Immunol 34:3039–3046

Park YC, Burkitt V, Villa AR, Tong L, Wu H (1999) Structural basis for self-association and receptor recognition of human TRAF2. Nature 398:533–538

Parry RV, Rumbley CA, Vandenberghe LH, June CH, Riley JL (2003) CD28 and inducible costimulatory protein Src homology 2 binding domains show distinct regulation of phosphatidylinositol 3-kinase, Bcl-xL, and IL-2 expression in primary human CD4 T lymphocytes. J Immunol 171:166–174

Parry RV, Chemnitz JM, Frauwirth KA, Lanfranco AR, Braunstein I, Kobayashi SV, Linsley PS, Thompson CB, Riley JL (2005) CTLA-4 and PD-1 receptors inhibit T-cell activation by distinct mechanisms. Mol Cell Biol 25:9543–9553

Patsoukis N, Brown J, Petkova V, Liu F, Li L, Boussiotis VA (2012) Selective effects of PD-1 on Akt and Ras pathways regulate molecular components of the cell cycle and inhibit T cell proliferation. Sci Signal 5:ra46

Patsoukis N, Li L, Sari D, Petkova V, Boussiotis VA (2013) PD-1 increases PTEN phosphatase activity while decreasing PTEN protein stability by inhibiting casein kinase 2. Mol Cell Biol 33:3091–3098

Patsoukis N, Bardhan K, Chatterjee P, Sari D, Liu B, Bell LN, Karoly ED, Freeman GJ, Petkova V, Seth P, Li L, Boussiotis VA (2015) PD-1 alters T-cell metabolic reprogramming by inhibiting glycolysis and promoting lipolysis and fatty acid oxidation. Nat Commun 6:6692

Pedros C, Zhang Y, Hu JK, Choi YS, Canonigo-Balancio AJ, Yates JR 3rd, Altman A, Crotty S, Kong KF (2016) A TRAF-like motif of the inducible costimulator ICOS controls development of germinal center TFH cells via the kinase TBK1. Nat Immunol 17:825–833

Pei Y, Zhu P, Dang Y, Wu J, Yang X, Wan B, Liu JO, Yi Q, Yu L (2008) Nuclear export of NF90 to stabilize IL-2 mRNA is mediated by AKT-dependent phosphorylation at Ser647 in response to CD28 costimulation. J Immunol 180:222–229

Pobezinskaya YL, Choksi S, Morgan MJ, Cao X, Liu ZG (2011) The adaptor protein TRADD is essential for TNF-like ligand 1A/death receptor 3 signaling. J Immunol 186:5212–5216

Porquet N, Poirier A, Houle F, Pin AL, Gout S, Tremblay PL, Paquet ER, Klinck R, Auger FA, Huot J (2011) Survival advantages conferred to colon cancer cells by E-selectin-induced activation of the PI3K-NFkappaB survival axis downstream of death receptor-3. BMC Cancer 11:285

Prasad KV, Cai YC, Raab M, Duckworth B, Cantley L, Shoelson SE, Rudd CE (1994) T-cell antigen CD28 interacts with the lipid kinase phosphatidylinositol 3-kinase by a cytoplasmic Tyr(P)-met-Xaa-met motif. Proc Natl Acad Sci U S A 91:2834–2838

Prasad KV, Ao Z, Yoon Y, Wu MX, Rizk M, Jacquot S, Schlossman SF (1997) CD27, a member of the tumor necrosis factor receptor family, induces apoptosis and binds to Siva, a proapoptotic protein. Proc Natl Acad Sci U S A 94:6346–6351

del Prete G, de Carli M, Almerigogna F, Daniel CK, D'elios MM, Zancuoghi G, Vinante F, Pizzolo G, Romagnani S (1995) Preferential expression of CD30 by human CD4+ T cells producing Th2-type cytokines. FASEB J 9:81–86

Py B, Slomianny C, Auberger P, Petit PX, Benichou S (2004) Siva-1 and an alternative splice form lacking the death domain, Siva-2, similarly induce apoptosis in T lymphocytes via a caspase-dependent mitochondrial pathway. J Immunol 172:4008–4017

Quigley M, Pereyra F, Nilsson B, Porichis F, Fonseca C, Eichbaum Q, Julg B, Jesneck JL, Brosnahan K, Imam S, Russell K, Toth I, Piechocka-Trocha A, Dolfi D, Angelosanto J, Crawford A, Shin H, Kwon DS, Zupkosky J, Francisco L, Freeman GJ, Wherry EJ, Kaufmann DE, Walker BD, Ebert B, Haining WN (2010) Transcriptional analysis of HIV-specific CD8+ T cells shows that PD-1 inhibits T cell function by upregulating BATF. Nat Med 16:1147–1151

Qureshi OS, Zheng Y, Nakamura K, Attridge K, Manzotti C, Schmidt EM, Baker J, Jeffery LE, Kaur S, Briggs Z, Hou TZ, Futter CE, Anderson G, Walker LS, Sansom DM (2011) Trans-endocytosis of CD80 and CD86: a molecular basis for the cell-extrinsic function of CTLA-4. Science 332:600–603

Raab M, Cai YC, Bunnell SC, Heyeck SD, Berg LJ, Rudd CE (1995) p56Lck and p59Fyn regulate CD28 binding to phosphatidylinositol 3-kinase, growth factor receptor-bound protein GRB-2, and T cell-specific protein-tyrosine kinase ITK: implications for T-cell costimulation. Proc Natl Acad Sci U S A 92:8891–8895

Rabot M, EL Costa H, Polgar B, Marie-Cardine A, Aguerre-Girr M, Barakonyi A, Valitutti S, Bensussan A, LE Bouteiller P (2007) CD160-activating NK cell effector functions depend on the phosphatidylinositol 3-kinase recruitment. Int Immunol 19:401–409

Rangachari M, Zhu C, Sakuishi K, Xiao S, Karman J, Chen A, Angin M, Wakeham A, Greenfield EA, Sobel RA, Okada H, Mckinnon PJ, Mak TW, Addo MM, Anderson AC, Kuchroo VK (2012) Bat3 promotes T cell responses and autoimmunity by repressing Tim-3-mediated cell death and exhaustion. Nat Med 18:1394–1400

Ritthipichai K, Haymaker C, Martinez-Paniagua M, Aschenbrenner A, Yi X, Zhang M, Kale C, Hailemichael Y, Overwijk WW, Vence L, Roszik J, Varadarajan N, Nurieva R, Radvanyi LG, Hwu P, Bernatchez C (2017) Multifaceted role of BTLA in the control of CD8+ T cell fate after antigen encounter. Clin Cancer Res

Rodriguez M, Cabal-Hierro L, Carcedo MT, Iglesias JM, Artime N, Darnay BG, Lazo PS (2011) NF-kappaB signal triggering and termination by tumor necrosis factor receptor 2. J Biol Chem 286:22814–22824

Rogers PR, Song J, Gramaglia I, Killeen N, Croft M (2001) OX40 promotes Bcl-xL and Bcl-2 expression and is essential for long-term survival of CD4 T cells. Immunity 15:445–455

Roncagalli R, Cucchetti M, Jarmuzynski N, Gregoire C, Bergot E, Audebert S, Baudelet E, Menoita MG, Joachim A, Durand S, Suchanek M, Fiore F, Zhang L, Liang Y, Camoin L, Malissen M, Malissen B (2016) The scaffolding function of the RLTPR protein explains its essential role for CD28 co-stimulation in mouse and human T cells. J Exp Med 213:2437–2457

Ronchetti S, Nocentini G, Bianchini R, Krausz LT, Migliorati G, Riccardi C (2007) Glucocorticoid-induced TNFR-related protein lowers the threshold of CD28 costimulation in CD8+ T cells. J Immunol 179:5916–5926

Rothe M, Pan MG, Henzel WJ, Ayres TM, Goeddel DV (1995) The TNFR2-TRAF signaling complex contains two novel proteins related to baculoviral inhibitor of apoptosis proteins. Cell 83:1243–1252

Ruan Q, Kameswaran V, Tone Y, Li L, Liou HC, Greene MI, Tone M, Chen YH (2009) Development of Foxp3(+) regulatory t cells is driven by the c-Rel enhanceosome. Immunity 31:932–940

Sabatos CA, Chakravarti S, Cha E, Schubart A, Sanchez-Fueyo A, Zheng XX, Coyle AJ, Strom TB, Freeman GJ, Kuchroo VK (2003) Interaction of Tim-3 and Tim-3 ligand regulates T helper type 1 responses and induction of peripheral tolerance. Nat Immunol 4:1102–1110

Sabbagh L, Pulle G, Liu Y, Tsitsikov EN, Watts TH (2008) ERK-dependent Bim modulation downstream of the 4-1BB-TRAF1 signaling axis is a critical mediator of CD8 T cell survival in vivo. J Immunol 180:8093–8101

Sabbagh L, Andreeva D, Laramee GD, Oussa NA, Lew D, Bisson N, Soumounou Y, Pawson T, Watts TH (2013) Leukocyte-specific protein 1 links TNF receptor-associated factor 1 to survival signaling downstream of 4-1BB in T cells. J Leukoc Biol 93:713–721

Sadra A, Cinek T, Arellano JL, Shi J, Truitt KE, Imboden JB (1999) Identification of tyrosine phosphorylation sites in the CD28 cytoplasmic domain and their role in the costimulation of Jurkat T cells. J Immunol 162:1966–1973

Sanchez-Fueyo A, Tian J, Picarella D, Domenig C, Zheng XX, Sabatos CA, Manlongat N, Bender O, Kamradt T, Kuchroo VK, Gutierrez-Ramos JC, Coyle AJ, Strom TB (2003) Tim-3 inhibits T helper type 1-mediated auto- and alloimmune responses and promotes immunological tolerance. Nat Immunol 4:1093–1101

Sanchez-Lockhart M, Miller J (2006) Engagement of CD28 outside of the immunological synapse results in up-regulation of IL-2 mRNA stability but not IL-2 transcription. J Immunol 176:4778–4784

Sanchez-Lockhart M, Marin E, Graf B, Abe R, Harada Y, Sedwick CE, Miller J (2004) Cutting edge: CD28-mediated transcriptional and posttranscriptional regulation of IL-2 expression are controlled through different signaling pathways. J Immunol 173:7120–7124

Saoulli K, Lee SY, Cannons JL, Yeh WC, Santana A, Goldstein MD, Bangia N, Debenedette MA, Mak TW, Choi Y, Watts TH (1998) CD28-independent, TRAF2-dependent costimulation of resting T cells by 4-1BB ligand. J Exp Med 187:1849–1862

Sarmento OF, Svingen PA, Xiong Y, Sun Z, Bamidele AO, Mathison AJ, Smyrk TC, Nair AA, Gonzalez MM, Sagstetter MR, Baheti S, Mcgovern DP, Friton JJ, Papadakis KA, Gautam G, Xavier RJ, Urrutia RA, Faubion WA (2017) The role of the histone Methyltransferase enhancer of Zeste homolog 2 (EZH2) in the Pathobiological mechanisms underlying inflammatory bowel disease (IBD). J Biol Chem 292:706–722

Saunders PA, Hendrycks VR, Lidinsky WA, Woods ML (2005) PD-L2:PD-1 involvement in T cell proliferation, cytokine production, and integrin-mediated adhesion. Eur J Immunol 35:3561–3569

Schneider H, Rudd CE (2008) CD28 and Grb-2, relative to gads or Grap, preferentially co-operate with Vav1 in the activation of NFAT/AP-1 transcription. Biochem Biophys Res Commun 369:616–621

Schneider H, Martin M, Agarraberes FA, Yin L, Rapoport I, Kirchhausen T, Rudd CE (1999) Cytolytic T lymphocyte-associated antigen-4 and the TCR zeta/CD3 complex, but not CD28, interact with clathrin adaptor complexes AP-1 and AP-2. J Immunol 163:1868–1879

Schneider H, Valk E, Leung R, Rudd CE (2008) CTLA-4 activation of phosphatidylinositol 3-kinase (PI 3-K) and protein kinase B (PKB/AKT) sustains T-cell anergy without cell death. PLoS One 3:e3842

Schober T, Magg T, Laschinger M, Rohlfs M, Linhares ND, Puchalka J, Weisser T, Fehlner K, Mautner J, Walz C, Hussein K, Jaeger G, Kammer B, Schmid I, Bahia M, Pena SD, Behrends U, Belohradsky BH, Klein C, Hauck F (2017) A human immunodeficiency syndrome caused by mutations in CARMIL2. Nat Commun 8:14209

Schreiber TH, Wolf D, Tsai MS, Chirinos J, Deyev VV, Gonzalez L, Malek TR, Levy RB, Podack ER (2010) Therapeutic Treg expansion in mice by TNFRSF25 prevents allergic lung inflammation. J Clin Invest 120:3629–3640

Sedy JR, Gavrieli M, Potter KG, Hurchla MA, Lindsley RC, Hildner K, Scheu S, Pfeffer K, Ware CF, Murphy TL, Murphy KM (2005) B and T lymphocyte attenuator regulates T cell activation through interaction with herpesvirus entry mediator. Nat Immunol 6:90–98

Sedy JR, Bjordahl RL, Bekiaris V, Macauley MG, Ware BC, Norris PS, Lurain NS, Benedict CA, Ware CF (2013) CD160 activation by herpesvirus entry mediator augments inflammatory cytokine production and cytolytic function by NK cells. J Immunol 191:828–836

Semple K, Nguyen A, Yu Y, Wang H, Anasetti C, Yu XZ (2011) Strong CD28 costimulation suppresses induction of regulatory T cells from naive precursors through Lck signaling. Blood 117:3096–3103

Seth S, Maier MK, Qiu Q, Ravens I, Kremmer E, Forster R, Bernhardt G (2007) The murine pan T cell marker CD96 is an adhesion receptor for CD155 and nectin-1. Biochem Biophys Res Commun 364:959–965

Shapiro VS, Truitt KE, Imboden JB, Weiss A (1997) CD28 mediates transcriptional upregulation of the interleukin-2 (IL-2) promoter through a composite element containing the CD28RE and NF-IL-2B AP-1 sites. Mol Cell Biol 17:4051–4058

Sheppard KA, Fitz LJ, Lee JM, Benander C, George JA, Wooters J, Qiu Y, Jussif JM, Carter LL, Wood CR, Chaudhary D (2004) PD-1 inhibits T-cell receptor induced phosphorylation of the ZAP70/CD3zeta signalosome and downstream signaling to PKCtheta. FEBS Lett 574:37–41

Shi CS, Kehrl JH (2003) Tumor necrosis factor (TNF)-induced germinal center kinase-related (GCKR) and stress-activated protein kinase (SAPK) activation depends upon the E2/E3 complex Ubc13-Uev1A/TNF receptor-associated factor 2 (TRAF2). J Biol Chem 278:15429–15434

Shibuya A, Campbell D, Hannum C, Yssel H, Franz-Bacon K, Mcclanahan T, Kitamura T, Nicholl J, Sutherland GR, Lanier LL, Phillips JH (1996) DNAM-1, a novel adhesion molecule involved in the cytolytic function of T lymphocytes. Immunity 4:573–581

Shibuya A, Lanier LL, Phillips JH (1998) Protein kinase C is involved in the regulation of both signaling and adhesion mediated by DNAX accessory molecule-1 receptor. J Immunol 161:1671–1676

Shibuya K, Lanier LL, Phillips JH, Ochs HD, Shimizu K, Nakayama E, Nakauchi H, Shibuya A (1999) Physical and functional association of LFA-1 with DNAM-1 adhesion molecule. Immunity 11:615–623

Shimizu J, Yamazaki S, Takahashi T, Ishida Y, Sakaguchi S (2002) Stimulation of CD25(+)CD4(+) regulatory T cells through GITR breaks immunological self-tolerance. Nat Immunol 3:135–142

Shinohara T, Taniwaki M, Ishida Y, Kawaichi M, Honjo T (1994) Structure and chromosomal localization of the human PD-1 gene (PDCD1). Genomics 23:704–706

Shirakawa J, Wang Y, Tahara-Hanaoka S, Honda S, Shibuya K, Shibuya A (2006) LFA-1-dependent lipid raft recruitment of DNAM-1 (CD226) in CD4+ T cell. Int Immunol 18:951–957

Shui JW, Larange A, Kim G, Vela JL, Zahner S, Cheroutre H, Kronenberg M (2012) HVEM signalling at mucosal barriers provides host defence against pathogenic bacteria. Nature 488:222–225

Smith CA, Gruss HJ, Davis T, Anderson D, Farrah T, Baker E, Sutherland GR, Brannan CI, Copeland NG, Jenkins NA et al (1993) CD30 antigen, a marker for Hodgkin's lymphoma, is a receptor whose ligand defines an emerging family of cytokines with homology to TNF. Cell 73:1349–1360

Snell LM, Mcpherson AJ, Lin GH, Sakaguchi S, Pandolfi PP, Riccardi C, Watts TH (2010) CD8 T cell-intrinsic GITR is required for T cell clonal expansion and mouse survival following severe influenza infection. J Immunol 185:7223–7234

So T, Choi H, Croft M (2011a) OX40 complexes with phosphoinositide 3-kinase and protein kinase B (PKB) to augment TCR-dependent PKB signaling. J Immunol 186:3547–3555

So T, Soroosh P, Eun SY, Altman A, Croft M (2011b) Antigen-independent signalosome of CARMA1, PKCtheta, and TNF receptor-associated factor 2 (TRAF2) determines NF-kappaB signaling in T cells. Proc Natl Acad Sci U S A 108:2903–2908

Soligo M, Camperio C, Caristi S, Scotta C, DEL Porto P, Costanzo A, Mantel PY, Schmidt-Weber CB, Piccolella E (2011) CD28 costimulation regulates FOXP3 in a RelA/NF-kappaB-dependent mechanism. Eur J Immunol 41:503–513

Song J, Salek-Ardakani S, Rogers PR, Cheng M, van Parijs L, Croft M (2004) The costimulation-regulated duration of PKB activation controls T cell longevity. Nat Immunol 5:150–158

Song J, So T, Croft M (2008) Activation of NF-kappaB1 by OX40 contributes to antigen-driven T cell expansion and survival. J Immunol 180:7240–7248

Soroosh P, Ine S, Sugamura K, Ishii N (2007) Differential requirements for OX40 signals on generation of effector and central memory CD4+ T cells. J Immunol 179:5014–5023

Soroosh P, Doherty TA, So T, Mehta AK, Khorram N, Norris PS, Scheu S, Pfeffer K, Ware C, Croft M (2011) Herpesvirus entry mediator (TNFRSF14) regulates the persistence of T helper memory cell populations. J Exp Med 208:797–809

Sorte HS, Osnes LT, Fevang B, Aukrust P, Erichsen HC, Backe PH, Abrahamsen TG, Kittang OB, Overland T, Jhangiani SN, Muzny DM, Vigeland MD, Samarakoon P, Gambin T, Akdemir ZH, Gibbs RA, Rodningen OK, Lyle R, Lupski JR, Stray-Pedersen A (2016) A potential founder variant in CARMIL2/RLTPR in three Norwegian families with warts, molluscum contagiosum, and T-cell dysfunction. Mol Genet Genomic Med 4:604–616

Spinicelli S, Nocentini G, Ronchetti S, Krausz LT, Bianchini R, Riccardi C (2002) GITR interacts with the pro-apoptotic protein Siva and induces apoptosis. Cell Death Differ 9:1382–1384

Stanietsky N, Rovis TL, Glasner A, Seidel E, Tsukerman P, Yamin R, Enk J, Jonjic S, Mandelboim O (2013) Mouse TIGIT inhibits NK-cell cytotoxicity upon interaction with PVR. Eur J Immunol 43:2138–2150

Stein PH, Fraser JD, Weiss A (1994) The cytoplasmic domain of CD28 is both necessary and sufficient for costimulation of interleukin-2 secretion and association with phosphatidylinositol 3′-kinase. Mol Cell Biol 14:3392–3402

Steinberg MW, Cheung TC, Ware CF (2011) The signaling networks of the herpesvirus entry mediator (TNFRSF14) in immune regulation. Immunol Rev 244:169–187

Stephens GL, Mchugh RS, Whitters MJ, Young DA, Luxenberg D, Carreno BM, Collins M, Shevach EM (2004) Engagement of glucocorticoid-induced TNFR family-related receptor on effector T cells by its ligand mediates resistance to suppression by CD4+CD25+ T cells. J Immunol 173:5008–5020

Stumpf M, Zhou X, Chikuma S, Bluestone JA (2014) Tyrosine 201 of the cytoplasmic tail of CTLA-4 critically affects T regulatory cell suppressive function. Eur J Immunol 44:1737–1746

Tai X, Cowan M, Feigenbaum L, Singer A (2005) CD28 costimulation of developing thymocytes induces Foxp3 expression and regulatory T cell differentiation independently of interleukin 2. Nat Immunol 6:152–162

Tai X, van Laethem F, Sharpe AH, Singer A (2007) Induction of autoimmune disease in CTLA-4−/− mice depends on a specific CD28 motif that is required for in vivo costimulation. Proc Natl Acad Sci U S A 104:13756–13761

Takeda K, Harada Y, Watanabe R, Inutake Y, Ogawa S, Onuki K, Kagaya S, Tanabe K, Kishimoto H, Abe R (2008) CD28 stimulation triggers NF-kappaB activation through the CARMA1-PKCtheta-Grb2/gads axis. Int Immunol 20:1507–1515

Tang Q, Henriksen KJ, Boden EK, Tooley AJ, Ye J, Subudhi SK, Zheng XX, Strom TB, Bluestone JA (2003) Cutting edge: CD28 controls peripheral homeostasis of CD4+CD25+ regulatory T cells. J Immunol 171:3348–3352

Tang ZS, Hao YH, Zhang EJ, Xu CL, Zhou Y, Zheng X, Yang DL (2016) CD28 family of receptors on T cells in chronic HBV infection: expression characteristics, clinical significance and correlations with PD-1 blockade. Mol Med Rep 14:1107–1116

Tavano R, Contento RL, Baranda SJ, Soligo M, Tuosto L, Manes S, Viola A (2006) CD28 interaction with filamin-A controls lipid raft accumulation at the T-cell immunological synapse. Nat Cell Biol 8:1270–1276

Teft WA, Chau TA, Madrenas J (2009) Structure-function analysis of the CTLA-4 interaction with PP2A. BMC Immunol 10:23

Tesselaar K, Xiao Y, Arens R, van Schijndel GM, Schuurhuis DH, Mebius RE, Borst J, van Lier RA (2003) Expression of the murine CD27 ligand CD70 in vitro and in vivo. J Immunol 170:33–40

Thaker YR, Schneider H, Rudd CE (2015) TCR and CD28 activate the transcription factor NF-kappaB in T-cells via distinct adaptor signaling complexes. Immunol Lett 163:113–119

Thomas RM, Gao L, Wells AD (2005) Signals from CD28 induce stable epigenetic modification of the IL-2 promoter. J Immunol 174:4639–4646

Thompson CB, Lindsten T, Ledbetter JA, Kunkel SL, Young HA, Emerson SG, Leiden JM, June CH (1989) CD28 activation pathway regulates the production of multiple T-cell-derived lymphokines/cytokines. Proc Natl Acad Sci U S A 86:1333–1337

Tian R, Wang H, Gish GD, Petsalaki E, Pasculescu A, Shi Y, Mollenauer M, Bagshaw RD, Yosef N, Hunter T, Gingras AC, Weiss A, Pawson T (2015) Combinatorial proteomic analysis of intercellular signaling applied to the CD28 T-cell costimulatory receptor. Proc Natl Acad Sci U S A 112:E1594–E1603

Tone M, Tone Y, Adams E, Yates SF, Frewin MR, Cobbold SP, Waldmann H (2003) Mouse glucocorticoid-induced tumor necrosis factor receptor ligand is costimulatory for T cells. Proc Natl Acad Sci U S A 100:15059–15064

Tseng SY, Otsuji M, Gorski K, Huang X, Slansky JE, Pai SI, Shalabi A, Shin T, Pardoll DM, Tsuchiya H (2001) B7-DC, a new dendritic cell molecule with potent costimulatory properties for T cells. J Exp Med 193:839–846

Tsujimura K, Obata Y, Matsudaira Y, Nishida K, Akatsuka Y, Ito Y, Demachi-Okamura A, Kuzushima K, Takahashi T (2006) Characterization of murine CD160+ CD8+ T lymphocytes. Immunol Lett 106:48–56

Tu TC, Brown NK, Kim TJ, Wroblewska J, Yang X, Guo X, Lee SH, Kumar V, Lee KM, Fu YX (2015) CD160 is essential for NK-mediated IFN-gamma production. J Exp Med 212:415–429

Valk E, Leung R, Kang H, Kaneko K, Rudd CE, Schneider H (2006) T cell receptor-interacting molecule acts as a chaperone to modulate surface expression of the CTLA-4 coreceptor. Immunity 25:807–821

Vang KB, Yang J, Pagan AJ, Li LX, Wang J, Green JM, Beg AA, Farrar MA (2010) Cutting edge: CD28 and c-Rel-dependent pathways initiate regulatory T cell development. J Immunol 184:4074–4077

Verhoeven DH, de Hooge AS, Mooiman EC, Santos SJ, Ten Dam MM, Gelderblom H, Melief CJ, Hogendoorn PC, Egeler RM, van Tol MJ, Schilham MW, Lankester AC (2008) NK cells recognize and lyse Ewing sarcoma cells through NKG2D and DNAM-1 receptor dependent pathways. Mol Immunol 45:3917–3925

Vigano S, Banga R, Bellanger F, Pellaton C, Farina A, Comte D, Harari A, Perreau M (2014) CD160-associated CD8 T-cell functional impairment is independent of PD-1 expression. PLoS Pathog 10:e1004380

Viola A, Schroeder S, Sakakibara Y, Lanzavecchia A (1999) T lymphocyte costimulation mediated by reorganization of membrane microdomains. Science 283:680–682

Wang PL, O'farrell S, Clayberger C, Krensky AM (1992) Identification and molecular cloning of tactile. A novel human T cell activation antigen that is a member of the Ig gene superfamily. J Immunol 148:2600–2608

Wang L, Rubinstein R, Lines JL, Wasiuk A, Ahonen C, Guo Y, Lu LF, Gondek D, Wang Y, Fava RA, Fiser A, Almo S, Noelle RJ (2011) VISTA, a novel mouse Ig superfamily ligand that negatively regulates T cell responses. J Exp Med 208:577–592

Wang L, Liu Y, Beier UH, Han R, Bhatti TR, Akimova T, Hancock WW (2013) Foxp3+ T-regulatory cells require DNA methyltransferase 1 expression to prevent development of lethal autoimmunity. Blood 121:3631–3639

Wang L, le Mercier I, Putra J, Chen W, Liu J, Schenk AD, Nowak EC, Suriawinata AA, Li J, Noelle RJ (2014) Disruption of the immune-checkpoint VISTA gene imparts a proinflammatory phenotype with predisposition to the development of autoimmunity. Proc Natl Acad Sci U S A 111:14846–14851

Wang XD, Gong Y, Chen ZL, Gong BN, Xie JJ, Zhong CQ, Wang QL, Diao LH, Xu A, Han J, Altman A, Li Y (2015) TCR-induced sumoylation of the kinase PKC-theta controls T cell synapse organization and T cell activation. Nat Immunol 16:1195–1203

Wang Y, Ma CS, Ling Y, Bousfiha A, Camcioglu Y, Jacquot S, Payne K, Crestani E, Roncagalli R, Belkadi A, Kerner G, Lorenzo L, Deswarte C, Chrabieh M, Patin E, Vincent QB, Muller-Fleckenstein I, Fleckenstein B, Ailal F, Quintana-Murci L, Fraitag S, Alyanakian MA, Leruez-Ville M, Picard C, Puel A, Bustamante J, Boisson-Dupuis S, Malissen M, Malissen B, Abel L, Hovnanian A, Notarangelo LD, Jouanguy E, Tangye SG, Beziat V, Casanova JL (2016) Dual T cell- and B cell-intrinsic deficiency in humans with biallelic RLTPR mutations. J Exp Med 213:2413–2435

Ware CF, Sedy JR (2011) TNF superfamily networks: bidirectional and interference pathways of the herpesvirus entry mediator (TNFSF14). Curr Opin Immunol 23:627–631

Watanabe N, Gavrieli M, Sedy JR, Yang J, Fallarino F, Loftin SK, Hurchla MA, Zimmerman N, Sim J, Zang X, Murphy TL, Russell JH, Allison JP, Murphy KM (2003) BTLA is a lymphocyte inhibitory receptor with similarities to CTLA-4 and PD-1. Nat Immunol 4:670–679

Watanabe R, Harada Y, Takeda K, Takahashi J, Ohnuki K, Ogawa S, Ohgai D, Kaibara N, Koiwai O, Tanabe K, Toma H, Sugamura K, Abe R (2006) Grb2 and gads exhibit different interactions with CD28 and play distinct roles in CD28-mediated costimulation. J Immunol 177:1085–1091

Wei F, Zhong S, Ma Z, Kong H, Medvec A, Ahmed R, Freeman GJ, Krogsgaard M, Riley JL (2013) Strength of PD-1 signaling differentially affects T-cell effector functions. Proc Natl Acad Sci U S A 110:E2480–E2489

Wen L, Zhuang L, Luo X, Wei P (2003) TL1A-induced NF-kappaB activation and c-IAP2 production prevent DR3-mediated apoptosis in TF-1 cells. J Biol Chem 278:39251–39258 van de Weyer PS, Muehlfeit M, Klose C, Bonventre JV, Walz G, Kuehn EW (2006) A highly conserved tyrosine of Tim-3 is phosphorylated upon stimulation by its ligand galectin-9. Biochem Biophys Res Commun 351:571–576

Whitbeck JC, Peng C, Lou H, Xu R, Willis SH, Ponce De Leon M, Peng T, Nicola AV, Montgomery RI, Warner MS, Soulika AM, Spruce LA, Moore WT, Lambris JD, Spear PG, Cohen GH, Eisenberg RJ (1997) Glycoprotein D of herpes simplex virus (HSV) binds directly to HVEM, a member of the tumor necrosis factor receptor superfamily and a mediator of HSV entry. J Virol 71:6083–6093

Wicovsky A, Henkler F, Salzmann S, Scheurich P, Kneitz C, Wajant H (2009) Tumor necrosis factor receptor-associated factor-1 enhances proinflammatory TNF receptor-2 signaling and modifies TNFR1-TNFR2 cooperation. Oncogene 28:1769–1781

Workman CJ, Vignali DA (2003) The CD4-related molecule, LAG-3 (CD223), regulates the expansion of activated T cells. Eur J Immunol 33:970–979

Workman CJ, Dugger KJ, Vignali DA (2002) Cutting edge: molecular analysis of the negative regulatory function of lymphocyte activation gene-3. J Immunol 169:5392–5395

Wright CW, Duckett CS (2009) The aryl hydrocarbon nuclear translocator alters CD30-mediated NF-kappaB-dependent transcription. Science 323:251–255

Wright CW, Rumble JM, Duckett CS (2007) CD30 activates both the canonical and alternative NF-kappaB pathways in anaplastic large cell lymphoma cells. J Biol Chem 282:10252–10262

Xiao X, Balasubramanian S, Liu W, Chu X, Wang H, Taparowsky EJ, Fu YX, Choi Y, Walsh MC, Li XC (2012) OX40 signaling favors the induction of T(H)9 cells and airway inflammation. Nat Immunol 13:981–990

Xu F, Liu J, Liu D, Liu B, Wang M, Hu Z, Du X, Tang L, He F (2014) LSECtin expressed on melanoma cells promotes tumor progression by inhibiting antitumor T-cell responses. Cancer Res 74:3418–3428

Yamamoto H, Kishimoto T, Minamoto S (1998) NF-kappaB activation in CD27 signaling: involvement of TNF receptor-associated factors in its signaling and identification of functional region of CD27. J Immunol 161:4753–4759

Yamazaki T, Akiba H, Iwai H, Matsuda H, Aoki M, Tanno Y, Shin T, Tsuchiya H, Pardoll DM, Okumura K, Azuma M, Yagita H (2002) Expression of programmed death 1 ligands by murine T cells and APC. J Immunol 169:5538–5545

Yang R, Qu C, Zhou Y, Konkel JE, Shi S, Liu Y, Chen C, Liu S, Liu D, Chen Y, Zandi E, Chen W, Zhou Y, Shi S (2015) Hydrogen sulfide promotes Tet1- and Tet2-mediated Foxp3 Demethylation to drive regulatory T cell differentiation and maintain immune homeostasis. Immunity 43:251–263

Yang L, Qiao G, Hassan Y, Li Z, Zhang X, Kong H, Zeng W, Yin F, Zhang J (2016) Program Death-1 suppresses autoimmune arthritis by inhibiting Th17 response. Arch Immunol Ther Exp 64:417–423

Yang W, Pan W, Chen S, Trendel N, Jiang S, Xiao F, Xue M, Wu W, Peng Z, Li X, Ji H, Liu X, Jiang H, Wang H, Shen H, Dushek O, Li H, Xu C (2017) Dynamic regulation of CD28 conformation and signaling by charged lipids and ions. Nat Struct Mol Biol

Ye H, Park YC, Kreishman M, Kieff E, Wu H (1999) The structural basis for the recognition of diverse receptor sequences by TRAF2. Mol Cell 4:321–330

Ye H, Arron JR, Lamothe B, Cirilli M, Kobayashi T, Shevde NK, Segal D, Dzivenu OK, Vologodskaia M, Yim M, Du K, Singh S, Pike JW, Darnay BG, Choi Y, Wu H (2002) Distinct molecular mechanism for initiating TRAF6 signalling. Nature 418:443–447

Yokosuka T, Kobayashi W, Sakata-Sogawa K, Takamatsu M, Hashimoto-Tane A, Dustin ML, Tokunaga M, Saito T (2008) Spatiotemporal regulation of T cell costimulation by TCR-CD28 microclusters and protein kinase C theta translocation. Immunity 29:589–601

Yokosuka T, Kobayashi W, Takamatsu M, Sakata-Sogawa K, Zeng H, Hashimoto-Tane A, Yagita H, Tokunaga M, Saito T (2010) Spatiotemporal basis of CTLA-4 costimulatory molecule-mediated negative regulation of T cell activation. Immunity 33:326–339

Yokosuka T, Takamatsu M, Kobayashi-Imanishi W, Hashimoto-Tane A, Azuma M, Saito T (2012) Programmed cell death 1 forms negative costimulatory microclusters that directly inhibit T cell receptor signaling by recruiting phosphatase SHP2. J Exp Med 209:1201–1217

Yoon KW, Byun S, Kwon E, Hwang SY, Chu K, Hiraki M, Jo SH, Weins A, Hakroush S, Cebulla A, Sykes DB, Greka A, Mundel P, Fisher DE, Mandinova A, Lee SW (2015) Control of signaling-mediated clearance of apoptotic cells by the tumor suppressor p53. Science 349:1261669

Yu X, Harden K, Gonzalez LC, Francesco M, Chiang E, Irving B, Tom I, Ivelja S, Refino CJ, Clark H, Eaton D, Grogan JL (2009) The surface protein TIGIT suppresses T cell activation by promoting the generation of mature immunoregulatory dendritic cells. Nat Immunol 10:48–57

Zhan Y, Funda DP, Every AL, Fundova P, Purton JF, Liddicoat DR, Cole TJ, Godfrey DI, Brady JL, Mannering SI, Harrison LC, Lew AM (2004) TCR-mediated activation promotes GITR upregulation in T cells and resistance to glucocorticoid-induced death. Int Immunol 16:1315–1321

Zhang X, Schwartz JC, Guo X, Bhatia S, Cao E, Lorenz M, Cammer M, Chen L, Zhang ZY, Edidin MA, Nathenson SG, Almo SC (2004) Structural and functional analysis of the costimulatory receptor programmed death-1. Immunity 20:337–347

Zhang Q, Cui F, Fang L, Hong J, Zheng B, Zhang JZ (2013a) TNF-alpha impairs differentiation and function of TGF-beta-induced Treg cells in autoimmune diseases through Akt and Smad3 signaling pathway. J Mol Cell Biol 5:85–98

Zhang R, Huynh A, Whitcher G, Chang J, Maltzman JS, Turka LA (2013b) An obligate cell-intrinsic function for CD28 in Tregs. J Clin Invest 123:580–593

Zhang Z, Wu N, Lu Y, Davidson D, Colonna M, Veillette A (2015) DNAM-1 controls NK cell activation via an ITT-like motif. J Exp Med 212:2165–2182

Zheng C, Kabaleeswaran V, Wang Y, Cheng G, Wu H (2010a) Crystal structures of the TRAF2: cIAP2 and the TRAF1: TRAF2: cIAP2 complexes: affinity, specificity, and regulation. Mol Cell 38:101–113

Zheng Y, Josefowicz S, Chaudhry A, Peng XP, Forbush K, Rudensky AY (2010b) Role of conserved non-coding DNA elements in the Foxp3 gene in regulatory T-cell fate. Nature 463:808–812

Zhou Z, Song X, Berezov A, Zhang G, Li Y, Zhang H, Murali R, Li B, Greene MI (2008a) Human glucocorticoid-induced TNF receptor ligand regulates its signaling activity through multiple oligomerization states. Proc Natl Acad Sci U S A 105:5465–5470

Zhou Z, Tone Y, Song X, Furuuchi K, Lear JD, Waldmann H, Tone M, Greene MI, Murali R (2008b) Structural basis for ligand-mediated mouse GITR activation. Proc Natl Acad Sci U S A 105:641–645

Zhu C, Anderson AC, Schubart A, Xiong H, Imitola J, Khoury SJ, Zheng XX, Strom TB, Kuchroo VK (2005) The Tim-3 ligand galectin-9 negatively regulates T helper type 1 immunity. Nat Immunol 6:1245–1252

Zhu P, Jiang W, Cao L, Yu W, Pei Y, Yang X, Wan B, Liu JO, Yi Q, Yu L (2010) IL-2 mRNA stabilization upon PMA stimulation is dependent on NF90-Ser647 phosphorylation by protein kinase CbetaI. J Immunol 185:5140–5149

Chapter 5
Molecular Dynamics of Co-signal Molecules in T-Cell Activation

Takashi Saito

Abstract T-cell activation is induced through the TCR microcluster (TCR-MC), which is generated by dynamically recruiting the TCR, kinases, and adaptors to trigger the full activation signal. Co-stimulation receptors also accumulate, mostly at the TCR-MC, and induce signals that positively and negatively modulate the direction and magnitude of T-cell activation. CD28 initially colocalizes with the TCR-MC but then migrates to a distinct region of the cSMAC called the signaling cSMAC, where it recruits and associates with PKCθ, CARMA1, and Rltpr to induce sustained co-stimulation signals leading to NF-kB activation. Although CTLA-4 and PD-1 mediate inhibitory functions in T-cell activation, their molecular dynamics are quite different. Both are expressed only after activation, when they function as feedback inhibition of T-cell activation. Whereas PD-1 initially accumulates in the TCR-MC and then moves to the cSMAC, CTLA-4 directly accumulates at the cSMAC. PD-1 inhibits activation by inducing dephosphorylation of TCR-upstream signaling molecules by transiently recruiting SHP2, whereas CTLA-4 competes with CD28 for CD80/86 binding within the signaling cSMAC. In general, for both positive and negative co-stimulation, these co-stimulation receptors are also clustered in a ligand-dependent fashion, and their colocalization with the TCR-MC is required to mediate co-stimulation signals.

Keywords Imaging · TCR signaling · Microclusters · Immune synapse · Co-stimulation · CD28 · CTLA-4 · PD-1

T. Saito (✉)
Laboratory for Cell Signaling, RIKEN Center for Integrative Medical Sciences,
Yokohama, Japan
e-mail: takashi.saito@riken.jp

© Springer Nature Singapore Pte Ltd. 2019
M. Azuma, H. Yagita (eds.), *Co-signal Molecules in T Cell Activation*,
Advances in Experimental Medicine and Biology 1189,
https://doi.org/10.1007/978-981-32-9717-3_5

5.1 Immunological Synapse and TCR- Microclusters

5.1.1 Immunological Synapse

T cells recognize antigen (Ag) as a peptide-MHC complex on Ag-presenting cells (APC) such as dendritic cells (DC) through direct cell-cell interactions. The T-cell antigen receptor (TCR) binds to the Ag peptide-MHC complex (pMHC) and triggers T-cell activation by recruiting various signaling molecules including the Src-family kinase Lck and the Syk-family kinase ZAP-70. Upon formation of the T cell-APC conjugate, T cells become polarized toward the APC and create a unique structure at the interface between the two cells called the immune or immunological synapse (IS). Upon Ag recognition/activation, the TCR-CD3 complex accumulates at the center of the IS as the central (c-) supramolecular activation complex (cSMAC) and is surrounded by the integrin LFA1 as the peripheral (p-) SMAC (Monks et al. 1998; Grakoui et al. 1999). When originally characterized, this structure appeared to support a model in which the cSMAC contained the TCR as the Ag recognition component and the pSMAC contained the integrin to promote cell-cell adhesion. Together with accumulated evidence that various signaling molecules are recruited to the IS, this structure appeared to be the site of Ag recognition and signal transduction for T-cell activation. However, the generation of the cSMAC and pSMAC takes 5–10 min after the interaction of T cells with APCs or with MHC-containing planar lipid bilayers, kinetics that did not correspond at all to those of early T-cell activation events such as tyrosine phosphorylation, and intracellular Ca^{2+} flux, which can occur within a few minutes (Lee et al. 2003).

In addition, early analysis of the signaling complex responsible for T-cell activation using Jurkat cells stimulated with immobilized anti-CD3 antibody (Ab) revealed that this intracellular complex, which includes the adaptor proteins LAT and SLP-76/Gads as well as effector molecules such as PLCγ (Bunnell et al. 2002), is formed immediately upon stimulation. Results of these imaging analyses using Jurkat cells were consistent with previous biochemical analyses of the well-established proximal signal transduction events upon TCR stimulation (Au-Yeung et al. 2009; Samelson 2002; Jordan et al. 2003): phosphorylation of the ITAMs of CD3 chains by Lck recruits ZAP-70 which induces phosphorylation of adaptor proteins LAT and SLP-76 followed by activation of further downstream effector molecules. Davis and Krummel first observed a small cluster of CD3ζ at the interface between normal T cells and cell line B cells prior to cSMAC formation (Krummel et al. 2000).

To precisely and dynamically analyze membrane proximal events upon stimulation of normal T cells with pMHC complexes, we have performed high-resolution imaging using a combination of total internal reflection fluorescence (TIRF) microscopy and a supported planar bilayer membrane containing mobile pMHC and ICAM-1 as a pseudo-APC membrane. Using this system, we found that the TCR complexes accumulate to form small clusters, termed TCR-microclusters (TCR-MCs), immediately after the T cells attached to the membrane, which is much faster than IS formation (Yokosuka et al. 2005; Bunnell et al. 2006; Sharpe and

5 Molecular Dynamics of Co-signal Molecules in T-Cell Activation

Freeman 2002). Analysis of the generation and regulation of TCR-MCs has provided new insights into the molecular mechanisms of T-cell activation.

In this article, we first highlight our current understanding of the spatiotemporal regulation of T-cell activation through TCR-MC and co-stimulation through CD28-MCs and then discuss modulation by inhibitory co-stimulation receptors.

5.1.2 TCR- Microclusters and Initial Activation Signals

When T cells attach to a planar membrane containing peptide-MHC and ICAM-1, the TCR-MCs are first generated at the contact site. As T cells start spreading on the membrane, TCR-MCs are formed over the entire interface. After maximum spreading, T cells then start to contract and all of the TCR-MCs move toward the center of the interface to form the cSMAC. Quantitative analysis of the fluorescence intensity of individual TCR-MC revealed that a single TCR-MC contains approximately 100 TCR-CD3 complexes (Yokosuka et al. 2005). Some of the MCs fuse with each other as they move to the center from the periphery during the contraction phase. By tracking the movement of TCR signaling molecules ZAP-70 and SLP-76, as representative kinase and adaptor proteins, respectively, two critical observations were made: Firstly, a single TCR-MC contains both ZAP-70 and SLP-76, indicating that a TCR-MC represents a functional signal some containing TCR, kinases, and adaptors and is responsible for transducing T-cell activation signals. Secondly, although ZAP-70 and SLP-76 accumulate within the same TCR-MCs, unlike TCR-CD3, they do not move to the center of the interface but instead disappear on the way to the center. Thus, only the TCR complex is transported to the center to form the cSMAC. TCR-MCs are continuously generated at the edge of the periphery of the contact site, where lamellipodia-like structures may be newly associated with peptide-MHC complexes. TCR-MC generation is not restricted to the artificial bilayer system, but was confirmed at the T cell-APC interface; therefore, it should reflect the physiological state, although the detection of the TCR-MC required further technical advances in microscopic analysis in vivo.

The idea that the TCR-MC is the unit responsible for generating TCR activation signals came initially from the finding that every TCR-MC is stained with anti-phospho-tyrosine and anti-phospho-ZAP-70 Abs upon stimulation. Analysis of individual T cells revealed that the Ca^{2+} influx is induced in parallel with TCR-MC generation, which is a much earlier event than cSMAC formation. Thus, TCR-MCs represent a unit to transduce TCR recognition signals for activation. When T cells were treated with the src-kinase inhibitor PP2 to compare kinetics of the known biochemical events in the TCR proximal signaling cascade, TCR-MCs were still induced even in the absence of Lck function; however, PP2 blocked the recruitment of ZAP-70 to the TCR-MCs and generation of the cSMAC (Yokosuka et al. 2005).

By analysis of the components of TCR-MCs using individual GFP-fused signaling molecules, we found that proximal signaling molecules, such as CD3s, Lck, ZAP-70, LAT, SLP-76, Gads, Grb2, Itk, PLCγ, PI3K, Carma1, IKK, Vav, Nck, and WASP, are contained within TCR-MCs, but other molecules such as Ras, Rac,

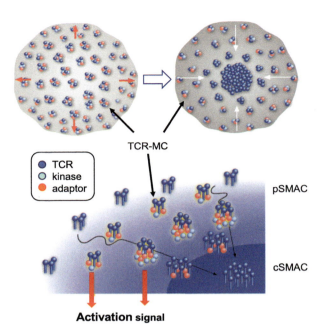

Fig. 5.1 Spatiotemporal regulation of TCR microcluster formation at immune synapse. A T cell exhibits sequential processes, spreading, contraction, and immune synapse formation, upon antigen/MHC recognition by TCR. A T cell generates TCR microcluster (MC) containing TCR, kinases, and adaptors immediately after a T cell attaches to APC or planar bilayer. Activation signals are induced through TCR-MCs. TCR-MCs move toward the center of the interface to generate cSMAC, whereas kinases and adaptors do not move to cSMAC and dissociate from MCs during the course to cSMAC

Sos, Erk, Akt, Pdk-1, and CD45 are not present. Therefore, consistent with the proposed role of TCR-MCs, the proximal signaling molecules to induce initial activation signals are the main components of the TCR-MCs. These findings are almost entirely consistent with those derived from analysis of the signaling complex in Jurkat cells (Bunnell et al. 2002, 2006), except that the TCR-CD3 complex is not involved within the signaling complex since the TCR complex on the cell surface is fixed and does not move in Jurkat cells stimulated with immobilized Ab (Fig. 5.1).

5.2 Dynamics of CD28 Co-stimulation in T-Cell Activation

5.2.1 Dynamics of CD28

T-cell activation is positively and negatively regulated by several co-stimulation signals through co-stimulation receptors, which consequently determine the fate of T cells. The major positive co-stimulation receptor is CD28, whose ligands on APCs are CD80 and CD86 (Sharpe and Freeman 2002; Rudd and Schneider 2003). It has been known for some time that when T cells are stimulated in the absence of CD28-mediated co-stimulation, they become unresponsive, a state termed "anergy" (Harding et al. 1992; Schwartz 2003). It has also been shown that the co-stimulation signal can be delivered independently of TCR signals, since TCR stimulation without co-ligation of these receptors significantly enhances T-cell activation. In spite of extensive analysis of CD28 signaling pathways, which have suggested a critical role of PI3K to mediate co-stimulation signals (Pages et al. 1994; Harada et al. 2003), the molecular nature and spatial relationship between CD28 and TCR remain unclear.

We analyzed the dynamics of CD28 and related signaling molecules, particularly to understand their spatial and temporal regulation and the signaling relationship between TCR-MCs and co-stimulation (Yokosuka et al. 2008). Upon initial Ag stimulation, CD28 generates microclusters that are completely colocalized with TCR-MCs. CD28-MCs moved to the center of the interface, similar to the TCR. When the cSMAC was formed, CD28 accumulated at the peripheral areas within the cSMAC, which was still within the cSMAC since the CD28 accumulated area was surrounded by the ring of LFA-1 representing the pSMAC. Therefore, after T-cell stimulation, CD28 as the major co-stimulation receptor is colocalized with TCR-MCs at the early phase and then later with the cSMAC. These CD28 dynamics suggested that the CD28-mediated signal should be transmitted together with TCR signals.

Accumulation of CD28 into the cSMAC is regulated by the strength of the co-stimulation and TCR signals (Fig. 5.2). We have defined two distinct sub-regions within the cSMAC based on high-resolution microscopic analysis, CD3^{hi} and CD3^{lo} (Fig. 5.2) (Saito et al. 2010). The CD3^{hi} region represents the classic cSMAC, in which TCR-CD3 robustly accumulated. When analyzed using fluorescent-labeled MHC-peptide (pMHC) molecules on a planar bilayer, this CD3^{hi} region did not overlap with the pMHC clusters, indicating that the CD3^{hi} region was not associated with pMHC on the cell surface, but was instead internalized within the cells by endocytosis for degradation. In contrast, the CD3^{lo} regions overlapped with pMHC, indicating that this region was associated with pMHC on the cell surface. Furthermore, we performed FLAP analysis, a technique that uses a strong laser to bleach fluorescence regionally and then analyzes dynamics of the molecule recovering. We observed that the CD3^{hi} region had a very rigid structure, whereas the CD3^{lo} region was dynamically regulated and the fluorescence immediately recovered. CD28-MCs overlapped with the CD3^{lo} region. As described later for CTLA-4, the CD3^{lo} region, where various co-stimulation receptors accumulate for regulation, is the target for both positive and negative co-stimulation; thus, we call this region the "signaling cSMAC." Therefore, the accumulation of CD28 in the cSMAC is dependent on the mutual strength of TCR and CD28 co-stimulation signaling. When both TCR and co-stimulation signals are weak, the cSMAC is very small, but is large and contains many CD3^{hi} as well as CD3^{lo} (signaling cSMAC) regions when both signals are strong. In this situation, strong activation signals as well as TCR degradation are induced. On the other hand, when a strong TCR signal

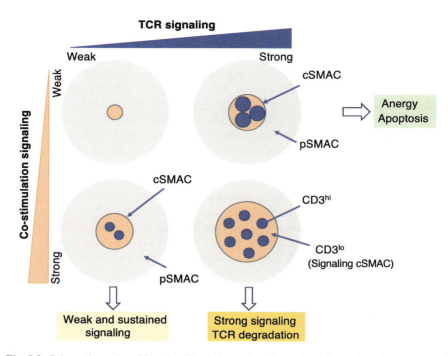

Fig. 5.2 Schematic model of functionally distinct sub-regions of cSMAC. cSMAC is segregated into two sub-regions according to the density of TCR-CD3: CD3^{hi} and CD3^{lo}. The size of cSMAC is determined by TCR signal strength. In the absence of CD28 co-stimulation, the majority of cSMAC are CD3^{hi} region where extensive internalization and degradation of TCR occurs. In contrast, in the presence of strong co-stimulation, CD3^{lo} region becomes dominant as "signaling cSMAC" which is responsible for sustained co-stimulation signaling. Therefore, the proportion of CD3^{hi} and CD3^{lo} regions are determined by the strength of TCR signal and co-stimulation signal. TCR signal strength depends on antigen concentration, while co-stimulation strength depends on the expression of CD28 on T cells and CD80/86 on APC

and a weak co-stimulation signal are induced, large CD3^{hi} but small CD3^{lo} regions are generated, which induces a rather anergic or apoptotic status in the T cells. Conversely, strong co-stimulation and weak TCR signals induce large CD3^{lo} and small CD3^{hi} regions within the cSMAC, which may result in weak and sustained activation signals (Fig. 5.2).

5.2.2 Dynamics of PKCθ in CD28 Co-stimulation

To identify molecule(s) mediating downstream events in CD28-mediated co-stimulation that function together with, and move similarly to, CD28, we have analyzed the dynamic movement of various signaling molecules as GFP-fusion proteins.

The molecules that are thought to be involved in CD28-mediated co-stimulation, including PI3K, Grb2, Gads, Itk, Vav, PP2A, and PKCθ (Raab et al. 1995; Watanabe et al. 2006; Villalba et al. 2000; Chuang et al. 2000), were chosen for these studies, although most of these molecules are also involved in the TCR-downstream signaling pathway. After analyzing the dynamics of these molecules individually, we found that only PKCθ accumulated into the cSMAC upon stimulation. Indeed, PKCθ was colocalized in TCR-MCs upon initial activation, then moved to the center of the interface together with the TCR, and then accumulated in the same region as CD28 in the cSMAC. CD28 and PKCθ not only move together, but more critically, they are also physically associated, since PKCθ was co-immunoprecipitated with CD28 in normal T cells upon TCR stimulation. The localization of CD28 in the signaling cSMAC is dynamically maintained. On the basis of the observation that clusters of both CD28 and PKCθ recovered soon after these regions were photobleached. In addition, blocking of the CD28-CD80 interaction by CTLA-4-Ig abrogated the accumulation of not only CD28 but also PKCθ in that region, indicating that CD28 recruits PKCθ to the signaling cSMAC probably to mediate sustained co-stimulation signals such as NF-κB activation. Indeed, we observed that Carma1, which forms the Carma1-Bcl10-Malt1(CBM) complex to induce NF-κB activation in lymphocytes, also accumulates in the same region as CD28 and PKCθ upon TCR stimulation (Yokosuka et al. 2010). We analyzed CD28 mutants to identify the regions of the molecule responsible for CD28 cluster formation and PKCθ recruitment. Mutant CD28 lacking CD80-binding capacity cannot form CD28-MCs, whereas a CD28 mutant lacking the cytoplasmic tail could induce clustering but failed to recruit and accumulate PKCθ, and this further correlated with defective co-stimulatory function.

Therefore, our imaging analysis of CD28-mediated co-stimulation revealed an important mode of signal regulation during co-stimulation: the CD28 co-stimulatory receptor initially accumulates in the TCR-MCs and then moves to the special region of the cSMAC. PKCθ is associated with, and co-translocate with, CD28 and mediates sustained co-stimulation signals, particularly for NF-κB activation.

5.2.3 Regulation of CARMA1 Clustering by CD28 Co-stimulation

CARMA1 (or CARD11) is a CARD domain-bearing scaffold protein that forms clusters with Bcl10 and Malt-1 to form the CBM complex upon T-cell activation (Good et al. 2011). The CBM complex has been shown to be critical for inducing NF-κB activation in both T and B cells (Thome 2004). If any component of the CBM complex is absent, T-cell activation events, such as proliferation and cytokine production, are not induced at all upon antigen stimulation. Activation of the CBM complex to induce NF-κB requires CD28 co-stimulation. As briefly described above, the dynamic behavior of CARMA1 is similar to CD28 and

PKCθ, namely, it accumulates in the TCR-MC at initial TCR activation and then moves and accumulates in the signaling cSMAC suggesting that the CD28-PKCθ-CARMA1 axis in the same region of the cSMAC may induce NF-kB activation as co-stimulation signals.

It has been shown that CARMA1 is the molecule with the most frequent mutations in diffuse large B-cell lymphoma (DLBCL) (Lenz et al. 2008). Such lymphoma-inducing mutant CARMA1, as an "oncogenic CARD11," forms spontaneous large clusters in B cells. If these mutants are expressed in T cells, spontaneous large clusters of CARMA1 were also observed, similar to those in the B-cell tumors. These B cells, and even T cells bearing spontaneous clusters of CARMA1, show strong activation of NF-kB, and such sustained activation induces tumorigenesis. In contrast to spontaneous cluster formation by the oncogenic mutant CARMA1, normal CARMA1 forms clusters only upon TCR-CD28 stimulation, which is critical for promoting the proper level of NF-kB activation for sustained co-stimulation signals (Hara et al. 2015; Hara and Saito 2009).

5.2.4   *Rltpr-Mediated Regulation of Co-stimulation*

Rltpr (CARMIL2) was identified as a mediator of CD28 co-stimulatory signals based on the analysis of mice with a mutant LAT (Thr136 to Phe), which lacks PLCγ association and exhibits abnormal activation of CD4+ T cells (Aguado et al. 2002; Sommers et al. 2002). The Malissen group developed an approach to identify molecules that repair the abnormal activation phenotype of the LAT mutant mice by screening mice on the LAT mutant background after random mutagenesis. They found a mutant mouse bearing a mutation of Rltpr, which showed normal T-cell activation. The Rltpr mutant as well as Rltpr-deficient mice phenocopied the CD28-deficient mice, indicating that Rltpr contributes to CD28 co-stimulation signaling. The dynamic behavior of Rltpr at the immune synapse upon stimulation is almost identical to that of CD28, PKCθ, and CARMA1, which colocalize with TCR-MC at the early activation phase and accumulate later into the cSMAC, as described above. This result also suggests that Rltpr is involved in CD28 cluster formation and signaling at the immune synapse (Liang et al. 2013). Indeed, T cells with the mutant Rltpr have defective clustering of PKCθ and CARMA1, although TCR-MC and CD28 clusters are generated similarly to wild-type T cells, indicating that Rltpr connects the CD28 and PKCθ/CARMA1 pathways. Recent LC-mass analysis demonstrated that Rltpr physically associates with CD28 and CARMA1 (Roncagalli et al. 2016).

Rltpr is known to bind the actin capping protein CAPZ (A, B), which induces remodeling of the cortical actin cytoskeleton and probably also induces endocytosis of CD28 upon activation. Therefore, Rltpr functions in CD28 signaling in two ways,

5 Molecular Dynamics of Co-signal Molecules in T-Cell Activation

first through the association/link to the PKCθ/CARMA1 pathway, probably to induce NF-kB activation, and second through association with the actin cytoskeleton for CD28 endocytosis (Sommers et al. 2002).

The similar behaviors of Rltpr and CD28/PKCθ/CARMA1 in imaging analysis have now been directly demonstrated by their biochemical as well as functional association for CD28 co-stimulatory signaling.

5.2.5 Spatial Regulation of Signal 1 Versus Signal 2

Regarding the spatial regulation of activation and co-stimulation signals, particularly in the cSMAC, we defined two distinct sub-regions in the cSMAC based on our high-resolution microscopic analysis. The distinction between the two regions is based on the density of CD3, i.e., CD3^{hi} and CD3^{lo} regions (Fig. 5.2); Yokosuka and Saito 2010). CD3^{hi} represents the well-known typical cSMAC where there are abundant TCR-CD3 complexes. When analyzed using fluorescently labeled probes for MHC class II, it became clear that there was no overlap between the CD3^{hi} region and the pMHC; however, the CD3^{lo} region correlated well with pMHC. This analysis indicates that TCRs in the CD3^{lo} region are associated with pMHC on the cell surface, whereas TCRs in the CD3^{hi} region appear to no longer be assembled with pMHC and are probably destined for internalization and degradation. Photobleaching experiments indicated that the CD3^{lo} region is dynamically regulated, whereas CD3^{hi} is very rigid and did not recover after photobleaching. Importantly, since CD28 and PKCθ as well as Carma-1 all accumulate in this CD3^{lo} region, it is the region mediating signal transduction, particularly for sustained co-stimulation signal, as the "signaling cSMAC."

The relative dimensions of the CD3^{lo} and CD3^{hi} regions are regulated by the strength of the TCR and co-stimulation signals as shown in Fig. 5.2. A high dose of Ag induces a larger proportion of CD3^{hi}, which will be internalized/degraded, whereas a low dose of Ag results in a larger CD3^{lo} region, which induces active signaling. Conversely, strong co-stimulation increases the CD3^{lo}, and weak co-stimulation increases the CD3^{hi} regions, respectively.

These studies lead to a new global and testable model for TCR signaling. Spatially differential regulation through the peripheral TCR-MC and the signaling cSMAC represent the site for "signal 1" and "signal 2" described in classic co-stimulation models (Schwartz 2003). TCR-MCs induce Ag recognition signals through the TCR as "signal 1," and the signaling cSMAC (CD3^{lo} cSMAC) induces sustained co-stimulatory signals as "signal 2" within a single T cell (Fig. 5.3).

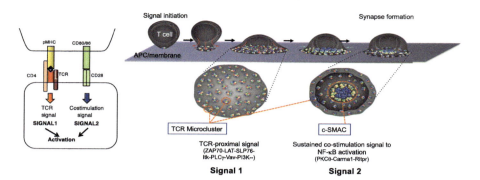

Fig. 5.3 Differential compartmentalization for antigen-recognition signal (signal 1) and co-stimulation signal (signal 2). Whereas peripheral TCR-MCs induce Ag recognition signal through activation of ZAP70, LAT, and SLP76, co-stimulation signals are induced in the localized specialized cSMAC regions "signaling cSMAC" through recruitment of CD28, PKCθ, and CARMA1. From the classical "two-signal" model of T-cell activation, these signals may represent "signal 1" and "signal 2," respectively, within a single cell basis. Therefore, these signals are generated by spatially distinct signaling modules

5.3 Dynamics of CTLA-4 in T-Cell Activation

5.3.1 Regulation of Cell Surface CTLA-4 Expression

After analyzing the dynamic regulation of CD28-mediated positive co-stimulation, we investigated the negative regulation mediated by CTLA-4, one of the major negative co-stimulatory receptors. CTLA-4 has the same ligands, CD80 and CD86, as CD28, but whereas CD28 is constitutively expressed on the cell surface, CTLA-4 is not expressed in resting normal T cells, except on regulatory T cells, which constitutively express high levels of CTLA-4, until its expression is induced by TCR stimulation (Linsley et al. 1996; Iida et al. 2000). The *ctla4* gene is transcribed and translated upon TCR stimulation, but in the absence of further stimulation, most of the protein is retained and degraded within lysosomes through endocytosis by assembly with the AP2 complex (Shiratori et al. 1997; Zhang and Allison 1997; Saito 1998). Upon TCR stimulation, endocytosis is inhibited by the disassembly from AP2, and CTLA-4 accumulates and is expressed on the cell surface. This regulation can be observed by microscopy as the dynamics of CTLA-4. Since CTLA-4 has a much higher affinity than CD28 for the same ligands, CD80/86, even low-level expression of CTLA-4 on the cell surface can compete for ligand binding with CD28, which is thought to be the main mechanism of CTLA-4-mediated inhibition of T-cell activation. Previous studies revealed that CTLA-4 is transported from storage in endosome/lysosomes to the plasma membrane (as a "secretory lysosome") upon further T-cell stimulation. The induction of cell surface CTLA-4 expression is only induced by strong TCR activation, whereas weak activation leads only to translocation of these vesicles to the vicinity of the plasma membrane (Egan and Allison 2002). However, exactly how CTLA-4 blocks T-cell activation had remained unclear.

5.3.2 Dynamics of CTLA-4 and Its Inhibitory Function

When we analyzed spatiotemporal regulation of CTLA-4 expression upon TCR stimulation on planar bilayer membrane, we found that CTLA-4 also forms microclusters upon stimulation, but these do not initially colocalize in TCR-MCs and instead directly accumulate in the cSMAC (Yokosuka et al. 2010). Consistent with previous functional data (Egan and Allison 2002), this accumulation into the cSMAC is only induced by strong and not by weak stimulation, such as stimulation with low concentrations of antigen or a weak agonist. The region of the cSMAC where the CTLA-4-MCs accumulate is exactly the same region where CD28 and PKCθ accumulate (signaling cSMAC). Thus, when CTLA-4-MCs accumulate into the cSMAC upon TCR stimulation, CD28 and PKCθ do not accumulate anymore at the same region. Therefore, CTLA-4 pushes CD28 and PKCθ away from the specific region of the cSMAC to the outside of the cSMAC, which results in the blockade of CD28-mediated sustained co-stimulation signals. This is at least a major inhibitory mechanism of the CTLA-4-CD28 axis, in addition to negative signal delivery by CTLA-4 binding to the ligand. To determine whether the accumulation of CTLA-4 in the cSMAC is required for CTLA-4-mediated inhibition of T-cell activation, we used a trick by preparing CTLA-4 chimeras with an unrelated surface protein CD22, which possess the first ligand-binding Ig domain of CTLA-4 together with various sizes of the CD22 ectodomain. The idea behind this experiment is that only short molecules because of their short extracellular Ig domains can accumulate in the cSMAC, whereas large molecules would be excluded and accumulate outside of the cSMAC. This is analogous to the exclusion of large molecules such as CD45 from the immunological synapse. Indeed, the short ectodomain (one or two Ig domains)-bearing CTLA-4 were colocalized with the TCR-MCs and accumulated later in the cSMAC, whereas molecules with longer ectodomains failed to localize in either the TCR-MCs or the cSMAC. Functionally, only CTLA-4 with short ectodomains, which colocalized with TCR-MCs, could inhibit T-cell activation. These results indicated the importance of CTLA-4 localization in the cSMAC to mediate its inhibitory function (Yokosuka et al. 2010).

5.4 Dynamics of PD-1 in T-Cell Activation

5.4.1 Dynamics of PD-1

PD-1 has been shown to mediate negative regulation of T-cell function. This was first evidenced in PD-1-deficient mice (KO), which develop autoimmune diseases with aging, the symptoms depending on the genetic background of the mice. PD-1 KO mice on a C57BL/6 background develop lupus-like arthritis and glomerulonephritis, whereas those on a BALB/c background have dilated cardiomyopathy (Nishimura et al. 2001). CTLA-4 deficiency results in acute lymphadenopathy within several weeks after birth (Waterhouse et al. 1995), and autoimmune diseases resulting from PD-1 deficiency develop at ~6 months, suggesting functional differences between these two inhibitory receptors. PD-1-KO mice exhibit enhanced T-cell activation and increase effector/memory T cells. Since PD-1 possesses ITIM and ITSM inhibitory motifs within its cytoplasmic tail, the mechanism of PD-1-mediated inhibition of T-cell activation has been suggested to be through its association with phosphatases SHP-1 and/or SHP-2 (Okazaki et al. 2001).

To gain precise insight into the inhibitory mechanism, we have analyzed the dynamic features of PD-1 and the recruitment of effector molecules, including phosphatases, upon T-cell activation (Yokosuka et al. 2012). PD-1 is not expressed on resting T cells and is only induced upon TCR stimulation. Activated/effector T cells, exhausted T cells resulting from chronic infection or multiple rounds of antigen stimulation, and regulatory T cells express cell surface PD-1. PD-1 generates microclusters upon TCR stimulation by interaction with its ligand PD-L1 or PD-L2 on the APC or the planar bilayer. No clustering at all was observed in the absence of the ligands. The ligand-dependent PD-1 microclusters colocalized with TCR-MCs at the initial activation phase, and later, after cSMACs formed, PD-1 accumulated into signaling cSMAC where CD28 and PKCθ accumulate.

5.4.2 Molecular Mechanism of PD-1-Mediated Suppression

Functional analysis of T cells expressing PD-1with ITIM or ITSM mutations showed that the ITSM has the dominant role in mediating inhibition of T-cell activation (Yokosuka et al. 2012). The analysis of the association of the PD-1 ITSM/ITIM with phosphatases revealed that PD-1 transiently associates with SHP2 but not SHP1 after TCR activation. This was also confirmed by FRET analysis, where PD-1 and SHP2 but not SHP1 generated a positive FRET signal. When PD-1 was directly fused with SHP1 or SHP2 at the C-terminus, both chimeric proteins could induce suppression of T-cell activation. Therefore, if PD-1 recruits either SHP1 or SHP2, either could be inhibitory. However, under physiological conditions, SHP2 is selectively recruited to PD-1 upon stimulation and mediates the inhibition of T-cell activation. The molecular basis of the specificity for SHP2 is unknown.

The target molecules for PD-1-recruited SHP2 to dephosphorylate were analyzed by both biochemical and imaging approaches. Very upstream molecules in TCR signaling, such as CD3ζ, ZAP70, and SLP76, as well as downstream effector molecules, such as Vav-1 and Erk, were dephosphorylated by SHP2 upon PD-1 stimulation. These data indicate that PD-1/SHP2-mediated dephosphorylation occurs very upstream in TCR activation signaling. A comparison of the dynamic features and the related inhibitory functions of CTLA-4 and PD-1 is summarized in (Fig. 5.4).

Receptor	PD-1	CTLA-4
Expression	Cell surface of activated T cells Constitutively on Tfh	Secretary lysosome in activated T cells Constitutively on Treg
Ligands	PD-L1 / PD-L2	CD80 / CD86
localization at Immune synapse	TCR-MC / c-SMAC	TCR/CD3^{lo} c-SMAC
Cytoplasmic tyrosine motif	ITIM / ITSM	ITIM-like
Phosphatase assembly	SHP2	PP2A / SHP1,2 ?
Inhibition of TCR signal	Dephosphorylation of proximal TCR signaling as CD3ζ. PLCγ, Erk	Compete ligand-binding with CD28, leading to disruption of CD28-PKCθ-CARMA1 clusters

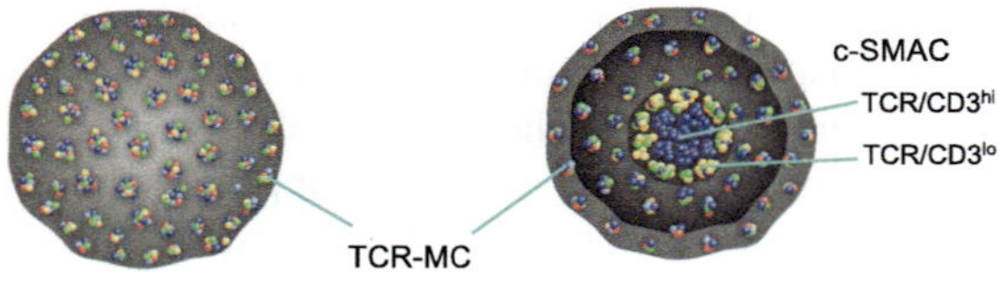

Fig. 5.4 Distinct mechanism of inhibitory signals mediated through PD-1 and CTLA-4. Although both PD-1 and CTLA-4 are expressed only upon T-cell activation, the majority of CTLA-4 in activated T cells is still stored in secretory lysosomes, while PD-1 is expressed on the cell surface. Both generate MCs in the ligand-dependent manner. While PD-1 is localized in TCR-MC and later in cSMAC, CTLA-4 is directly recruited into cSMAC. PD-1 recruits specifically SHP-2 to its ITIM/ITSM regions and induces dephosphorylation of the upstream TCR signal molecules. In contrast, CTLA-4 competes the ligand binding with CD28 at cSMAC which lead the disruption of CD28-PKCθ-CARMA1 axis for sustained co-stimulation signal. These two inhibitory receptors induce quite different mechanism to mediate inhibitory functions

5.4.3 Colocalization of PD-1 and TCR Microclusters

Since PD-1 colocalizes with TCR-MCs to mediate inhibition of T-cell activation, we addressed whether the colocalization between PD-1 and TCR-MC is required for this inhibition. We used a trick similar to the one used in the CTLA-4 studies, constructing PD-1 chimeras with the unrelated surface protein CD22 that all possess the first ligand-binding Ig domain of PD-1 but have various sizes of the CD22 ectodomain. We could use this strategy because we previously showed that the TCR-MC is surrounded by adhesion molecules such as LFA1 and Pyk2, which we call a "microsynapse," since its structure is similar to the immune synapse in microscale (Hashimoto-Tane et al. 2016). Indeed, we found that whereas the short ectodomain (one or two Ig domains)-bearing PD-1 colocalized well with the TCR-MCs,

PD-1 chimeras with larger ectodomains failed to colocalize there. Functionally, the short PD-1 chimeras inhibited phosphorylation of signaling molecules such as Erk and Vav, but the larger PD-1 chimeras failed to do so. Consequently, the short PD-1 induced inhibition of T-cell activation and cytokine secretion, whereas the longer PD-1 s could not. Therefore, colocalization of PD-1 clusters with TCR-MCs coincides with the ability to inhibit T-cell activation, and the colocalization of PD-1 with TCR-MC is required to mediate suppression of T-cell activation (Yokosuka et al. 2012).

It is well known that PD-1^{hi} T cells are induced as exhausted T cells by chronic virus infection or by multiple rounds of antigen stimulation (Barber et al. 2006). Such exhausted T cells can be restored to normal function by blocking the PD-1-PD-ligand interaction by the addition of anti-PD-1 (or anti-PD-L) Ab. Anti-cancer immunotherapy has been started to apply for cancer patients with anti-PD-1 or PD-L Ab (Topalian et al. 2012). Parallel to the functional restoration, the colocalization of PD-1 with TCR-MC in exhausted T cells, which induces inhibitory signals, is also inhibited by the addition of anti-PD-1 Ab. Therefore, checkpoint Ab treatment induces separation of the colocalized PD-1 cluster from TCR-MC, which results in potentiation of T-cell activation and further anti-cancer immunity.

Conversely, if the TCR-MC could be colocalized with PD-1 independently of its ligands by some special method such as bi-specific antibodies crosslinking of the TCR and PD-1, this treatment should induce specific suppression of activation/function of antigen-specific T cells, particularly in diseases with abnormally activated T cells such as autoimmunity. This could be one applicable intervention to translate the basic finding that colocalization of TCR-MC and PD-1 induces suppression of the T-cell activation/response into clinical practice.

5.5 Dynamics of Other Co-signal Receptors

There are many known co-stimulatory receptors on T cells and their ligands on APCs. Only major co-stimulatory receptors in the B7 family are described in this article from the imaging/dynamic point of view. There are other critical families of positive and negative co-stimulatory receptors, for example, TNF-family receptors, and their dynamics in the immune synapse and their relationship with TCR-MCs should be analyzed further.

A prototypical positive co-stimulation receptor is ICOS, which belongs to the CD28 superfamily and is expressed on the surface of activated/memory-type T cells but not by naïve T cells. ICOS is structurally and functionally related to CD28 (Hutloff et al. 1999). Preliminary experiments on the dynamic features of ICOS on activated T cells demonstrate that it also accumulates in the TCR-MC upon TCR stimulation and recruits PI3K in a similar relationship to that of CD28, which accumulates in the TCR-MC and recruits PKCθ. The ICOS-PI3K axis mediates co-stimulatory signals in activated/memory T cells (Fos et al. 2008).

Another prototypical co-stimulation inhibitory receptor is LAG3 (CD223). LAG3 belongs to the Ig superfamily and contains four Ig-like domains in its extracellular region. LAG3 binds to MHC class II with higher affinity than CD4 (Triebel et al. 1990). Functional analysis revealed that LAG3 inhibits T-cell activation in a manner similar to CTLA-4 and PD-1 (Nguyen and Ohashi 2015; Lui and Davis 2018). When the dynamic features of LAG3 were analyzed, LAG3 also accumulated in TCR-MCs upon TCR stimulation. Whether colocalization between LAG3 and TCR-MC is required for LAG3-mediated suppression of T-cell activation, similar to PD-1, and the mechanism of LAG3 suppression of T-cell activation needs to be addressed further.

5.6 Conclusion Remarks and Future Perspectives

In this article, we summarize the findings/knowledge on the dynamic features of TCR and co-stimulation signals which is accumulated during a decade. T-cell activation is induced upon antigen/MHC recognition by TCR. Activation signals are generated initially at the site of TCR microcluster and then at cSMAC for sustained co-stimulation signals. High-resolution microscopic study revealed the existence of a signaling region within cSMAC where dominant co-stimulation molecules we analyzed (CD28, CTLA-4, and PD-1) accumulate and regulate for sustained co-stimulation signals. In this region, CD28 and CTLA-4 compete for the ligand binding, which determines positive vs. negative fate/direction of T-cell activation, and PD-1 associates close to TCR and dephosphorylates TCR-upstream signaling molecules. Activation signals are induced and regulated by molecular clustering as shown by TCR, CD28, CARMA1, CTLA-4, and PD-1. Generation and dissociation of the cluster formation determine the direction and fate of particular activation signals. When these clusters localize close enough to TCR-MC, TCR activation signal is regulated by the clusters positively or negatively. This seems to be a general rule for T-cell activation regulation. From this point of view, several other co-stimulatory and coinhibitory receptors are also the candidate for modulating T-cell activation as have already been studied as checkpoint inhibitors. Not only activation of T cells by checkpoint inhibitors, but also it is possible to suppress antigen-specific T cells as discussed above by crosslinking between TCR-MC and inhibitory receptors (independent of its ligand binding). Not only CTLA-4 and PD-1 but also several critical inhibitory receptors have to be extensively studied for both positive and negative regulation of T-cell activation.

Acknowledgments We thank M.L. Dustin, M. Tokunaga, H. Yagita, M. Azuma, and T. Honjo for the collaboration; T. Yokosuka and A. Hashimoto-Tane for the main study; W. Kobayashi, M. Takamatsu, M. Sakuma, and M. Unno for the technical help; and M. Yoshioka and H. Yamaguchi for the secretarial help.

References

Aguado E, Richelme S, Nuñez-Cruz S, Miazek A, Mura AM, Richelme M, Guo XJ, Sainty D, He HT, Malissen B, Malissen M (2002) Induction of T helper type 2 immunity by a point mutation in the LAT adaptor. Science 296:2036–2040

Au-Yeung BB, Deindl S, Hwu LY, Palacios EH, Levin SE, Kuriyan J, Weiss A (2009 Mar) The structure, regulation and function of ZAP-70. Immunol Rev 228:41–57

Barber DL, Wherry EJ, Masopust D, Zhu B, Allison JP, Sharpe AH, Freeman GJ, Ahmed R (2006) Restoring function in exhausted CD8 T cells during chronic viral infection. Nature 439:682–687

Bunnell SC, Hong DI, Kardon JR, Yamazaki T, McGlade CJ, Bar VA, Samelson LE (2002) T cell receptor ligation induces the formation of dynamically regulated signaling assemblies. J Cell Biol 158:1263–1275

Bunnell SC, Singer AL, Hong DI, Jacque BH, Jordan MS, Seminario MC, Barr VA, Koretzky GA, Samelson LE (2006) Persistence of cooperatively stabilized signaling clusters derives T-cell activation. Mol Cell Biol 26:7155–7166

Chuang E, Fisher TS, Morgan RW, Robbins MD, Duerr JM, Vander Heiden MG, Gardner JP, Hambor JE, Neveu MJ, Thompson CB (2000) The CD28 and CTLA-4 receptors associate with the serine/threonine phosphatase PP2A. Immunity 13:313–322

Egan JG, Allison JP (2002) Cytotoxic T lymphocyte antigen-4 accumulation in the immunological synapse is regulated by TCR signal strength. Immunity 16:23–35

Fos C, Salles A, Lang V, Carrette F, Audebert S, Pastor S, Ghiotto M, Olive D, Bismuth G, Nunès JA (2008) ICOS ligation recruits the p50alpha PI3K regulatory subunit to the immunological synapse. J Immunol 181:1969–1977

Good MC, Zalatan JG, Lim WA (2011) Scaffold proteins: hubs for controlling the flow of cellular information. Science 332:680–686

Grakoui A, Bromley SK, Sumen C, Davis MM, Shaw AS, Allen PM, Dustin ML (1999) The immunological synapse: a molecular machine controlling T cell activation. Science 285:221–227

Hara H, Saito T (2009) CARD9 vs. CARMA1 in innate and adaptive immunities. Trends Immunol 30:234–242

Hara H, Yokosuka T, Hirakawa H, Ishihara C, Yasukawa S, Yamazaki M, Koseki H, Yoshida H, Saito T (2015) Clustering of CARMA1 through SH3-GUK domain interactions is required for its activation of NF-kB signaling. Nat Commun 6:5555

Harada Y, Ohgai D, Watanabe R, Okano K, Koiwai O, Tanabe K, Toma H, Altman A, Abe R (2003) A single amino acid alteration in cytoplasmic domain determines IL-2 promoter activation by ligation of CD28 but not inducible costimulator (ICOS). J Exp Med 197:257–162

Harding FA, McArthur JG, Gross JA, Raulet DH, Allison JP (1992) CD28-mediated signaling co-stimulates murine T cells and prevents induction of anergy in T-cell clones. Nature 356:607–609

Hashimoto-Tane A, Sakuma M, Ike H, Yokosuka T, Kimura Y, Ohara O, Saito T (2016) Micro adhesion-ring surrounding TCR microclusters are essential for T cell activation. J Exp Med 213:1609–1625

Hutloff A, Dittrich AM, Beier KC, Eljaschewitsch B, Kraft R, Anagnostopoulos I, Kroczek RA (1999) ICOS is an inducible T-cell co-stimulator structurally and functionally related to CD28. Nature 397:263–266

Iida T, Ohno H, Nakaseko C, Sakuma M, Takeda-Ezaki M, Arase H, Kominami E, Fujisawa T, Saito T (2000) Regulation of cell surface expression of CTLA-4 by secretion of CTLA-4-containing lysosomes upon activation of CD4+ T cells. J Immunol 165:5062–5068

Jordan MS, Singer AL, Koretzky GA (2003) Adaptors as central mediators of signal transduction in immune cells. Nat Immunol 4:110–116

Krummel MF, Sjaastad MD, Wulfin D, Davis MM (2000) Differential clustering of CD4 and CD3zeta during T cell recognition. Science 289:1349–1352

5 Molecular Dynamics of Co-signal Molecules in T-Cell Activation

Lee KH, Dinner AR, Tu C, Campi F, Rachaudhuri S, Verma R, Sims TN, Burack WR, Wu H, Wang J, Kanagawa O, Markiewicz M, Allen PM, Dustin ML, Chakraborty AK, Shaw AS (2003) The immunological synapse balances T cell receptor signaling and degradation. Science 302:1218–1222

Lenz G, Davis RE, Ngo VN, Lam L, George TC, Wright GW, Dave SS, Zhao H, Xu W, Rosenwald A, Ott G, Muller-Hermelink HK, Gascoyne RD, Connors JM, Rimsza LM, Campo E, Jaffe ES, Delabie J, Smeland EB, Fisher RI, Chan WC, Staudt LM (2008) Oncogenic CARD11 mutations in human diffuse large B cell lymphoma. Science 319:1676–1679

Liang Y, Cucchetti M, Roncagalli R, Yokosuka T, Malzac A, Bertosio E, Imbert J, Nijman IJ, Suchanek M, Saito T, Wülfing C, Malissen B, Malissen M (2013) The lymphoid lineage-specific actin-uncapping protein Rltpr is essential for costimulation via CD28 and the development of regulatory T cells. Nat Immunol 14:858–866

Linsley PS, Bradshaw J, Greene J, Peach R, Bennett KL, Mittler RS (1996) Intracellular trafficking of CTLA-4 and focal localization towards sites of TCR engagement. Immunity 4:535–543

Lui Y, Davis SJ (2018) LAG-3: a very singular immune checkpoint. Nat Immunol 19:1278–1279

Monks CR, Freiburg BA, Kupfer H, Sciaky N, Kupfer A (1998) Three-dimensional segregation of supramolecular activation clusters in T cells. Nature 395:82–86

Nguyen LT, Ohashi PS (2015) Clinical blockage of PD1 and LAG3 – potential mechanisms of action. Nat Rev Immunol 15:45–56

Nishimura H, Okazaki T, Tanaka Y, Nakatani K, Hara M, Matsumori A, Sasayama S, Mizoguchi A, Hiai H, Minato N, Honjo T (2001) Autoimmune dilated cardiomyopathy in PD-1 receptor-deficient mice. Science 291:319–322

Okazaki T, Maeda A, Nishimura H, Kurosaki T, Honjo T (2001) PD-1 immunoreceptor inhibits B cell receptor-mediated signaling by recruiting src homology 2-domain-containing tyrosine phosphatase 2 to phosphotyrosine. Proc Natl Acad Sci U S A 98:13866–13871

Pages F, Ragueneau M, Rottapel R, Truneh A, Nunes J, Imbert J, Olive D (1994) Binding of phosphatidylinositol-3-OH kinase to CD28 is required for T cell signaling. Nature 369:327–329

Raab M, Cai YC, Bunnell SC, Heyeck SD, Berg LJ, Rudd CE (1995) p56Lck and p59Fyn regulate CD28 binding to phosphatidylinositol-3-kinase, growth factor receptor-bound protein GRB-2, and T cell-specific protein-tyrosine kinase ITK: implications for T cell costimulation. Proc Natl Acad Sci U S A 92:8891–8895

Roncagalli R, Cucchetti M, Jarmuzynski N, Grégoire C, Bergot E, Audebert S, Baudelet E, Menoita MG, Joachim A, Durand S, Suchanek M, Fiore F, Zhang L, Liang Y, Camoin L, Malissen M, Malissen B (2016) The scaffolding function of the RLTPR protein explains its essential role for CD28 co-stimulation in mouse and human T cells. J Exp Med 213:2437–2457

Rudd CE, Schneider H (2003) Unifying concepts in CD28, ICOS and CTLA4 co-receptor signaling. Nat Rev Immunol 3:544–556

Saito T (1998) Negative regulation of T cell activation. Curr Opin Immunol 10:313–321

Saito T, Yokosuka T, Hashimoto-Tane A (2010) Dynamic regulation of T cell activation and co-stimulation through TCR-microclusters. FEBS Lett 584:4865–4871

Samelson LE (2002) Signal transduction mediated by the T cell antigen receptor: the role of adapter proteins. Annu Rev Immunol 20:371–394

Schwartz RH (2003) T cell anergy. Annu Rev Immunol 21:305–334

Sharpe AH, Freeman GJ (2002) The B7-CD28 superfamily. Nat Rev Immunol 2:116–126

Shiratori T, Miyatake S, Ohno H, Nakaseko C, Isono K, Bonifatino JS, Saito T (1997) Tyrosine phosphorylation controls internalization of CTLA-4 by regulating its interaction with clathrin-associated adaptor complex AP-2. Immunity 6:583–589

Sommers CL, Park CS, Lee J, Feng C, Fuller CL, Grinberg A, Hildebrand JA, Lacaná E, Menon RK, Shores EW, Samelson LE, Love PE (2002) A LAT mutation that inhibits T cell development yet induces lymphoproliferation. Science 296:2040–2043

Thome M (2004) CARMA1, BCL-10 and MALT1 in lymphocyte development and activation. Nat Rev Immunol 4:348–359

Topalian SL, Hodi FS, Brahmer JR, Gettinger SN, Smith DC, McDermott DF, Powderly JD, Carvajal RD, Sosman JA, Atkins MB, Leming PD, Spigel DR, Antonia SJ, Horn L, Drake CG, Pardoll DM, Chen L, Sharfman WH, Anders RA, Taube JM, McMiller TL, Xu H, Korman AJ, Jure-Kunkel M, Agrawal S, McDonald D, Kollia GD, Gupta A, Wigginton JM, Sznol M (2012) Safety, activity, and immune correlates of anti-PD-1 antibody in cancer. N Engl J Med 366:2443–2454

Triebel F, Jitsukawa S, Baixeras E, Roman-Roman S, Genevee C, Viegas-Pequignot E, Hercend T (1990) LAG-3, a novel lymphocyte activation gene closely related to CD4. J Exp Med 171:1393–1405

Villalba M, Coudronniere N, Deckert M, Teixeiro E, Mas P, Altman A (2000) A novel functional interaction between Vav and PKCtheta is required for TCR-induced T cell activation. Immunity 12:151–160

Watanabe R, Harada Y, Takeda K, Takahashi J, Ohnuki K, Ogawa S, Ohgai D, Kaibara N, Koiwai O, Tanabe K et al (2006) Grb2 and Gads exhibit different interactions with CD28 and play distinct roles in CD28-medaited costimulation. J Immunol 177:1085–1091

Waterhouse P, Penninger JM, Timms E, Wakeham A, Shahinian A, Lee KP, Thompson CB, Griesser H, Mak TW (1995) Lymphoproliferative disorders with early lethality in mice deficient in Ctla-4. Science 270:985–988

Yokosuka T, Saito T (2010) The immunological synapse, TCR microclusters, and T cell activation. Curr Top Microbiol Immunol 340:81–108

Yokosuka T, Sakata-Sogawa K, Kobayashi W, Hiroshima M, Hashimoto-Tane A, Tokunaga M, Dustin ML, Saito T (2005) Newly generated T cell receptor microclusters initiate and sustain T cell activation by recruitment of Zap70 and SLP-76. Nat Immunol 6:1253–1262

Yokosuka T, Kobayashi W, Sakata-Sogawa K, Takamatsu M, Hashimoto-Tane A, Dustin M, Tokunaga M, Saito T (2008) Spatiotemporal regulation of T cell costimulation by TCR-CD28 microclusters and protein kinase c-θ translocation. Immunity 29:589–601

Yokosuka T, Kobayashi W, Takamatsu M, Sakata-Sogawa K, Zeng H, Yagita H, Takunaga M, Saito T (2010) Spatiotemporal basis of CTLA-4 costimulatory molecule-mediated negative regulation of T cell activation. Immunity 33:1–14

Yokosuka T, Takamatsu M, Kobayashi-Imanishi W, Hashimoto-Tane A, Azuma M, Saito T (2012) Programmed cell death 1 forms negative costimulatory microclusters that directly inhibit T cell receptor signaling by recruiting phosphatase SHP2. J Exp Med 209:1201–1217

Zhang Y, Allison JP (1997) Interaction of CTLA-4 with AP50, a clathrin-coated pit adaptor protein. Proc Natl Acad Sci U S A 94:9273–9278

Chapter 6
Role of Co-stimulatory Molecules in T Helper Cell Differentiation

Michelle Schorer, Vijay K. Kuchroo, and Nicole Joller

Abstract $CD4^+$ T cells play a central role in orchestrating the immune response to a variety of pathogens but also regulate autoimmune responses, asthma, allergic responses, as well as tumor immunity. To cover this broad spectrum of responses, naïve $CD4^+$ T cells differentiate into one of several lineages of T helper cells, including Th1, Th2, Th17, and T_{FH}, as defined by their cytokine pattern and function. The fate decision of T helper cell differentiation integrates signals delivered through the T cell receptor, cytokine receptors, and the pattern of co-stimulatory signals received. In this review, we summarize the contribution of co-stimulatory and co-inhibitory receptors to the differentiation and maintenance of T helper cell responses.

Keywords Co-stimulatory molecules · T cell differentiation · Th1 · Th2 · Th17 · T_{FH}

6.1 Introduction

$CD4^+$ T helper (Th) cells orchestrate the adaptive immune response and play a central role in immune protection. They do this by acting on a multitude of other immune compartments – they help B cells make antibodies, they license antigen-presenting cells (APCs) to prime cytotoxic immune responses, they enhance the function of innate cells and contribute to their maturation, and they recruit various

---

M. Schorer · N. Joller (✉)
Institute for Experimental Immunology, University of Zurich, Zurich, Switzerland
e-mail: schorer@immunology.uzh.ch; nicole.joller@immunology.uzh.ch

V. K. Kuchroo
Evergrande Center for Immunologic Diseases, Harvard Medical School and Brigham & Women's Hospital, Boston, MA, USA

Klarman Cell Observatory, Broad Institute of MIT and Harvard, Cambridge, MA, USA
e-mail: vkuchroo@evergrande.hms.harvard.edu

© Springer Nature Singapore Pte Ltd. 2019
M. Azuma, H. Yagita (eds.), *Co-signal Molecules in T Cell Activation*,
Advances in Experimental Medicine and Biology 1189,
https://doi.org/10.1007/978-981-32-9717-3_6

cell populations to the site of infection and inflammation. The seminal work of Mosmann and Coffman 30 years ago (Mosmann et al. 1986) made it clear that these diverse functions are not achieved by a homogenous cell population but that distinct functional subsets exist within the Th compartment that allow for the breath of immune responses necessary to react to the broad spectrum of threats the immune system faces. Mosmann and Coffman initially described two distinct lineages: Th1 cells, which are characterized by the expression of IFN-γ and promote immune responses against intracellular viruses and bacteria, and Th2 cells, which are marked by IL-4 production and drive protective immune responses against multicellular pathogens such as parasites and helminthes. With the discovery of Th17 cells, which orchestrate immune responses against fungi and extracellular bacteria (Harrington et al. 2005; Langrish et al. 2005; Park et al. 2005); T follicular helper (T_{FH}) cells, which are specialized to promote B cell responses (Breitfeld et al. 2000; Kim et al. 2001; Schaerli et al. 2000); and Th9 cells (Dardalhon et al. 2008; Veldhoen et al. 2008), the diversity of Th subsets has further increased. Although detailed subset descriptions allow for further subdivision of these lineages, this chapter will focus on the four most intensely studied effector lineages, Th1, Th2, Th17, and T_{FH} cells.

Apart from natural Foxp3[+] regulatory T cells, which already differentiate in the thymus, naïve CD4[+] T cells differentiate into the different Th lineages when they become activated in the periphery, and their lineage is determined by the pattern of signals they receive during initial antigen encounter. Three signals are required to fully activate naïve CD4[+] T cells, and all three signals contribute to their lineage decision: (i) T cell receptor stimulation through the recognition of peptide antigen in the context of MHC II is required as a first signal for T cell activation, (ii) co-stimulatory signals provided by one or more surface molecules on APCs are required to prevent the induction of anergy, and (iii) cytokines secreted mostly by APCs are required for optimal generation of effector and memory T cells and their survival. Lineage-instructing cytokines have the most dominant effect on CD4[+] T cell differentiation into different Th lineages and induce the expression of their lineage transcription factors (Table 6.1). Th1 cells express T-bet and are generated in the presence of IL-12 and IFN-γ (Hsieh et al. 1993; Manetti et al. 1993; Szabo et al. 2000), Th2 cells express GATA-3 and are induced by IL-4 (Kopf et al. 1993; Zheng and Flavell 1997), and Th17 cells express RORγt and are generated in the presence of TGF-β and IL-6 (Bettelli et al. 2006; Mangan et al. 2006; Veldhoen et al. 2006; Ivanov et al. 2006).

However, Th responses can also be generated in the absence of these lineage-instructing cytokines. In particular Th1 responses elicited upon viral infection are in many cases IL-12-independent (Oxenius et al. 1999; Schijns et al. 1998). Similarly, some anti-parasite Th2 responses are elicited in the absence of IL-4 (Jankovic et al. 2000). Strengths and duration of signal during T cell activation thus also play an important role in determining the lineage fate as highlighted by a number of studies showing that TCR affinity and antigen dose affect the differentiation of naïve CD4[+] T cells into the Th1 or Th2 lineage. Altered peptide ligands were used to test the effect of altered TCR affinity on Th differentiation and revealed that higher-affinity TCRs promote Th1 differentiation, while lower TCR affinity results in a bias toward

Table 6.1 Overview of the T helper lineages

Lineage	Transcription factor	Differentiating cytokines	Pathogen control	Disease involvement	Co-stimulatory molecules		
					Promote	Inhibit	Alter function
Th1	T-bet	IFN-γ, IL-12	Viruses, intracellular bateria	Autoimmunity	CD40L, ICOS, CD226	Tim-3, TIGIT	
Th2	GATA-3	IL-4	Parasites, helminths	Allergies, athma	CD28, ICOS, OX40, Tim-1	CD226	
Th17	RORγt	IL-6 + TGF-β; IL-1β + IL-6 + IL-23	Fungi, extracellular bacteria	Autoimmunity	ICOS, CD40L, OX40	PD-1, TIGIT, Tim-3	CD5L, PROCR
T$_{FH}$	Bcl6	Unknown	Antibody-mediated control (germinal center reaction)		CD28, ICOS, PD-1		

The table summarizes the most important characteristics of the different T helper lineages and the co-stimulatory and co-inhibitory receptors affecting their development and function

Th2 differentiation (Chaturvedi et al. 1996; Kumar et al. 1995; Pfeiffer et al. 1995; Tao et al. 1997b). Similar results were obtained when the antigen dose was altered, as low antigen promoted Th2 differentiation, while high antigen favored Th1 cells (Constant et al. 1995; Hosken et al. 1995). In addition to the interaction of the TCR with the peptide/MHC complex, the signal delivered during T cell activation is strongly influenced by co-stimulatory or co-inhibitory signals, which are the focus of this chapter. Co-stimulatory molecules affect the strength as well as the nature of the signal delivered and thereby greatly impact the lineage fate decision of Th cells. Signals delivered by co-signaling molecules can directly modulate signal strength and thereby affect Th differentiation; they can alter the nature of the signal to initiate a transcriptional program that will favor or inhibit differentiation of a specific lineage. Moreover, they can indirectly modulate the environment by altering the cytokine production by APCs, or they can have an impact on the survival of already differentiated Th cells. We will highlight the most important co-signaling molecules affecting differentiation and function of Th1, Th2, Th17, and T_{FH} cells and outline how they contribute to shaping the immune response.

6.2 Th1 Cells

Ligation of the constitutively expressed co-stimulatory molecule CD28 is essential during early T cell activation as it is required for T cell proliferation and survival and cytokine production. CD28 engagement is closely linked to TCR signaling strength, and as differentiation into the Th1 lineage is favored by strong antigenic stimulation, CD28 engagement in the presence of high antigen doses or a high-affinity TCR results in Th1 differentiation (Fig. 6.1) (Tao et al. 1997a; Rogers and Croft 2000). However, prolonged engagement of CD28 is supportive of Th2 differentiation (Jorritsma et al. 2003). In vitro, T cell activation with high but not low antigen doses was shown to induce expression of CD40L, which binds to CD40 on DCs and thereby induces them to produce IL-12 (Cella et al. 1996; Koch et al. 1996). This mechanism was also effective in vivo, and CD40-CD40L interaction enhanced IL-12 production in DCs and thus promoted Th1 responses in *Leishmania major* infection and a model of colitis (Stuber et al. 1996; Campbell et al. 1996).

CD28 stimulation also induces expression of the inducible co-stimulator (ICOS), which is expressed on activated T cells (Hutloff et al. 1999). Early work suggested that ICOS ligation on T cells promotes secretion of both Th1- and Th2-associated cytokines and thus does not affect the lineage decision (Dong et al. 2001; Kopf et al. 2000; McAdam et al. 2001; Yoshinaga et al. 1999). However, a multitude of studies since then have shed more light on the role of ICOS in Th differentiation and revealed that the effect of ICOS on Th responses seems to be strongly dependent on the timing and context. Overall, ICOS appears to favor Th1 differentiation as the absence of ICOS or its ligand results in defective Th1 responses in several disease settings. As such, ICOS KO mice are unable to mount a Th1 response upon *Salmonella enterica* (serovar Typhimurium) infection, leading to higher bacterial burden in

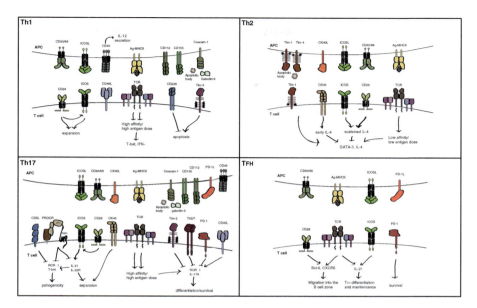

Fig. 6.1 Co-stimulatory molecules in Th1, Th2, Th17, and T$_{FH}$ cells. The most important co-stimulatory and co-inhibitory molecules that play a role in Th1 (top left), Th2 (top right), Th17 (bottom left), and T$_{FH}$ (bottom right) differentiation and their ligands are summarized graphically

these mice and unresolved infection even at late time points (Vidric et al. 2006). Similarly, disruption of ICOS signaling by ICOS-Ig treatment during oral *Listeria monocytogenes* infection dampens the pathogen-specific Th1 response, hampering pathogen control and enhancing lethality (Mittrucker et al. 2002). Furthermore, ICOS-deficient NOD mice do not develop diabetes due to a diminished Th1 response (Hawiger et al. 2008). In the context of a strong Th1-polarizing environment, CD28 and ICOS seem to play synergistic and partially redundant roles. CD28- and ICOS-deficient mice mount normal Th1 responses upon *Toxoplasma gondii* infection, a strong inducer of Th1 immunity (Villegas et al. 2002; Wilson et al. 2006). However, treatment of CD28$^{-/-}$ mice with anti-ICOSL antibodies reduces this Th1 response and results in an increased parasite burden (Villegas et al. 2002). Similarly, the reduction in the Th1 response observed upon ICOS-Ig treatment during LCMV infection is potentiated in CD28$^{-/-}$ mice (Kopf et al. 2000). Some reports, however, suggest that ICOS might dampen Th1 responses. ICOS$^{-/-}$ mice mount an enhanced Th1 response upon *Mycobacterium tuberculosis* or *Plasmodium chabaudi chabaudi* infection, leading to improved pathogen control (Nouailles et al. 2011; Wikenheiser et al. 2016). It is important to note that in these settings the regulatory response was also strongly inhibited due to the ability of ICOS to promote IL-10 production and Treg function (Busse et al. 2012; Lohning et al. 2003; Burmeister et al. 2008; Ito et al. 2008) and as such the enhanced Th1 response is most likely a secondary effect. Overall, ICOS seems to promote Th1 responses, but due to its expression on all Th subsets, this effect is not exclusive for Th1 responses.

In contrast, the co-stimulatory receptor CD226 was identified to be specifically expressed on Th1 but not Th2 cells and thus likely specifically regulates Th1 responses (Dardalhon et al. 2005). CD226 (also called DNAM-1) is an activating receptor and binds to the ligands CD155 (PVR) and CD112 (nectin-2), which it shares with the co-inhibitory receptor TIGIT forming a pathway that is reminiscent of the CD28/CTLA-4 pathway (Levin et al. 2011; Stanietsky et al. 2009; Yu et al. 2009; Bottino et al. 2003). In the absence of CD28, co-stimulation through LFA-1 becomes dominant, which binds to CD226 for inducing its co-stimulatory activity (Gaglia et al. 2000; Shibuya et al. 2003). LFA-1 itself has been shown to promote Th1 differentiation through induction of T-bet, while downregulating GATA-3 and CD226 signaling is a critical step in this process (Verma et al. 2016; Smits et al. 2002; Salomon and Bluestone 1998; Shibuya et al. 2003). Furthermore, blocking of CD226 results in decreased Th1 responses due to reduced T cell expansion and survival (Dardalhon et al. 2005). Indeed, CD226 has been suggested to act as an anti-apoptotic molecule involved in positive selection of T cells in the thymus (Fang et al. 2009). CD226 could therefore be involved in the selective expansion of Th1 cells by acting as an anti-apoptotic molecule in a subset-specific manner. More recently, CD226 was shown to promote in vitro differentiation of human Th1 as well as Th17 cells, while its co-inhibitory counterpart TIGIT had the opposite effect (Lozano et al. 2012; Lozano et al. 2013). Indeed, CD226 has been genetically linked to susceptibility to multiple Th1- and/or Th17-driven autoimmune diseases, including type 1 diabetes, rheumatoid arthritis, and multiple sclerosis (MS), supporting an important role for CD226 in regulating Th1 (and Th17) responses (Hafler et al. 2009).

Like CD226, Tim-3 is specifically expressed on Th1 cells, but unlike CD226 it acts as a negative regulator of the Th1 response (Monney et al. 2002; Khademi et al. 2004; Hastings et al. 2009). Tim-3 binding to its ligand galectin-9 induces cell death in Th1 cells and thereby effectively limits the Th1 response (Zhu et al. 2005). The absence of Tim-3 or its functional blockade strongly enhanced Th1 responses in vivo and resulted in exacerbated experimental autoimmune encephalomyelitis (EAE, a T cell-mediated autoimmune disease that serves as an animal model for MS), accelerated type 1 diabetes, and impaired tolerance induction (Monney et al. 2002; Sabatos et al. 2003; Sanchez-Fueyo et al. 2003). In subsequent studies, administration of the Tim-3 ligand galectin-9 was shown to ameliorate skin inflammation and experimental autoimmune arthritis, suggesting that Tim-3 ligation attenuates Th1 as well as Th17 responses (Niwa et al. 2009; Seki et al. 2008). Thus, although Th17 cells only express low levels of Tim-3 (Chen et al. 2006), Tim-3 may also play a role in attenuating Th17 responses. Importantly, the regulatory role of Tim-3 in Th1 responses is also observed in humans as Tim-3 is dysregulated in MS patients but its expression is regained in patients responding to IFN-β treatment (Koguchi et al. 2006; Yang et al. 2008; Ottoboni et al. 2012). Similarly, reduced expression of Tim-3 is observed in rheumatoid arthritis patients, but responsiveness to treatment (methotrexate or tocilizumab) is associated with restored Tim-3 expression (Liu et al. 2010). Moreover, the negative regulatory role for Tim-3 in T cells has been extended to exhausted T cells in chronic viral infections such as LCMV or HIV, where Tim-3 blockade could partially restore T cell function (Jin et al. 2010;

Grabmeier-Pfistershammer et al. 2017). Collectively, these data highlight the importance of Tim-3 as a negative regulator of Th1 responses and its relevance in human diseases.

6.3 Th2 Cells

Th2 cells arise in response to extracellular parasites, including helminthes, but also play an important role in the induction of asthma and allergic diseases (Hotez et al. 2008; Licona-Limon et al. 2013). Th2 priming and maturation is dependent on the availability of high levels of IL-4, which not only facilitates the differentiation of Th2 cells in an autocrine manner but also directly blocks the generation of Th1 cells from naïve T cells (Choi and Reiser 1998). Importantly, IL-4 signaling in T cells induces the expression of GATA-3, the master transcription factor of Th2 cells (Rodriguez-Palmero et al. 1999; Ouyang et al. 2000). Besides the stimulation by polarizing cytokines, the differentiation of Th2 cells is largely directed by co-stimulatory signals (Fig. 6.1). Sustained CD28 co-stimulation plays an important role in Th2 differentiation, as it was shown to enhance IL-4 mediated Th2 differentiation by increasing IL-4 responsiveness (McArthur and Raulet 1993; Rulifson et al. 1997; Kubo et al. 1999).

Additionally, CD28 was shown to induce the expression of ICOS, which regulates Th2 development. Th2 cells express significantly higher levels of ICOS than Th1 cells, and ICOS blockade markedly decreases the production of IL-4 and IL-10 and inhibits the differentiation of Th2 cells (McAdam et al. 2000). Importantly, inhibition of ICOS was demonstrated to attenuate airway hyper-responsiveness in vivo in an adoptive transfer model using differentiated Th2 cells (Coyle et al. 2000). The significance of the ICOS-ICOSL pathway in preventing Th2-driven airway inflammation is further supported by another study showing that ICOS limits T cell proliferation and increases IL-10 production in T cells (Gonzalo et al. 2001; Akbari et al. 2002). Furthermore, ICOS blockade also significantly inhibits the differentiation of Th2 cells in *Nippostrongylus brasiliensis* infection, a parasitic model pathogen whose in vivo clearance is critically dependent on an IL-4R-mediated Th2 immune response. Of note, although the treatment was shown to impair the generation of Th2 cells in this model, it had no significant impact on the clearance of the worms (Kopf et al. 2000). Given its importance in guiding Th1/Th2 differentiation during allergic and parasitic immune responses, ICOS blockade was also successfully tested in models of acute and chronic allograft rejection. In both acute and chronic graft rejection, ICOS was significantly upregulated and anti-ICOS therapy allowed for permanent engraftment in a fully MHC-mismatched mouse model (Ozkaynak et al. 2001; Harada et al. 2003). Interestingly, ICOS is not exclusively associated with the production of typical Th2 cytokines. Single-cell analysis on ICOS^{low}, ICOS^{medium}, and ICOS^{high} T cells revealed an even stronger link to IL-10 production, as T cells with high ICOS expression mainly secreted IL-10 (Lohning et al. 2003). Collectively these findings indicate that ICOS is involved in the regulation of various

Th lineages as well as regulatory processes but seems to have a preferential role in the generation of Th2 cells, since ICOS signaling during early T cell activation enhances IL-4 production, thereby promoting Th2 lineage decision and inhibiting Th1 cell generation (Nurieva et al. 2003; Watanabe et al. 2005).

Another co-stimulatory pathway that was shown to be involved in the regulation of Th differentiation is OX40-OX40L. OX40 is induced upon T cell activation on both $CD4^+$ and $CD8^+$ T cells (Paterson et al. 1987; Mallett et al. 1990). Early studies on isolated human $CD4^+$ T cells revealed that OX40 ligation in combination with CD28 co-stimulation increased the release of IL-4 and IL-13, classic Th2 cytokines, which nurtured the idea that OX40 co-stimulation could be involved in augmenting Th2 differentiation (Ohshima et al. 1998). Later findings however indicated that the Th1 vs. Th2 differentiation was not affected by the OX40-OX40L pathway. Both polarized Th1 and Th2 cells were demonstrated to express OX40, suggesting an important role of the pathway for both types of responses (Gramaglia et al. 1998). In the $OX40L^{-/-}$ mouse model, $CD4^+$ T cells displayed a defect in the production of both IFN-γ and IL-4 in vitro (Chen et al. 1999) and failed to produce Th1 as well as Th2 cytokines in response to allergen sensitization, suggesting that the OX40-OX40L pathway augments an ongoing immune response and T cell activation in general, regardless of the Th lineage (Rogers and Croft 2000; Arestides et al. 2002). Nevertheless, it is now known that OX40 ligation is critical for naïve T cells to initially transcribe IL-4 (So et al. 2006), since in the absence of IL-4, OX40 engagement mediates the early production of IL-4, which promotes Th2 commitment. Therefore, OX40 ligation certainly favors a Th2 phenotype. However, the co-stimulatory activity of OX40 on T cell activation, proliferation, and survival is dominant in most settings and will augment all types of effector responses.

More recently, Tim molecules have emerged as important regulators of immune activation and tolerance in models of autoimmunity and cancer (Anderson et al. 2016). The Tim proteins were originally identified during a screening for asthma susceptibility genes, which revealed a gene locus named *Tapr* that contains the *Tim* genes (McIntire et al. 2001). The *Tapr* locus was demonstrated to be involved in the early differentiation of Th2 cells by regulating the production of IL-4 and IL-13 during primary antigen-specific responses to OVA sensitization. Of the different Tim proteins that are encoded by the *Tapr* locus, Tim-1 is expressed on $CD4^+$ T cells that contribute to atopic and asthmatic disease (Kuchroo et al. 2003). Tim-1 is readily upregulated on naïve T cells after activation and highly expressed on differentiated Th2 cells (Umetsu et al. 2005). An initial study using an antagonistic anti-Tim-1 antibody reported that anti-Tim-1 treatment suppressed the development of allergic airway inflammation. In the study, the decreased frequency of inflammatory cells after anti-Tim-1 blockade coincided with the significantly decreased production of Th2 cytokines like IL-13, IL-4, IL-5, and IL-10 (Encinas et al. 2005). Strikingly, Tim-1 blockade did not affect Th1 differentiation, seeing that the levels of IFN-γ did not increase, which strengthened the hypothesis that Tim-1 mainly regulates Th2 immune responses. More recent experiments however found that the administration of an inhibitory anti-Tim-1 antibody also decreased the production of Th1/Th17 cytokines and inhibited the antigen-specific expansion of pathogenic CD4$^+$ T cells in EAE (Xiao et al. 2007). In the same study, the authors showed that the antibody affinity critically determines the functional outcome of the T cell response, which supports the notion that signal strength rather than binding itself dictates the differentiation faith of T cells. While Tim-1 ligation with a lower-affinity antibody promoted Th2 responses, administration of a high-affinity antibody during EAE induction enhanced pathogenic Th1 and Th17. Surprisingly, genetic ablation of Tim-1 in Tim-1$^{-/-}$ mice resulted in a similar degree of airway inflammation as displayed by wild-type mice after OVA and alum immunization (Curtiss et al. 2012). Moreover, in vitro re-stimulation of Tim-1-deficient splenocytes lead to the enhanced secretion of IL-5 and IL-13, as well as IL-4, IL-10, and IL-17, which suggested that Tim-1 promotes Th2 responses during allergen sensitization. This striking discrepancy between the earlier studies using antibodies and the genetic knockout model highlights the fact that in addition to the Tim-1 signal strength, also the timing of signal engagement/blockade might greatly influence the differentiation decision of T cells. The enhanced inflammation in Tim-1-deficient mice could be the consequence of a dysregulated negative control of T cell responses. This notion is underlined by the finding that Tim-1 is also expressed on dendritic cells, where Tim-1 signaling regulates co-stimulatory molecule expression and pro-inflammatory cytokine production (Xiao et al. 2011). This process promotes T cell responses in general and negatively regulates the generation of regulatory T cells. In addition, cross-linking of Tim-1 de-stabilizes regulatory T cells and thereby indirectly promotes pro-inflammatory immune responses (Degauque et al. 2008).

6.4 Th17

Fifteen years ago, the discovery that IL-23 rather than IL-12 is the major driver of many autoimmune diseases has paved the way for the identification of the Th17 lineage (Harrington et al. 2005; Langrish et al. 2005; Park et al. 2005; Cua et al. 2003; Murphy et al. 2003). It is, however, not IL-23 but a combination of IL-6 and TGF-β that induces differentiation of naïve CD4$^+$ T cells into Th17 cells (Bettelli et al. 2006; Mangan et al. 2006; Veldhoen et al. 2006; Ivanov et al. 2006). Nevertheless, IL-23 plays a central role in Th17 biology as it is required to expand and stabilize the Th17 lineage and confer it with its autopathogenic properties (Jager et al. 2009; Veldhoen et al. 2006; Awasthi et al. 2009). The discovery of Th17 cells initiated a major revision of the Th1/Th2 paradigm, and it is now clear that the Th compartment is much more complex than the initially proposed dual system. As Th17 can be highly autopathogenic, many of the initial studies on Th17 cells were performed in autoimmune settings, and Th17 cells were identified as the main drivers of numerous autoimmune disorders, including MS, rheumatoid arthritis, inflammatory bowel disease, and psoriasis (Patel and Kuchroo 2015). Indeed, therapeutic interventions targeting components of the Th17 pathway have since proven successful in many of these conditions (Patel and Kuchroo 2015). However, in healthy individuals, the primary function of Th17 cells is to mediate protective immunity against infections with fungi and extracellular bacteria (Sallusto 2016). In addition to inducing tissue inflammation, Th17 cells also promote B cell responses and the formation of ectopic lymphoid follicles in the tissues (Mitsdoerffer et al. 2010; Peters et al. 2011; Ota et al. 2011; Rangel-Moreno et al. 2011).

Like Th1 cells, Th17 cells develop after strong antigenic stimulation and CD28 favors their differentiation (Fig. 6.1) (Gomez-Rodriguez et al. 2009; Iezzi et al. 2009; Park et al. 2005). However, the main function of CD28 in Th17 development might be its ability to induce ICOS (Hutloff et al. 1999; McAdam et al. 2001; Aicher et al. 2000). Indeed, Th17 cells have been shown to express higher levels of ICOS than Th1 cells (Nakae et al. 2007), and ICOS strongly enhances Th17 differentiation of human CD4[+] T cells in vitro (Paulos et al. 2010). Interestingly, CD28 co-stimulation counteracted ICOS stimulation in this setting, dampening RORγt and cytokine expression (Paulos et al. 2010), which supports the induction of ICOS expression as the primary role of CD28 in Th17 differentiation. Several genetically modified mouse models have confirmed the importance of ICOS for Th17 cells in vivo in that overexpression of ICOS due to a mutation in its negative regulator Roquin in sanroque mice causes a lupus-like autoimmune syndrome (Yu et al. 2007). Conversely, ICOS-deficient mice have been reported to show impaired Th17 responses (Park et al. 2005). Furthermore, mice with an ICOS signaling defect that prevents interaction of ICOS with PI3K mount impaired Th17 responses upon *Chlamydia muridarum* infection, resulting in decreased pathogen control (Gao et al. 2012). However, other studies found ICOS KO mice to mount normal or even enhanced Th17 responses and develop slightly more severe EAE (Bauquet et al. 2009; Galicia et al. 2009). These discrepancies were resolved when the mechanism by which ICOS contributes to Th17 responses was elucidated. An earlier study had already suggested that ICOS might play distinct roles during different phases of the immune response as inhibition of ICOS during the priming phase of EAE exacerbated diseases but ICOS blockade during the effector phase had a protective effect (Rottman et al. 2001). Indeed, primary differentiation of Th17 cells is independent of ICOS (Bauquet et al. 2009). However, ICOS ligation results in the activation of c-Maf, which in turn augments IL-23R expression and IL-21 production allowing for a paracrine and autocrine expansion of the Th17 response (Bauquet et al. 2009). ICOS thus does not affect the differentiation of Th17 cells per se but plays an essential role in the population expansion of Th17 cells.

Another function of ICOS is its ability to induce expression of CD40L on T cells (McAdam et al. 2001). CD40L ligation is important for Th17 induction with high antigen doses, and the absence of the CD40-CD40L interaction prevents the development of EAE by specifically reducing the Th17 but not the Th1 response (Grewal et al. 1996; Iezzi et al. 2009). Studies showing that the CD40-CD40L interaction induces enhanced IL-6 and IL-23 production in DCs suggest that CD40L does not affect Th17 differentiation in a cell-intrinsic manner but indirectly conditions DCs to provide a cytokine environment that promotes Th17 differentiation (Perona-Wright et al. 2009; Iezzi et al. 2009). OX40 has also been implicated in Th17-driven diseases such as EAE and MS (Ndhlovu et al. 2001; Carboni et al. 2003), and the reported induction of IL-6 in mast cells by OX40L ligation suggests

6 Role of Co-stimulatory Molecules in T Helper Cell Differentiation 163

that OX40 promotes Th17 differentiation in a similar manner as CD40L (Piconese et al. 2009).

In addition to co-stimulatory molecules, co-inhibitory receptors such as PD-1 also regulate the Th17 lineage. Absence or blockade of PD-1 and PD-L1 resulted in more severe EAE, a phenotype that was not observed when PD-L2 was targeted (Carter et al. 2007; Salama et al. 2003). Early studies in EAE and *Mycobacterium tuberculosis* infection in humans, which are characterized by mixed Th1 and Th17 responses, suggested that the PD-1/PD-L1 interaction specifically suppressed the Th1 and not the Th17 response (Babu et al. 2009; Schreiner et al. 2008). However, a series of recent reports points in the opposite direction. Hirahara and colleagues showed that IL-27-mediated inhibition of Th17 responses is in part achieved through the ability of IL-27 to induce PD-L1 expression on T cells, which inhibits the differentiation of Th17 cells in *trans* through the PD-1-PD-L1 interaction (Hirahara et al. 2012). This *trans* suppression of Th17 cells also played a functional role during EAE in vivo. Furthermore, recombinant PD-L1 was suggested to selectively block Th17 but not Th1 and Th2 differentiation (Herold et al. 2015), and PD-L1 transgenic mice are less susceptible to EAE because of a reduced Th17 (but not Th1) response (Shi et al. 2017). Importantly, overexpression of PD-L1 did not affect the regulatory T cell response in these mice, supporting the notion that it specifically influences the Th17 response.

In addition to affecting the differentiation of Th17 cells, co-signaling molecules have most recently also been shown to affect the phenotype and immunological function of Th17 cells. Th17 cells come in (at least) two flavors: so-called pathogenic Th17 cells are induced in the presence of IL-6, IL-1β, and IL-23, co-express both RORγt and T-bet, secrete GM-CSF, and are highly pathogenic in inducing EAE, while non-pathogenic Th17 cells are induced by TGF-β1 and IL-6, are negative for T-bet, but express IL-10 in addition to IL-17 (Ghoreschi et al. 2010; Lee et al. 2012). These two Th17 subsets appear to be functionally and transcriptionally distinct and might have evolved to combat different types of pathogens. Based on studies with human Th17 cell clones, it appears that "pathogenic" Th17 cells are induced to combat fungal infections, while "non-pathogenic" Th17 cells seem to be generated in response to infections with extracellular bacteria (Zielinski et al. 2012). The transcriptional characterization of these two Th17 subsets formed the basis for the identification of two surface receptors – PROCR (protein C receptor) and CD5L (CD5 antigen-like or AIM) – that act as regulators of Th17 pathogenicity (Kishi et al. 2016; Wang et al. 2015). CD5L, a member of the cysteine-rich scavenger receptor superfamily involved in regulation of lipid metabolism (Miyazaki et al. 1999; Sarrias et al. 2004), is specifically expressed in non-pathogenic Th17 cells. CD5L has no effect on Th17 differentiation itself but inhibits Th17 pathogenicity by modulating the intracellular lipid composition. The CD5L-induced restriction of cholesterol synthesis reduces ligand availability for RORγt and thereby limits its activity and enforces the non-pathogenic Th17 phenotype (Wang et al. 2015). Like CD5L, PROCR is also specifically expressed on non-pathogenic Th17 cells (Kishi et al. 2016). PROCR inhibits IL-23R and IL-1R expression, which are critical for the generation of pathogenic Th17 cells (Awasthi et al. 2009; Chung et al. 2009; Cua et al. 2003; Sutton et al. 2006). Interestingly, PROCR expression is induced by transcription factors that also drive the differentiation of Th17 cells (Kishi et al. 2016), suggesting that it acts as a built-in break to control Th17 pathogenicity under steady-state conditions. Given that Th17 cells are abundantly present at mucosal sites and barrier tissues, default PROCR expression might serve to maintain tissue homeostasis and prevent chronic inflammation at these sites. Although PROCR is expressed at much lower levels in non-pathogenic Th17 cells, its engagement through its ligand activated protein C (aPC) induces functional conversion of pathogenic to non-pathogenic Th17 cells (Kishi et al. 2016). Indeed, administration of aPC was shown to ameliorate EAE, and aPC is detectable in chronic active plaques of MS patients (Han et al. 2008), supporting an active regulatory role for PROCR and its ligand in Th17 pathogenicity. Co-signaling molecules thus not only affect Th17 differentiation but also serve to regulate their functional state.

6.5 T_{FH} Cells

T follicular helper cells (T_{FH}) are a subset of CD4$^+$ T cells located in lymph nodes, and their main function is to provide help for B cells during the germinal center reaction, which ensures the generation of high-affinity antibodies (Crotty 2011). In contrast to the other Th subsets, T_{FH} differentiation follows a multifaceted pathway that involves not only the upregulation of specific chemokine receptors but also direct interaction with B cells in secondary lymphoid organs (Crotty 2014). T_{FH} cells are characterized by the expression of their master transcription factor Bcl-6, as well as the surface receptors CXCR5, ICOS, and PD-1 (Fazilleau et al. 2009a). Similarly to other Th lineages, early T_{FH} differentiation is highly dependent on CD28 engagement and TCR signal strength. Weber and colleagues recently showed that CD28-deficient T cells are unable to induce Bcl-6, which is necessary for the migration of T_{FH} cells into the B cell zone where they undergo further differentiation steps (Weber et al. 2015) (Fig. 6.1). Besides CD28 signaling, it was found that T cell precursors with a high-affinity TCR preferentially differentiate into CXCR5$^+$ T_{FH} cells that display a tissue-resident phenotype (Fazilleau et al. 2009b). At the same time, greater TCR signal strength also induced higher levels of IL-21 in vitro, a cytokine that is fundamental for both T_{FH} generation and subsequent germinal center formation (Vogelzang et al. 2008; Nurieva et al. 2008). During the later stages of T_{FH} differentiation, ICOS signaling is key in ensuring the maintenance of T_{FH} cells in the germinal center. Indeed, abrogation of ICOS signaling results in the loss of T_{FH} cells and the collapse of the already formed germinal center response (Weber et al. 2015; Bossaller et al. 2006; Warnatz et al. 2006). B cells express high levels of ICOSL in the secondary lymphoid organs, and the ICOS-ICOSL binding interaction is required for proper T_{FH} differentiation not only under steady-state conditions but also during acute infections or immunization (Xu et al. 2013; Haynes et al. 2007). As a consequence, ICOS deficiency leads to profound defects in antibody production and immunoglobulin isotype switching in both mice and humans (Akiba et al. 2005; Bentebibel et al. 2016). Furthermore, ICOS engagement also induces IL-21 production by Th cells, which is crucial for germinal center maintenance and T_{FH} development (Bauquet et al. 2009).

T$_{FH}$ cells were also shown to express the highest levels of PD-1 compared to other T cell subsets under homeostatic conditions. Follicular regulatory T cells (T$_{FR}$), which restrain T$_{FH}$ responses, are negatively regulated by PD-1, as PD-1$^{-/-}$ and PD-L1$^{-/-}$ mice have a greater abundance of T$_{FR}$ (Sage et al. 2013). PD-1 expression by T$_{FH}$ cells is also important in mediating their function in that the interaction of PD-1 with PD-L1 on germinal center B cells delivers important survival signals to the B cells and regulates the generation and affinity maturation of long-lived plasma cells in the germinal center (Good-Jacobson et al. 2010). Mice deficient in PD-L2, PD-L1, or PD-1 displayed defects in the number of long-lived plasma cells, which support the notion that the PD-1/PD-1 L pathway represents an important signaling pathway that provides T cell-dependent B cell help.

6.6 Conclusion

The integration of signals from co-stimulatory and inhibitory molecules is a key step in the activation of naïve CD4$^+$ T cells as it not only allows for full activation of T cells but based on its composition also influences Th differentiation and thus shapes the ensuing immune response (Fig. 6.2). The signals delivered through co-stimulatory receptors in this context are threefold: (i) they directly act on Th cells to

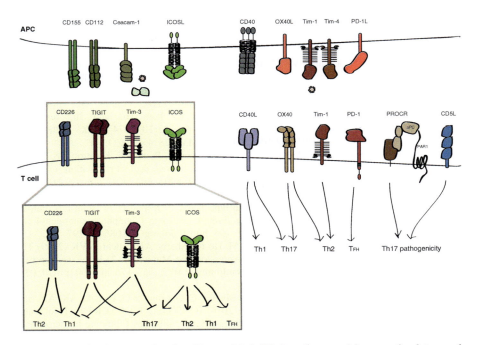

Fig. 6.2 Co-stimulatory molecules affect multiple T helper lineages. Many co-stimulatory and co-inhibitory receptors affect the differentiation, expansion, and maintenance of more than one T helper lineage. This graph summarizes the function of the receptors in a receptor-centric fashion, highlighting their diverse effects

modulate TCR signal strength and affect the transcriptional program of a specific lineage, (ii) they engage ligands on APC and thereby may alter their function and cytokine pattern, and (iii) they influence the function and survival of already differentiated Th cells. The composition of co-stimulatory signals thus substantially influences the differentiation and maintenance of different Th lineages and represents a carefully orchestrated tool by which the interaction of Th cells and APCs can optimize the immune response to the encountered threat.

Acknowledgments This work was supported by the Swiss National Science Foundation (PP00P3_150663 and PP00P3_ 181037 to N.J.), the European Research Council (677200 to N.J.), the Zuercher Universitaetsverein (ZUNIV-FAN to N.J.), the Olga Mayenfisch Stiftung (to N.J.), and the Novartis Foundation for medical-biological research (17A027 to N.J.).

References

Aicher A, Hayden-Ledbetter M, Brady WA, Pezzutto A, Richter G, Magaletti D, Buckwalter S, Ledbetter JA, Clark EA (2000) Characterization of human inducible costimulator ligand expression and function. J Immunol 164(9):4689–4696

Akbari O, Freeman GJ, Meyer EH, Greenfield EA, Chang TT, Sharpe AH, Berry G, DeKruyff RH, Umetsu DT (2002) Antigen-specific regulatory T cells develop via the ICOS-ICOS-ligand pathway and inhibit allergen-induced airway hyperreactivity. Nat Med 8(9):1024–1032. https://doi.org/10.1038/nm745

Akiba H, Takeda K, Kojima Y, Usui Y, Harada N, Yamazaki T, Ma J, Tezuka K, Yagita H, Okumura K (2005) The role of ICOS in the CXCR5+ follicular B helper T cell maintenance in vivo. J Immunol 175(4):2340–2348

Anderson AC, Joller N, Kuchroo VK (2016) Lag-3, Tim-3, and TIGIT: co-inhibitory receptors with specialized functions in immune regulation. Immunity 44(5):989–1004. https://doi.org/10.1016/j.immuni.2016.05.001

Arestides RS, He H, Westlake RM, Chen AI, Sharpe AH, Perkins DL, Finn PW (2002) Costimulatory molecule OX40L is critical for both Th1 and Th2 responses in allergic inflammation. Eur J Immunol 32(10):2874–2880. https://doi.org/10.1002/1521-4141(2002010)32:10<2874::AID-IMMU2874>3.0.CO;2-4

Awasthi A, Riol-Blanco L, Jager A, Korn T, Pot C, Galileos G, Bettelli E, Kuchroo VK, Oukka M (2009) Cutting edge: IL-23 receptor gfp reporter mice reveal distinct populations of IL-17-producing cells. J Immunol 182 (10):5904–5908. 182/10/5904 [pii] 74049/jimmunol.0900732

Babu S, Bhat SQ, Kumar NP, Jayantasri S, Rukmani S, Kumaran P, Gopi PG, Kolappan C, Kumaraswami V, Nutman TB (2009) Human type 1 and 17 responses in latent tuberculosis are modulated by coincident filarial infection through cytotoxic T lymphocyte antigen-4 and programmed death-1. J Infect Dis 200(2):288–298. https://doi.org/10.1086/599797

Bauquet AT, Jin H, Paterson AM, Mitsdoerffer M, Ho IC, Sharpe AH, Kuchroo VK (2009) The costimulatory molecule ICOS regulates the expression of c-Maf and IL-21 in the development of follicular T helper cells and TH-17 cells. Nat Immunol 10(2):167–175. ni.1690 [pii]101038/ni.1690

Bentebibel SE, Khurana S, Schmitt N, Kurup P, Mueller C, Obermoser G, Palucka AK, Albrecht RA, Garcia-Sastre A, Golding H, Ueno H (2016) ICOS(+)PD-1(+)CXCR3(+) T follicular helper cells contribute to the generation of high-avidity antibodies following influenza vaccination. Sci Rep 6:26494. https://doi.org/10.1038/srep26494

Bettelli E, Carrier Y, Gao W, Korn T, Strom TB, Oukka M, Weiner HL, Kuchroo VK (2006) Reciprocal developmental pathways for the generation of pathogenic effector TH17 and regulatory T cells. Nature 441(7090):235–238. nature04753 [pii]131038/nature04753

Bossaller L, Burger J, Draeger R, Grimbacher B, Knoth R, Plebani A, Durandy A, Baumann U, Schlesier M, Welcher AA, Peter HH, Warnatz K (2006) ICOS deficiency is associated with a severe reduction of CXCR5+CD4 germinal center Th cells. J Immunol 177(7):4927–4932

Bottino C, Castriconi R, Pende D, Rivera P, Nanni M, Carnemolla B, Cantoni C, Grassi J, Marcenaro S, Reymond N, Vitale M, Moretta L, Lopez M, Moretta A (2003) Identification of PVR (CD155) and Nectin-2 (CD112) as cell surface ligands for the human DNAM-1 (CD226) activating molecule. J Exp Med 198(4):557–567. https://doi.org/10.1084/jem.20030788 jem.20030788 [pii]

Breitfeld D, Ohl L, Kremmer E, Ellwart J, Sallusto F, Lipp M, Forster R (2000) Follicular B helper T cells express CXC chemokine receptor 5, localize to B cell follicles, and support immunoglobulin production. J Exp Med 192(11):1545–1552

Burmeister Y, Lischke T, Dahler AC, Mages HW, Lam KP, Coyle AJ, Kroczek RA, Hutloff A (2008) ICOS controls the pool size of effector-memory and regulatory T cells. J Immunol 180(2):774–782

Busse M, Krech M, Meyer-Bahlburg A, Hennig C, Hansen G (2012) ICOS mediates the generation and function of CD4+CD25+Foxp3+ regulatory T cells conveying respiratory tolerance. J Immunol 189(4):1975–1982. https://doi.org/10.4049/jimmunol.1103581

Campbell KA, Ovendale PJ, Kennedy MK, Fanslow WC, Reed SG, Maliszewski CR (1996) CD40 ligand is required for protective cell-mediated immunity to Leishmania major. Immunity 4(3):283–289

Carboni S, Aboul-Enein F, Waltzinger C, Killeen N, Lassmann H, Pena-Rossi C (2003) CD134 plays a crucial role in the pathogenesis of EAE and is upregulated in the CNS of patients with multiple sclerosis. J Neuroimmunol 145(1–2):1–11

Carter LL, Leach MW, Azoitei ML, Cui J, Pelker JW, Jussif J, Benoit S, Ireland G, Luxenberg D, Askew GR, Milarski KL, Groves C, Brown T, Carito BA, Percival K, Carreno BM, Collins M, Marusic S (2007) PD-1/PD-L1, but not PD-1/PD-L2, interactions regulate the severity of experimental autoimmune encephalomyelitis. J Neuroimmunol 182(1–2):124–134. https://doi.org/10.1016/j.jneuroim.2006.10.006

Cella M, Scheidegger D, Palmer-Lehmann K, Lane P, Lanzavecchia A, Alber G (1996) Ligation of CD40 on dendritic cells triggers production of high levels of interleukin-12 and enhances T cell stimulatory capacity: T-T help via APC activation. J Exp Med 184(2):747–752

Chaturvedi P, Yu Q, Southwood S, Sette A, Singh B (1996) Peptide analogs with different affinities for MHC alter the cytokine profile of T helper cells. Int Immunol 8(5):745–755

Chen AI, McAdam AJ, Buhlmann JE, Scott S, Lupher ML Jr, Greenfield EA, Baum PR, Fanslow WC, Calderhead DM, Freeman GJ, Sharpe AH (1999) Ox40-ligand has a critical costimulatory role in dendritic cell: T cell interactions. Immunity 11(6):689–698

Chen Y, Langrish CL, McKenzie B, Joyce-Shaikh B, Stumhofer JS, McClanahan T, Blumenschein W, Churakovsa T, Low J, Presta L, Hunter CA, Kastelein RA, Cua DJ (2006) Anti-IL-23 therapy inhibits multiple inflammatory pathways and ameliorates autoimmune encephalomyelitis. J Clin Invest 116(5):1317–1326. https://doi.org/10.1172/JCI25308

Choi P, Reiser H (1998) IL-4: role in disease and regulation of production. Clin Exp Immunol 113(3):317–319

Chung Y, Chang SH, Martinez GJ, Yang XO, Nurieva R, Kang HS, Ma L, Watowich SS, Jetten AM, Tian Q, Dong C (2009) Critical regulation of early Th17 cell differentiation by interleukin-1 signaling. Immunity 30(4):576–587. https://doi.org/10.1016/j.immuni.2009.02.007. S1074-7613(09)00142-3 [pii]

Constant S, Pfeiffer C, Woodard A, Pasqualini T, Bottomly K (1995) Extent of T cell receptor ligation can determine the functional differentiation of naive CD4+ T cells. J Exp Med 182(5):1591–1596

Coyle AJ, Lehar S, Lloyd C, Tian J, Delaney T, Manning S, Nguyen T, Burwell T, Schneider H, Gonzalo JA, Gosselin M, Owen LR, Rudd CE, Gutierrez-Ramos JC (2000) The CD28-related molecule ICOS is required for effective T cell-dependent immune responses. Immunity 13(1):95–105

Crotty S (2011) Follicular helper CD4 T cells (TFH). Annu Rev Immunol 29:621–663. https://doi.org/10.1146/annurev-immunol-031210-101400

Crotty S (2014) T follicular helper cell differentiation, function, and roles in disease. Immunity 41(4):529–542. https://doi.org/10.1016/j.immuni.2014.10.004

Cua DJ, Sherlock J, Chen Y, Murphy CA, Joyce B, Seymour B, Lucian L, To W, Kwan S, Churakova T, Zurawski S, Wiekowski M, Lira SA, Gorman D, Kastelein RA, Sedgwick JD (2003) Interleukin-23 rather than interleukin-12 is the critical cytokine for autoimmune inflammation of the brain. Nature 421(6924):744–748. https://doi.org/10.1038/nature01355. nature01355 [pii]

Curtiss ML, Gorman JV, Businga TR, Traver G, Singh M, Meyerholz DK, Kline JN, Murphy AJ, Valenzuela DM, Colgan JD, Rothman PB, Cassel SL (2012) Tim-1 regulates Th2 responses in an airway hypersensitivity model. Eur J Immunol 42(3):651–661. https://doi.org/10.1002/eji.201141581

Dardalhon V, Schubart AS, Reddy J, Meyers JH, Monney L, Sabatos CA, Ahuja R, Nguyen K, Freeman GJ, Greenfield EA, Sobel RA, Kuchroo VK (2005) CD226 is specifically expressed on the surface of Th1 cells and regulates their expansion and effector functions. J Immunol 175(3):1558–1565. 175/3/1558 [pii]

Dardalhon V, Awasthi A, Kwon H, Galileos G, Gao W, Sobel RA, Mitsdoerffer M, Strom TB, Elyaman W, Ho IC, Khoury S, Oukka M, Kuchroo VK (2008) IL-4 inhibits TGF-beta-induced Foxp3+ T cells and, together with TGF-beta, generates IL-9+ IL-10+ Foxp3(−) effector T cells. Nat Immunol 9 (12):1347–1355. ni.1677 [pii] 381038/ni.1677

Degauque N, Mariat C, Kenny J, Zhang D, Gao W, Vu MD, Alexopoulos S, Oukka M, Umetsu DT, DeKruyff RH, Kuchroo V, Zheng XX, Strom TB (2008) Immunostimulatory Tim-1-specific antibody deprograms Tregs and prevents transplant tolerance in mice. J Clin Invest 118(2):735–741. https://doi.org/10.1172/JCI32562

Dong C, Juedes AE, Temann UA, Shresta S, Allison JP, Ruddle NH, Flavell RA (2001) ICOS co-stimulatory receptor is essential for T-cell activation and function. Nature 409(6816):97–101. https://doi.org/10.1038/35051100

Encinas JA, Janssen EM, Weiner DB, Calarota SA, Nieto D, Moll T, Carlo DJ, Moss RB (2005) Anti-T-cell Ig and mucin domain-containing protein 1 antibody decreases TH2 airway inflammation in a mouse model of asthma. J Allergy Clin Immunol 116(6):1343–1349. https://doi.org/10.1016/j.jaci.2005.08.031

Fang L, Zhang X, Miao J, Zhao F, Yang K, Zhuang R, Bujard H, Wei Y, Yang A, Chen L, Jin B (2009) Expression of CD226 antagonizes apoptotic cell death in murine thymocytes. J Immunol 182 (9):5453-5460. 182/9/5453 [pii] 444049/jimmunol.0803090

Fazilleau N, Mark L, McHeyzer-Williams LJ, McHeyzer-Williams MG (2009a) Follicular helper T cells: lineage and location. Immunity 30(3):324–335. https://doi.org/10.1016/j.immuni.2009.03.003

Fazilleau N, McHeyzer-Williams LJ, Rosen H, McHeyzer-Williams MG (2009b) The function of follicular helper T cells is regulated by the strength of T cell antigen receptor binding. Nat Immunol 10(4):375–384. https://doi.org/10.1038/ni.1704

Gaglia JL, Greenfield EA, Mattoo A, Sharpe AH, Freeman GJ, Kuchroo VK (2000) Intercellular adhesion molecule 1 is critical for activation of CD28-deficient T cells. J Immunol 165(11):6091–6098

Galicia G, Kasran A, Uyttenhove C, De Swert K, Van Snick J, Ceuppens JL (2009) ICOS deficiency results in exacerbated IL-17 mediated experimental autoimmune encephalomyelitis. J Clin Immunol 29(4):426–433. https://doi.org/10.1007/s10875-009-9287-7

Gao X, Gigoux M, Yang J, Leconte J, Yang X, Suh WK (2012) Anti-chlamydial Th17 responses are controlled by the inducible costimulator partially through phosphoinositide 3-kinase signaling. PLoS One 7(12):e52657. https://doi.org/10.1371/journal.pone.0052657

Ghoreschi K, Laurence A, Yang XP, Tato CM, McGeachy MJ, Konkel JE, Ramos HL, Wei L, Davidson TS, Bouladoux N, Grainger JR, Chen Q, Kanno Y, Watford WT, Sun HW, Eberl G, Shevach EM, Belkaid Y, Cua DJ, Chen W, O'Shea JJ (2010) Generation of pathogenic T(H)17 cells in the absence of TGF-beta signalling. Nature 467(7318):967–971. nature09447 [pii] 511038/nature09447

Gomez-Rodriguez J, Sahu N, Handon R, Davidson TS, Anderson SM, Kirby MR, August A, Schwartzberg PL (2009) Differential expression of interleukin-17A and -17F is coupled to T cell receptor signaling via inducible T cell kinase. Immunity 31(4):587–597. https://doi.org/10.1016/j.immuni.2009.07.009

Gonzalo JA, Tian J, Delaney T, Corcoran J, Rottman JB, Lora J, Al-garawi A, Kroczek R, Gutierrez-Ramos JC, Coyle AJ (2001) ICOS is critical for T helper cell-mediated lung mucosal inflammatory responses. Nat Immunol 2(7):597–604. https://doi.org/10.1038/89739

Good-Jacobson KL, Szumilas CG, Chen L, Sharpe AH, Tomayko MM, Shlomchik MJ (2010) PD-1 regulates germinal center B cell survival and the formation and affinity of long-lived plasma cells. Nat Immunol 11(6):535–542. https://doi.org/10.1038/ni.1877

Grabmeier-Pfistershammer K, Stecher C, Zettl M, Rosskopf S, Rieger A, Zlabinger GJ, Steinberger P (2017) Antibodies targeting BTLA or TIM-3 enhance HIV-1 specific T cell responses in combination with PD-1 blockade. Clin Immunol 183:167–173. https://doi.org/10.1016/j.clim.2017.09.002

Gramaglia I, Lemon M, Weinberg AD, Croft M (1998) Ox40 ligand, a potent costimulator of effector CD4(+) T cells. FASEB J 12(5):A941–A941

Grewal IS, Foellmer HG, Grewal KD, Xu J, Hardardottir F, Baron JL, Janeway CA Jr, Flavell RA (1996) Requirement for CD40 ligand in costimulation induction, T cell activation, and experimental allergic encephalomyelitis. Science 273(5283):1864–1867

Hafler JP, Maier LM, Cooper JD, Plagnol V, Hinks A, Simmonds MJ, Stevens HE, Walker NM, Healy B, Howson JM, Maisuria M, Duley S, Coleman G, Gough SC, Worthington J, Kuchroo VK, Wicker LS, Todd JA (2009) CD226 Gly307Ser association with multiple autoimmune diseases. Genes Immun 10(1):5–10. gene200882 [pii] 591038/gene.2008.82

Han MH, Hwang SI, Roy DB, Lundgren DH, Price JV, Ousman SS, Fernald GH, Gerlitz B, Robinson WH, Baranzini SE, Grinnell BW, Raine CS, Sobel RA, Han DK, Steinman L (2008) Proteomic analysis of active multiple sclerosis lesions reveals therapeutic targets. Nature 451(7182):1076–1081. https://doi.org/10.1038/nature06559. nature06559 [pii]

Harada H, Salama AD, Sho M, Izawa A, Sandner SE, Ito T, Akiba H, Yagita H, Sharpe AH, Freeman GJ, Sayegh MH (2003) The role of the ICOS-B7h T cell costimulatory pathway in transplantation immunity. J Clin Invest 112(2):234–243. https://doi.org/10.1172/JCI17008

Harrington LE, Hatton RD, Mangan PR, Turner H, Murphy TL, Murphy KM, Weaver CT (2005) Interleukin 17-producing CD4+ effector T cells develop via a lineage distinct from the T helper type 1 and 2 lineages. Nat Immunol 6(11):1123–1132. https://doi.org/10.1038/ni1254

Hastings WD, Anderson DE, Kassam N, Koguchi K, Greenfield EA, Kent SC, Zheng XX, Strom TB, Hafler DA, Kuchroo VK (2009) TIM-3 is expressed on activated human CD4+ T cells and regulates Th1 and Th17 cytokines. Eur J Immunol 39(9):2492–2501. https://doi.org/10.1002/eji.200939274

Hawiger D, Tran E, Du W, Booth CJ, Wen L, Dong C, Flavell RA (2008) ICOS mediates the development of insulin-dependent diabetes mellitus in nonobese diabetic mice. J Immunol 180(5):3140–3147

Haynes NM, Allen CD, Lesley R, Ansel KM, Killeen N, Cyster JG (2007) Role of CXCR5 and CCR7 in follicular Th cell positioning and appearance of a programmed cell death gene-1high germinal center-associated subpopulation. J Immunol 179(8):5099–5108

Herold M, Posevitz V, Chudyka D, Hucke S, Gross C, Kurth F, Leder C, Loser K, Kurts C, Knolle P, Klotz L, Wiendl H (2015) B7-H1 selectively controls TH17 differentiation and central nervous system autoimmunity via a novel non-PD-1-mediated pathway. J Immunol 195(8):3584–3595. https://doi.org/10.4049/jimmunol.1402746

Hirahara K, Ghoreschi K, Yang XP, Takahashi H, Laurence A, Vahedi G, Sciume G, Hall AO, Dupont CD, Francisco LM, Chen Q, Tanaka M, Kanno Y, Sun HW, Sharpe AH, Hunter CA, O'Shea JJ (2012) Interleukin-27 priming of T cells controls IL-17 production in trans via induction of the ligand PD-L1. Immunity 36(6):1017–1030. https://doi.org/10.1016/j.immuni.2012.03.024. S1074-7613(12)00235-X [pii]

Hosken NA, Shibuya K, Heath AW, Murphy KM, O'Garra A (1995) The effect of antigen dose on CD4+ T helper cell phenotype development in a T cell receptor-alpha beta-transgenic model. J Exp Med 182(5):1579–1584

Hotez PJ, Brindley PJ, Bethony JM, King CH, Pearce EJ, Jacobson J (2008) Helminth infections: the great neglected tropical diseases. J Clin Invest 118(4):1311–1321. https://doi.org/10.1172/JCI34261

Hsieh CS, Macatonia SE, Tripp CS, Wolf SF, O'Garra A, Murphy KM (1993) Development of TH1 CD4+ T cells through IL-12 produced by listeria-induced macrophages. Science 260(5107):547–549

Hutloff A, Dittrich AM, Beier KC, Eljaschewitsch B, Kraft R, Anagnostopoulos I, Kroczek RA (1999) ICOS is an inducible T-cell co-stimulator structurally and functionally related to CD28. Nature 397(6716):263–266. https://doi.org/10.1038/16717

Iezzi G, Sonderegger I, Ampenberger F, Schmitz N, Marsland BJ, Kopf M (2009) CD40-CD40L cross-talk integrates strong antigenic signals and microbial stimuli to induce development of IL-17-producing CD4+ T cells. Proc Natl Acad Sci U S A 106(3):876–881. https://doi.org/10.1073/pnas.0810769106

Ito T, Hanabuchi S, Wang YH, Park WR, Arima K, Bover L, Qin FX, Gilliet M, Liu YJ (2008) Two functional subsets of FOXP3+ regulatory T cells in human thymus and periphery. Immunity 28(6):870–880. https://doi.org/10.1016/j.immuni.2008.03.018

Ivanov II, McKenzie BS, Zhou L, Tadokoro CE, Lepelley A, Lafaille JJ, Cua DJ, Littman DR (2006) The orphan nuclear receptor RORgammat directs the differentiation program of proinflammatory IL-17+ T helper cells. Cell 126(6):1121–1133. https://doi.org/10.1016/j.cell.2006.07.035

Jager A, Dardalhon V, Sobel RA, Bettelli E, Kuchroo VK (2009) Th1, Th17, and Th9 effector cells induce experimental autoimmune encephalomyelitis with different pathological phenotypes. J Immunol 183(11):7169–7177. jimmunol.0901906 [pii] 784049/jimmunol.0901906

Jankovic D, Kullberg MC, Noben-Trauth N, Caspar P, Paul WE, Sher A (2000) Single cell analysis reveals that IL-4 receptor/Stat6 signaling is not required for the in vivo or in vitro development of CD4+ lymphocytes with a Th2 cytokine profile. J Immunol 164(6):3047–3055

Jin HT, Anderson AC, Tan WG, West EE, Ha SJ, Araki K, Freeman GJ, Kuchroo VK, Ahmed R (2010) Cooperation of Tim-3 and PD-1 in CD8 T-cell exhaustion during chronic viral infection. Proc Natl Acad Sci U S A 107(33):14733–14738. 1009731107 [pii] 811073/pnas.1009731107

Jorritsma PJ, Brogdon JL, Bottomly K (2003) Role of TCR-induced extracellular signal-regulated kinase activation in the regulation of early IL-4 expression in naive CD4+ T cells. J Immunol 170(5):2427–2434

Khademi M, Illes Z, Gielen AW, Marta M, Takazawa N, Baecher-Allan C, Brundin L, Hannerz J, Martin C, Harris RA, Hafler DA, Kuchroo VK, Olsson T, Piehl F, Wallstrom E (2004) T cell Ig- and mucin-domain-containing molecule-3 (TIM-3) and TIM-1 molecules are differentially expressed on human Th1 and Th2 cells and in cerebrospinal fluid-derived mononuclear cells in multiple sclerosis. J Immunol 172(11):7169–7176

Kim CH, Rott LS, Clark-Lewis I, Campbell DJ, Wu L, Butcher EC (2001) Subspecialization of CXCR5+ T cells: B helper activity is focused in a germinal center-localized subset of CXCR5+ T cells. J Exp Med 193(12):1373–1381

Kishi Y, Kondo T, Xiao S, Yosef N, Gaublomme J, Wu C, Wang C, Chihara N, Regev A, Joller N, Kuchroo VK (2016) Protein C receptor (PROCR) is a negative regulator of Th17 pathogenicity. J Exp Med 213(11):2489–2501. https://doi.org/10.1084/jem.20151118

Koch F, Stanzl U, Jennewein P, Janke K, Heufler C, Kampgen E, Romani N, Schuler G (1996) High level IL-12 production by murine dendritic cells: upregulation via MHC class II and CD40 molecules and downregulation by IL-4 and IL-10. J Exp Med 184(2):741–746

Koguchi K, Anderson DE, Yang L, O'Connor KC, Kuchroo VK, Hafler DA (2006) Dysregulated T cell expression of TIM3 in multiple sclerosis. J Exp Med 203(6):1413–1418. jem.20060210 [pii] 891084/jem.20060210

Kopf M, Le Gros G, Bachmann M, Lamers MC, Bluethmann H, Kohler G (1993) Disruption of the murine IL-4 gene blocks Th2 cytokine responses. Nature 362(6417):245–248. https://doi.org/10.1038/362245a0

Kopf M, Coyle AJ, Schmitz N, Barner M, Oxenius A, Gallimore A, Gutierrez-Ramos JC, Bachmann MF (2000) Inducible costimulator protein (ICOS) controls T helper cell subset polarization after virus and parasite infection. J Exp Med 192(1):53–61

Kubo M, Yamashita M, Abe R, Tada T, Okumura K, Ransom JT, Nakayama T (1999) CD28 costimulation accelerates IL-4 receptor sensitivity and IL-4-mediated Th2 differentiation. J Immunol 163(5):2432–2442

Kuchroo VK, Umetsu DT, DeKruyff RH, Freeman GJ (2003) The TIM gene family: emerging roles in immunity and disease. Nat Rev Immunol 3(6):454–462. https://doi.org/10.1038/nri1111

Kumar V, Bhardwaj V, Soares L, Alexander J, Sette A, Sercarz E (1995) Major histocompatibility complex binding affinity of an antigenic determinant is crucial for the differential secretion of interleukin 4/5 or interferon gamma by T cells. Proc Natl Acad Sci U S A 92(21):9510–9514

Langrish CL, Chen Y, Blumenschein WM, Mattson J, Basham B, Sedgwick JD, McClanahan T, Kastelein RA, Cua DJ (2005) IL-23 drives a pathogenic T cell population that induces autoimmune inflammation. J Exp Med 201(2):233–240. https://doi.org/10.1084/jem.20041257

Lee Y, Awasthi A, Yosef N, Quintana FJ, Xiao S, Peters A, Wu C, Kleinewietfeld M, Kunder S, Hafler DA, Sobel RA, Regev A, Kuchroo VK (2012) Induction and molecular signature of pathogenic TH17 cells. Nat Immunol 13(10):991–999. ni.2416 [pii] 971038/ni.2416

Levin SD, Taft DW, Brandt CS, Bucher C, Howard ED, Chadwick EM, Johnston J, Hammond A, Bontadelli K, Ardourel D, Hebb L, Wolf A, Bukowski TR, Rixon MW, Kuijper JL, Ostrander CD, West JW, Bilsborough J, Fox B, Gao Z, Xu W, Ramsdell F, Blazar BR, Lewis KE (2011) Vstm3 is a member of the CD28 family and an important modulator of T-cell function. Eur J Immunol 41(4):902–915. https://doi.org/10.1002/eji.201041136

Licona-Limon P, Kim LK, Palm NW, Flavell RA (2013) TH2, allergy and group 2 innate lymphoid cells. Nat Immunol 14(6):536–542. https://doi.org/10.1038/ni.2617

Liu Y, Shu Q, Gao L, Hou N, Zhao D, Liu X, Zhang X, Xu L, Yue X, Zhu F, Guo C, Liang X, Ma C (2010) Increased Tim-3 expression on peripheral lymphocytes from patients with rheumatoid arthritis negatively correlates with disease activity. Clin Immunol 137(2):288–295. https://doi.org/10.1016/j.clim.2010.07.012

Lohning M, Hutloff A, Kallinich T, Mages HW, Bonhagen K, Radbruch A, Hamelmann E, Kroczek RA (2003) Expression of ICOS in vivo defines CD4+ effector T cells with high inflammatory potential and a strong bias for secretion of interleukin 10. J Exp Med 197(2):181–193

Lozano E, Dominguez-Villar M, Kuchroo V, Hafler DA (2012) The TIGIT/CD226 Axis Regulates Human T Cell Function. J Immunol jimmunol.1103627 [pii] https://doi.org/10.4049/jimmunol.1103627

Lozano E, Joller N, Cao Y, Kuchroo V, Hafler DA (2013) The CD226/CD155 interaction regulates the proinflammatory (Th1/Th17)/anti-inflammatory (Th2) balance in humans. J Immunol. jimmunol.1300945 [pii] https://doi.org/10.4049/jimmunol.1300945

Mallett S, Fossum S, Barclay AN (1990) Characterization of the MRC OX40 antigen of activated CD4 positive T lymphocytes--a molecule related to nerve growth factor receptor. EMBO J 9(4):1063–1068

Manetti R, Parronchi P, Giudizi MG, Piccinni MP, Maggi E, Trinchieri G, Romagnani S (1993) Natural killer cell stimulatory factor (interleukin 12 [IL-12]) induces T helper type 1 (Th1)-specific immune responses and inhibits the development of IL-4-producing Th cells. J Exp Med 177(4):1199–1204

Mangan PR, Harrington LE, O'Quinn DB, Helms WS, Bullard DC, Elson CO, Hatton RD, Wahl SM, Schoeb TR, Weaver CT (2006) Transforming growth factor-beta induces development of the T(H)17 lineage. Nature 441 (7090):231–234. nature04754 [pii] https://doi.org/10.1038/nature04754

McAdam AJ, Chang TT, Lumelsky AE, Greenfield EA, Boussiotis VA, Duke-Cohan JS, Chernova T, Malenkovich N, Jabs C, Kuchroo VK, Ling V, Collins M, Sharpe AH, Freeman GJ (2000) Mouse inducible costimulatory molecule (ICOS) expression is enhanced by CD28 costimulation and regulates differentiation of CD4+ T cells. J Immunol 165(9):5035–5040

McAdam AJ, Greenwald RJ, Levin MA, Chernova T, Malenkovich N, Ling V, Freeman GJ, Sharpe AH (2001) ICOS is critical for CD40-mediated antibody class switching. Nature 409(6816):102–105. https://doi.org/10.1038/35051107

McArthur JG, Raulet DH (1993) CD28-induced costimulation of T helper type 2 cells mediated by induction of responsiveness to interleukin 4. J Exp Med 178(5):1645–1653

McIntire JJ, Umetsu SE, Akbari O, Potter M, Kuchroo VK, Barsh GS, Freeman GJ, Umetsu DT, DeKruyff RH (2001) Identification of Tapr (an airway hyperreactivity regulatory locus) and the linked Tim gene family. Nat Immunol 2(12):1109–1116. https://doi.org/10.1038/ni739

Mitsdoerffer M, Lee Y, Jager A, Kim HJ, Korn T, Kolls JK, Cantor H, Bettelli E, Kuchroo VK (2010) Proinflammatory T helper type 17 cells are effective B-cell helpers. Proc Natl Acad Sci U S A 107(32):14292–14297. 1009234107 [pii] https://doi.org/10.1073/pnas.1009234107

Mittrucker HW, Kursar M, Kohler A, Yanagihara D, Yoshinaga SK, Kaufmann SH (2002) Inducible costimulator protein controls the protective T cell response against Listeria monocytogenes. J Immunol 169(10):5813–5817

Miyazaki T, Hirokami Y, Matsuhashi N, Takatsuka H, Naito M (1999) Increased susceptibility of thymocytes to apoptosis in mice lacking AIM, a novel murine macrophage-derived soluble factor belonging to the scavenger receptor cysteine-rich domain superfamily. J Exp Med 189(2):413–422

Monney L, Sabatos CA, Gaglia JL, Ryu A, Waldner H, Chernova T, Manning S, Greenfield EA, Coyle AJ, Sobel RA, Freeman GJ, Kuchroo VK (2002) Th1-specific cell surface protein Tim-3 regulates macrophage activation and severity of an autoimmune disease. Nature 415(6871):536–541. https://doi.org/10.1038/415536a. 415536a [pii]

Mosmann TR, Cherwinski H, Bond MW, Giedlin MA, Coffman RL (1986) Two types of murine helper T cell clone. I. Definition according to profiles of lymphokine activities and secreted proteins. J Immunol 136(7):2348–2357

Murphy CA, Langrish CL, Chen Y, Blumenschein W, McClanahan T, Kastelein RA, Sedgwick JD, Cua DJ (2003) Divergent pro- and antiinflammatory roles for IL-23 and IL-12 in joint autoimmune inflammation. J Exp Med 198(12):1951–1957. https://doi.org/10.1084/jem.20030896

Nakae S, Iwakura Y, Suto H, Galli SJ (2007) Phenotypic differences between Th1 and Th17 cells and negative regulation of Th1 cell differentiation by IL-17. J Leukoc Biol 81(5):1258–1268. https://doi.org/10.1189/jlb.1006610

Ndhlovu LC, Ishii N, Murata K, Sato T, Sugamura K (2001) Critical involvement of OX40 ligand signals in the T cell priming events during experimental autoimmune encephalomyelitis. J Immunol 167(5):2991–2999

Niwa H, Satoh T, Matsushima Y, Hosoya K, Saeki K, Niki T, Hirashima M, Yokozeki H (2009) Stable form of galectin-9, a Tim-3 ligand, inhibits contact hypersensitivity and psoriatic reactions: a potent therapeutic tool for Th1- and/or Th17-mediated skin inflammation. Clin Immunol 132(2):184–194. https://doi.org/10.1016/j.clim.2009.04.012

Nouailles G, Day TA, Kuhlmann S, Loewe D, Dorhoi A, Gamradt P, Hurwitz R, Jorg S, Pradl L, Hutloff A, Koch M, Kursar M, Kaufmann SH (2011) Impact of inducible co-stimulatory molecule (ICOS) on T-cell responses and protection against Mycobacterium tuberculosis infection. Eur J Immunol 41(4):981–991. https://doi.org/10.1002/eji.201040608

Nurieva RI, Treuting P, Duong J, Flavell RA, Dong C (2003) Inducible costimulator is essential for collagen-induced arthritis. J Clin Invest 111(5):701–706. https://doi.org/10.1172/JCI17321

Nurieva RI, Chung Y, Hwang D, Yang XO, Kang HS, Ma L, Wang YH, Watowich SS, Jetten AM, Tian Q, Dong C (2008) Generation of T follicular helper cells is mediated by interleukin-21 but independent of T helper 1, 2, or 17 cell lineages. Immunity 29(1):138–149. https://doi.org/10.1016/j.immuni.2008.05.009

Ohshima Y, Yang LP, Uchiyama T, Tanaka Y, Baum P, Sergerie M, Hermann P, Delespesse G (1998) OX40 costimulation enhances interleukin-4 (IL-4) expression at priming and promotes the differentiation of naive human CD4(+) T cells into high IL-4-producing effectors. Blood 92(9):3338–3345

Ota N, Wong K, Valdez PA, Zheng Y, Crellin NK, Diehl L, Ouyang W (2011) IL-22 bridges the lymphotoxin pathway with the maintenance of colonic lymphoid structures during infection with Citrobacter rodentium. Nat Immunol 12(10):941–948. https://doi.org/10.1038/ni.2089

Ottoboni L, Keenan BT, Tamayo P, Kuchroo M, Mesirov JP, Buckle GJ, Khoury SJ, Hafler DA, Weiner HL, De Jager PL (2012) An RNA profile identifies two subsets of multiple sclerosis patients differing in disease activity. Sci Transl Med 4(153):153ra131. https://doi.org/10.1126/scitranslmed.3004186

Ouyang W, Lohning M, Gao Z, Assenmacher M, Ranganath S, Radbruch A, Murphy KM (2000) Stat6-independent GATA-3 autoactivation directs IL-4-independent Th2 development and commitment. Immunity 12(1):27–37

Oxenius A, Karrer U, Zinkernagel RM, Hengartner H (1999) IL-12 is not required for induction of type 1 cytokine responses in viral infections. J Immunol 162(2):965–973

Ozkaynak E, Gao W, Shemmeri N, Wang C, Gutierrez-Ramos JC, Amaral J, Qin S, Rottman JB, Coyle AJ, Hancock WW (2001) Importance of ICOS-B7RP-1 costimulation in acute and chronic allograft rejection. Nat Immunol 2(7):591–596. https://doi.org/10.1038/89731

Park H, Li Z, Yang XO, Chang SH, Nurieva R, Wang YH, Wang Y, Hood L, Zhu Z, Tian Q, Dong C (2005) A distinct lineage of CD4 T cells regulates tissue inflammation by producing interleukin 17. Nat Immunol 6(11):1133–1141. https://doi.org/10.1038/ni1261

Patel DD, Kuchroo VK (2015) Th17 cell pathway in human immunity: Lessons from genetics and therapeutic interventions. Immunity 43(6):1040–1051. https://doi.org/10.1016/j.immuni.2015.12.003

Paterson DJ, Jefferies WA, Green JR, Brandon MR, Corthesy P, Puklavec M, Williams AF (1987) Antigens of activated rat T lymphocytes including a molecule of 50,000 Mr detected only on CD4 positive T blasts. Mol Immunol 24(12):1281–1290

Paulos CM, Carpenito C, Plesa G, Suhoski MM, Varela-Rohena A, Golovina TN, Carroll RG, Riley JL, June CH (2010) The inducible costimulator (ICOS) is critical for the development of human T(H)17 cells. Sci Transl Med 2(55):55ra78. https://doi.org/10.1126/scitranslmed.3000448

Perona-Wright G, Jenkins SJ, O'Connor RA, Zienkiewicz D, McSorley HJ, Maizels RM, Anderton SM, MacDonald AS (2009) A pivotal role for CD40-mediated IL-6 production by dendritic cells during IL-17 induction in vivo. J Immunol 182(5):2808–2815. https://doi.org/10.4049/jimmunol.0803553

Peters A, Pitcher LA, Sullivan JM, Mitsdoerffer M, Acton SE, Franz B, Wucherpfennig K, Turley S, Carroll MC, Sobel RA, Bettelli E, Kuchroo VK (2011) Th17 cells induce ectopic lymphoid follicles in central nervous system tissue inflammation. Immunity 35(6):986–996. S1074-7613(11)00503-6 [pii] https://doi.org/10.1016/j.immuni.2011.10.015

Pfeiffer C, Stein J, Southwood S, Ketelaar H, Sette A, Bottomly K (1995) Altered peptide ligands can control CD4 T lymphocyte differentiation in vivo. J Exp Med 181(4):1569–1574

Piconese S, Gri G, Tripodo C, Musio S, Gorzanelli A, Frossi B, Pedotti R, Pucillo CE, Colombo MP (2009) Mast cells counteract regulatory T-cell suppression through interleukin-6 and OX40/OX40L axis toward Th17-cell differentiation. Blood 114(13):2639–2648. https://doi.org/10.1182/blood-2009-05-220004

Rangel-Moreno J, Carragher DM, de la Luz G-HM, Hwang JY, Kusser K, Hartson L, Kolls JK, Khader SA, Randall TD (2011) The development of inducible bronchus-associated lymphoid tissue depends on IL-17. Nat Immunol 12(7):639–646. https://doi.org/10.1038/ni.2053

Rodriguez-Palmero M, Hara T, Thumbs A, Hunig T (1999) Triggering of T cell proliferation through CD28 induces GATA-3 and promotes T helper type 2 differentiation in vitro and in vivo. Eur J Immunol 29(12):3914–3924. https://doi.org/10.1002/(SICI)1521-4141(199912)29:12<3914::AID-IMMU3914>3.0.CO;20-#

Rogers PR, Croft M (2000) CD28, Ox-40, LFA-1, and CD4 modulation of Th1/Th2 differentiation is directly dependent on the dose of antigen. J Immunol 164(6):2955–2963. https://doi.org/10.4049/jimmunol.164.6.2955

Rottman JB, Smith T, Tonra JR, Ganley K, Bloom T, Silva R, Pierce B, Gutierrez-Ramos JC, Ozkaynak E, Coyle AJ (2001) The costimulatory molecule ICOS plays an important role in the immunopathogenesis of EAE. Nat Immunol 2(7):605–611. https://doi.org/10.1038/89750

Rulifson IC, Sperling AI, Fields PE, Fitch FW, Bluestone JA (1997) CD28 costimulation promotes the production of Th2 cytokines. J Immunol 158(2):658–665

Sabatos CA, Chakravarti S, Cha E, Schubart A, Sanchez-Fueyo A, Zheng XX, Coyle AJ, Strom TB, Freeman GJ, Kuchroo VK (2003) Interaction of Tim-3 and Tim-3 ligand regulates T helper type 1 responses and induction of peripheral tolerance. Nat Immunol 4(11):1102–1110. https://doi.org/10.1038/ni988. ni988 [pii]

Sage PT, Francisco LM, Carman CV, Sharpe AH (2013) The receptor PD-1 controls follicular regulatory T cells in the lymph nodes and blood. Nat Immunol 14(2):152–161. https://doi.org/10.1038/ni.2496

Salama AD, Chitnis T, Imitola J, Ansari MJ, Akiba H, Tushima F, Azuma M, Yagita H, Sayegh MH, Khoury SJ (2003) Critical role of the programmed death-1 (PD-1) pathway in regulation of experimental autoimmune encephalomyelitis. J Exp Med 198(1):71–78. https://doi.org/10.1084/jem.20022119. jem.20022119 [pii]

Sallusto F (2016) Heterogeneity of Human CD4(+) T Cells Against Microbes. Annu Rev Immunol 34:317–334. https://doi.org/10.1146/annurev-immunol-032414-112056

Salomon B, Bluestone JA (1998) LFA-1 interaction with ICAM-1 and ICAM-2 regulates Th2 cytokine production. J Immunol 161(10):5138–5142

Sanchez-Fueyo A, Tian J, Picarella D, Domenig C, Zheng XX, Sabatos CA, Manlongat N, Bender O, Kamradt T, Kuchroo VK, Gutierrez-Ramos JC, Coyle AJ, Strom TB (2003) Tim-3 inhibits T helper type 1-mediated auto- and alloimmune responses and promotes immunological tolerance. Nat Immunol 4(11):1093–1101. https://doi.org/10.1038/ni987

Sarrias MR, Padilla O, Monreal Y, Carrascal M, Abian J, Vives J, Yelamos J, Lozano F (2004) Biochemical characterization of recombinant and circulating human Spalpha. Tissue Antigens 63(4):335–344

Schaerli P, Willimann K, Lang AB, Lipp M, Loetscher P, Moser B (2000) CXC chemokine receptor 5 expression defines follicular homing T cells with B cell helper function. J Exp Med 192(11):1553–1562

Schijns VE, Haagmans BL, Wierda CM, Kruithof B, Heijnen IA, Alber G, Horzinek MC (1998) Mice lacking IL-12 develop polarized Th1 cells during viral infection. J Immunol 160(8):3958–3964

Schreiner B, Bailey SL, Shin T, Chen L, Miller SD (2008) PD-1 ligands expressed on myeloid-derived APC in the CNS regulate T-cell responses in EAE. Eur J Immunol 38(10):2706–2717. https://doi.org/10.1002/eji.200838137

Seki M, Oomizu S, Sakata KM, Sakata A, Arikawa T, Watanabe K, Ito K, Takeshita K, Niki T, Saita N, Nishi N, Yamauchi A, Katoh S, Matsukawa A, Kuchroo V, Hirashima M (2008) Galectin-9 suppresses the generation of Th17, promotes the induction of regulatory T cells, and regulates experimental autoimmune arthritis. Clin Immunol 127(1):78–88. https://doi.org/10.1016/j.clim.2008.01.006

Shi SJ, Ding ML, Wang LJ, Wu JH, Han DH, Zheng GX, Guo ZY, Xi WJ, Qin WJ, Yang AG, Wen WH (2017) CD4(+)T cell specific B7-H1 selectively inhibits proliferation of naive T cells and Th17 differentiation in experimental autoimmune encephalomyelitis. Oncotarget 8(52):90028–90036. https://doi.org/10.18632/oncotarget.21357

Shibuya K, Shirakawa J, Kameyama T, Honda S, Tahara-Hanaoka S, Miyamoto A, Onodera M, Sumida T, Nakauchi H, Miyoshi H, Shibuya A (2003) CD226 (DNAM-1) is involved in lymphocyte function-associated antigen 1 costimulatory signal for naive T cell differentiation and proliferation. J Exp Med 198(12):1829–1839. https://doi.org/10.1084/jem.20030958. jem.20030958 [pii]

Smits HH, de Jong EC, Schuitemaker JH, Geijtenbeek TB, van Kooyk Y, Kapsenberg ML, Wierenga EA (2002) Intercellular adhesion molecule-1/LFA-1 ligation favors human Th1 development. J Immunol 168(4):1710–1716

So T, Song J, Sugie K, Altman A, Croft M (2006) Signals from OX40 regulate nuclear factor of activated T cells c1 and T cell helper 2 lineage commitment. Proc Natl Acad Sci U S A 103(10):3740–3745. https://doi.org/10.1073/pnas.0600205103

Stanietsky N, Simic H, Arapovic J, Toporik A, Levy O, Novik A, Levine Z, Beiman M, Dassa L, Achdout H, Stern-Ginossar N, Tsukerman P, Jonjic S, Mandelboim O (2009) The interaction of TIGIT with PVR and PVRL2 inhibits human NK cell cytotoxicity. Proc Natl Acad Sci U S A 106(42):17858–17863. https://doi.org/10.1073/pnas.0903474106

Stuber E, Strober W, Neurath M (1996) Blocking the CD40L-CD40 interaction in vivo specifically prevents the priming of T helper 1 cells through the inhibition of interleukin 12 secretion. J Exp Med 183(2):693–698

Sutton C, Brereton C, Keogh B, Mills KH, Lavelle EC (2006) A crucial role for interleukin (IL)-1 in the induction of IL-17-producing T cells that mediate autoimmune encephalomyelitis. J Exp Med 203(7):1685–1691. jem.20060285 [pii] https://doi.org/10.1084/jem.20060285

Szabo SJ, Kim ST, Costa GL, Zhang X, Fathman CG, Glimcher LH (2000) A novel transcription factor, T-bet, directs Th1 lineage commitment. Cell 100(6):655–669

Tao X, Constant S, Jorritsma P, Bottomly K (1997a) Strength of TCR signal determines the costimulatory requirements for Th1 and Th2 CD4+ T cell differentiation. J Immunol 159(12):5956–5963

Tao X, Grant C, Constant S, Bottomly K (1997b) Induction of IL-4-producing CD4+ T cells by antigenic peptides altered for TCR binding. J Immunol 158(9):4237–4244

Umetsu SE, Lee WL, McIntire JJ, Downey L, Sanjanwala B, Akbari O, Berry GJ, Nagumo H, Freeman GJ, Umetsu DT, DeKruyff RH (2005) TIM-1 induces T cell activation and inhibits the development of peripheral tolerance. Nat Immunol 6(5):447–454. https://doi.org/10.1038/ni1186

Veldhoen M, Hocking RJ, Atkins CJ, Locksley RM, Stockinger B (2006) TGFbeta in the context of an inflammatory cytokine milieu supports de novo differentiation of IL-17-producing T cells. Immunity 24(2):179–189. S1074-7613(06)00004-5 [pii] https://doi.org/10.1016/j.immuni.2006.01.001

Veldhoen M, Uyttenhove C, van Snick J, Helmby H, Westendorf A, Buer J, Martin B, Wilhelm C, Stockinger B (2008) Transforming growth factor-beta 'reprograms' the differentiation of T helper 2 cells and promotes an interleukin 9-producing subset. Nat Immunol 9(12):1341–1346. https://doi.org/10.1038/ni.1659

Verma NK, Fazil MH, Ong ST, Chalasani ML, Low JH, Kottaiswamy APP, Kizhakeyil A, Kumar S, Panda AK, Freeley M, Smith SM, Boehm BO, Kelleher D (2016) LFA-1/ICAM-1 ligation in human T cells promotes Th1 polarization through a GSK3beta signaling-dependent notch pathway. J Immunol 197(1):108–118. https://doi.org/10.4049/jimmunol.1501264

Vidric M, Bladt AT, Dianzani U, Watts TH (2006) Role for inducible costimulator in control of Salmonella enterica serovar Typhimurium infection in mice. Infect Immun 74(2):1050–1061. https://doi.org/10.1128/IAI.74.2.1050-1061.2006

Villegas EN, Lieberman LA, Mason N, Blass SL, Zediak VP, Peach R, Horan T, Yoshinaga S, Hunter CA (2002) A role for inducible costimulator protein in the CD28- independent mechanism of resistance to Toxoplasma gondii. J Immunol 169(2):937–943

Vogelzang A, McGuire HM, Yu D, Sprent J, Mackay CR, King C (2008) A fundamental role for interleukin-21 in the generation of T follicular helper cells. Immunity 29(1):127–137. https://doi.org/10.1016/j.immuni.2008.06.001

Wang C, Yosef N, Gaublomme J, Wu C, Lee Y, Clish CB, Kaminski J, Xiao S, Meyer Zu Horste G, Pawlak M, Kishi Y, Joller N, Karwacz K, Zhu C, Ordovas-Montanes M, Madi A, Wortman I, Miyazaki T, Sobel RA, Park H, Regev A, Kuchroo VK (2015) CD5L/AIM regulates lipid biosynthesis and restrains Th17 Cell pathogenicity. Cell 163(6):1413–1427. https://doi.org/10.1016/j.cell.2015.10.068

Warnatz K, Bossaller L, Salzer U, Skrabl-Baumgartner A, Schwinger W, van der Burg M, van Dongen JJ, Orlowska-Volk M, Knoth R, Durandy A, Draeger R, Schlesier M, Peter HH, Grimbacher B (2006) Human ICOS deficiency abrogates the germinal center reaction and provides a monogenic model for common variable immunodeficiency. Blood 107(8):3045–3052. https://doi.org/10.1182/blood-2005-07-2955

Watanabe M, Hara Y, Tanabe K, Toma H, Abe R (2005) A distinct role for ICOS-mediated co-stimulatory signaling in CD4+ and CD8+ T cell subsets. Int Immunol 17(3):269–278. https://doi.org/10.1093/intimm/dxh206

Weber JP, Fuhrmann F, Feist RK, Lahmann A, Al Baz MS, Gentz LJ, Vu Van D, Mages HW, Haftmann C, Riedel R, Grun JR, Schuh W, Kroczek RA, Radbruch A, Mashreghi MF, Hutloff A (2015) ICOS maintains the T follicular helper cell phenotype by down-regulating Kruppel-like factor 2. J Exp Med 212(2):217–233. https://doi.org/10.1084/jem.20141432

Wikenheiser DJ, Ghosh D, Kennedy B, Stumhofer JS (2016) The costimulatory molecule ICOS regulates Host Th1 and follicular Th cell differentiation in response to plasmodium chabaudi chabaudi AS infection. J Immunol 196(2):778–791. https://doi.org/10.4049/jimmunol.1403206

Wilson EH, Zaph C, Mohrs M, Welcher A, Siu J, Artis D, Hunter CA (2006) B7RP-1-ICOS interactions are required for optimal infection-induced expansion of CD4+ Th1 and Th2 responses. J Immunol 177(4):2365–2372

Xiao S, Najafian N, Reddy J, Albin M, Zhu C, Jensen E, Imitola J, Korn T, Anderson AC, Zhang Z, Gutierrez C, Moll T, Sobel RA, Umetsu DT, Yagita H, Akiba H, Strom T, Sayegh MH, DeKruyff RH, Khoury SJ, Kuchroo VK (2007) Differential engagement of Tim-1 during activation can positively or negatively costimulate T cell expansion and effector function. J Exp Med 204(7):1691–1702. https://doi.org/10.1084/jem.20062498

Xiao S, Zhu B, Jin H, Zhu C, Umetsu DT, DeKruyff RH, Kuchroo VK (2011) Tim-1 stimulation of dendritic cells regulates the balance between effector and regulatory T cells. Eur J Immunol 41(6):1539–1549. https://doi.org/10.1002/eji.201040993

Xu H, Li X, Liu D, Li J, Zhang X, Chen X, Hou S, Peng L, Xu C, Liu W, Zhang L, Qi H (2013) Follicular T-helper cell recruitment governed by bystander B cells and ICOS-driven motility. Nature 496(7446):523–527. https://doi.org/10.1038/nature12058

Yang L, Anderson DE, Kuchroo J, Hafler DA (2008) Lack of TIM-3 immunoregulation in multiple sclerosis. J Immunol 180(7):4409–4414

Yoshinaga SK, Whoriskey JS, Khare SD, Sarmiento U, Guo J, Horan T, Shih G, Zhang M, Coccia MA, Kohno T, Tafuri-Bladt A, Brankow D, Campbell P, Chang D, Chiu L, Dai T, Duncan G, Elliott GS, Hui A, McCabe SM, Scully S, Shahinian A, Shaklee CL, Van G, Mak TW, Senaldi G (1999) T-cell co-stimulation through B7RP-1 and ICOS. Nature 402(6763):827–832. https://doi.org/10.1038/45582

Yu D, Tan AH, Hu X, Athanasopoulos V, Simpson N, Silva DG, Hutloff A, Giles KM, Leedman PJ, Lam KP, Goodnow CC, Vinuesa CG (2007) Roquin represses autoimmunity by limiting inducible T-cell co-stimulator messenger RNA. Nature 450(7167):299–303. https://doi.org/10.1038/nature06253

6 Role of Co-stimulatory Molecules in T Helper Cell Differentiation

Yu X, Harden K, Gonzalez LC, Francesco M, Chiang E, Irving B, Tom I, Ivelja S, Refino CJ, Clark H, Eaton D, Grogan JL (2009) The surface protein TIGIT suppresses T cell activation by promoting the generation of mature immunoregulatory dendritic cells. Nat Immunol 10(1):48–57. https://doi.org/10.1038/ni.1674

Zheng W, Flavell RA (1997) The transcription factor GATA-3 is necessary and sufficient for Th2 cytokine gene expression in CD4 T cells. Cell 89(4):587–596

Zhu C, Anderson AC, Schubart A, Xiong H, Imitola J, Khoury SJ, Zheng XX, Strom TB, Kuchroo VK (2005) The Tim-3 ligand galectin-9 negatively regulates T helper type 1 immunity. Nat Immunol 6(12):1245–1252. https://doi.org/10.1038/ni1271

Zielinski CE, Mele F, Aschenbrenner D, Jarrossay D, Ronchi F, Gattorno M, Monticelli S, Lanzavecchia A, Sallusto F (2012) Pathogen-induced human TH17 cells produce IFN-gamma or IL-10 and are regulated by IL-1beta. Nature 484(7395):514–518. nature10957 [pii] https://doi.org/10.1038/nature10957

Chapter 7
Control of Regulatory T Cells by Co-signal Molecules

James Badger Wing, Christopher Tay, and Shimon Sakaguchi

Abstract Foxp3-expressing regulatory T cells (Tregs) perform a vital function in the maintenance of immune homeostasis. A large part of Treg suppressive function is derived from their ability to control and restrict the availability of co-signal molecules to other T cells. However, Tregs themselves also depend on many of the same co-signals for their own homeostasis, making this a complex system of feedback. In this chapter, we discuss the critical role of co-signaling in Treg cell biology.

Keywords Tregs · CTLA-4 · PD-1 · CD28 · OX40 · GITR · CD27 · CD30 · TIGIT · DR3 · TNFR2 · ICOS · Tim-3

7.1 Tregs

The first indications that some thymically derived cells had a critical suppressive function came from early work by Nishizuka and colleagues who demonstrated that day 3 thymectomy of mice led to severe autoimmunity, suggesting that cells produced after 3 days were responsible for the maintenance of immune homeostasis (Nishizuka and Sakakura 1969). However, it was not until 1995 when Tregs (Tregs), as we now know them, were definitively described on the basis of their expression of the IL2 receptor alpha chain (CD25) and that transfer of these cells could prevent

J. B. Wing · C. Tay
Laboratory of Experimental Immunology, WPI Immunology Frontier Research Center (IFReC), Osaka University, Osaka, Japan

S. Sakaguchi (✉)
Laboratory of Experimental Immunology, WPI Immunology Frontier Research Center (IFReC), Osaka University, Osaka, Japan

Department of Experimental Pathology, Institute for Frontier Medical Sciences, Kyoto University, Kyoto, Japan
e-mail: shimon@ifrec.osaka-u.ac.jp

© Springer Nature Singapore Pte Ltd. 2019
M. Azuma, H. Yagita (eds.), *Co-signal Molecules in T Cell Activation*,
Advances in Experimental Medicine and Biology 1189,
https://doi.org/10.1007/978-981-32-9717-3_7

autoimmunity (Sakaguchi et al. 1995). Shortly afterward, it was also found that in the neonatal period, Tregs develop in a slightly delayed fashion in comparison to effector T cells, explaining why thymectomy at day 3 allows the development of effector T cells but not Tregs (Asano et al. 1996).

Tregs are dependent on the master transcription factor Foxp3, and ectopic expression of Foxp3 into Foxp3 T cells induces suppressive function (Ramsdell and Ziegler 2014). Conversely, disruption of Foxp3 function results in the development of severe autoimmunity in both mice and humans as characterized by the scurfy mouse strain and immunodysregulation polyendocrinopathy enteropathy X-linked (IPEX) syndrome (Wildin et al. 2001). IPEX is characterized by severe allergy with hyper-IgE production, autoimmune disease such as type 1 diabetes mellitus, and inflammatory bowel disease (Wildin et al. 2001; Ramsdell and Ziegler 2014). While Foxp3 is critical for the function of Tregs, it is not alone responsible for all Treg-type gene expression as its transfection only causes partial reproduction of the Treg cell gene signature (Sugimoto et al. 2006). Treg gene expression is also stably maintained by epigenetic programming. Demethylation of key Treg genes such as CTLA-4 and Foxp3 itself allows their constitutive expression (Ohkura et al. 2013). Tregs are critical for prevention of autoimmunity throughout life, and depletion of Tregs in adult mice leads to catastrophic autoimmunity (Kim et al. 2007). In addition to the severe fatal inflammation associated with total loss of Treg function, more subtle defects of Treg number and function have been implicated in a wide range of autoimmune diseases such as SLE, Sjögren's syndrome, psoriasis, autoimmune hepatitis, myasthenia gravis, and inflammatory bowel disease (Grant et al. 2015).

Tregs can be split into two primary categories, thymically derived Tregs (tTregs) and peripherally derived Tregs (pTregs). tTregs are essential for the maintenance of immune self-tolerance and make up the majority of Tregs in circulation. pTregs are formed from Foxp3-negative non-Tregs exposed to signals such as TGFβ and IL-2 in peripheral organs; they have a critical and overlapping role with tTregs, being particularly important for the control of inflammation at barrier sites such as the gastrointestinal tract and lungs (Josefowicz et al. 2012). A third group also exists, in vitro derived Tregs (iTregs), consisting of originally Foxp3-negative conventional CD4 T cells (Tconv) that have been induced to convert to Foxp3$^+$ cells by in vitro treatment with antigen, IL-2, and TGF-β. While iTregs have proven a valuable tool for understanding Treg function, they cannot be considered the exact equivalent of in vivo derived pTregs since they lack the proper epigenetic programming and as a result are unstable, tending to lose Foxp3 expression without its active maintenance (Ohkura et al. 2013). In the past, the terms pTregs and iTregs have been used interchangeably, while tTregs were also often described as natural Tregs (nTregs), leading to a certain amount of confusion. Recent recommendations to clarify the nomenclature aim to address this and should be observed where possible (Abbas et al. 2013). In addition to differences in their site of origin, Tregs also display a high level of functional diversity with tissue-resident Tregs in areas such as the visceral adipose tissue, tumor environment, and muscles, showing characteristic phenotypes (Burzyn et al. 2013). Further, Tregs may mirror effector T-cell subtypes

7 Control of Regulatory T Cells by Co-signal Molecules

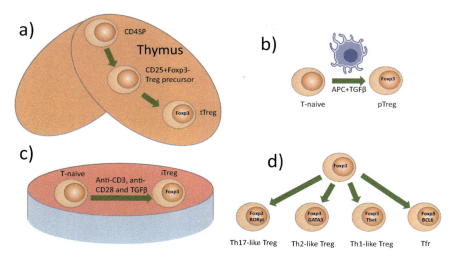

Fig. 7.1 Diversity of Treg cells. Tregs can be broadly divided into the key subgroups of (**a**) thymically derived tTregs. (**b**) Peripheral Tregs (pTregs) converted from Foxp3-negative cells outside the thymus in vivo. (**c**) In vitro Tregs (iTregs) converted from Foxp3-negative T cells in vitro. (**d**) Tregs can also mirror effector T-cell subsets by gaining expression of key transcription factors and chemokine receptors but not inflammatory cytokines. These cells may be derived from either mainly tTregs (e.g., Tfr) or mainly pTregs (e.g., Th17-like Tregs)

gaining expression of Th17-, Th1-, Th2-, and Tfh-associated transcription factors (RORγt, T-bet, Gata3, and BCL6, respectively) to form functionally specialized subpopulations of Tregs. These cells gain expression of matching chemokine receptors allowing them to track the matching effector subtype to the site of inflammation to deliver suppression in situ (Wing and Sakaguchi 2012) (Fig. 7.1).

While in most circumstances prevention of autoimmune responses to self-antigens is desirable, the presence of Tregs also suppresses responses to tumor antigens. As a result, Treg depletion or functional blockade leads to tumor regression in many cases. A number of therapies aimed at exploiting negative or positive co-signal molecules expressed by Tregs have been developed with the aim of enhancing antitumor immunity, forming an important part of antitumor immunotherapy (Tanaka and Sakaguchi 2017).

7.2 Control of Tregs by Co-signal Molecules

7.2.1 Two Signals Required for T-Cell Activation

During the immune response, antigens are processed and presented to Tregs by antigen-presenting cells (APCs) such as dendritic cells (DCs). Recognition of antigens by the T-cell receptor is essential for both the development and activation of T cells.

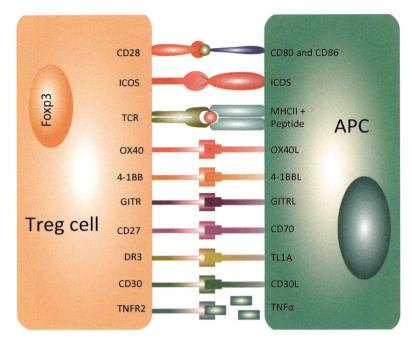

Fig. 7.2 Costimulatory molecules expressed by Tregs and their ligands. Tregs express a range of costimulatory molecules of the Ig superfamily (CD28 and ICOS) and the TNF-receptor superfamily (OX40, 4-1BB, GITR, CD27, CD30, DR3, and TNFR2)

However, TCR signals alone are not sufficient to fully activate T cells, often leading to anergy or cell death when presented without a second signal. The two-signal model of T-cell activation was initially described by Bretscher and Cohn in 1970 (Bretscher and Cohn 1970). In this model, T cells require both the recognition of a presented antigen via the TCR but also a second co-signal. The requirement for the co-signal prevents the activation of T cells by recognition of their antigen alone, and the availability of the second signal to be is closely regulated to prevent autoimmunity. Initially, CD28 signaling was considered to be the sole second signal, and while it remains of utmost importance, it has now become clear that a range of other co-signals have roles in T-cell activation and differentiation (Fig. 7.2). While the two-signal model provides a useful conceptual framework, it is also important to consider that the various second signals are not necessarily equivalent to one another and may have roles that vary at different stages of T-cell activation. The different roles may be sequential with CD28 required for initial signaling of naïve T cells, causing the upregulation of other co-signal molecules of the immunoglobulin family and tumor necrosis factor receptor superfamily (TNFRSF) members. These co-signal molecules then play important roles in the differentiation of the T cells into specialized subsets and their survival in the periphery (Watts 2005). Not all co-signal molecules are stimulatory; in some cases, they act to suppress the T cell expressing them in a

7 Control of Regulatory T Cells by Co-signal Molecules

cell-intrinsic manner and dampen their activation. In addition, some Treg co-signal molecules act in a cell-extrinsic manner to allow the Treg to exert control over the local cellular environment. The interplay between these positive and negative co-signals, received and given by the Tregs, allows a fine level of balance and homeostatic feedback that prevents both autoimmunity and the development of an overly immunosuppressed environment by unchecked expansion of Tregs.

7.2.2 Costimulators in Treg Biology

7.2.2.1 CD28

CD28 is a cell surface homodimer and a member of the Ig superfamily. It is constitutively expressed by almost all T cells and has a critical role in the initial activation of both naïve Tconvs and naïve Tregs (Sharpe and Freeman 2002). CD28's ligands CD80 and CD86 (also known as B7-1 and B7-2) are expressed by activated APCs such as DCs and B cells. To a lesser extent, they are also expressed by activated T cells. Expression of CD28 by Tregs is essential for their development in the thymus with mice lacking CD28 or CD80 and CD86 having severe defects in the thymic development of Tregs and a resultant lack of Tregs in the periphery (Tang et al. 2003). CD28 signaling is required for the production of IL-2 by Tconvs in the thymus, which is in turn essential for conversion of Treg thymic precursors into mature Tregs (Tai et al. 2005). CD28 also has a cell-intrinsic role in Tregs themselves as CD28 signaling into a potential Treg cell is essential for their upregulation of Foxp3. This effect applies early in the Treg differentiation process as thymic development of both Treg precursor populations, i.e., $CD25^+Foxp3^-$ and $CD25^-Foxp3^+CD4$ single positive thymocytes, are severely impaired in CD28-deficient mice (Lio and Hsieh 2008; Tai et al. 2005). Similar to its role in the thymus, CD28 is also essential for the formation of both in vivo pTregs and in vitro iTregs from $CD4^+Foxp3^-$ T cells (Guo et al. 2008).

Apart from its role in the formation of Tregs, CD28 signaling is also required by Tregs for their full activation and proliferation in the periphery. Genetic deficiency of CD80 and CD86 or CD28 results in a severe defect in the numbers of peripheral Tregs; in part this is due to the loss of thymic production of Tregs, but experiments inhibiting CD80 and CD86 via CTLA-4Ig (a solubilized form of CTLA-4) in adult mice demonstrate that loss of peripheral CD28 signaling causes a similar reduction in Treg number even in mice with adult thymectomy (Salomon et al. 2000; Tang et al. 2003). Similar to the thymus, at least part of the loss of Treg cell numbers in the peripheral organs of mice lacking CD28 signaling is indirect due to a loss of IL-2 production by CD28-deficient Tconvs; however, a clear cell-intrinsic role for CD28 in Tregs was demonstrated by the finding that CD28-deficient Tregs transferred into a wild-type mouse failed to proliferate (Tang et al. 2003). In addition to mouse studies, human Tregs also respond in a similar manner as Treg cell proliferation in vitro is dependent on the availability of CD28 signaling (Hombach et al. 2007). While loss of CD28 signaling affects both Tregs and Tconvs, overall the loss of CD28 shifts the balance of immune homeostasis toward autoimmunity. Genetic deficiency of CD28, CD80, and CD86 or their blockade by CTLA-4Ig in the diabetes-prone NOD mouse model results in accelerated development of diabetes and autoimmune exocrine pancreatitis due to the deficiency of functional Tregs. This can be reversed by transfer of Tregs from a CD28-sufficient mouse (Salomon et al. 2000; Meagher et al. 2008). Loss of tolerance to a self-antigen similar to that seen in Treg-depleted mice was also found to occur in CD80- and CD86-deficient mice upon reconstitution with CD80- and CD86-sufficient dendritic cells, demonstrating that a lack of Tregs was unable to control the self-reactive response once CD80 and CD86 signaling was made available to self-reactive T cells (Lohr et al. 2003).

While experiments examining the effect of blocking antibodies or CTLA-Ig on Tregs are compelling, they struggle to precisely separate the effects of these same reagents on Tconvs, which indirectly affect Treg homeostasis via IL-2 production. Recent work addressed this longstanding issue by the conditional depletion of CD28 in mature Foxp3[+] Tregs, allowing the examination of the role of CD28 after its role in the initial differentiation of Tregs (Zhang et al. 2013). These mice have a normal number of Tregs in the peripheral lymphoid organs, and these Tregs have normal in vitro suppressive capacity. However, despite this the mice develop autoimmunity at multiple sites with particular foci in the skin and lungs. Additionally, CD28-deficient Tregs were found to have a defect in their proliferation and maturation and a resulting loss of expression of activation markers such as CTLA-4, PD1, and CCR6, suggesting a defect in the generation of effector Tregs. Additionally, CD28-deficient Tregs were unable to prevent colitis induced by Treg depletion; and the autoimmunity seen in these conditional knockout mice was preventable by the transfer of CD28-sufficient Tregs (Zhang et al. 2013).

Due to its critical role in Treg function and homeostasis, therapies to selectively expand Tregs by stimulation of CD28 have attracted significant interest. Initial experiments in mice demonstrated that superagonists against CD28 selectively expanded Tregs in vitro and in vivo and were expected to be a promising therapy in the treatment of autoimmune disease (Beyersdorf et al. 2006; Lin and Hunig 2003). However, this field has been set back by the unexpected results of a phase 1 trial in which the superagonistic anti-CD28 antibody TGH1412 triggered severe cytokine storms in healthy volunteers (Suntharalingam et al. 2006). In summation, it is clear that CD28 signaling plays a critical role at all points of Treg development and function.

7.2.2.2 Inducible T-Cell Costimulator (ICOS)

ICOS (CD278) is a member of the CD28 family of the immunoglobulin superfamily. As its name suggests, ICOS expression is not found on naïve T cells but is induced by TCR and CD28 signaling and as a result expressed on activated CD8 and CD4 T cells, including Tregs (Wikenheiser and Stumhofer 2016). ICOS has a high level of sequence homology with CD28, but despite this their roles are not redundant. While CD28 is essential for initial T-cell activation, ICOS plays a more specialized function in the differentiation of effector T cells, having an important role in the formation of Th2 cells during infection and particularly a key role in antibody responses due to the dependence of T-follicular helper cells on ICOS signaling (Wikenheiser and Stumhofer 2016). ICOS also plays a role in Treg cell biology. Knockout of ICOS reveals no change to the number of thymic Tregs but a significant reduction in the number of Tregs in peripheral sites such as the spleen. This does not result in autoimmunity since the loss of Tregs is partial (from approximately 12% to 8% of CD4 T cells) and is also balanced by a loss of ICOS in effector memory T cells (Burmeister et al. 2008). Cell transfer experiments demonstrate that this is a cell-intrinsic effect dependent on a loss of proliferation and increased sensitivity to activation-induced apoptosis in ICOS-deficient Tregs (Burmeister et al. 2008). Similar to its lack of a role in the thymus, ICOS also has no clear role in the formation of pTregs from $CD25^-CD4^+$ Tconvs in vivo (Guo et al. 2008).

While loss of ICOS on Tregs does not result in the development of spontaneous autoimmunity in wild-type mice, it does increase sensitivity in already autoimmune-prone models. In two strains of mice susceptible to the induction of diabetes, NOD mice and BDC2.5 T cell receptor transgenic mice, knockout of ICOS or its blockade by antibodies results in loss of Treg protective functions and increased disease progression (Kornete et al. 2012; Herman et al. 2004). This is because Tregs resident in the pancreas express high levels of ICOS, and loss of ICOS leads to a loss of their proliferative potential and suppressive capability (Kornete et al. 2012). ICOS also plays a key role in the maintenance of mucosal tolerance. Mice given intranasal doses of myelin basic protein (MOG) peptides develop resistance to experimental autoimmune encephalomyelitis (EAE) in an ICOS-dependent and cell transferable manner (Miyamoto et al. 2005). In the lung mucosa, 50% of Tregs express ICOS, and this rises to 70–80% following exposure to inhaled antigens such as Ova. Genetic knockout of ICOS results in both lower initial levels of Tregs in the lung mucosa and a failure to expand following antigen challenge. As a result, in contrast to wild-type Tregs, ICOS-deficient Tregs are unable to induce tolerance to respiratory allergens when transferred to previously sensitized mice (Busse et al. 2012; Akbari et al. 2002). As a result, it seems that ICOS is primarily important for the maintenance and function of specialized tissue-resident Tregs.

7.2.2.3 Tumor Necrosis Factor Receptor Superfamily (TNFRSF)

The tumor necrosis factor receptor superfamily is a class of co-signal molecules with varied and to some extent redundant functions in Treg cell biology. Here we will focus on members of the TNFRSF with well-described roles in Treg cell biology, namely, OX40, glucocorticoid-induced tumor necrosis factor-related receptor (GITR), CD27, CD30, DR3, TNFR2, and 4-1BB (Watts 2005; Croft 2014).

GITR

Glucocorticoid-induced tumor necrosis factor-related receptor (GITR) is constitutively expressed at a high level by Tregs and can be upregulated by activated Foxp3[-] CD4 and CD8 T cells. Previously we found that anti-GITR antibodies could break self-tolerance, leading to the induction of autoimmune gastritis (Shimizu et al. 2002), and also overcome Treg cell-mediated suppression of the antitumor response, leading to tumor eradication (Ko et al. 2005). Furthermore, anti-GITR antibodies are also capable of abrogating Treg suppressive function in vitro (Shimizu et al. 2002). However, since GITR can also be expressed by effector T cells, it was initially unclear whether it was acting primarily to block Treg function or to stimulate effector T cells to the extent that they became resistant to Treg cell suppression (Stephens et al. 2004). A further factor is the possibility of Treg depletion by antibody-dependent cell death. While initial reports suggested that Treg depletion was not occurring, this is often a difficult factor to rule out since it is known that in some cases (such as anti-CTLA-4) an antibody that does not deplete, or even expands, Treg cell numbers in the lymphoid organs has the ability to deplete Tregs in certain microenvironments such as the colon and the tumor (Simpson et al. 2013). To address some of these issues, Shevach and colleagues used Fc-GITR-L, which mimics engagement of GITR without causing antibody-dependent cell depletion. They found that GITR stimulation induces the proliferation of both Tconvs and Tregs in naïve mice and that these Tregs retained their full suppressive capacity. However, when GITR-sufficient Tregs were co-transferred into T-cell-deficient mice with GITR-deficient effector T cells, treatment with Fc-GITR-L caused severe loss of Tregs and abrogation of the ability of the Tregs to prevent colitis. In contrast, GITR engagement by Fc-GITR-L preferentially enhances Treg proliferation in lymphoid organs (Liao et al. 2010). These findings emphasize the different roles of co-signaling pathways in different cellular contexts with the same signals resulting in either Treg expansion or loss of Tregs depending on the context. The mechanisms underlying these divergent roles are unclear but may depend on overstimulation of Tregs in highly inflammatory conditions, such as those seen in colitis induced by Treg depletion, leading to activation-induced cell death (Ephrem et al. 2013).

Genetic knockout of GITR reveals that the numbers of peripheral Tregs in the lymph nodes and spleen are reduced by around 30–50%. No spontaneous autoimmunity is seen, and the Tregs taken from these mice retain their full functional capacity, demonstrating that GITR is not essential for Treg function (Stephens et al. 2004; Ronchetti et al. 2004). GITR may also have a role in the thymic differentiation of Tregs. It is expressed by thymic Treg precursors and acts to enhance conversion of Treg precursors to mature Tregs and a resulting mild loss of thymic Tregs. Loss of GITR leads to mild defects in the production of Tregs in a competitive setting such as GITR-deficient bone marrow chimera mixed with wild-type bone marrow (Mahmud et al. 2014). In addition to quantitative changes to thymic output, competition for GITR signaling also drives the selection of Treg precursors with high-affinity TCRs. As a result, excessive GITR signaling provided by high doses of Fc-GITR-L leads to a broadening of the Treg cell TCR repertoire with the results that cells bearing lower-affinity TCRs are able to receive sufficient signaling to become Tregs (Mahmud et al. 2014).

OX40

OX40 (CD134) is a costimulatory molecule expressed on activation by Tconvs but constitutively expressed by Tregs. Its ligand OX40L is expressed by a range of APCs (DCs, B cells) and to a lesser extent by NK cells and activated T cells (Chen et al. 1999). OX40 is broadly considered to be a costimulatory molecule since blockade of OX40 signaling ameliorates autoimmunity (Redmond and Weinberg 2007). However, this overall effect masks a difference in its function on Tconvs and Tregs. OX40 signaling in Tconvs leads to an increase in cytokine production and proliferation while its role in Tregs is more complex (Webb et al. 2016). Knockout of OX40 does not lead to a severe loss of Treg cell numbers or function at most lymphoid sites; yet a mild reduction in Treg cellularity can be seen in younger mice, recovering to normal levels in older mice (Vu et al. 2007; Griseri et al. 2010; Takeda et al. 2004). OX40 also aids the proliferation of mature Tregs in vitro, suggesting that it may also have a role in the homoeostasis of mature Tregs (Takeda et al. 2004). OX40 also has a role in the conversion of Foxp3⁻ T cells to pTregs (Vu et al. 2007).

However, despite these roles in the formation and maintenance of Tregs, OX40 also appears to suppress certain aspects of Treg cell function. Several studies have demonstrated that engagement of OX40 appears to inhibit the suppressive function of Tregs, at least partly by interfering with Foxp3 gene expression (Kinnear et al. 2013; Vu et al. 2007; Valzasina et al. 2005). More recent work demonstrates that OX40 stimulation induces initial Treg proliferation at multiple organ sites, T-cell infiltration of the lungs, and downregulation of Foxp3 expression levels in Foxp3-expressing cells, driving Tregs to an apparently exhausted phenotype. However, in the presence of additional IL-2, this can be prevented as Tregs expanded by both OX40-ligand and IL-2 in vivo proliferate well and maintain strong suppressive function. Together, these results suggest that the effect of OX40 is also dependent on the availability of cytokines since OX40 alone expands Tregs but pushes them into a relatively exhausted state unless additional supplementation with IL-2 is provided (Xiao et al. 2012).

OX40 is highly expressed by Tregs within the tumor microenvironment (Piconese et al. 2008). As a result, a number of studies have examined the effects of OX40 blockade on the antitumor response. Here, agonistic OX40 antibodies enhance immunological rejection of tumors by a combination of its stimulatory effects on Tconvs, reducing the suppressive capacity of tumor-resident Tregs, and by direct depletion of OX40 high Tregs. A number of clinical trials of anti-OX40 as an anti-cancer agent are now underway (Sanmamed et al. 2015). In addition to its cell-intrinsic effects, there is some evidence of a cell-extrinsic role for Treg OX40 affecting OX40 ligand-expressing cells. Tregs suppress the activation and degranulation of mast cells via engagement of Treg OX40 with OX40L expressed by mast cells (Piconese et al. 2009).

In contrast to its Treg inhibiting role in many other sites, OX40 has an important role in the ability of Tregs to maintain gut homeostasis. OX40-deficient mice have a reduction in the number of Tregs found in the lamina propria due to a cell-intrinsic defect in their ability to accumulate in the gut (Griseri et al. 2010). Upon adoptive transfer, OX40-deficient Tregs are unable to prevent colitis induced by co-transferred effector T cells. OX40-deficient mice do not spontaneously develop colitis, but this may be due to the dependence of effector T cells on OX40 for their ability to cause colitis (Griseri et al. 2010). Notably, mice expressing high levels of transgenic OX40L on T cells spontaneously develop colitis, while OX40-sufficient Tregs co-transferred alongside effector T cells into T- and B-cell-deficient RAG-KO mice expressing transgenic OX40L in many tissues under the control of chicken β-actin promoter are unable to prevent colitis (Murata et al. 2002; Takeda et al. 2004). Together these results suggest that OX40 expression on Tregs is critical for their suppression of colitis but that excessive OX40L signaling is capable of tipping the balance toward autoimmunity, either by excessive stimulation of effector T cells or by suppression of Treg cell function. As a result, the role of OX40 in Treg cells seems highly complex since it aids thymic development of Tregs and their proliferation, has an inhibitory effect on Treg suppressive activity in many situations, but also plays an important role in the maintenance and trafficking of Tregs into the gut.

4-1BB

4-1BB ((CD137) is not constitutively expressed by human Tregs found in peripheral blood but is rapidly upregulated on their activation, and as a result, following antigen-specific stimulation in vivo, almost all 4-1BB-positive cells are Tregs at 5 hours poststimulation, while at 20 hours Tconv also upregulates 4-1BB (Schoenbrunn et al. 2012). In mouse Tregs, 4-1BB is expressed at low levels in the resting state, but similar to human Tregs, it is rapidly upregulated following stimulation (McHugh et al. 2002).

Genetic deficiency of 4-1BB does not lead to overt autoimmunity or clear abnormalities in T-cell responses (Kwon et al. 2002). 4-1BB signaling enhances the proliferation of Tregs both in vitro and in vivo (Zheng et al. 2004), and anti-4-1BBL treatment allows the large-scale expansion of Tregs ex vivo while retaining their suppressive functions and ability to prevent allogeneic pancreatic islet rejection and resulting diabetes (Elpek et al. 2007). In contrast to OX40, loss of 4-1BB on either adoptively transferred effector T cells or Tregs had no clear effect on the ability of the cells to induce or control colitis, respectively (Maerten et al. 2006).

Similar to a number of other co-signal molecules, there is significant interest in the manipulation of 4-1BB in the context of antitumor immunotherapy. Treatment with anti-4-1BB effectively enhances antitumor immunity either alone or in combination with other treatments such as anti-CTLA-4 (Kocak et al. 2006). Since 4-1BB is expressed by intratumoral Tregs and CD4 and CD8 effector T cells, it is important to understand which cells are being affected by its engagement. A more recent study found that intratumoral Treg proliferation was slightly reduced following treatment with anti-4-1BB. This was seen in conjunction with a reduction in the absolute number of Tregs infiltrating the tumor and a reduction in their expression of both PD-1 and CTLA-4, suggesting that the Tregs may have been less activated and suppressive (Curran et al. 2011). It is thus likely that anti-4-1BB enhances antitumor responses by reducing both the number and function of tumor-infiltrating Tregs.

CD27

CD27 is another member of the TNFR superfamily expressed by Tregs and activated Tconvs in the periphery and developing thymocytes. The signaling cascade resulting from CD27 stimulation is partially characterized with TRAF-mediated activation of JNK- and NIK-dependent activation of the NFκB pathway (Bullock 2017).

CD70, the ligand for CD27, is constitutively expressed by medullary thymic epithelial cells and thymic DCs, suggesting a role in the thymic development of T cells (Coquet et al. 2013). Mice lacking either CD27 or CD70 expression have a partial loss of Treg cell numbers in both the thymus and the periphery but no loss of suppressive function by the remaining Tregs. Mechanistically, it appears that CD27 co-signals in developing Tregs suppress their apoptosis by suppressing the expression of proapoptotic BCL-2 family members such as Puma and Bak, allowing them to survive positive selection (Coquet et al. 2013). Expression of CD27 by tumor-infiltrating Tregs may also have a role on their survival and function. CD27-deficient Tregs fail to accumulate in the tumor environment, and as a result, antitumor responses are enhanced. Similar to the situation in the thymus, this appears to primarily be a defect in the survival of Tregs (Claus et al. 2012).

Tregs may also possess the cell-extrinsic ability to regulate CD70 expression on DCs via CD27. CD27-expressing Tregs cause the loss of surface CD70 from interacting DCs in a contact-dependent manner. In a mirror image of the transendocytosis central to the function of CTLA-4, in this case the DC internalizes both CD70 and bound CD27 from the Treg cell (Dhainaut et al. 2015).

CD30, DR3, and TNFR2

CD30 is expressed by activated effector T cells and Tregs, while CD30L (CD154) is expressed by DCs, thymic epithelia cells, B cells, eosinophils, and neutrophils. The role of CD30 in Treg biology is not well characterized, but several groups have reported that CD30 expression by Tregs plays a role in transplantation tolerance. CD30-deficient Tregs are not capable of suppressing CD8 T-cell memory responses responsible for the rejection of allogenic skin grafts. In this case, CD30 expressed by Tregs is required for their contact-dependent suppressive function. Whether this is by direct cell-extrinsic function of CD30 or indirectly via a requirement for CD30 signaling to activate the full suppressive function of the Tregs is unclear, although the latter seems more credible (Dai et al. 2004). Tregs lacking CD30 expression also have a significantly weakened ability to prevent graft versus host disease (GvHD), while antibody blockade of CD30L in the early but not late stages of GvHD induction prevents Treg control of the disease (Zeiser et al. 2007).

DR3 (TNFRSF25) is selectively expressed on Tregs in mice with little expression seen in Foxp3⁻ Tconvs. Agonistic antibodies to DR3 preferentially cause the proliferation of Tregs in a TCR- and IL-2-dependent manner. Interestingly due to its more Treg-specific expression profile, anti-DR3 seems better able to specifically expand Tregs than other TNFRSF molecules such as GITR, CD27, OX40, and 4-1BB, making it a good candidate immunotherapeutic agent (Schreiber et al. 2010). Accordingly, mice treated with anti-DR3 are resistant to allergic lung inflammation and have delayed rejection of allogenic heart transplantation; and T cells from anti-DR3-treated hosts mediate reduced GvHD (Kim et al. 2015; Schreiber et al. 2010).

TNFR2 is expressed by both resting and activated Tregs. TNFR2 signaling induced by its ligand TNF-α causes the expansion of both mouse and human Tregs (Okubo et al. 2013; Chen et al. 2007). Murine Tregs expanded in this manner have enhanced in vitro suppressive function; however, contrasting results have been reported by different groups as to the effect of TNF on human Treg suppressive function, although the majority suggest that Tregs treated with TNF-α have reduced suppressive function (Nie et al. 2016). Genetic deficiency of TNFR2 results in a reduction in the number of Tregs in both the thymus and the spleen, a phenotype also seen in mice with triple knockout of the TNFR2 ligands: TNF, lymphotoxin-α, and lymphotoxin-β (Chen et al. 2013). Further to this, addition of TNF, to cultures containing pre-Tregs, enhances their conversion to mature Tregs in comparison to IL-2 alone (Mahmud et al. 2014). A role for TNFR2 in the in vivo suppressive function of Tregs was demonstrated as Tregs lacking TNFR2 are unable to prevent colitis due to a deficiency in their stability and competitive fitness (Chen et al. 2013).

Redundancy of TNFRSF Members in Treg Cell Function

Some redundancy between different members of the TNFR family is seen. While the magnitude of the reductions of Treg numbers in GITR-, OX40-, or TNFR2-deficient mice is relatively mild, combining OX40 genetic depletion with tailless dominant negative forms of GITR or TNFR reveals a much more severe defect in Treg cell numbers with all the combination of all three leading to a near total loss of thymic Treg production. This role for TNFR family members is in turn dependent on CD28 signaling for the induction of their initial expression (Mahmud et al. 2014).

Many of the TNFRSF members have signaling cascades that terminate in activation of the transcription factor NF-κB family of transcription factors. In particular, cRel and RelA have vital roles in the thymic production, maintenance, and suppressive function of Tregs (Li and Jacks 2017). Engagement of GITR, OX40, and 4-1BB induces the phosphorylation of RelA, which anti-CD3 and anti-CD28 fail to do, suggesting they are acting via distinct signaling pathways. While individual knockouts of GITR, OX40, and 4-1BB result in relatively mild defects in Treg formation and function, conditional knockout of RelA in mature Tregs results in serious autoimmune pathology, resulting in the death of the mice at around 100 days of age. The Treg cell defect was cell intrinsic and seems to primarily result from a loss of the ability of naïve/central Tregs to differentiate into highly suppressive effector Tregs (Vasanthakumar et al. 2017). As a result, it seems that loss of one TNFRSF member expressed by Tregs can be compensated for by the action of others, but loss of multiple receptors or of the downstream signaling molecules they share leads to severe defects in either Treg formation in the thymus or the differentiation and function of Tregs in the periphery, demonstrating that TNFRSF members, as a group, have an essential role in Treg cell function.

7.2.3 Coinhibitors in Treg Biology

7.2.3.1 Coinhibitory Molecules

Coinhibitory receptors are integral to the synchrony of immune responses. They provide a means for the immune system to coordinate its defense mechanisms to achieve sustainable immunity without development of autoimmunity. Their expression generally coincides with the activation of immune cells; however, each is highly dependent on the availability of their respective ligands to elicit immunomodulatory signals. From a therapeutic viewpoint, coinhibitory receptors and ligands present avenues for the development of antagonists to counter their effects in chronic viral infections and cancer, diseases that capitalize on the immune checkpoint receptors as Achilles heels of viral- and tumor antigen-specific T cells to restrain their responses. This strategy has produced promising results in recent years with certain limitations that are potentially due to the lack of understanding of coinhibitory molecules in immune cells other than conventional T cells. In this section, we discuss the roles of coinhibitory receptors in Tregs, which are known to express them in substantial amounts (Fig. 7.3).

7.2.3.2 PD-1

Programmed cell death-1 (PD-1 or CD279)) is a coinhibitory surface receptor belonging to the CD28 superfamily. It is a 50–55 kDa type 1 transmembrane glycoprotein with a single IgV domain in its extracellular region that shares 21–33% sequence homology with CTLA-4, CD28, and ICOS. One key feature of PD-1 that distinguishes it from other CD28 family members is its inability to homodimerize due to a lack of membrane cysteine (Zhang et al. 2004). The intracellular cytoplasmic region of PD-1 consists of two tyrosine-based residues – tyrosine-based inhibitory motif (ITIM) and immunoreceptor tyrosine-based switch motif (ITSM); the latter is responsible for transducing negative signaling (Long 1999; Sidorenko and

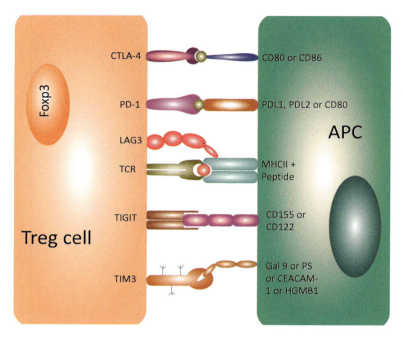

Fig. 7.3 Coinhibitory molecules expressed by Tregs and their ligands on antigen-presenting cells. Suppressive function may be mainly either cell intrinsic (TIM3, PD1, Lag-3), cell extrinsic (ligand capture by CTLA-4), or a mixture of both (cell-intrinsic signaling by TIGIT and TIGIT triggered release of the suppressive molecule Fgl2)

Clark 2003). PD-1 is expressed on activated T cells, B cells, NK cells, NKT cells, dendritic cells, and monocytes. The level of PD-1 expression increases with constant antigen exposure and stimulation. High PD-1 expression is a characteristic feature of exhausted unresponsive T cells (Freeman et al. 2006); however, it is also expressed by highly activated T cells, making PD-1 alone unable to differentiate between these contrasting cell types. Upon activation in T cells, the nuclear factor of activated T cells c1 (NFATc1) translocates to the promoter region of PD-1 to drive PD-1 expression (Oestreich et al. 2008). Interestingly, a recent study suggested that this may be epigenetically repressed by the chromatin organizer special AT-rich sequence-binding protein-1 (Satb1) through its recruitment of nucleosome remodeling deacetylase (NURD) complex to the PD-1 promoter, a process that is partly counterbalanced by Smad proteins competing for the same promoter-binding region (Stephen et al. 2017). The exact mechanism which dictates PD-1 expression remains to be determined.

PD-1 binds to two ligands, namely, PD-L1 and PD-L2, with stronger binding to PD-L2 (Freeman et al. 2000; Latchman et al. 2001; Tseng et al. 2001; Karunarathne et al. 2016). In mice, while PD-L1 is constitutively expressed on a wide variety of immune cells including T and B cells, dendritic cells, macrophages, and bone-marrow-derived mast cells, PD-L2 expression is mainly limited to primed professional antigen-presenting cells such as DCs, macrophages, peritoneal B1 B cells, and germinal center B cells (Freeman et al. 2000; Yamazaki et al. 2002; Zhong et al. 2007). Additionally, PD-L1 can be induced on cells of nonhematopoietic origin (e.g., vascular endothelial cells) (Eppihimer et al. 2002). In humans, PD-L2 is also present on T cells and vascular endothelial cells (Tseng et al. 2001; Messal et al. 2011). PD-L1 expression is preferentially enhanced by IFNγ, whereas PD-L2 is upregulated by IL-4 and GM-CSF (Yamazaki et al. 2002; Loke and Allison 2003). Besides PD-1, PD-L1 serves as a ligand for CD80/B7-1 for which the effect of this interaction leans toward inhibition of T-cell responses (Butte et al. 2007). An alternative binding partner for PD-L2 has also been proposed with contrasting properties to PD-1 (Shin et al. 2003). This is supported by the increased killing of PD-L2-expressing tumor cells compared to non-PD-L2-expressing tumor cells by PD-1$^{-/-}$ cytotoxic T cells (Liu et al. 2003). Identifying the receptor is paramount to make further inroads into this pathway.

Upon ligation to PD-Ls, ITSM of PD-1 becomes phosphorylated and recruits SHP-2 (SH2 domain-containing tyrosine phosphatase 2) which in turn dephosphorylates other signaling molecules in the TCR complex, for example, CD3, ZAP70 (ζ-associated protein of 70 kDa), and PI3K (phosphatidylinositol-3-kinase) (Parry et al. 2005). Consequently, T cells have reduced capacity to proliferate and produce cytokines as well as the transcription factors – T-bet, Eomes, and GATA3 – required for specialized Th1/Th2 functions (Nurieva et al. 2006). In the event of strong TCR and CD28 stimulation, PD-1-mediated inhibitory effects can be overcome (Freeman et al. 2000). This can also occur through the STAT5-dependent cytokine pathways of IL-2, IL-7, and IL-15 (Bennett et al. 2003). Mice rendered genetically deficient in PD-1 are susceptible to strain-specific autoimmune diseases. PD-1KO C57Bl6 mice sustain mild lupus-like nephritis and arthritis with late onset, while PD-1KO BALB/c and NOD mice develop cardiomyopathy and type 1 diabetes, respectively (Nishimura et al. 1999; Nishimura et al. 2001; Wang et al. 2005). The strain- and tissue-specific nature of the observed autoimmunity suggests a loss of peripheral tolerance rather than central tolerance in PD-1KO mice. Nevertheless, it is not known whether autoimmunity in PD-1KO mice results from increased activation of T cells per se or whether DCs and macrophages, which have been shown to secrete larger amounts of cytokines when deficient in PD-1 (Rui et al. 2013), also contribute through the promotion of inflammation.

Alternatively, the breakdown in peripheral versus central tolerance in PD-1KO mice may be explained by the role that PD-1 plays in T-cell development. Given that PD-1 is first expressed in early CD4-CD8- thymocytes and is upregulated upon TCR recognition in CD4+CD8+ thymocytes, PD-1 can affect the maturation of T cells by calibrating the TCR signal threshold for positive and negative selection (Nishimura et al. 1996; Blank et al. 2003). Hence, it is likely that thymic emigrants in mice lacking inhibitory PD-1 contain less self-recognizing Tconvs and perhaps more Tregs. Indeed, the percentage and number of thymic CD4$^+$Foxp3$^+$ cells in young PD-1KO mice are higher compared to wild-type controls. The authors also demonstrated reduced total CD4 single positive PD-1KO thymic T cells specific for MJ23, a native prostate antigen, in chimeric mice containing a mixture of MJ23

TCR transgenic Rag1$^{-/-}$ PD-1-deficient and PD-1-sufficient bone marrow cells, indicative of possible increased negative selection of PD-1KO immature CD4 T cells. On the other hand, there was increased differentiation of PD-1KO MJ23-specific thymic T cells into Tregs. Nevertheless, studies have yet to be performed to determine whether the TCR repertoire of mature Tconvs has decreased affinity for self-antigens and that of Tregs has increased affinity in PD-1KO mice.

Although PD-1 is highly expressed by activated Tregs, there is limited knowledge on its exact function in Tregs. In comparison to PD-1$^-$ Tregs, PD-1^{hi}-expressing Tregs have reduced demethylation in the Foxp3 locus, are less proliferative in vitro, exert weaker suppression on Tconvs, and have shorter telomeres, traits consistent with terminal differentiation and exhaustion (Lowther et al. 2016). This observation also raises two important questions pertaining to dormancy and memory of Tregs since the graded manner which PD-1 is expressed could be associated with activation status. On this note, the effect of blocking PD-1 signaling during activation of Tregs needs to be carefully assessed in future studies. According to current evidence, it is likely that PD-1 blockade on Tregs would bring about increased immunosuppression. This stems from a study that found T-follicular regulatory cells, a subtype of Tregs residing within lymphoid follicular zones, derived from PD-1KO mice are more efficient in preventing Tconv proliferation in vitro (Sage et al. 2013). A second study made a similar finding in vivo by transferring CD4$^+$Foxp3$^+$ Tregs from either wild-type or PD-1KO mice into mice that were rendered susceptible to pancreatitis by partial impairment of Foxp3 expression (Zhang et al. 2016). Not only did the transfer of PD-1KO Tregs result in decreased conventional CD4 and CD8 T-cell activation; there were also less cellular infiltrates and pathological damage in the pancreas. Nonetheless, one caveat with assessing Tregs from PD-1KO mice is the possibility that whole Treg activity is enhanced as a compensatory response to the global increase in T-cell activation and not directly due to PD-1 deficiency itself.

Another area of interest in PD-1 that is related to Tregs is its role in the conversion of Tconvs to peripheral Tregs (pTregs). PD-L1 expression on antigen-presenting cells has been shown to be critical for TGFβ-induced development of pTregs from Tconvs (Francisco et al. 2009). Furthermore, transfer of naïve CD4 Tconvs into RagKO mice deficient in both PD-L1 and PD-L2 produced less pTregs and caused more severe inflammatory disease. Downregulation of Akt/mTOR signaling is believed to facilitate PD-L1-mediated generation of pTregs. However, it should be noted that these data cannot definitively link the PD-L1:PD-1 axis to pTreg development as PD-L1, in addition to PD-1, binds to CD80 which is expressed on Tconvs as well. This could be inferred by an apparent increase in number, but not frequency which remained unchanged, of pTregs converted from PD-1KO Tconvs in RagKO mice (Ellestad et al. 2014). Here, due consideration must also be given to the analysis and interpretation of pTreg frequency, and absolute number in the various organs (i.e., blood and lymph nodes) for PD-1KO Tconvs is inherently more proliferative and readily mobilized. Therefore, an increase in pTregs may merely be a consequence of increased expansion and activation of PD-1KO Tconvs rather than an absence of PD-1-mediated regulation of pTreg conversion. Despite this, the results clearly suggest that PD-1 may not be absolutely essential for Tconvs to differentiate

7 Control of Regulatory T Cells by Co-signal Molecules

into pTregs. More stringent experimental designs are required to investigate the effect of PD-1 on this aspect of immune regulation.

Due to its high expression in Tconv, Treg, and CD8 cells in the tumor environment, targeting the PD-1 pathway has been considered a key candidate for antitumor immunotherapy (Iwai et al. 2017). Early experiments in mice demonstrated that either anti-PD-1 or anti-PD-L1 is effective at inducing antitumor immune responses and anti-PD-1 agents such as Nivolumab have proven a relative success in the clinic either alone or in combination with other immunotherapeutic agents such as anti-CTLA-4 (Callahan et al. 2014).

7.2.3.3 CTLA-4

Cytotoxic T-cell lymphocyte antigen-4 (CTLA-4, CD152)) is a close relative of CD28 and shares the same ligands, CD80 and CD86. However, while CD28 is a critical costimulatory molecule, CTLA-4 is known for its suppressive function. CTLA-4 is constitutively expressed by Tregs and can also be expressed by activated Tconvs. Genetic knockout of CTLA-4 results in severe fatal autoimmunity and lymphoproliferation in a manner similar to that seen in Foxp3-deficient scurfy mice (Tivol et al. 1995). Correspondingly genetic knockout of both CD80 and CD86 or CD28 prevents the autoimmunity seen in CTLA-4-deficient mice demonstrating the opposing roles of CTLA-4 inhibition and CD28 stimulation (Mandelbrot et al. 1999; Tai et al. 2007). Conditional knockout of CTLA-4 specifically on Tregs results in severe inflammation with similar consequences but slightly delayed fatality to fully CTLA-4-deficient mice (Wing et al. 2008). Surprisingly, in contrast to germline or Treg conditional knockout, CTLA-4 depletion in adult mice is not fatal and even leads to resistance to EAE. Despite this, CTLA-4 depletion in adult mice does result in severe autoimmunity (pneumonitis, gastritis, insulitis, and sialadenitis) (Klocke et al. 2016). These findings suggest that while CTLA-4 is critical for Treg cell suppressive function during the neonatal period, if depleted in the mature immune system, other Treg suppressive mechanisms are able to partially compensate for this to prevent fatal autoimmunity. This partial redundancy of other suppressive molecules replacing CTLA-4 function is also demonstrated by the finding that highly activated CTLA-4 KO Tregs taken from CTLA-4-deficient mice are suppressive in vitro while CTLA-4 KO Tregs taken from bone marrow chimera or mosaic mice are not. This is because strong activation of Tregs, which occurs in a mouse with a total lack of CTLA-4, allows upregulation of other suppressive molecules. This does not occur in the marrow chimera where immune homeostasis is retained (Wing et al. 2008). The key role of CTLA-4 in the maintenance of immune homeostasis in humans has recently been demonstrated by the discovery of a rare patient group suffering from severe autoimmunity due to heterozygous loss of function mutations of the CTLA-4 gene (Schubert et al. 2014; Kuehn et al. 2014). In contrast, heterozygous loss of CTLA-4 in mice has little measurable effect, possibly due to the unchallenging clean conditions that specific pathogen-free mice are kept in.

CTLA-4 has been demonstrated to have both cell-extrinsic and cell-intrinsic functions (Wing et al. 2011). The key cell-extrinsic function of CTLA-4 is to control availability of its ligands CD80 and CD86 on antigen-presenting cells in a contact-dependent manner (Onishi et al. 2008). This ability to deplete CD80 and CD86 can be blocked by anti-CTLA-4 antibodies and is also lost in Tregs with genetic deficiency of CTLA-4 (Wing et al. 2008). CTLA-4 rapidly cycles on and off the cell membrane into intracellular pools, where the majority of CTLA-4 is located. As it engages with CD80 and CD86, it is able to pull them off the surface of APCs, sequestering them into the Treg where they are then degraded; as a result, Tregs rapidly remove CD80 and CD86 from APCs in a contact-dependent manner (Walker and Sansom 2015).

CTLA-4 has also been reported to have cell-intrinsic functions. Recent work suggests that CTLA-4 may affect the motility of Tregs via interaction of its cytoplasmic tail with the protein kinase C isoform PKC-η. This complex recruits a GIT2–αPIX–PAK complex that controls the disassembly of focal adhesion points between the Treg and APCs and as a result affects the ability of the Treg to disengage from an APC in order to seek new targets. This results in a partial loss of suppressive function in Tregs lacking PKC-η, causing a loss of ability to prevent antitumor responses, but still retaining the capacity to prevent colitis following cell transfer into RAG-deficient mice (Kong et al. 2014). Several other reports have also suggested that CTLA-4 may play a role in the arrest or enhancement of T cell and Treg mobility on contact with APCs; however, this has proven controversial with different studies providing conflicting evidence (Walker and Sansom 2015). While cell-intrinsic mechanisms may play a role in the fine-tuning of CTLA-4 function, they appear dispensable for the main role of CTLA-4 in the control of immune homeostasis since bone marrow chimera experiments and use of conditional knockout mice where half of Tregs express CTLA-4 demonstrate that CTLA-4-deficient Tconvs and Tregs do not have a clear phenotype as long as they are in the presence of CTLA-4-sufficient Tregs (Bachmann et al. 1999; Wing et al. 2008).

CTLA-4 expression by Tregs is also critical for their ability to prevent antitumor responses, and as a result, CTLA-4 cKO mice rapidly clear tumors (Wing et al. 2008). Treatment of tumor-bearing mice with anti-CTLA-4 leads to tumor regression. In the clinic, anti-CTLA-4 is already in use with compounds such as ipilimumab, already showing efficacy in the treatment of human melanoma. Treatment attempts at other cancers such as prostate and non-small cell lung cancer have not been initially successful, but combination therapies with Nivolumab (anti-PD-1) have yielded promising initial results (Callahan et al. 2014). Due to its importance in regulation of the immune system, other reagents targeting the CTLA-4 pathway have been developed. CTLA-4Ig, in which CTLA-4 has been fused with the Fc region of IgG1 to create a solubilized form of CTLA-4 that blocks CD80 and CD86, is a currently licensed drug (abatacept) for the treatment of rheumatoid arthritis and has been shown to have significant benefit to this patient group. However, trials in other autoimmune/inflammatory conditions such as asthma, lupus, and ulcerative colitis have been less successful (Adams et al. 2016).

7.2.3.4 Lag-3

Lymphocyte activation gene-3 (Lag-3) is a transmembrane protein with a conformation reminiscent of the CD4 coreceptor. It mainly binds to major histocompatibility complex II (MHCII) and has greater affinity compared to the binding of CD4 to MHCII (Huard et al. 1995). In spite of this, Lag-3 can also regulate MHCI-restricted CD8 T cells intrinsically (Grosso et al. 2007), suggesting a role of other Lag-3 ligands such as LSECtin, a member of the C-type lectin receptor superfamily, found predominantly in dendritic cells in blockade of T-effector responses (Xu et al. 2014). It is notable that deficiency in Lag-3 leads to spontaneous autoimmunity only in autoimmune-prone mice stains such as the NOD background (Bettini et al. 2011). During T-cell activation, Lag-3 cross-links with CD3 and modulates T-cell activity through a pathway that has yet to be uncovered (Hannier et al. 1998). To date, it is only known that Lag-3 depends on the KIEELE motif of its intracellular domain to transduce inhibitory signals in CD4 Tcons (Workman et al. 2002). Whether Lag-3 requires the other two motifs, one containing serine-phosphorylation sites and the other containing glutamic acid-proline repeats, for its function in other T-cell subsets remains to be determined (Workman et al. 2002). This is worth consideration particularly for Tregs where Lag-3 may either act as a cell-intrinsic inhibitory coreceptor or serve as a cell-extrinsic immune suppressive arm as discussed below.

Within the activated population of whole CD4 T cells, Lag-3 is preferentially expressed and maintained on pTregs. Using a Lag-3 blocking antibody, it was found that Lag-3 was crucial for pTregs to mount efficient suppression on Tconvs and protect mice from death in a model of lethal pneumonitis (Huang et al. 2004). A similar finding was obtained for tTregs although this was debatable due to the ambiguous nature of identifying tTregs as CD4$^+$CD25$^+$ cells in earlier studies (Huang et al. 2004). This controversy is compounded by another study that showed wild-type and Lag-3KO CD4$^+$CD25^{hi} Tregs did not differ in their ability to prevent allogeneic GvHD (Sega et al. 2014). As GvHD is only preventable by the transfer of CD62L$^+$ naïve Tregs, which are essentially tTregs, into host mice (Ermann et al. 2005), the initial claim that Lag-3 is indispensable for tTreg function may not be completely true. On a similar note, one must account for differences, if any, in the proportion of CD62L$^+$ naïve Tregs within the CD4$^+$CD25^{hi} cells in wild-type and Lag-3KO mice. A recent study addressed some of these issues by generating NOD mice with a conditional knockout of Lag-3 specifically in Foxp3$^+$ Tregs. It was found that such mice had a lower incidence of diabetes, which may be attributed to Lag-3 restricting the maintenance and proliferation of islet-infiltrating Tregs through downregulation of Eos and IL-2-Stat5 signaling (Zhang et al. 2017). Importantly, the inhibition of Eos by Lag-3 likely subjects Tregs to become unstable and disposed to reprogramming, a typical feature of pTregs (Sharma et al. 2013).

7.2.3.5 TIGIT

The coinhibitory T-cell immunoreceptor with Ig and ITIM domains (TIGIT)) and its partner costimulatory receptor CD226 can be deemed to regulate T-cell responses in ways similar to CD28/CTLA-4 (Joller et al. 2011). Both TIGIT and CD226 bind to CD155 and CD112 with the former exhibiting stronger affinity (Anderson et al. 2016). The intracellular domain of TIGIT consists of an ITIM motif and an immunoglobulin tail tyrosine (ITT)-like motif (Yu et al. 2009). The cell-intrinsic inhibitory function of TIGIT hinges on its ITT-like motif which becomes phosphorylated and recruits SHIP1 to dampen NF-κB signaling upon ligation of TIGIT to its ligand (Li et al. 2014). Besides, TIGIT has been shown to exert cell-extrinsic immunoregulatory effects by stimulating IL-10 and blocking IL-12 production by DCs through its interaction with CD155, hence repressing Th1 immunity (Yu et al. 2009). This can also be achieved by TIGIT-expressing Tregs (Joller et al. 2014). In humans, TIGIT[+] T cells are particularly enriched in the Foxp3[+]Helios[+] thymic Treg fraction. Moreover, while level of TIGIT expression is markedly higher, CD226 expression is lower in Helios[+] compared to Helios[-] Tregs and Tconvs (Joller et al. 2014). It is currently postulated that TIGIT is a late activation marker and limits the proliferative capacity of tTregs. In contrast, TIGIT[-]CD226[+] Tregs harbor properties that are synonymous to iTregs such as higher IFNγ and IL-10 production and reduced Foxp3-TSDR demethylation (Fuhrman et al. 2015; Joller et al. 2014). Intriguingly, TIGIT was found to be highly necessary for the conversion of murine Tconvs into iTregs in vitro.

Due to the novel identification of TIGIT[+] Tregs, the function of this particular Treg subset is still unclear. It was earlier shown that upregulation of TIGIT during Treg activation was hindered in an IL-12-mediated Th1 environment, suggesting a possible role in counterbalancing T-helper effector responses (Fuhrman et al. 2015). This concept has been validated in mice where, as in humans, tTregs are the major source of TIGIT[+] Tregs which coexpress neuropilin-1 and Helios and are distinctly more activated and suppressive in comparison to TIGIT[-] Tregs (Joller et al. 2014). Elevated expression of costimulatory (e.g., ICOS) and coinhibitory molecules (e.g., PD-1, CTLA-4, Tim3, Lag3) and Treg signature genes (e.g., Foxp3, CD25, GITR, IL-10) bear testament to the highly immunosuppressive phenotype of TIGIT[+] Tregs (Joller et al. 2014). This was similarly observed in tumor-infiltrating TIGIT[+] Tregs, which were behind the suppression of antitumor CD8 T-cell responses (Kurtulus et al. 2015). Perhaps, one peculiar trait of TIGIT[+] Tregs is their preferential expression of Th1- and Th17-specific genes over those of Th2 (Joller et al. 2014). This includes the respective chemokine receptors. In line with their gene expression profile, TIGIT[+] Tregs suppress Th1 and Th17 but not Th2 responses. Mechanistically, this particular function of TIGIT[+] Tregs owes to their increased propensity to secrete soluble fibrinogen-like protein 2 (Fgl2) in addition to IL-10 (Joller et al. 2014). It is conceivable that the combined effect of Fgl2 and IL-10 from TIGIT[+] Tregs tilts the T-helper balance from Th1/Th17 to Th2. Interestingly, in comparison to other activated Tregs, TIGIT has twofold greater expression by highly differentiated

CD25-negative T-follicular regulatory cells located in germinal centers, suggesting that it may have a role in the regulation of antibody responses (Wing et al. 2017).

7.2.3.6 Tim-3

T-cell immunoglobulin-3 (Tim-3) is the first among the Tim family of proteins that was discovered (Anderson et al. 2016). As a coinhibitory molecule, any compromise on Tim-3 function unleashes activated T cells, particularly Th1, to instigate immune-mediated diseases. This can be brought about by modifications to the Tim-3 gene or blocking Tim-3 with anti-Tim3 antibody (Monney et al. 2002; Koguchi et al. 2006). The spontaneity of autoimmune development from antagonizing Tim-3 firmly underlines Tim-3 as a major immune regulator. Reversion of Tim-3[+] T cells from a dysfunctional state to a highly autoreactive state has been shown to account for the effect of Tim-3 blockade (Koguchi et al. 2006), though it is necessary to recognize that Tim-3 is expressed in multiple other cells such as Tregs, NK cells, NKT cells, and APCs (Anderson et al. 2016).

Several ligands have been identified for Tim-3, one of which is galactin-9 (GAL-9). Engagement of GAL-9 leads to cell death in Tim-3[+] Th1 cells and protects mice from experimental autoimmune encephalomyelitis. Other ligands include phosphatidylserine (PS), high mobility group protein B1 (HGMB1), and carcinoembryonic antigen cell adhesion molecule-1 (Ceacam-1) (Anderson et al. 2016). Since T cells do not possess any ability to phagocytose apoptotic cell function, the PS:Tim-3 pathway has not been examined in T cells. As for HMGB-1 whose role is to chaperone DNA from apoptotic cells to dendritic cells and macrophages, it is proposed that Tim-3 sequesters it to keep inflammatory responses under control (Chiba et al. 2012). Lately, Ceacam-1 has emerged as an interesting candidate that is coexpressed with Tim-3 in activated T cells. Both Ceacam-1 and Tim-3 interact with each other in cis and trans through their N-terminal domains to mediate Tim-3-dependent inhibition. Heterodimerization of the molecules in cis is especially vital for Tim-3 maturation and maintenance on the cell surface. This is evidently manifested in Ceacam-1-deficient T cells which are low in Tim-3 expression and are highly pathogenic.

Clearly, Tim-3 is important to immune tolerance, and the degree of redundancy it shares with Tregs ought to be ascertained. Thus far, it is known that Tim-3[+] Tregs belong to a specific PD-1-expressing activated Treg subset that is almost exclusively found within inflamed tissues (Sakuishi et al. 2013). The same can be assumed for human Tim-3[+] Tregs which are not immediately detectable ex vivo but only after stimulation with anti-CD3 and anti-CD28 (Gautron et al. 2014). The in vitro activated Tim-3[+] Tregs are more suppressive against Th1 and Th17 responses compared to their Tim-3[-] counterparts which are barely effective in Th17 suppression. In mice, Tim-3[+]PD-1[+] Tregs were reported to have high expression of the classic regulatory genes (e.g., CD25, CTLA-4, and IL-10) and display strong in vitro immunosuppression (Sakuishi et al. 2013). Notwithstanding these traits, the short-term survival of

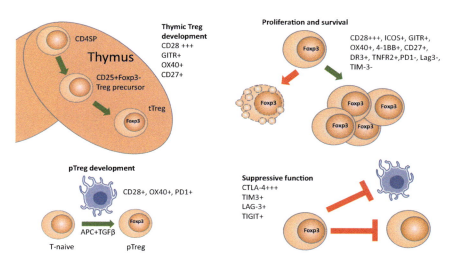

Fig. 7.4 The role of diverse suppressive and coinhibitory signals in key checkpoints in Treg development and function. Plus or minus signs denote a positive or negative contribution to the noted function

Tim-3⁺PD-1⁺ Tregs allows them to only delay but not prevent allograft rejection (Gupta et al. 2012). On a more positive note, future cancer treatment can leverage combined blockade of Tim-3 and PD-1, which abrogates much of the enhanced immunoregulatory functions of Tim-3⁺ Tregs, in particular IL-10 production (Sakuishi et al. 2013). This would facilitate a two-pronged approach to relive anti-tumor T cells from checkpoint blockade as well as suppression by Tregs (Fig. 7.4).

7.3 Conclusion

One notable similarity between a range of the co-signal molecules discussed here is the strongly context-dependent nature of their function. Many positive co-signal molecules are capable of enhancing Treg proliferation when given in the context of an environment with relatively low inflammatory milieu. On the other hand, these same signals cause the death or loss of function of the Tregs in more activated environments, notably inside tumors. The exact mechanisms underlying this phenomenon are not fully clear but may be the result of either overstimulation leading to activation-induced cell death or alterations to intracellular conditions of the Tregs leading to different co-factors becoming involved in the downstream signaling events following engagement of the co-signal molecule. For example, the TNFRSF members CD27, GITR, OX40, and 4-1BB can bind to TRAF2, which leads to activation of canonical NF-κB signaling and proliferation and activation of Tregs. Alternatively, the proapoptotic molecule Siva can also interact with the signaling domains of CD27 and GITR, resulting in increased apoptosis of Tregs via the TRAF pathway (Spinicelli et al. 2002; Nocentini and Riccardi 2005). The choice of these opposing pathways may be the result of the environment and signaling through other ligands or cytokines resulting in changes to the availability of downstream adaptor molecules.

Tregs are critical for the prevention of autoimmunity while also being capable of preventing beneficial responses such as antitumor immunity. As a result, their function must be tightly regulated by a range of co-signals either enhancing or suppressing their proliferation and function dependent on context. Further Tregs themselves control the availability of co-signals to other T cells, most notably by their ability to regulate CD80 and CD86 expression by CTLA-4 and thus restrict the availably of CD28 signals to Tconv. These different costimulatory and coinhibitory factors intertwine to result in a fine-tuned system to control immune homeostasis with multiple levels of feedback and redundancy and balance the need for protective immune responses with reducing the likelihood of autoimmunity.

References

Abbas AK, Benoist C, Bluestone JA, Campbell DJ, Ghosh S, Hori S, Jiang S, Kuchroo VK, Mathis D, Roncarolo MG, Rudensky A, Sakaguchi S, Shevach EM, Vignali DA, Ziegler SF (2013) Regulatory T cells: recommendations to simplify the nomenclature. Nat Immunol 14(4):307–308. https://doi.org/10.1038/ni.2554

Adams AB, Ford ML, Larsen CP (2016) Costimulation blockade in autoimmunity and transplantation: the CD28 pathway. J Immunol 197(6):2045–2050. https://doi.org/10.4049/jimmunol.1601135

Akbari O, Freeman GJ, Meyer EH, Greenfield EA, Chang TT, Sharpe AH, Berry G, DeKruyff RH, Umetsu DT (2002) Antigen-specific regulatory T cells develop via the ICOS-ICOS-ligand pathway and inhibit allergen-induced airway hyperreactivity. Nat Med 8(9):1024–1032. https://doi.org/10.1038/nm745

Anderson AC, Joller N, Kuchroo VK (2016) Lag-3, Tim-3, and TIGIT: co-inhibitory receptors with specialized functions in immune regulation. Immunity 44(5):989–1004. https://doi.org/10.1016/j.immuni.2016.05.001

Asano M, Toda M, Sakaguchi N, Sakaguchi S (1996) Autoimmune disease as a consequence of developmental abnormality of a T cell subpopulation. J Exp Med 184(2):387–396

Bachmann MF, Kohler G, Ecabert B, Mak TW, Kopf M (1999) Cutting edge: lymphoproliferative disease in the absence of CTLA-4 is not T cell autonomous. J Immunol 163(3):1128–1131

Bennett F, Luxenberg D, Ling V, Wang IM, Marquette K, Lowe D, Khan N, Veldman G, Jacobs KA, Valge-Archer VE, Collins M, Carreno BM (2003) Program death-1 engagement upon TCR activation has distinct effects on costimulation and cytokine-driven proliferation: attenuation of ICOS, IL-4, and IL-21, but not CD28, IL-7, and IL-15 responses. J Immunol 170(2):711–718

Bettini M, Szymczak-Workman AL, Forbes K, Castellaw AH, Selby M, Pan X, Drake CG, Korman AJ, Vignali DA (2011) Cutting edge: accelerated autoimmune diabetes in the absence of LAG-3. J Immunol 187(7):3493–3498. https://doi.org/10.4049/jimmunol.1100714

Beyersdorf N, Hanke T, Kerkau T, Hunig T (2006) CD28 superagonists put a break on autoimmunity by preferentially activating CD4+CD25+ regulatory T cells. Autoimmun Rev 5(1):40–45. https://doi.org/10.1016/j.autrev.2005.06.001

Blank C, Brown I, Marks R, Nishimura H, Honjo T, Gajewski TF (2003) Absence of programmed death receptor 1 alters thymic development and enhances generation of CD4/CD8 double-negative TCR-transgenic T cells. J Immunol 171(9):4574–4581

Bretscher P, Cohn M (1970) A theory of self-nonself discrimination. Science 169(3950):1042–1049

Bullock TN (2017) Stimulating CD27 to quantitatively and qualitatively shape adaptive immunity to cancer. Curr Opin Immunol 45:82–88. https://doi.org/10.1016/j.coi.2017.02.001

Burmeister Y, Lischke T, Dahler AC, Mages HW, Lam KP, Coyle AJ, Kroczek RA, Hutloff A (2008) ICOS controls the pool size of effector-memory and regulatory T cells. J Immunol 180(2):774–782

Burzyn D, Benoist C, Mathis D (2013) Regulatory T cells in nonlymphoid tissues. Nat Immunol 14(10):1007–1013. https://doi.org/10.1038/ni.2683

Busse M, Krech M, Meyer-Bahlburg A, Hennig C, Hansen G (2012) ICOS mediates the generation and function of CD4+CD25+Foxp3+ regulatory T cells conveying respiratory tolerance. J Immunol 189(4):1975–1982. https://doi.org/10.4049/jimmunol.1103581

Butte MJ, Keir ME, Phamduy TB, Sharpe AH, Freeman GJ (2007) Programmed death-1 ligand 1 interacts specifically with the B7-1 costimulatory molecule to inhibit T cell responses. Immunity 27(1):111–122. https://doi.org/10.1016/j.immuni.2007.05.016

Callahan MK, Postow MA, Wolchok JD (2014) CTLA-4 and PD-1 pathway blockade: combinations in the clinic. Front Oncol 4:385. https://doi.org/10.3389/fonc.2014.00385

Chen AI, McAdam AJ, Buhlmann JE, Scott S, Lupher ML Jr, Greenfield EA, Baum PR, Fanslow WC, Calderhead DM, Freeman GJ, Sharpe AH (1999) Ox40-ligand has a critical costimulatory role in dendritic cell: T cell interactions. Immunity 11(6):689–698

Chen X, Baumel M, Mannel DN, Howard OM, Oppenheim JJ (2007) Interaction of TNF with TNF receptor type 2 promotes expansion and function of mouse CD4+CD25+ T regulatory cells. J Immunol 179(1):154–161

Chen X, Wu X, Zhou Q, Howard OM, Netea MG, Oppenheim JJ (2013) TNFR2 is critical for the stabilization of the CD4+Foxp3+ regulatory T. cell phenotype in the inflammatory environment. J Immunol 190(3):1076–1084. https://doi.org/10.4049/jimmunol.1202659

Chiba S, Baghdadi M, Akiba H, Yoshiyama H, Kinoshita I, Dosaka-Akita H, Fujioka Y, Ohba Y, Gorman JV, Colgan JD, Hirashima M, Uede T, Takaoka A, Yagita H, Jinushi M (2012) Tumor-infiltrating DCs suppress nucleic acid-mediated innate immune responses through interactions between the receptor TIM-3 and the alarmin HMGB1. Nat Immunol 13(9):832–842. https://doi.org/10.1038/ni.2376

Claus C, Riether C, Schurch C, Matter MS, Hilmenyuk T, Ochsenbein AF (2012) CD27 signaling increases the frequency of regulatory T cells and promotes tumor growth. Cancer Res 72(14):3664–3676. https://doi.org/10.1158/0008-5472.CAN-11-2791

Coquet JM, Ribot JC, Babala N, Middendorp S, van der Horst G, Xiao Y, Neves JF, Fonseca-Pereira D, Jacobs H, Pennington DJ, Silva-Santos B, Borst J (2013) Epithelial and dendritic cells in the thymic medulla promote CD4+Foxp3+ regulatory T cell development via the CD27-CD70 pathway. J Exp Med 210(4):715–728. https://doi.org/10.1084/jem.20112061

Croft M (2014) The TNF family in T cell differentiation and function – unanswered questions and future directions. Semin Immunol 26(3):183–190. https://doi.org/10.1016/j.smim.2014.02.005

Curran MA, Kim M, Montalvo W, Al-Shamkhani A, Allison JP (2011) Combination CTLA-4 blockade and 4-1BB activation enhances tumor rejection by increasing T-cell infiltration, proliferation, and cytokine production. PLoS One 6(4):e19499. https://doi.org/10.1371/journal.pone.0019499

Dai Z, Li Q, Wang Y, Gao G, Diggs LS, Tellides G, Lakkis FG (2004) CD4+CD25+ regulatory T cells suppress allograft rejection mediated by memory CD8+ T cells via a CD30-dependent mechanism. J Clin Invest 113(2):310–317. https://doi.org/10.1172/JCI19727

Dhainaut M, Coquerelle C, Uzureau S, Denoeud J, Acolty V, Oldenhove G, Galuppo A, Sparwasser T, Thielemans K, Pays E, Yagita H, Borst J, Moser M (2015) Thymus-derived regulatory T cells restrain pro-inflammatory Th1 responses by downregulating CD70 on dendritic cells. EMBO J 34(10):1336–1348. https://doi.org/10.15252/embj.201490312

Ellestad KK, Thangavelu G, Ewen CL, Boon L, Anderson CC (2014) PD-1 is not required for natural or peripherally induced regulatory T cells: severe autoimmunity despite normal production of regulatory T cells. Eur J Immunol 44(12):3560–3572. https://doi.org/10.1002/eji.201444688

Elpek KG, Yolcu ES, Franke DD, Lacelle C, Schabowsky RH, Shirwan H (2007) Ex vivo expansion of CD4+CD25+FoxP3+ T regulatory cells based on synergy between IL-2 and 4-1BB signaling. J Immunol 179(11):7295–7304

Ephrem A, Epstein AL, Stephens GL, Thornton AM, Glass D, Shevach EM (2013) Modulation of Treg cells/T effector function by GITR signaling is context-dependent. Eur J Immunol 43(9):2421–2429. https://doi.org/10.1002/eji.201343451

Eppihimer MJ, Gunn J, Freeman GJ, Greenfield EA, Chernova T, Erickson J, Leonard JP (2002) Expression and regulation of the PD-L1 immunoinhibitory molecule on microvascular endothelial cells. Microcirculation 9(2):133–145. https://doi.org/10.1038/sj/mn/7800123

Ermann J, Hoffmann P, Edinger M, Dutt S, Blankenberg FG, Higgins JP, Negrin RS, Fathman CG, Strober S (2005) Only the CD62L+ subpopulation of CD4+CD25+ regulatory T cells protects from lethal acute GVHD. Blood 105(5):2220–2226. https://doi.org/10.1182/blood-2004-05-2044

Francisco LM, Salinas VH, Brown KE, Vanguri VK, Freeman GJ, Kuchroo VK, Sharpe AH (2009) PD-L1 regulates the development, maintenance, and function of induced regulatory T cells. J Exp Med 206(13):3015–3029. https://doi.org/10.1084/jem.20090847

Freeman GJ, Long AJ, Iwai Y, Bourque K, Chernova T, Nishimura H, Fitz LJ, Malenkovich N, Okazaki T, Byrne MC, Horton HF, Fouser L, Carter L, Ling V, Bowman MR, Carreno BM, Collins M, Wood CR, Honjo T (2000) Engagement of the PD-1 immunoinhibitory receptor by a novel B7 family member leads to negative regulation of lymphocyte activation. J Exp Med 192(7):1027–1034

Freeman GJ, Wherry EJ, Ahmed R, Sharpe AH (2006) Reinvigorating exhausted HIV-specific T cells via PD-1-PD-1 ligand blockade. J Exp Med 203(10):2223–2227. https://doi.org/10.1084/jem.20061800

Fuhrman CA, Yeh WI, Seay HR, Saikumar Lakshmi P, Chopra G, Zhang L, Perry DJ, McClymont SA, Yadav M, Lopez MC, Baker HV, Zhang Y, Li Y, Whitley M, von Schack D, Atkinson MA, Bluestone JA, Brusko TM (2015) Divergent phenotypes of human regulatory T cells expressing the receptors TIGIT and CD226. J Immunol 195(1):145–155. https://doi.org/10.4049/jimmunol.1402381

Gautron AS, Dominguez-Villar M, de Marcken M, Hafler DA (2014) Enhanced suppressor function of TIM-3+ FoxP3+ regulatory T cells. Eur J Immunol 44(9):2703–2711. https://doi.org/10.1002/eji.201344392

Grant CR, Liberal R, Mieli-Vergani G, Vergani D, Longhi MS (2015) Regulatory T-cells in autoimmune diseases: challenges, controversies and--yet--unanswered questions. Autoimmun Rev 14(2):105–116. https://doi.org/10.1016/j.autrev.2014.10.012

Griseri T, Asquith M, Thompson C, Powrie F (2010) OX40 is required for regulatory T cell-mediated control of colitis. J Exp Med 207(4):699–709. https://doi.org/10.1084/jem.20091618

Grosso JF, Kelleher CC, Harris TJ, Maris CH, Hipkiss EL, De Marzo A, Anders R, Netto G, Getnet D, Bruno TC, Goldberg MV, Pardoll DM, Drake CG (2007) LAG-3 regulates CD8+ T cell accumulation and effector function in murine self- and tumor-tolerance systems. J Clin Invest 117(11):3383–3392. https://doi.org/10.1172/JCI31184

Guo F, Iclozan C, Suh WK, Anasetti C, Yu XZ (2008) CD28 controls differentiation of regulatory T cells from naive CD4 T cells. J Immunol 181(4):2285–2291

Gupta S, Thornley TB, Gao W, Larocca R, Turka LA, Kuchroo VK, Strom TB (2012) Allograft rejection is restrained by short-lived TIM-3+PD-1+Foxp3+ Tregs. J Clin Invest 122(7):2395–2404. https://doi.org/10.1172/JCI45138

Hannier S, Tournier M, Bismuth G, Triebel F (1998) CD3/TCR complex-associated lymphocyte activation gene-3 molecules inhibit CD3/TCR signaling. J Immunol 161(8):4058–4065

Herman AE, Freeman GJ, Mathis D, Benoist C (2004) CD4+CD25+ T regulatory cells dependent on ICOS promote regulation of effector cells in the prediabetic lesion. J Exp Med 199(11):1479–1489. https://doi.org/10.1084/jem.20040179

Hombach AA, Kofler D, Hombach A, Rappl G, Abken H (2007) Effective proliferation of human regulatory T cells requires a strong costimulatory CD28 signal that cannot be substituted by IL-2. J Immunol 179(11):7924–7931

Huang CT, Workman CJ, Flies D, Pan X, Marson AL, Zhou G, Hipkiss EL, Ravi S, Kowalski J, Levitsky HI, Powell JD, Pardoll DM, Drake CG, Vignali DA (2004) Role of LAG-3 in regulatory T cells. Immunity 21(4):503–513. https://doi.org/10.1016/j.immuni.2004.08.010

Huard B, Prigent P, Tournier M, Bruniquel D, Triebel F (1995) CD4/major histocompatibility complex class II interaction analyzed with CD4- and lymphocyte activation gene-3 (LAG-3)-Ig fusion proteins. Eur J Immunol 25(9):2718–2721. https://doi.org/10.1002/eji.1830250949

Iwai Y, Hamanishi J, Chamoto K, Honjo T (2017) Cancer immunotherapies targeting the PD-1 signaling pathway. J Biomed Sci 24(1):26. https://doi.org/10.1186/s12929-017-0329-9

Joller N, Hafler JP, Brynedal B, Kassam N, Spoerl S, Levin SD, Sharpe AH, Kuchroo VK (2011) Cutting edge: TIGIT has T cell-intrinsic inhibitory functions. J Immunol 186(3):1338–1342. https://doi.org/10.4049/jimmunol.1003081

Joller N, Lozano E, Burkett PR, Patel B, Xiao S, Zhu C, Xia J, Tan TG, Sefik E, Yajnik V, Sharpe AH, Quintana FJ, Mathis D, Benoist C, Hafler DA, Kuchroo VK (2014) Treg cells expressing the coinhibitory molecule TIGIT selectively inhibit proinflammatory Th1 and Th17 cell responses. Immunity 40(4):569–581. https://doi.org/10.1016/j.immuni.2014.02.012

Josefowicz SZ, Niec RE, Kim HY, Treuting P, Chinen T, Zheng Y, Umetsu DT, Rudensky AY (2012) Extrathymically generated regulatory T cells control mucosal TH2 inflammation. Nature 482(7385):395–399. https://doi.org/10.1038/nature10772

Karunarathne DS, Horne-Debets JM, Huang JX, Faleiro R, Leow CY, Amante F, Watkins TS, Miles JJ, Dwyer PJ, Stacey KJ, Yarski M, Poh CM, Lee JS, Cooper MA, Rénia L, Richard D, McCarthy JS, Sharpe AH, Wykes MN (2016) Programmed death-1 ligand 2-mediated regulation of the PD-L1 to PD-1 axis is essential for establishing CD4(+) T cell immunity. Immunity 45(2):333–345. https://doi.org/10.1016/j.immuni.2016.07.017

Kim JM, Rasmussen JP, Rudensky AY (2007) Regulatory T cells prevent catastrophic autoimmunity throughout the lifespan of mice. Nat Immunol 8(2):191–197. https://doi.org/10.1038/ni1428

Kim BS, Nishikii H, Baker J, Pierini A, Schneidawind D, Pan Y, Beilhack A, Park CG, Negrin RS (2015) Treatment with agonistic DR3 antibody results in expansion of donor Tregs and reduced graft-versus-host disease. Blood 126(4):546–557. https://doi.org/10.1182/blood-2015-04-637587

Kinnear G, Wood KJ, Fallah-Arani F, Jones ND (2013) A diametric role for OX40 in the response of effector/memory CD4+ T cells and regulatory T cells to alloantigen. J Immunol 191(3):1465–1475. https://doi.org/10.4049/jimmunol.1300553

Klocke K, Sakaguchi S, Holmdahl R, Wing K (2016) Induction of autoimmune disease by deletion of CTLA-4 in mice in adulthood. Proc Natl Acad Sci U S A 113(17):E2383–E2392. https://doi.org/10.1073/pnas.1603892113

Ko K, Yamazaki S, Nakamura K, Nishioka T, Hirota K, Yamaguchi T, Shimizu J, Nomura T, Chiba T, Sakaguchi S (2005) Treatment of advanced tumors with agonistic anti-GITR mAb and its effects on tumor-infiltrating Foxp3+CD25+CD4+ regulatory T cells. J Exp Med 202(7):885–891. https://doi.org/10.1084/jem.20050940

Kocak E, Lute K, Chang X, May KF Jr, Exten KR, Zhang H, Abdessalam SF, Lehman AM, Jarjoura D, Zheng P, Liu Y (2006) Combination therapy with anti-CTL antigen-4 and anti-4-1BB antibodies enhances cancer immunity and reduces autoimmunity. Cancer Res 66(14):7276–7284. https://doi.org/10.1158/0008-5472.CAN-05-2128

Koguchi K, Anderson DE, Yang L, O'Connor KC, Kuchroo VK, Hafler DA (2006) Dysregulated T cell expression of TIM3 in multiple sclerosis. J Exp Med 203(6):1413–1418. https://doi.org/10.1084/jem.20060210

Kong K-F, Fu G, Zhang Y, Yokosuka T, Casas J, Canonigo-Balancio AJ, Becart S, Kim G, Yates JR, Kronenberg M, Saito T, Gascoigne NRJ, Altman A (2014) Protein kinase C-η controls CTLA-4-mediated regulatory T cell function. Nat Immunol 15(5):465–472. https://doi.org/10.1038/ni.2866

Kornete M, Sgouroudis E, Piccirillo CA (2012) ICOS-dependent homeostasis and function of Foxp3+ regulatory T cells in islets of nonobese diabetic mice. J Immunol 188(3):1064–1074. https://doi.org/10.4049/jimmunol.1101303

Kuehn HS, Ouyang W, Lo B, Deenick EK, Niemela JE, Avery DT, Schickel JN, Tran DQ, Stoddard J, Zhang Y, Frucht DM, Dumitriu B, Scheinberg P, Folio LR, Frein CA, Price S, Koh C, Heller T, Seroogy CM, Huttenlocher A, Rao VK, Su HC, Kleiner D, Notarangelo LD, Rampertaap Y, Olivier KN, McElwee J, Hughes J, Pittaluga S, Oliveira JB, Meffre E, Fleisher TA, Holland SM, Lenardo MJ, Tangye SG, Uzel G (2014) Immune dysregulation in human subjects with heterozygous germline mutations in CTLA4. Science 345(6204):1623–1627. https://doi.org/10.1126/science.1255904

Kurtulus S, Sakuishi K, Ngiow SF, Joller N, Tan DJ, Teng MW, Smyth MJ, Kuchroo VK, Anderson AC (2015) TIGIT predominantly regulates the immune response via regulatory T cells. J Clin Invest 125(11):4053–4062. https://doi.org/10.1172/JCI81187

Kwon BS, Hurtado JC, Lee ZH, Kwack KB, Seo SK, Choi BK, Koller BH, Wolisi G, Broxmeyer HE, Vinay DS (2002) Immune responses in 4-1BB (CD137)-deficient mice. J Immunol 168(11):5483–5490

Latchman Y, Wood CR, Chernova T, Chaudhary D, Borde M, Chernova I, Iwai Y, Long AJ, Brown JA, Nunes R, Greenfield EA, Bourque K, Boussiotis VA, Carter LL, Carreno BM, Malenkovich N, Nishimura H, Okazaki T, Honjo T, Sharpe AH, Freeman GJ (2001) PD-L2 is a second ligand for PD-1 and inhibits T cell activation. Nat Immunol 2(3):261–268. https://doi.org/10.1038/85330

Li A, Jacks T (2017) Driving Rel-iant Tregs toward an identity crisis. Immunity 47(3):391–393. https://doi.org/10.1016/j.immuni.2017.08.014

Li M, Xia P, Du Y, Liu S, Huang G, Chen J, Zhang H, Hou N, Cheng X, Zhou L, Li P, Yang X, Fan Z (2014) T-cell immunoglobulin and ITIM domain (TIGIT) receptor/poliovirus receptor (PVR) ligand engagement suppresses interferon-γ production of natural killer cells via β-arrestin 2-mediated negative signaling. J Biol Chem 289(25):17647–17657. https://doi.org/10.1074/jbc.M114.572420

Liao G, Nayak S, Regueiro JR, Berger SB, Detre C, Romero X, de Waal Malefyt R, Chatila TA, Herzog RW, Terhorst C (2010) GITR engagement preferentially enhances proliferation of functionally competent CD4+CD25+FoxP3+ regulatory T cells. Int Immunol 22(4):259–270. https://doi.org/10.1093/intimm/dxq001

Lin CH, Hunig T (2003) Efficient expansion of regulatory T cells in vitro and in vivo with a CD28 superagonist. Eur J Immunol 33(3):626–638. https://doi.org/10.1002/eji.200323570

Lio CW, Hsieh CS (2008) A two-step process for thymic regulatory T cell development. Immunity 28(1):100–111. https://doi.org/10.1016/j.immuni.2007.11.021

Liu X, Gao JX, Wen J, Yin L, Li O, Zuo T, Gajewski TF, Fu YX, Zheng P, Liu Y (2003) B7DC/PDL2 promotes tumor immunity by a PD-1-independent mechanism. J Exp Med 197(12):1721–1730. https://doi.org/10.1084/jem.20022089

Lohr J, Knoechel B, Jiang S, Sharpe AH, Abbas AK (2003) The inhibitory function of B7 costimulators in T cell responses to foreign and self-antigens. Nat Immunol 4(7):664–669. https://doi.org/10.1038/ni939

Loke P, Allison JP (2003) PD-L1 and PD-L2 are differentially regulated by Th1 and Th2 cells. Proc Natl Acad Sci U S A 100(9):5336–5341. https://doi.org/10.1073/pnas.0931259100

Long EO (1999) Regulation of immune responses through inhibitory receptors. Annu Rev Immunol 17:875–904. https://doi.org/10.1146/annurev.immunol.17.1.875

Lowther DE, Goods BA, Lucca LE, Lerner BA, Raddassi K, van Dijk D, Hernandez AL, Duan X, Gunel M, Coric V, Krishnaswamy S, Love JC, Hafler DA (2016) PD-1 marks dysfunctional regulatory T cells in malignant gliomas. JCI Insight 1(5). https://doi.org/10.1172/jci.insight.85935

Maerten P, Kwon BS, Shen C, De Hertogh G, Cadot P, Bullens DM, Overbergh L, Mathieu C, Van Assche G, Geboes K, Rutgeerts P, Ceuppens JL (2006) Involvement of 4-1BB (CD137)-4-1BBligand interaction in the modulation of CD4 T cell-mediated inflammatory colitis. Clin Exp Immunol 143(2):228–236. https://doi.org/10.1111/j.1365-2249.2005.02991.x

Mahmud SA, Manlove LS, Schmitz HM, Xing Y, Wang Y, Owen DL, Schenkel JM, Boomer JS, Green JM, Yagita H, Chi H, Ka H, Ma F (2014) Costimulation via the tumor-necrosis factor receptor superfamily couples TCR signal strength to the thymic differentiation of regulatory T cells. Nat Immunol 15(5):473–481. https://doi.org/10.1038/ni.2849

Mandelbrot DA, McAdam AJ, Sharpe AH (1999) B7-1 or B7-2 is required to produce the lympho-proliferative phenotype in mice lacking cytotoxic T lymphocyte-associated antigen 4 (CTLA-4). J Exp Med 189(2):435–440

McHugh RS, Whitters MJ, Piccirillo CA, Young DA, Shevach EM, Collins M, Byrne MC (2002) CD4(+)CD25(+) immunoregulatory T cells: gene expression analysis reveals a functional role for the glucocorticoid-induced TNF receptor. Immunity 16(2):311–323

Meagher C, Tang Q, Fife BT, Bour-Jordan H, Wu J, Pardoux C, Bi M, Melli K, Bluestone JA (2008) Spontaneous development of a pancreatic exocrine disease in CD28-deficient NOD mice. J Immunol 180(12):7793–7803

Messal N, Serriari NE, Pastor S, Nunès JA, Olive D (2011) PD-L2 is expressed on activated human T cells and regulates their function. Mol Immunol 48(15-16):2214–2219. https://doi.org/10.1016/j.molimm.2011.06.436

Miyamoto K, Kingsley CI, Zhang X, Jabs C, Izikson L, Sobel RA, Weiner HL, Kuchroo VK, Sharpe AH (2005) The ICOS molecule plays a crucial role in the development of mucosal tolerance. J Immunol 175(11):7341–7347

Monney L, Sabatos CA, Gaglia JL, Ryu A, Waldner H, Chernova T, Manning S, Greenfield EA, Coyle AJ, Sobel RA, Freeman GJ, Kuchroo VK (2002) Th1-specific cell surface protein Tim-3 regulates macrophage activation and severity of an autoimmune disease. Nature 415(6871):536–541. https://doi.org/10.1038/415536a

Murata K, Nose M, Ndhlovu LC, Sato T, Sugamura K, Ishii N (2002) Constitutive OX40/OX40 ligand interaction induces autoimmune-like diseases. J Immunol 169(8):4628–4636

Nie H, Zheng Y, Li R, Zhang J (2016) Reply to Suppressive activity of human regulatory T cells is maintained in the presence of TNF. Nat Med 22(1):18–19. https://doi.org/10.1038/nm.4018

Nishimura H, Agata Y, Kawasaki A, Sato M, Imamura S, Minato N, Yagita H, Nakano T, Honjo T (1996) Developmentally regulated expression of the PD-1 protein on the surface of double-negative (CD4-CD8-) thymocytes. Int Immunol 8(5):773–780

Nishimura H, Nose M, Hiai H, Minato N, Honjo T (1999) Development of lupus-like autoimmune diseases by disruption of the PD-1 gene encoding an ITIM motif-carrying immunoreceptor. Immunity 11(2):141–151

Nishimura H, Okazaki T, Tanaka Y, Nakatani K, Hara M, Matsumori A, Sasayama S, Mizoguchi A, Hiai H, Minato N, Honjo T (2001) Autoimmune dilated cardiomyopathy in PD-1 receptor-deficient mice. Science 291(5502):319–322. https://doi.org/10.1126/science.291.5502.319

Nishizuka Y, Sakakura T (1969) Thymus and reproduction: sex-linked dysgenesia of the gonad after neonatal thymectomy in mice. Science 166(3906):753–755

Nocentini G, Riccardi C (2005) GITR: a multifaceted regulator of immunity belonging to the tumor necrosis factor receptor superfamily. Eur J Immunol 35(4):1016–1022. https://doi.org/10.1002/eji.200425818

Nurieva R, Thomas S, Nguyen T, Martin-Orozco N, Wang Y, Kaja MK, Yu XZ, Dong C (2006) T-cell tolerance or function is determined by combinatorial costimulatory signals. EMBO J 25(11):2623–2633. https://doi.org/10.1038/sj.emboj.7601146

Oestreich KJ, Yoon H, Ahmed R, Boss JM (2008) NFATc1 regulates PD-1 expression upon T cell activation. J Immunol 181(7):4832–4839

Ohkura N, Kitagawa Y, Sakaguchi S (2013) Development and maintenance of regulatory T cells. Immunity 38(3):414–423. https://doi.org/10.1016/j.immuni.2013.03.002

Okubo Y, Mera T, Wang L, Faustman DL (2013) Homogeneous expansion of human T-regulatory cells via tumor necrosis factor receptor 2. Sci Rep 3:3153. https://doi.org/10.1038/srep03153

Onishi Y, Fehervari Z, Yamaguchi T, Sakaguchi S (2008) Foxp3(+) natural regulatory T cells preferentially form aggregates on dendritic cells in vitro and actively inhibit their maturation. Proc Natl Acad Sci U S A 105(29):10113–10118. https://doi.org/10.1073/Pnas.0711106105

Parry RV, Chemnitz JM, Frauwirth KA, Lanfranco AR, Braunstein I, Kobayashi SV, Linsley PS, Thompson CB, Riley JL (2005) CTLA-4 and PD-1 receptors inhibit T-cell activation by distinct mechanisms. Mol Cell Biol 25(21):9543–9553. https://doi.org/10.1128/MCB.25.21.9543-9553.2005

Piconese S, Valzasina B, Colombo MP (2008) OX40 triggering blocks suppression by regulatory T cells and facilitates tumor rejection. J Exp Med 205(4):825–839. https://doi.org/10.1084/jem.20071341

Piconese S, Gri G, Tripodo C, Musio S, Gorzanelli A, Frossi B, Pedotti R, Pucillo CE, Colombo MP (2009) Mast cells counteract regulatory T-cell suppression through interleukin-6 and OX40/OX40L axis toward Th17-cell differentiation. Blood 114(13):2639–2648. https://doi.org/10.1182/blood-2009-05-220004

Ramsdell F, Ziegler SF (2014) FOXP3 and scurfy: how it all began. Nat Rev Immunol 14(5):343–349. https://doi.org/10.1038/nri3650

Redmond WL, Weinberg AD (2007) Targeting OX40 and OX40L for the treatment of autoimmunity and cancer. Crit Rev Immunol 27(5):415–436

Ronchetti S, Zollo O, Bruscoli S, Agostini M, Bianchini R, Nocentini G, Ayroldi E, Riccardi C (2004) GITR, a member of the TNF receptor superfamily, is costimulatory to mouse T lymphocyte subpopulations. Eur J Immunol 34(3):613–622. https://doi.org/10.1002/eji.200324804

Rui Y, Honjo T, Chikuma S (2013) Programmed cell death 1 inhibits inflammatory helper T-cell development through controlling the innate immune response. Proc Natl Acad Sci U S A 110(40):16073–16078. https://doi.org/10.1073/pnas.1315828110

Sage PT, Francisco LM, Carman CV, Sharpe AH (2013) The receptor PD-1 controls follicular regulatory T cells in the lymph nodes and blood. Nat Immunol 14(2):152–161. https://doi.org/10.1038/ni.2496

Sakaguchi S, Sakaguchi N, Asano M, Itoh M, Toda M (1995) Immunologic self-tolerance maintained by activated T cells expressing IL-2 receptor alpha-chains (CD25). Breakdown of a single mechanism of self-tolerance causes various autoimmune diseases. J Immunol 155(3):1151–1164

Sakuishi K, Ngiow SF, Sullivan JM, Teng MW, Kuchroo VK, Smyth MJ, Anderson AC (2013) TIM3(+)FOXP3(+) regulatory T cells are tissue-specific promoters of T-cell dysfunction in cancer. Oncoimmunology 2(4):e23849. https://doi.org/10.4161/onci.23849

Salomon B, Lenschow DJ, Rhee L, Ashourian N, Singh B, Sharpe A, Bluestone JA (2000) B7/CD28 costimulation is essential for the homeostasis of the CD4+CD25+ immunoregulatory T cells that control autoimmune diabetes. Immunity 12(4):431–440

Sanmamed MF, Pastor F, Rodriguez A, Perez-Gracia JL, Rodriguez-Ruiz ME, Jure-Kunkel M, Melero I (2015) Agonists of Co-stimulation in cancer immunotherapy directed against CD137, OX40, GITR, CD27, CD28, and ICOS. Semin Oncol 42(4):640–655. https://doi.org/10.1053/j.seminoncol.2015.05.014

Schoenbrunn A, Frentsch M, Kohler S, Keye J, Dooms H, Moewes B, Dong J, Loddenkemper C, Sieper J, Wu P, Romagnani C, Matzmohr N, Thiel A (2012) A converse 4-1BB and CD40 ligand expression pattern delineates activated regulatory T cells (Treg) and conventional T cells enabling direct isolation of alloantigen-reactive natural Foxp3+ Treg. J Immunol 189(12):5985–5994. https://doi.org/10.4049/jimmunol.1201090

Schreiber TH, Wolf D, Tsai MS, Chirinos J, Deyev VV, Gonzalez L, Malek TR, Levy RB, Podack ER (2010) Therapeutic Treg expansion in mice by TNFRSF25 prevents allergic lung inflammation. J Clin Invest 120(10):3629–3640. https://doi.org/10.1172/JCI42933

Schubert D, Bode C, Kenefeck R, Hou TZ, Wing JB, Kennedy A, Bulashevska A, Petersen BS, Schaffer AA, Gruning BA, Unger S, Frede N, Baumann U, Witte T, Schmidt RE, Dueckers G, Niehues T, Seneviratne S, Kanariou M, Speckmann C, Ehl S, Rensing-Ehl A, Warnatz K, Rakhmanov M, Thimme R, Hasselblatt P, Emmerich F, Cathomen T, Backofen R, Fisch P, Seidl M, May A, Schmitt-Graeff A, Ikemizu S, Salzer U, Franke A, Sakaguchi S, Walker LS, Sansom DM, Grimbacher B (2014) Autosomal dominant immune dysregulation syndrome in humans with CTLA4 mutations. Nat Med 20(12):1410–1416. https://doi.org/10.1038/nm.3746

Sega EI, Leveson-Gower DB, Florek M, Schneidawind D, Luong RH, Negrin RS (2014) Role of lymphocyte activation gene-3 (Lag-3) in conventional and regulatory T cell function in allogeneic transplantation. PLoS One 9(1):e86551. https://doi.org/10.1371/journal.pone.0086551

Sharma MD, Huang L, Choi JH, Lee EJ, Wilson JM, Lemos H, Pan F, Blazar BR, Pardoll DM, Mellor AL, Shi H, Munn DH (2013) An inherently bifunctional subset of Foxp3+ T helper cells is controlled by the transcription factor eos. Immunity 38(5):998–1012. https://doi.org/10.1016/j.immuni.2013.01.013

Sharpe AH, Freeman GJ (2002) The B7-CD28 superfamily. Nat Rev Immunol 2(2):116–126. https://doi.org/10.1038/nri727

Shimizu J, Yamazaki S, Takahashi T, Ishida Y, Sakaguchi S (2002) Stimulation of CD25(+)CD4(+) regulatory T cells through GITR breaks immunological self-tolerance. Nat Immunol 3(2):135–142. https://doi.org/10.1038/ni759

Shin T, Kennedy G, Gorski K, Tsuchiya H, Koseki H, Azuma M, Yagita H, Chen L, Powell J, Pardoll D, Housseau F (2003) Cooperative B7-1/2 (CD80/CD86) and B7-DC costimulation of CD4+ T cells independent of the PD-1 receptor. J Exp Med 198(1):31–38. https://doi.org/10.1084/jem.20030242

Sidorenko SP, Clark EA (2003) The dual-function CD150 receptor subfamily: the viral attraction. Nat Immunol 4(1):19–24. https://doi.org/10.1038/ni0103-19

Simpson TR, Li F, Montalvo-Ortiz W, Sepulveda MA, Bergerhoff K, Arce F, Roddie C, Henry JY, Yagita H, Wolchok JD, Peggs KS, Ravetch JV, Allison JP, Quezada SA (2013) Fc-dependent depletion of tumor-infiltrating regulatory T cells co-defines the efficacy of anti-CTLA-4 therapy against melanoma. J Exp Med 210(9):1695–1710. https://doi.org/10.1084/jem.20130579

Spinicelli S, Nocentini G, Ronchetti S, Krausz LT, Bianchini R, Riccardi C (2002) GITR interacts with the pro-apoptotic protein Siva and induces apoptosis. Cell Death Differ 9(12):1382–1384. https://doi.org/10.1038/sj.cdd.4401140

Stephen TL, Payne KK, Chaurio RA, Allegrezza MJ, Zhu H, Perez-Sanz J, Perales-Puchalt A, Nguyen JM, Vara-Ailor AE, Eruslanov EB, Borowsky ME, Zhang R, Laufer TM, Conejo-Garcia JR (2017) SATB1 expression governs epigenetic repression of PD-1 in tumor-reactive T cells. Immunity 46(1):51–64. https://doi.org/10.1016/j.immuni.2016.12.015

Stephens GL, McHugh RS, Whitters MJ, Young DA, Luxenberg D, Carreno BM, Collins M, Shevach EM (2004) Engagement of glucocorticoid-induced TNFR family-related receptor on effector T cells by its ligand mediates resistance to suppression by CD4+CD25+ T cells. J Immunol 173(8):5008–5020

Sugimoto N, Oida T, Hirota K, Nakamura K, Nomura T, Uchiyama T, Sakaguchi S (2006) Foxp3-dependent and -independent molecules specific for CD25+CD4+ natural regulatory T cells revealed by DNA microarray analysis. Int Immunol 18(8):1197–1209. https://doi.org/10.1093/intimm/dxl060

Suntharalingam G, Perry MR, Ward S, Brett SJ, Castello-Cortes A, Brunner MD, Panoskaltsis N (2006) Cytokine storm in a phase 1 trial of the anti-CD28 monoclonal antibody TGN1412. N Engl J Med 355(10):1018–1028. https://doi.org/10.1056/NEJMoa063842

Tai X, Cowan M, Feigenbaum L, Singer A (2005) CD28 costimulation of developing thymocytes induces Foxp3 expression and regulatory T cell differentiation independently of interleukin 2. Nat Immunol 6(2):152–162. https://doi.org/10.1038/ni1160

Tai X, Van Laethem F, Sharpe AH, Singer A (2007) Induction of autoimmune disease in CTLA-4-/- mice depends on a specific CD28 motif that is required for in vivo costimulation. Proc Natl Acad Sci U S A 104(34):13756–13761. https://doi.org/10.1073/pnas.0706509104

Takeda I, Ine S, Killeen N, Ndhlovu LC, Murata K, Satomi S, Sugamura K, Ishii N (2004) Distinct roles for the OX40-OX40 ligand interaction in regulatory and nonregulatory T cells. J Immunol 172(6):3580–3589

Tanaka A, Sakaguchi S (2017) Regulatory T cells in cancer immunotherapy. Cell Res 27(1):109–118. https://doi.org/10.1038/cr.2016.151

Tang Q, Henriksen KJ, Boden EK, Tooley AJ, Ye J, Subudhi SK, Zheng XX, Strom TB, Bluestone JA (2003) Cutting edge: CD28 controls peripheral homeostasis of CD4+CD25+ regulatory T cells. J Immunol 171(7):3348–3352

Tivol EA, Borriello F, Schweitzer AN, Lynch WP, Bluestone JA, Sharpe AH (1995) Loss of CTLA-4 leads to massive lymphoproliferation and fatal multiorgan tissue destruction, revealing a critical negative regulatory role of CTLA-4. Immunity 3(5):541–547

Tseng SY, Otsuji M, Gorski K, Huang X, Slansky JE, Pai SI, Shalabi A, Shin T, Pardoll DM, Tsuchiya H (2001) B7-DC, a new dendritic cell molecule with potent costimulatory properties for T cells. J Exp Med 193(7):839–846

Valzasina B, Guiducci C, Dislich H, Killeen N, Weinberg AD, Colombo MP (2005) Triggering of OX40 (CD134) on CD4(+)CD25+ T cells blocks their inhibitory activity: a novel regulatory role for OX40 and its comparison with GITR. Blood 105(7):2845–2851. https://doi.org/10.1182/blood-2004-07-2959

Vasanthakumar A, Liao Y, Teh P, Pascutti MF, Oja AE, Garnham AL, Gloury R, Tempany JC, Sidwell T, Cuadrado E, Tuijnenburg P, Kuijpers TW, Lalaoui N, Mielke LA, Bryant VL, Hodgkin PD, Silke J, Smyth GK, Nolte MA, Shi W, Kallies A (2017) The TNF receptor superfamily-NF-kappaB axis is critical to maintain effector regulatory T cells in lymphoid and non-lymphoid tissues. Cell Rep 20(12):2906–2920. https://doi.org/10.1016/j.celrep.2017.08.068

Vu MD, Xiao X, Gao W, Degauque N, Chen M, Kroemer A, Killeen N, Ishii N, Li XC (2007) OX40 costimulation turns off Foxp3+ Tregs. Blood 110(7):2501–2510. https://doi.org/10.1182/blood-2007-01-070748

Walker LSK, Sansom DM (2015) Confusing signals: recent progress in CTLA-4 biology. Trends Immunol:1–8. https://doi.org/10.1016/j.it.2014.12.001

Wang J, Yoshida T, Nakaki F, Hiai H, Okazaki T, Honjo T (2005) Establishment of NOD-Pdcd1-/-mice as an efficient animal model of type I diabetes. Proc Natl Acad Sci U S A 102(33):11823–11828. https://doi.org/10.1073/pnas.0505497102

Watts TH (2005) TNF/TNFR family members in costimulation of T cell responses. Annu Rev Immunol 23:23–68. https://doi.org/10.1146/annurev.immunol.23.021704.115839

Webb GJ, Hirschfield GM, Lane PJ (2016) OX40, OX40L and autoimmunity: a comprehensive review. Clin Rev Allergy Immunol 50(3):312–332. https://doi.org/10.1007/s12016-015-8498-3

Wikenheiser DJ, Stumhofer JS (2016) ICOS co-stimulation: friend or foe? Front Immunol 7:304. https://doi.org/10.3389/fimmu.2016.00304

Wildin RS, Ramsdell F, Peake J, Faravelli F, Casanova JL, Buist N, Levy-Lahad E, Mazzella M, Goulet O, Perroni L, Bricarelli FD, Byrne G, McEuen M, Proll S, Appleby M, Brunkow ME (2001) X-linked neonatal diabetes mellitus, enteropathy and endocrinopathy syndrome is the human equivalent of mouse scurfy. Nat Genet 27(1):18–20. https://doi.org/10.1038/83707

Wing JB, Sakaguchi S (2012) Multiple treg suppressive modules and their adaptability. Front Immunol 3:178. https://doi.org/10.3389/fimmu.2012.00178

Wing K, Onishi Y, Prieto-Martin P, Yamaguchi T, Miyara M, Fehervari Z, Nomura T, Sakaguchi S (2008) CTLA-4 control over Foxp3+ regulatory T cell function. Science 322(5899):271–275. https://doi.org/10.1126/science.1160062

Wing K, Yamaguchi T, Sakaguchi S (2011) Cell-autonomous and -non-autonomous roles of CTLA-4 in immune regulation. Trends Immunol 32(9):428–433. https://doi.org/10.1016/j.it.2011.06.002

Wing JB, Kitagawa Y, Locci M, Hume H, Tay C, Morita T, Kidani Y, Matsuda K, Inoue T, Kurosaki T, Crotty S, Coban C, Ohkura N, Sakaguchi S (2017) A distinct subpopulation of CD25- T-follicular regulatory cells localizes in the germinal centers. Proc Natl Acad Sci U S A 114(31):E6400–E6409. https://doi.org/10.1073/pnas.1705551114

Workman CJ, Dugger KJ, Vignali DA (2002) Cutting edge: molecular analysis of the negative regulatory function of lymphocyte activation gene-3. J Immunol 169(10):5392–5395

Xiao X, Gong W, Demirci G, Liu W, Spoerl S, Chu X, Bishop DK, Turka LA, Li XC (2012) New insights on OX40 in the control of T cell immunity and immune tolerance in vivo. J Immunol 188(2):892–901. https://doi.org/10.4049/jimmunol.1101373

Xu F, Liu J, Liu D, Liu B, Wang M, Hu Z, Du X, Tang L, He F (2014) LSECtin expressed on melanoma cells promotes tumor progression by inhibiting antitumor T-cell responses. Cancer Res 74(13):3418–3428. https://doi.org/10.1158/0008-5472.CAN-13-2690

Yamazaki T, Akiba H, Iwai H, Matsuda H, Aoki M, Tanno Y, Shin T, Tsuchiya H, Pardoll DM, Okumura K, Azuma M, Yagita H (2002) Expression of programmed death 1 ligands by murine T cells and APC. J Immunol 169(10):5538–5545

Yu X, Harden K, Gonzalez LC, Francesco M, Chiang E, Irving B, Tom I, Ivelja S, Refino CJ, Clark H, Eaton D, Grogan JL (2009) The surface protein TIGIT suppresses T cell activation by promoting the generation of mature immunoregulatory dendritic cells. Nat Immunol 10(1):48–57. https://doi.org/10.1038/ni.1674

Zeiser R, Nguyen VH, Hou JZ, Beilhack A, Zambricki E, Buess M, Contag CH, Negrin RS (2007) Early CD30 signaling is critical for adoptively transferred CD4+CD25+ regulatory T cells in prevention of acute graft-versus-host disease. Blood 109(5):2225–2233. https://doi.org/10.1182/blood-2006-07-038455

Zhang X, Schwartz JC, Guo X, Bhatia S, Cao E, Lorenz M, Cammer M, Chen L, Zhang ZY, Edidin MA, Nathenson SG, Almo SC (2004) Structural and functional analysis of the costimulatory receptor programmed death-1. Immunity 20(3):337–347

Zhang R, Huynh A, Whitcher G, Chang J, Maltzman JS, Turka LA (2013) An obligate cell-intrinsic function for CD28 in Tregs. J Clin Invest 123(2):580–593. https://doi.org/10.1172/JCI65013

Zhang B, Chikuma S, Hori S, Fagarasan S, Honjo T (2016) Nonoverlapping roles of PD-1 and FoxP3 in maintaining immune tolerance in a novel autoimmune pancreatitis mouse model. Proc Natl Acad Sci U S A 113(30):8490–8495. https://doi.org/10.1073/pnas.1608873113

Zhang Q, Chikina M, Szymczak-Workman AL, Horne W, Kolls JK, Vignali KM, Normolle D, Bettini M, Workman CJ, Vignali DAA (2017) LAG3 limits regulatory T cell proliferation and function in autoimmune diabetes. Sci Immunol 2(9). https://doi.org/10.1126/sciimmunol.aah4569

Zheng G, Wang B, Chen A (2004) The 4-1BB costimulation augments the proliferation of CD4+CD25+ regulatory T cells. J Immunol 173(4):2428–2434

Zhong X, Tumang JR, Gao W, Bai C, Rothstein TL (2007) PD-L2 expression extends beyond dendritic cells/macrophages to B1 cells enriched for V(H)11/V(H)12 and phosphatidylcholine binding. Eur J Immunol 37(9):2405–2410. https://doi.org/10.1002/eji.200737461

Part II
Co-signal Molecules in Health and Disease

Chapter 8
Stimulatory and Inhibitory Co-signals in Autoimmunity

Taku Okazaki and Il-mi Okazaki

Abstract Co-receptors cooperatively regulate the function of immune cells to optimize anti-infectious immunity while limiting autoimmunity by providing stimulatory and inhibitory co-signals. Among various co-receptors, those in the CD28/ CTLA-4 family play fundamental roles in the regulation of lymphocytes by modulating the strength, quality, and/or duration of the antigen receptor signal. The development of the lethal lymphoproliferative disorder and various tissue-specific autoimmune diseases in mice deficient for CTLA-4 and PD-1, respectively, clearly demonstrates their pivotal roles in the development and the maintenance of immune tolerance. The recent success of immunotherapies targeting CTLA-4 and PD-1 in the treatment of various cancers highlights their critical roles in the regulation of cancer immunity in human. In addition, the development of multifarious autoimmune diseases as immune-related adverse events of anti-CTLA-4 and anti-PD-1/ PD-L1 therapies and the successful clinical application of the CD28 blocking therapy using CTLA-4-Ig to the treatment of arthritis assure their crucial roles in the regulation of autoimmunity in human. Accumulating evidences in mice and humans indicate that genetic and environmental factors strikingly modify effects of the targeted inhibition and potentiation of co-signals. In this review, we summarize our current understanding of the roles of CD28, CTLA-4, and PD-1 in autoimmunity. Deeper understandings of the context-dependent and context-independent functions of co-signals are essential for the appropriate usage and the future development of innovative immunomodulatory therapies for a diverse array of diseases.

Keywords PD-1 · CTLA-4 · CD28 · Animal model · Cancer immunotherapy · irAE · SNV · Strain · Susceptibility · Tolerance

---

T. Okazaki (✉) · I.-m. Okazaki
Division of Immune Regulation, Institute of Advanced Medical Sciences, Tokushima University, Tokushima, Japan
e-mail: tokazaki@genome.tokushima-u.ac.jp

© Springer Nature Singapore Pte Ltd. 2019
M. Azuma, H. Yagita (eds.), *Co-signal Molecules in T Cell Activation*,
Advances in Experimental Medicine and Biology 1189,
https://doi.org/10.1007/978-981-32-9717-3_8

8.1 PD-1 and its Ligands

Programmed cell death 1 (PD-1, CD279, *Pdcd1*) was identified as a molecule whose expression was induced by apoptotic stimuli in 1992 (Ishida et al. 1992). The function of PD-1 as a negative regulator of immune responses was recognized by the spontaneous development of lupus-like arthritis and glomerulonephritis by PD-1 knockout mice on the C57BL/6 background (C57BL/6-*Pdcd1*$^{-/-}$ mice) (Nishimura et al. 1999). Later, PD-1 is classified in the CD28/CLTA-4 family based on the structural and functional characteristics. PD-1 has two ligands (PD-Ls), PD-L1 (programmed cell death 1 ligand 1, B7-H1, CD274, *Cd274*) and PD-L2 (programmed cell death 1 ligand 2, B7-DC, CD273, *Pdcd1lg2*). Upon interacting with either of PD-Ls together with antigen stimulation, PD-1 recruits SHP-2 (SH2 domain-containing tyrosine phosphatase 2), and SHP-2 dephosphorylates signaling molecules to suppress antigen receptor signal (Hui et al. 2017; Mizuno et al. 2019; Okazaki et al. 2001; Parry et al. 2005; Yokosuka et al. 2012). In addition to autoimmunity, PD-1 is involved in various immune responses such as tumor immunity, infectious immunity, transplant rejection, and allergy (Okazaki et al. 2013; Schildberg et al. 2016; Zhang and Vignali 2016).

PD-1 is expressed on double-negative αβ and γδ T cells in the thymus, on progenitors of innate lymphoid cells (ILCs) in the bone marrow, and on activated T, B, NK, ILC, and myeloid cells in the periphery. PD-L1 is expressed on T, B, and dendritic cells as well as many types of non-hematopoietic cells, while the expression of PD-L2 is more restricted and found mainly on dendritic cells, monocytes, and B-1 cells (Okazaki et al. 2013; Schildberg et al. 2016; Yu et al. 2016; Zhong et al. 2007). The expression of PD-Ls can be upregulated or induced by activation. PD-Ls are also expressed on some tumor cells and suppress antitumor immunity by inhibiting the activation and the effector function of tumor-specific T cells by eliciting the inhibitory function of PD-1 (Iwai et al. 2002). PD-L1 on tumor cells are also reported to suppress antitumor immunity by inducing apoptosis of T cells through non-PD-1 receptor, which has not been identified yet (Curiel et al. 2003; Dong et al. 2002).

Based on basic researches, cancer immunotherapies using anti-PD-1/PD-L1 blocking Abs were developed. Although the anti-PD-1/PD-L1 therapy provided unprecedented therapeutic benefits, they also revealed a new class of toxicities related to immune activation, which are called immune-related adverse events (irAEs) (Brahmer et al. 2010; Callahan et al. 2016; Michot et al. 2016; Topalian et al. 2012).

8.2 PD-1 in Autoimmunity

As mentioned above, PD-1 and PD-Ls play pivotal roles in the regulation of various immune responses. In this section, we summarize our current understanding of the roles of PD-1 and PD-Ls in autoimmunity.

8 Stimulatory and Inhibitory Co-signals in Autoimmunity

8.2.1 Autoimmunity in PD-1-Deficient Mice

Pdcd1$^{-/-}$ mice spontaneously develop different types of autoimmune diseases on different genetic backgrounds, suggesting that PD-1 deficiency exaggerates a strain-specific autoimmune susceptibility to induce strain-specific autoimmune phenotypes (Table 8.1). C57BL/6-*Pdcd1*$^{-/-}$ mice spontaneously develop glomerulonephritis with depositions of IgG3 and C3 in the glomeruli and arthritis with an extensive granulomatous inflammation as they age (Nishimura et al. 1999). Unlike other lupus-prone mice, common autoAbs such as anti-dsDNA Ab and rheumatoid factor are rarely detected in C57BL/6-*Pdcd1*$^{-/-}$ mice. The introduction of the loss of function mutation in Fas gene (*lpr*, C57BL/6-*lpr-Pdcd1*$^{-/-}$ mice) accelerates these phenotypes. Liu et al. reported the spontaneous activation of both CD4 and CD8 T cells and the development of chronic inflammation in multiple organs such as the liver, lung, and pancreas but not kidney and joint in aged C57BL/6-*Pdcd1*$^{-/-}$ mice, suggesting the effect of environmental factors on the phenotype of *Pdcd1*$^{-/-}$ mice (Liu et al. 2015). Dong et al. reported the accumulation of activated CD8 but not CD4 T cells in the liver of C57BL/6-*Cd274*$^{-/-}$ mice, which was reported to be dependent on an unidentified non-PD-1 receptor for PD-L1(Dong et al. 2004).

On the BALB/c background, *Pdcd1*$^{-/-}$ mice spontaneously develop gastritis and dilated cardiomyopathy (DCM) (Nishimura et al. 2001; Okazaki et al. 2005). These phenotypes are dependent on tissue-specific autoAbs that have undergone class switching and/or affinity maturation induced by AID (activation-induced cytidine

Table 8.1 Spontaneous autoimmune diseases in mice deficient for PD-1 and PD-Ls

Strain	Gene/treatment	Disease	Onset	Frequency
C57BL/6	PD-1	Glomerulonephritis, arthritis	$\geq$ 6 months	50%
		Pneumonitis, hepatitis, pancreatitis	12 months	15–25%
	PD-1/Fas	Glomerulonephritis, arthritis	$\geq$ 6 months	$\geq$80%
	PD-1/VISTA	Pneumonitis, hepatitis, pancreatitis	12 months	30–90%
BALB/c	PD-1	DCM	5–25 weeks	0–60%[1]
		Gastritis	10–25 weeks	20–100%[1]
	PD-1/FcγRIIB	Hydronephrosis	10–20 weeks	35%
		Cystitis	10 weeks	50%
	PD-1/LAG-3	Myocarditis	$\leq$ 10 weeks	100%
	PD-1/nTx[2]	Hepatitis, gastritis	$\leq$ 3 weeks	100%
MRL	PD-1	Myocarditis, pneumonitis, hepatitis	4–8 weeks	$\geq$90%
		Gastritis, sialoadenitis	4–8 weeks	50%
	PD-L1	Myocarditis, pneumonitis	4–7 weeks	100%
NOD	PD-1	T1DM, sialoadenitis	4–10 weeks	100%
	PD-L1	T1DM	4–10 weeks	100%
NOD.H2[b]	PD-1	Peripheral neuritis	15–25 weeks	100% (female)
		Gastritis, sialoadenitis	15–25 weeks	100%

[1]The penetrance of DCM and gastritis in BALB/c-*Pdcd1*$^{-/-}$ differs among different colonies
[2]Neonatal thymectomy

deaminase) (Okazaki et al. 2011). The development of DCM is shown to be dependent on autoAbs recognizing cTnI (cardiac troponin I). Although cTnI is known to regulate muscle contraction in the sarcomere, cTnI is also expressed on the surface of cardiomyocytes. Anti-cTnI Abs augment the voltage-dependent Ca^{2+} current of cardiomyocytes, suggesting that cTnI on the surface of cardiomyocytes plays unidentified roles to regulate the magnitude of Ca^{2+} current and that anti-cTnI Abs induce DCM by chronic enhancement of Ca^{2+} current of cardiomyocytes (Okazaki et al. 2003). Later, Goser et al. reported that immunization with cTnI but not with cTnT induced severe myocarditis in BALB/c and A/J mice, confirming the pathogenic role of autoimmune response against cTnI (Goser et al. 2006).

PD-1 deficiency drastically exaggerates Type I diabetes (T1DM) and sialoadenitis in non-obese diabetic (NOD) mouse, which is a widely used animal model of T1DM and Sjogren's syndrome (SS) (Wang et al. 2005). Interestingly, PD-L1 but not PD-L2 is highly expressed on β-cells in pancreatic islets with insulitis. In PD-1-sufficient NOD mice, lymphocytes form a cluster surrounding islets as though there is a barrier between the islets and lymphocytes. Because β-cells adjacent to lymphocytes express PD-L1 especially at high levels, PD-L1 on β-cells likely serves as a barrier to suppress the invasion of diabetogenic T cells. In NOD-$Pdcd1^{-/-}$ mice, this barrier is lost, and lymphocytes invade inside islets despite augmented PD-L1 expression on β-cells. Keir et al. clearly demonstrated that PD-L1 on β-cells but not on lymphoid cells was responsible for delaying diabetes using NOD-$Cd274^{-/-}$ mice, which also developed fulminant diabetes like NOD-$Pdcd1^{-/-}$ mice (Keir et al. 2006). In addition, the administration of Abs against PD-1 or PD-L1 to prediabetic NOD mice leads to the development of rapid and exacerbated diabetes (Ansari et al. 2003; Okamura et al. 2019).

NOD-$Pdcd1^{-/-}$ mice with a T1DM-resistant MHC haplotype (H2^b, NOD.H2^b-$Pdcd1^{-/-}$ mice) are protected from T1DM but develop peripheral polyneuropathy reminiscent of human Guillain-Barre syndrome (GBS) and chronic inflammatory demyelinating polyradiculoneuropathy (CIDP), sialoadenitis, pancreatitis, and gastritis (Yoshida et al. 2008). In addition, [(C57BL/6 x NOD.H2^b)$_{F1}$ x NOD.H2^b]$_{BC1}$-$Pdcd1^{-/-}$ mice develop polyneuritis, insulitis, sialoadenitis, gastritis, and vasculitis to a variable degree (Jiang et al. 2009).

MRL-lpr mouse is a common animal model of human lupus erythematosus, whose major genetic determinant is the lpr mutation of Fas gene. Besides the lpr mutation, MRL chromosomes harbor additional genetic factors that promote autoimmunity because Fas-intact MRL mice also develop lupus-like phenotypes in later life and the lpr mutation does not induce severe autoimmune diseases in other strains of mice such as C3H/HeJ, AKR, and C57BL/6. About 70% of MRL-$Pdcd1^{-/-}$ mice die of myocarditis by 10 weeks of age (Wang et al. 2010). In addition to myocarditis, MRL-$Pdcd1^{-/-}$ mice spontaneously develop pneumonitis, hepatitis, gastritis, and sialoadenitis. MRL-$Cd274^{-/-}$ mice also show similar but more severe phenotypes (Lucas et al. 2008).

The strain-specific autoimmune susceptibility relies on inherent genetic variances of the strain. Roles of several genes in the phenotypes of $Pdcd1^{-/-}$ mice have been examined. Mice deficient for the FcγRIIB (low-affinity-type IIb Fc receptor for IgG, *Fcgr2b*), an inhibitory Fc receptor, spontaneously develop lupus-like disease on the C57BL/6 but not on the BALB/c background (Nimmerjahn and Ravetch 2008). BALB/c-*Fcgr2b$^{-/-}$Pdcd1$^{-/-}$* mice develop autoimmune hydronephrosis and cystitis with concomitant production of autoAbs against urothelial antigens such as uroplakin IIIa, which is an essential component of urinary plaques regulating the apical surface area of the transitional cells (Okazaki et al. 2005; Sugino et al. 2012). In contrast, the frequency of DCM and gastritis of BALB/c-*Pdcd1$^{-/-}$* mice are not affected by the additional FcγRIIB deficiency. Therefore, PD-1 seems to regulate autoimmune responses synergistically with or independently of FcγRIIB depending on the target antigens.

PD-1 also collaborates with another inhibitory co-receptor, lymphocyte-activation gene 3 (LAG-3), in the regulation of autoimmunity and antitumor immunity (Maruhashi et al. 2018; Okazaki et al. 2011; Woo et al. 2012). Mice deficient for LAG-3 and PD-1 die of autoimmune myocarditis by 5 weeks of age. Because PD-1 and LAG-3 synergistically inhibit the activation of T cells, autoimmunity is likely due to the robust activation of autoreactive T cells in the absence of these inhibitory co-receptors.

VISTA (V-domain immunoglobulin suppressor of T-cell activation, *Vsir*) is a newly identified molecule that bears homology to PD-L1. VISTA on antigen-presenting cells (APCs) may suppress activation of T cells by binding to its unidentified receptor or VISTA on T cells may function as an inhibitory receptor to suppress their activation. Aged C57BL/6-*Vsir$^{-/-}$* mice develop mild hepatitis, pneumonitis, and pancreatitis, and these phenotypes are exaggerated by the concurrent deficiency of PD-1. Further analyses are needed to understand how PD-1 and VISTA collaborate to regulate autoimmunity (Liu et al. 2015).

In addition to effects of genetic variances and ablations, the effect of Treg depletion on phenotypes of *Pdcd1$^{-/-}$* mice has also been analyzed. Watanabe and colleagues reported that BALB/c-*Pdcd1$^{-/-}$* mice developed fatal hepatitis by neonatal thymectomy, which is known to induce oophoritis and gastritis in BALB/c mice by attenuating the production of thymic Treg cells (Kido et al. 2008). Therefore, PD-1 and Treg cells function in a nonredundant manner at least in part.

The role of PD-1 in autoimmunity has also been analyzed using antigen-induced models of autoimmunity (Table 8.2). In the experimental autoimmune encephalomyelitis (EAE), an animal model of human multiple sclerosis (MS), the relative contribution of PD-L1 and PD-L2, seems to differ depending on the genetic background of the mice and the timing of the blockade. Latchman et al. and Carter et al. reported that 129/Sv-*Pdcd1$^{-/-}$* and -*Cd274$^{-/-}$* mice developed more severe symptoms of EAE compared with wild-type mice (Carter et al. 2007; Latchman et al. 2004). On the other hand, Salama et al. and Zhu et al. reported that the blockade of PD-1 or PD-L2 but not PD-L1 augmented the severity of EAE on the C57BL/6 and NOD backgrounds (Salama et al. 2003; Zhu et al. 2006). Intriguingly, Zhu et al. found that the blockade of PD-L1 but not PD-L2 augmented the severity of EAE on the BALB/c background and the blockade of either PD-L1 or PD-L2 augmented the severity of EAE on the B10.S background (Zhu et al. 2006). *Pdcd1$^{-/-}$* and *Cd274$^{-/-}$* mice are also reported to develop more severe collagen-induced arthritis (CIA) and proteoglycan-induced arthritis (PGIA), respectively (Hamel et al. 2010; Raptopoulou

Table 8.2 Roles of PD-1, PD-L1, and PD-L2 in experimental models of autoimmune diseases in mice

Model	Disease	Gene/treatment	Strain	Effect
EAE	Encephalomyelitis	Anti-PD-1 Ab	C57BL/6	worse[1]
		Anti-PD-L1 Ab	C57BL/6	NS[1,2]
		Anti-PD-L2 Ab	C57BL/6	worse[1,2]
		Anti-PD-L1 Ab	BALB/c	NS[2]
		Anti-PD-L2 Ab	BALB/c	worse[2]
		Anti-PD-L1 Ab	B10.S	worse[2]
		Anti-PD-L2 Ab	B10.S	worse[2]
		Anti-PD-L1 Ab	NOD	NS[2]
		Anti-PD-L2 Ab	NOD	worse[2]
		Anti-PD-L1 Ab	SJL/J	worse[2]
		Anti-PD-L2 Ab	SJL/J	NS[2]
		$Pdcd1^{-/-}$	129/Sv	worse[3]
		$Cd274^{-/-}$	129/Sv	worse[3,4]
		$Pdcd1lg2^{-/-}$	129/Sv	NS[3]
CIA	Arthritis	$Pdcd1^{-/-}$	C57BL/6	worse[5]
PGIA	Arthritis	$Cd274^{-/-}$	BALB/c	worse[6]
EAM	Myocarditis	$Pdcd1^{-/-}$	BALB/c	worse[7]
		$Cd274^{-/-}$	BALB/c	NS[7]
EAD	Diabetes	Anti-PD-L1 Ab	C57BL/6	susceptible[8]
		$Pdcd1^{-/-}$	C57BL/6	susceptible[8]
		$Cd274^{-/-}$	C57BL/6	susceptible[8]
NSN	Nephritis	$Cd274^{-/-}$	C57BL/6	worse[9]
		$Pdcd1lg2^{-/-}$	C57BL/6	worse[9]

NS not significant, [1]Salama et al. 2003, [2]Zhu et al. 2006, [3]Carter et al. 2007, [4]Latchman et al. 2004, [5]Raptopoulou et al. 2010, [6]Hamel et al. 2010, [7]Tarrio et al. 2012, [8]Rajasalu et al. 2010, [9]Menke et al. 2007

et al. 2010). In addition, the administration of the dimeric PD-L1 protein composing of the extracellular region of PD-L1 and Fc portion of IgG (PD-L1-Ig) has been shown to ameliorate CIA and PGIA probably by eliciting PD-1-mediated inhibitory signal (Raptopoulou et al. 2010; Wang et al. 2011). Inhibitory effects of PD-1, PD-L1, and PD-L2 have also been reported in other animal models such as experimental autoimmune diabetes (EAD) and myocarditis (EAM) and nephrotoxic serum nephritis (NSN)(Menke et al. 2007; Rajasalu et al. 2010; Tarrio et al. 2012).

8.2.2 *Immune-Related Adverse Events of Anti-PD-1/PD-L1 Therapy*

As mentioned above, the understanding of the molecular mechanisms and biological significances of co-signals has propelled the rational development of cancer immunotherapies. To date, Abs against PD-1 (nivolumab and pembrolizumab), PD-L1 (atezolizumab, durvalumab, and avelumab), and CTLA-4 (ipilimumab) have been approved in one or more countries for the treatment of one or more cancers including melanoma, lung cancer, renal cell carcinoma, head and neck cancer, urothelial cancer, Merkel cell carcinoma, lymphoma, gastric cancer, and mismatch repair-deficient cancers (Brahmer et al. 2010; Callahan et al. 2016; Garassino et al. 2018; Kang et al. 2017; Kaufman et al. 2018; Topalian et al. 2012). However, anti-CTLA-4 and anti-PD-1/PD-L1 therapies accompanied various forms of irAEs in numerous organs including the gut, skin, endocrine organs, liver, heart, liver, kidney, and lung (Barroso-Sousa et al. 2018; Cukier et al. 2017; Michot et al. 2016; Naidoo et al. 2015). Interestingly, many of the autoimmune phenotypes observed in *Pdcd1*$^{-/-}$ and *Cd274*$^{-/-}$ mice and irAEs of anti-PD-1/PD-L1 therapy are shared (Table 8.3). These include T1DM (NOD-*Pdcd1*$^{-/-}$ and NOD-*Cd274*$^{-/-}$ mice), myocarditis (MRL-*Pdcd1*$^{-/-}$ mice, MRL-*Cd274*$^{-/-}$, BALB/c-*Pdcd1*$^{-/-}$*Lag3*$^{-/-}$ mice), pneumonitis (MRL-*Pdcd1*$^{-/-}$, MRL-*Cd274*$^{-/-}$, NOD.H2^b-*Pdcd1*$^{-/-}$, and C57BL/6-*Pdcd1*$^{-/-}$ *Vsir*$^{-/-}$ mice), GBS/CIDP (NOD.H2^b-*Pdcd1*$^{-/-}$ mice), hepatitis (MRL-*Pdcd1*$^{-/-}$ and C57BL/6-*Pdcd1*$^{-/-}$*Vsir*$^{-/-}$ mice and BALB/c-*Pdcd1*$^{-/-}$ mice with neonatal thymectomy), gastritis (BALB/c-*Pdcd1*$^{-/-}$, MRL-*Pdcd1*$^{-/-}$, and NOD.H2^b-*Pdcd1*$^{-/-}$ mice and BALB/c-*Pdcd1*$^{-/-}$ mice with neonatal thymectomy), cystitis (BALB/c-*Pdcd1*$^{-/-}$*Fcgr2b*$^{-/-}$ mice), glomerulonephritis (C57BL/6-*Pdcd1*$^{-/-}$ mice), pancreatitis (NOD.H2^b-*Pdcd1*$^{-/-}$ and C57BL/6-*Pdcd1*$^{-/-}$*Vsir*$^{-/-}$ mice), SS/sialoadenitis (NOD-*Pdcd1*$^{-/-}$, NOD.H2^b-*Pdcd1*$^{-/-}$, and MRL-*Pdcd1*$^{-/-}$ mice), arthritis (C57BL/6-*Pdcd1*$^{-/-}$ mice and CIA and PGIA in *Pdcd1*$^{-/-}$ and *Cd274*$^{-/-}$ mice, respectively), and encephalomyelitis (EAE in *Pdcd1*$^{-/-}$ and *Cd274*$^{-/-}$ mice) (Boike and Dejulio 2017;

Table 8.3 Immune-related adverse events of anti-PD-1/PD-L1 therapy that have been observed in *Pdcd1*$^{-/-}$, *Cd274*$^{-/-}$, and *Pdcd1lg2*$^{-/-}$ mice

irAE	Mice
T1DM	NOD-*Pdcd1*$^{-/-}$, NOD-*Cd274*$^{-/-}$, C57BL/6-*Pdcd1*$^{-/-}$ (EAD), C57BL/6-*Cd274*$^{-/-}$ (EAD)
Myocarditis	MRL-*Pdcd1*$^{-/-}$, MRL-*Cd274*$^{-/-}$, BALB/c-*Pdcd1*$^{-/-}$*Lag3*$^{-/-}$, BALB/c-*Pdcd1*$^{-/-}$ (EAM)
Pneumonitis	MRL-*Pdcd1*$^{-/-}$,MRL-*Cd274*$^{-/-}$,NOD.H2^b-*Pdcd1*$^{-/-}$,C57BL/6-*Pdcd1*$^{-/-}$*Vsir*$^{-/-}$
GBS/CIDP	NOD.H2^b-*Pdcd1*$^{-/-}$
Hepatitis	MRL-*Pdcd1*$^{-/-}$, C57BL/6-*Pdcd1*$^{-/-}$*Vsir*$^{-/-}$, BALB/c-*Pdcd1*$^{-/-}$ (nTx)
Gastritis	BALB/c-*Pdcd1*$^{-/-}$, MRL-*Pdcd1*$^{-/-}$, NOD.H2^b-*Pdcd1*$^{-/-}$, BALB/c-*Pdcd1*$^{-/-}$ (nTx)
Cystitis	BALB/c-*Pdcd1*$^{-/-}$*Fcgr2b*$^{-/-}$
Glomerulonephritis	C57BL/6-*Pdcd1*$^{-/-}$, C57BL/6-*Cd274*$^{-/-}$ (NSN), C57BL/6-*Pdcd1lg2*$^{-/-}$ (NSN)
Pancreatitis	NOD.H2^b-*Pdcd1*$^{-/-}$, C57BL/6-*Pdcd1*$^{-/-}$*Vsir*$^{-/-}$
SS/sialoadenitis	NOD-*Pdcd1*$^{-/-}$, MRL-*Pdcd1*$^{-/-}$, NOD.H2^b-*Pdcd1*$^{-/-}$
Arthritis	C57BL/6-*Pdcd1*$^{-/-}$, C57BL/6-*Pdcd1*$^{-/-}$ (CIA), C57BL/6-*Cd274*$^{-/-}$ (PGIA)
Encephalomyelitis	C57BL/6-*Pdcd1*$^{-/-}$ (EAE), C57BL/6-*Cd274*$^{-/-}$ (EAE)

Cappelli et al. 2017; de Maleissye et al. 2016; Haikal et al. 2018; Hughes et al. 2015; Ikeuchi et al. 2016; Larkin et al. 2017; Shimatani et al. 2018; Varricchi et al. 2017).

Of note, more diverse irAEs have been reported for anti-PD-1/PD-L1 therapy in human patients. These include irAEs in the skin (e.g., rash, vitiligo, lichenoid dermatitis, bullous pemphigoid, Stevens Johnson syndrome, and toxic epidermal necrolysis), mucosa (e.g., oral mucositis, gingivitis), endocrine glands (e.g., hypophysitis, hypothyroidism, hyperthyroidism, thyroiditis, and adrenal insufficiency), colon (e.g., colitis), neuromuscular junction (myasthenia gravis), and eye (e.g., uveitis, keratitis) (Michot et al. 2016; Naidoo et al. 2015). These observations indicate that irAEs of anti-PD-1/PD-L1 therapy are strongly affected by the genetic autoimmune susceptibility of patients just like the genetic background of the mice strongly affects autoimmune phenotypes of $Pdcd1^{-/-}$ and $Cd274^{-/-}$ mice. Thus, preclinical studies should be performed on various genetic backgrounds and conditions to obtain substantial information for the safe and efficient application of upcoming immunomodulatory therapies to human patients.

8.2.3 Genetic Variants of PD-1 Gene and Autoimmunity

Several single-nucleotide variants (SNVs) in PD-1 (*PDCD1*), PD-L1 (*CD274*), and PD-L2 (*PDCD1LG2*) genes have been reported to associate with human autoimmune diseases (Table 8.4). Prokunina and colleagues first reported the association of PD-1 genetic variants with human autoimmune diseases in 2002 (Prokunina et al. 2002). They found that the allele A of an SNV named PD1.3 (PD1.3A, rs111568821) was associated with the higher risk of systemic lupus erythematosus (SLE) in Europeans (relative risk = 2.6) and Mexicans (relative risk = 3.5) but not African Americans. The PD1.3A alters the expression level of PD-1 by disrupting the binding of RUNX1 (runt-related transcription factor 1) to the enhancer in the intron 4 of PD-1 gene (Bertsias et al. 2009). PD1.3 and/or several other SNVs on PD-1 gene have been reported to associate with the development of various autoimmune diseases such as T1DM, MS, subacute sclerosing panencephalitis, rheumatoid arthritis (RA), and ankylosing spondylitis (AS), juvenile onset of SLE, chronic idiopathic thrombocytopenic purpura, sympathetic ophthalmia, extraocular manifestations of Vogt-Koyanagi-Harada syndrome, antisperm Ab-related infertility, and Rasmussen syndrome (Cooper et al. 2007; Deng et al. 2017; Ishizaki et al. 2010; Kasamatsu et al. 2018; Meng et al. 2009; Okazaki and Honjo 2007; Pawlak-Adamska et al. 2017; Takahashi et al. 2013; Yang et al. 2011; Zamani et al. 2015). SNVs on PD-L1 and PD-L2 genes have also been found to associate with the development of several autoimmune diseases such as T1DM, Graves' disease, Addison's disease, SLE, and AS (Hayashi et al. 2008; Huang et al. 2011; Mitchell et al. 2009; Okazaki and Honjo 2007; Pizarro et al. 2014; Yang et al. 2011). In addition to autoimmune diseases, the association of SNVs on PD-1 and PD-L1 genes with the development of cancer has also been reported, which likely reflects the involvement of immune responses in the development of cancer (Hua et al. 2011; Kataoka et al. 2016; Mojtahedi et al. 2012).

8 Stimulatory and Inhibitory Co-signals in Autoimmunity

Table 8.4 Association of SNVs in PD-1, PD-L1, and PD-L2 genes with human autoimmune diseases

Disease	Gene	rs number
Systemic lupus erythematosus	*PDCD1*	rs111568821, rs2227981, rs6705653, rs41386349
	PDCD1LG2	rs7854303
Rheumatoid arthritis	*PDCD1*	rs36084323
Multiple sclerosis	*PDCD1*	rs111568821, rs2227981, rs2227982
Subacute sclerosing panencephalitis	*PDCD1*	rs36084323, rs34819629, rs2227982
Type 1 diabetes	*PDCD1*	rs34819629, rs111568821, rs2227981, rs10204525,
		rs2227982, rs36084323, rs35214377
	CD274	*rs2297137, rs4143815*
Ankylosing spondylitis	*PDCD1*	rs2227981, rs2227982
	PDCD1LG2	rs7854303
Idiopathic thrombocytopenic purpura	*PDCD1*	rs36084323, rs41386349, rs2227982
Sympathetic ophthalmia	*PDCD1*	rs2227981
Vogt-Koyanagi-Harada syndrome	*PDCD1*	rs2227981
Antisperm Ab-related infertility	*PDCD1*	rs111568821
Rasmussen syndrome	*PDCD1*	rs2227982
Graves' disease	*CD274*	rs1970000, rs822339, rs2282055, rs1411262, rs2297137
Addison' disease	*CD274*	rs822339, rs2282055, rs1411262

8.3 CD28, CTLA-4, and their Ligands

The activation of lymphocytes is tightly controlled by stimulatory and inhibitory co-signals in addition to the antigen receptor signal. CD28 provides the stimulatory co-signal that is required for the optimal activation of T cells upon interacting with either of two ligands, CD80 (B7.1) or CD86 (B7.2), as evidenced by the markedly impaired T-cell immunity in $Cd28^{-/-}$ mice (Shahinian et al. 1993). CD80/86 also bind to an inhibitory co-receptor, CTLA-4 that suppresses T-cell activation by transducing inhibitory signal and/or hampering the binding of CD28 with CD80/86 with its 10–20 times higher affinity to CD80/86 compared with CD28 (Collins et al. 2002; Linsley et al. 1991). While CD28 is constitutively expressed on T cells, CTLA-4 is not expressed on naive T cells, but its expression is rapidly induced upon T-cell activation. Thereby, CTLA-4 provides the negative feedback mechanism for T-cell activation, the absence of which results in the promiscuous activation of T cells and premature death of multiorgan lymphocytic infiltration (Tivol et al. 1995; Waterhouse et al. 1995).

Due to its critical role in the T-cell activation, CD28 represents a unique target for the therapy of autoimmunity. A soluble recombinant fusion protein comprising the extracellular domain of CTLA-4 and the Fc domain of IgG as a CD28 blocker (CTLA-4-Ig, abatacept) is now in clinical use for the therapy of arthritis (Cutolo and Nadler 2013; Kremer et al. 2003).

In contrast, CTLA-4 represents a preeminent target for the therapy of tumors. Allison and colleagues revealed the critical role of CTLA-4 in the tumor immunity in 1996, which leads to the clinical application of anti-CTLA-4 blocking Ab (ipilimumab) for the therapy of melanoma (Hodi et al. 2010; Leach et al. 1996; Phan et al. 2003). As the autoimmune phenotypes of $Ctla4^{-/-}$ mice are more intense compared with those of $Pdcd1^{-/-}$ mice, anti-CTLA-4 therapy generally induces more severe irAEs than anti-PD-1/PD-L1 therapy.

8.4 CD28, CTLA-4, and their Ligands in Autoimmunity

As mentioned above, CTLA-4 provides the critical inhibitory co-signal that restrains autoreactivity. In this section, we summarize our current understanding of the roles of CD28, CTLA-4, and CD80/86 in autoimmunity.

8.4.1 Autoimmunity in Mice Deficient for CTLA-4, CD28, and their Ligands

The essential role of CTLA-4 on immune tolerance was unraveled by the development of a lethal lymphoproliferative disorder in $Ctla4^{-/-}$ mice (Tivol et al. 1995; Waterhouse et al. 1995). In the absence of CTLA-4, T cells are nonspecifically activated and infiltrate various organs such as the heart, pancreas, lung, salivary gland, liver, joint, and vessels. Unlike $Pdcd1^{-/-}$ mice, the genetic background of the mice does not affect phenotypes of $Ctla4^{-/-}$ mice substantially (Luhder et al. 2000; Oosterwegel et al. 1999). Because the introduction of the truncated mutant of CTLA-4 lacking the cytoplasmic region can rescue the lethal lymphoproliferation in $Ctla4^{-/-}$ mice, the suppression of promiscuous activation of T cell by CTLA-4 does not require the signal mediated by its cytoplasmic region (Masteller et al. 2000; Takahashi et al. 2005). The polyclonal activation of T cells in $Ctla4^{-/-}$ mice has been reported to be cell non-autonomous based on the observation that CTLA-4-sufficient T cells could suppress the promiscuous activation and autoaggressiveness of $Ctla4^{-/-}$ T cells (Bachmann et al. 1999; Tivol and Gorski 2002). Later, the selective deletion of $Ctla4$ in Treg cells has been shown to recapitulate the lethal lymphoproliferative disorder, indicating that the functional impairment of Treg cells is responsible for the deadly disease (Wing et al. 2008). CTLA-4 on Treg cells has been reported to induce the expression of immunoregulatory molecules such as IDO (indoleamine 2,3-dioxigenase) on APCs and reduce CD80/86 expression on APCs by inducing the expression of cytokines that downmodulate their expression and/or by trogocytosing CD80/86 molecules from APCs, which make APCs defective in providing co-stimulation (Okazaki et al. 2013; Schildberg et al. 2016; Walker and Sansom 2015; Wing et al. 2011).

Besides cell non-autonomous function, CTLA-4 has cell-autonomous function as well. CTLA-4 has been reported to modulate various signaling pathways by recruiting multiple molecules including SHP-2, PP2A (protein phosphatase 2A), and PKCη (protein kinase C-η). Ise et al. showed that different tissue-specific T cells infiltrated into different target organs in $Ctla4^{-/-}$ mice with DO11.10 TCRβ transgene. In addition, they identified PDIA2 as an autoantigen of pancreatitis and showed that CTLA-4 suppressed the activation of PDIA2-specific T cells in a cell-autonomous manner (Ise et al. 2010).

The effect of inducible deletion of CTLA-4 in adult mice is controversial. Paterson et al. reported that the inducible deletion of CTLA-4 during adulthood did not induce lymphoproliferative disorder but resulted in the expansion of Treg cells that highly expressed inhibitory molecules other than CTLA-4, thereby conferring resistance to EAE (Paterson et al. 2015). On the other hand, Klocke et al. found that the conditional deletion of CTLA-4 in adult mice resulted in the spontaneous development of lymphoproliferation, hypergammaglobulinemia, pneumonitis, gastritis, insulitis, and sialoadenitis (Klocke et al. 2016). They also observed the preferential expansion of Treg cells and the resistance to the peptide-induced but not protein-induced EAE. The discrepancy is likely due to the difference in the MHC haplotype of mice used. The former and the latter studies use mice with H2^b (C57BL/6) and H2^q (C57BL/10Q) MHC haplotypes, respectively.

While CTLA-4 suppresses autoimmunity, CD28 promotes autoimmunity by potentiating autoreactive T cells. CD28 deficiency ameliorates renal vasculitis and arthritis of MRL-lpr mice (Tada et al. 1999). CD28 deficiency or CD28 blockade has been shown to prevent or alleviate antigen-induced models of autoimmunity such as CIA, EAE, myocarditis, thyroiditis, nephritis, and myasthenia gravis (Nishikawa et al. 1994; Perrin et al. 1995; Schildberg et al. 2016; Zhang and Vignali 2016). On the other hand, CD28 deficiency, compound deficiency of CD80/86, and the transgenic expression of CTLA-4-Ig increase the severity of T1DM in NOD mice. In these mice, the number of Treg cells is substantially reduced, and Th1 response is augmented because CD28 signal is required for the development and the maintenance of Treg cells (Lenschow et al. 1996; Salomon et al. 2000; Tang et al. 2003). CD80 plays the primary role in the protection of T1DM in NOD mice as the Ab-mediated blockade or genetic ablation of CD80 but not CD86 results in the exacerbation of T1DM. Interestingly, although NOD-$Cd86^{-/-}$ mice are protected from T1DM, they develop peripheral polyneuropathy like NOD.H2^b-$Pdcd1^{-/-}$ mice (Salomon et al. 2001). The differential role of CD80 and CD86 is also observed in MRL-lpr mice, in which the deficiency of CD80 but not CD86 aggravates glomerulonephritis (Liang et al. 1999). Therefore, CD80 and CD86 seem to have different functions depending on the context.

8.4.2 Immune-Related Adverse Events of Anti-CTLA-4 Therapy

The development of anti-CTLA-4 therapy clearly demonstrated that the modulation of T-cell function by deactivating inhibitory co-signal could result in effective anticancer therapy and opened a new era of cancer immunotherapy. However, it also revealed that cancer immunotherapies inevitably accompany irAEs. As $Ctla4^{-/-}$ mice develop much severe autoimmune phenotypes compared with $Pdcd1^{-/-}$ mice, more diverse and severe irAEs have been reported for anti-CTLA-4 therapy compared with anti-PD-1/PD-L1 therapy. The frequency of irAEs with any grade is up to 90% and 70% for anti-CTLA-4 and anti-PD-1/PD-L1 therapies, respectively. Grade III and IV irAEs are observed in 10–18%, and 7–12% of patients received anti-CTLA-4 and anti-PD-1/PD-L1 therapies, respectively (Michot et al. 2016; Naidoo et al. 2015).

The direct comparison of ipilimumab (anti-CTLA-4 Ab) with pembrolizumab (anti-PD-1 Ab) demonstrated a higher incidence of vitiligo in pembrolizumab-treated patients (10%) compared with ipilimumab-treated patients (2%) (Robert et al. 2015). Whereas the frequency of diarrhea/colitis is higher in anti-CTLA-4 therapy than anti-PD-1/PD-L1 therapy. The frequencies of hypothyroidism and hyperthyroidism are higher in anti-PD-1/PD-L1 therapy, while the frequency of hypophysitis is much higher in anti-CTLA-4 therapy. The frequencies of hypothyroidism, hyperthyroidism, and hypophysitis drastically increase in the anti-CTLA-4 and anti-PD-1/PD-L1 combinatorial therapy (Barroso-Sousa et al. 2018; Cukier et al. 2017). Iwama et al. reported that CTLA-4 was ectopically expressed on a subset of prolactin- and thyrotropin-secreting cells in pituitary glands and that anti-CTLA-4 Ab directly bound to CTLA-4 on these cells and induced inflammation by activating complement cascade *in situ* (Iwama et al. 2014). On the other hand, pneumonitis is less common with anti-CTLA-4 therapy compared with anti-PD-1/PD-L1 therapy.

8.4.3 Genetic Variants of CTLA-4 Gene and Autoimmunity

Since Yanagawa et al. first reported the association of the CTLA-4 genetic variant with Graves' diseases in 1995, several SNVs in CTLA-4 gene have been reported to associate with various autoimmune diseases such as RA, SLE, MS, systemic sclerosis, Hashimoto's thyroiditis, and T1DM (Ghaderi 2011; Romo-Tena et al. 2013; Yanagawa et al. 1995). These SNVs also associate with the development of various cancers such as breast cancer, bone tumor, bladder cancer, cervical cancer, hepatocellular carcinoma, MALT lymphoma, relapse of AML, and nasopharyngeal carcinoma (Cheng et al. 2006; Erfani et al. 2006; Hu et al. 2010). The association of the same SNVs to autoimmunity and cancer indicates that immune responses to tumor cells critically regulate the development of tumor. In addition to SNVs in CTLA-4 gene, some SNVs in CD28 and CD80/86 genes have also been reported to associate with autoimmunity (Hegab et al. 2016; Tanasilovic et al. 2017; Wagner et al. 2015).

Four splicing variants of CTLA-4 have been identified (full-length CTLA-4 with all four exons, soluble CTLA-4 lacking exon 3, ligand-independent CTLA-4 lacking exon 2, and soluble ligand nonbinding CTLA-4 lacking exons 2 and 3). Full-length CTLA-4 consists of the IgV-like domain that is involved in ligand binding, the transmembrane region, and the cytoplasmic domain. The soluble CTLA-4 lacks the transmembrane region. The ligand-independent CTLA-4 lacks the ligand-binding domain and is reported to transduce inhibitory signal in a ligand-independent manner (Schildberg et al. 2016; Zhang and Vignali 2016). SNVs that increase soluble CTLA-4 have been found to associate with Graves' disease, T1DM, and autoimmune hypothyroidism (Ueda et al. 2003). In NOD mice, an SNV in exon 2 has been reported to regulate the expression of ligand-independent CTLA-4 and affects diabetes susceptibility (Ueda et al. 2003; Vijayakrishnan et al. 2004). The restoration of ligand-independent CTLA4 expression in NOD mice has been shown to alleviate T1DM (Araki et al. 2009; Stumpf et al. 2013).

Later, heterozygous mutations in CTLA-4 gene that result in the reduced CTLA-4 expression have been found in patients with common variable immunodeficiency (CVID) (Kuehn et al. 2014; Schubert et al. 2014). Individuals with CTLA-4 mutations exhibit diverse symptoms of autoimmunity such as autoimmune cytopenia, arthritis, thyroiditis, enteropathy, and lymphadenopathy despite the high incidence of hypogammaglobulinemia with a gradual loss of B cells. Treg cells from these patients express lower amount of CTLA-4, have reduced capacities to trans-endocytose CD80/86 from APCs, and elicit weaker suppressive function.

8.4.4 Manipulation of CD28/CTLA-4 for the Treatment of Autoimmunity

Based on the findings that CD28 deficiency or CD28 blockade prevented or alleviated various spontaneous and antigen-induced models of autoimmunity, a soluble protein that comprises the extracellular domain of human CTLA-4 and the Fc domain of human IgG1 with modification to prevent complement fixation (abatacept) was developed as CD28 blocker (Adams et al. 2016; Cutolo and Nadler 2013). Abatacept is now in clinical use for the therapy of RA, juvenile idiopathic arthritis, and psoriatic arthritis. Clinical trials of abatacept for the treatment of other autoimmune diseases such as polymyositis and dermatomyositis are currently underway (Tjarnlund et al. 2018). In addition, belatacept which has two- and four-fold higher affinity to CD80 and CD86, respectively, with two amino acid substitutions (A29Y and L104E) in the ligand-binding domain of CTLA-4 has also been developed and is now in clinical use for the kidney transplantation as an immunosuppressant (Vincenti et al. 2016).

CTLA-4-Ig inhibits not only the stimulatory co-signal of CD28 but also the inhibitory co-signal of CTLA-4, which may result in the attenuation of the suppressive function of Treg cells. The selective inhibition of CD28 by monovalent anti-CD28 Ab has been shown to be effective in several experimental models of autoimmunity and transplantation and is now in early clinical development (Laurent et al. 2017; Suchard et al. 2013; Yang et al. 2015).

As mentioned above, CD28 signal is required for the development and the maintenance of Treg cells. Superagonistic anti-CD28 Ab (TGN1412) that activates T cells in the absence of T-cell receptor signal shows suppressive effects in multiple experimental models of autoimmunity by preferentially activating and expanding Treg cells. However, in the phase I clinical trial of TGN1412, all six volunteers experienced a cytokine release syndrome with multiorgan failure in 2006 (Tyrsin et al. 2016). After the careful examination of the event and the reevaluation of the Ab, the clinical trial of the same Ab (but with different name, TAB08) with reduced dosage has been started again in 2011 (Tabares et al. 2014). By reducing the amount of the Ab from 15- to 1000-folds, TAB08 was well tolerated and proinflammatory cytokine release was not observed. In the subsequent phase Ib clinical trial with RA patients, the majority of patients showed the improvements of clinical scores more than 20% with an acceptable level of adverse events (Tyrsin et al. 2016). Further clinical trials are expected to reveal its efficacy and safety in human autoimmunity.

8.5 Concluding Remarks

The unprecedented clinical efficacies and the occasional involvements of irAEs by cancer immunotherapies targeting CTLA-4 and PD-1 highlighted their pivotal roles in the regulation of immune responses against tumors and self tissues. Although we focused on CD28, CTLA-4, and PD-1 in the current article, other stimulatory and inhibitory co-receptors in the CD28/CTLA-4 family and those in the other families such as the TNF receptor superfamily and the leukocyte immunoglobulin-like receptor family also play unique roles in the regulation of autoimmunity. The function of individual co-receptors has been extensively studied, and the developments of immunomodulatory therapies targeting these receptors are actively explored worldwide. However, functional differences, redundancies, or co-operations among these receptors remain poorly understood. Future studies are expected to unravel the molecular network of stimulatory and inhibitory co-receptors that underlies the exquisite immunoregulatory system in which protective immunity is promoted while autoimmunity is prevented.

References

Adams AB, Ford ML, Larsen CP (2016) Costimulation blockade in autoimmunity and transplantation: the CD28 pathway. J Immunol 197:2045–2050

Ansari MJ et al (2003) The programmed death-1 (PD-1) pathway regulates autoimmune diabetes in nonobese diabetic (NOD) mice. J Exp Med 198:63–69

Araki M et al (2009) Genetic evidence that the differential expression of the ligand-independent isoform of CTLA-4 is the molecular basis of the Idd5.1 type 1 diabetes region in nonobese diabetic mice. J Immunol 183:5146–5157

Bachmann MF, Kohler G, Ecabert B, Mak TW, Kopf M (1999) Cutting edge: lymphoproliferative disease in the absence of CTLA-4 is not T cell autonomous. J Immunol 163:1128–1131

Barroso-Sousa R, Ott PA, Hodi FS, Kaiser UB, Tolaney SM, Min L (2018) Endocrine dysfunction induced by immune checkpoint inhibitors: practical recommendations for diagnosis and clinical management. Cancer 124:1111–1121

Bertsias GK et al (2009) Genetic, immunologic, and immunohistochemical analysis of the programmed death 1/programmed death ligand 1 pathway in human systemic lupus erythematosus. Arthritis Rheum 60:207–218

Boike J, Dejulio T (2017) Severe esophagitis and gastritis from nivolumab therapy ACG case. Rep J 4:e57

Brahmer JR et al (2010) Phase I study of single-agent anti-programmed death-1 (MDX-1106) in refractory solid tumors: safety, clinical activity, pharmacodynamics, and immunologic correlates. J Clin Oncol 28:3167–3175

Callahan MK, Postow MA, Wolchok JD (2016) Targeting T cell co-receptors for cancer therapy. Immunity 44:1069–1078

Cappelli LC et al (2017) Inflammatory arthritis and sicca syndrome induced by nivolumab and ipilimumab. Ann Rheum Dis 76:43–50

Carter LL et al (2007) PD-1/PD-L1, but not PD-1/PD-L2, interactions regulate the severity of experimental autoimmune encephalomyelitis. J Neuroimmunol 182:124–134

Cheng TY et al (2006) Association of T-cell regulatory gene polymorphisms with susceptibility to gastric mucosa-associated lymphoid tissue lymphoma. J Clin Oncol 24:3483–3489

Collins AV et al (2002) The interaction properties of costimulatory molecules revisited. Immunity 17:201–210

Cooper JD et al (2007) The candidate genes TAF5L, TCF7, PDCD1, IL6 and ICAM1 cannot be excluded from having effects in type 1 diabetes. BMC Med Genet 8:71

Cukier P, Santini FC, Scaranti M, Hoff AO (2017) Endocrine side effects of cancer immunotherapy. Endocr Relat Cancer 24:T331–T347

Curiel TJ et al (2003) Blockade of B7-H1 improves myeloid dendritic cell-mediated antitumor immunity. Nat Med 9:562–567

Cutolo M, Nadler SG (2013) Advances in CTLA-4-Ig-mediated modulation of inflammatory cell and immune response activation in rheumatoid arthritisx. Nat Med 9:562–567

de Maleissye MF, Nicolas G, Saiag P (2016) Pembrolizumab-induced demyelinating polyradiculoneuropathy. N Engl J Med 375:296–297

Deng J et al (2017) Association of a PDCD1 polymorphism with sympathetic ophthalmia in Han Chinese. Invest Ophthalmol Vis Sci 58:4218–4222

Dong H et al (2002) Tumor-associated B7-H1 promotes T-cell apoptosis: a potential mechanism of immune evasion. Nat Med 8:793–800

Dong H, Zhu G, Tamada K, Flies DB, van Deursen JM, Chen L (2004) B7-H1 determines accumulation and deletion of intrahepatic CD8(+) T lymphocytes. Immunity 20:327–336

Erfani N, Razmkhah M, Talei AR, Pezeshki AM, Doroudchi M, Monabati A, Ghaderi A (2006) Cytotoxic T lymphocyte antigen-4 promoter variants in breast cancer. Cancer Genet Cytogenet 165:114–120

Garassino MC et al (2018) Durvalumab as third-line or later treatment for advanced non-small-cell lung cancer (ATLANTIC): an open-label, single-arm, phase 2 study. Lancet Oncol 19:521–536

Ghaderi A (2011) CTLA4 gene variants in autoimmunity and cancer: a comparative review. Iran J Immunol 8:127–149

Goser S et al (2006) Cardiac troponin I but not cardiac troponin T induces severe autoimmune inflammation in the myocardium. Circulation 114:1693–1702

Haikal A, Borba E, Khaja T, Doolittle G, Schmidt P (2018) Nivolumab-induced new-onset seronegative rheumatoid arthritis in a patient with advanced metastatic melanoma: A case report and literature review. Avicenna J Med 8:34–36

Hamel KM, Cao Y, Wang Y, Rodeghero R, Kobezda T, Chen L, Finnegan A (2010) B7-H1 expression on non-B and non-T cells promotes distinct effects on T- and B-cell responses in autoimmune arthritis. Eur J Immunol 40:3117–3127

Hayashi M, Kouki T, Takasu N, Sunagawa S, Komiya I (2008) Association of an A/C single nucleotide polymorphism in programmed cell death-ligand 1 gene with Graves' disease in Japanese patients. Eur J Endocrinol 158:817–822

Hegab MM et al (2016) CD28 and PTPN22 are associated with susceptibility to rheumatoid arthritis in Egyptians. Hum Immunol 77:522–526

Hodi FS et al (2010) Improved survival with ipilimumab in patients with metastatic melanoma. N Engl J Med 363:711–723

Hu L et al (2010) CTLA-4 gene polymorphism +49 A/G contributes to genetic susceptibility to two infection-related cancers-hepatocellular carcinoma and cervical cancer. Hum Immunol 71:888–891

Hua Z et al (2011) PD-1 polymorphisms are associated with sporadic breast cancer in Chinese Han population of Northeast China. Breast Cancer Res Treat 129:195–201

Huang CH et al (2011) Effects of genetic polymorphisms of programmed cell death 1 and its ligands on the development of ankylosing spondylitis. Rheumatology (Oxford) 50:1809–1813

Hughes J, Vudattu N, Sznol M, Gettinger S, Kluger H, Lupsa B, Herold KC (2015) Precipitation of autoimmune diabetes with anti-PD-1 immunotherapy. Diabetes Care 38:e55–e57

Hui E et al. (2017) T cell costimulatory receptor CD28 is a primary target for PD-1-mediated inhibition Science 355:1428-1433

Ikeuchi K, Okuma Y, Tabata T (2016) Immune-related pancreatitis secondary to nivolumab in a patient with recurrent lung adenocarcinoma: A case report. Lung Cancer 99:148–150

Ise W et al (2010) CTLA-4 suppresses the pathogenicity of self antigen-specific T cells by cell-intrinsic and cell-extrinsic mechanisms. Nat Immunol 11:129–135

Ishida Y, Agata Y, Shibahara K, Honjo T (1992) Induced expression of PD-1, a novel member of the immunoglobulin gene superfamily, upon programmed cell death. Embo J 11:3887–3895

Ishizaki Y et al (2010) PD1 as a common candidate susceptibility gene of subacute sclerosing panencephalitis. Hum Genet 127:411–419

Iwai Y, Ishida M, Tanaka Y, Okazaki T, Honjo T, Minato N (2002) Involvement of PD-L1 on tumor cells in the escape from host immune system and tumor immunotherapy by PD-L1 blockade. Proc Natl Acad Sci U S A 99:12293–12297

Iwama S, De Remigis A, Callahan MK, Slovin SF, Wolchok JD, Caturegli P (2014) Pituitary expression of CTLA-4 mediates hypophysitis secondary to administration of CTLA-4 blocking antibody. Sci Transl Med 6:230ra245

Jiang F et al (2009) Identification of QTLs that modify peripheral neuropathy in NOD.H2b-Pdcd1−/− mice. Int Immunol 21:499–509

Kang YK et al (2017) Nivolumab in patients with advanced gastric or gastro-oesophageal junction cancer refractory to, or intolerant of, at least two previous chemotherapy regimens (ONO-4538-12, ATTRACTION-2): a randomised, double-blind, placebo-controlled, phase 3 trial. Lancet 390:2461–2471

Kasamatsu T et al (2018) PDCD1 and CTLA4 polymorphisms affect the susceptibility to, and clinical features of, chronic immune thrombocytopenia. Br J Haematol 180:705–714

Kataoka K et al (2016) Aberrant PD-L1 expression through 3'-UTR disruption in multiple cancers. Nature 534:402–406

Kaufman HL et al (2018) Updated efficacy of avelumab in patients with previously treated metastatic Merkel cell carcinoma after >/=1 year of follow-up: JAVELIN Merkel 200, a phase 2 clinical trial. J Immunother Cancer 6:7

Keir ME et al (2006) Tissue expression of PD-L1 mediates peripheral T cell tolerance. J Exp Med 203:883–895

Kido M et al (2008) Fatal autoimmune hepatitis induced by concurrent loss of naturally arising regulatory T cells and PD-1-mediated signaling. Gastroenterology 135:1333–1343

Klocke K, Sakaguchi S, Holmdahl R, Wing K (2016) Induction of autoimmune disease by deletion of CTLA-4 in mice in adulthood. Proc Natl Acad Sci U S A 113:E2383–E2392

Kremer JM et al (2003) Treatment of rheumatoid arthritis by selective inhibition of T-cell activation with fusion protein CTLA4Ig. N Engl J Med 349:1907–1915

Kuehn HS et al (2014) Immune dysregulation in human subjects with heterozygous germline mutations in CTLA4. Science 345:1623–1627

Larkin J et al (2017) Neurologic serious adverse events associated with Nivolumab plus Ipilimumab or Nivolumab alone in advanced melanoma, including a case series of encephalitis. Oncologist 22:709–718

Latchman YE et al (2004) PD-L1-deficient mice show that PD-L1 on T cells, antigen-presenting cells, and host tissues negatively regulates T cells. Proc Natl Acad Sci U S A 101:10691–10696

Laurent L et al (2017) Prevention of lupus nephritis development in NZB/NZW mice by selective blockade of CD28. Eur J Immunol 47:1368–1376

Leach DR, Krummel MF, Allison JP (1996) Enhancement of antitumor immunity by CTLA-4 blockade. Science 271:1734–1736

Lenschow DJ et al (1996) CD28/B7 regulation of Th1 and Th2 subsets in the development of autoimmune diabetes. Immunity 5:285–293

Liang B, Gee RJ, Kashgarian MJ, Sharpe AH, Mamula MJ (1999) B7 costimulation in the development of lupus: autoimmunity arises either in the absence of B7.1/B7.2 or in the presence of anti-b7.1/B7.2 blocking antibodies. J Immunol 163:2322–2329

Linsley PS, Brady W, Urnes M, Grosmaire LS, Damle NK, Ledbetter JA (1991) CTLA-4 is a second receptor for the B cell activation antigen B7. J Exp Med 174:561–569

Liu J et al (2015) Immune-checkpoint proteins VISTA and PD-1 nonredundantly regulate murine T-cell responses. Proc Natl Acad Sci U S A 112:6682–6687

Lucas JA, Menke J, Rabacal WA, Schoen FJ, Sharpe AH, Kelley VR (2008) Programmed death ligand 1 regulates a critical checkpoint for autoimmune myocarditis and pneumonitis in MRL mice. J Immunol 181:2513–2521

Luhder F, Chambers C, Allison JP, Benoist C, Mathis D (2000) Pinpointing when T cell costimulatory receptor CTLA-4 must be engaged to dampen diabetogenic T cells. Proc Natl Acad Sci U S A 97:12204–12209

Maruhashi T, Okazaki IM, Sugiura D, Takahashi S, Maeda TK, Shimizu K, Okazaki T (2018) LAG-3 inhibits the activation of CD4(+) T cells that recognize stable pMHCII through its conformation-dependent recognition of pMHCII. Nat Immunol 19:1415–1426

Masteller EL, Chuang E, Mullen AC, Reiner SL, Thompson CB (2000) Structural analysis of CTLA-4 function in vivo. J Immunol 164:5319–5327

Meng Q, Liu X, Yang P, Hou S, Du L, Zhou H, Kijlstra A (2009) PDCD1 genes may protect against extraocular manifestations in Chinese Han patients with Vogt-Koyanagi-Harada syndrome. Mol Vis 15:386–392

Menke J et al (2007) Programmed death 1 ligand (PD-L) 1 and PD-L2 limit autoimmune kidney disease: distinct roles. J Immunol 179:7466–7477

Michot JM et al (2016) Immune-related adverse events with immune checkpoint blockade: a comprehensive review. Eur J Cancer 54:139–148

Mitchell AL et al. (2009) Programmed death ligand 1 (PD-L1) gene variants contribute to autoimmune Addison's disease and Graves' disease susceptibility J Clin Endocrinol Metab 94:5139-5145

Mizuno R, Sugiura D, Shimizu K, Maruhashi T, Watada M, Okazaki I-m, Okazaki T (2019) PD-1 primarily targets TCR signal in the inhibition of functional T cell activation. Front Immunol 10:630. https://doi.org/10.3389/fimmu.2019.00630. eCollection 2019

Mojtahedi Z, Mohmedi M, Rahimifar S, Erfani N, Hosseini SV, Ghaderi A (2012) Programmed death-1 gene polymorphism (PD-1.5 C/T) is associated with colon cancer. Gene 508:229–232

Naidoo J et al (2015) Toxicities of the anti-PD-1 and anti-PD-L1 immune checkpoint antibodies. Ann Oncol 26:2375–2391

Nimmerjahn F, Ravetch JV (2008) Fcgamma receptors as regulators of immune responses. Nat Rev Immunol 8:34–47

Nishikawa K, Linsley PS, Collins AB, Stamenkovic I, McCluskey RT, Andres G (1994) Effect of CTLA-4 chimeric protein on rat autoimmune anti-glomerular basement membrane glomerulonephritis. Eur J Immunol 24:1249–1254

Nishimura H, Nose M, Hiai H, Minato N, Honjo T (1999) Development of lupus-like autoimmune diseases by disruption of the PD-1 gene encoding an ITIM motif-carrying immunoreceptor. Immunity 11:141–151

Nishimura H et al (2001) Autoimmune dilated cardiomyopathy in PD-1 receptor-deficient mice. Science 291:319–322

Okamura H, Okazaki I-m, Shimizu K, Maruhashi T, Sugiura D, Mizuno R, Okazaki T (2019) PD-1 aborts the activation trajectory of autoreactive CD8+ T cells to prohibit their acquisition of effector functions. J Autoimmun:102296. https://doi.org/10.1016/j.jaut.2019.06.007. [Epub ahead of print]

Okazaki T, Honjo T (2007) PD-1 and PD-1 ligands: from discovery to clinical application. Int Immunol 19:813–824

Okazaki T, Maeda A, Nishimura H, Kurosaki T, Honjo T (2001) PD-1 immunoreceptor inhibits B cell receptor-mediated signaling by recruiting src homology 2-domain-containing tyrosine phosphatase 2 to phosphotyrosine. Proc Natl Acad Sci U S A 98:13866–13871

Okazaki T et al (2003) Autoantibodies against cardiac troponin I are responsible for dilated cardiomyopathy in PD-1-deficient mice. Nat Med 9:1477–1483

Okazaki T, Otaka Y, Wang J, Hiai H, Takai T, Ravetch JV, Honjo T (2005) Hydronephrosis associated with antiurothelial and antinuclear autoantibodies in BALB/c-Fcgr2b−/-Pdcd1−/− mice. J Exp Med 202:1643–1648

Okazaki T et al (2011) PD-1 and LAG-3 inhibitory co-receptors act synergistically to prevent autoimmunity in mice. J Exp Med 208:395–407

Okazaki T, Chikuma S, Iwai Y, Fagarasan S, Honjo T (2013) A rheostat for immune responses: the unique properties of PD-1 and their advantages for clinical application. Nat Immunol 14:1212–1218

Oosterwegel MA, Mandelbrot DA, Boyd SD, Lorsbach RB, Jarrett DY, Abbas AK, Sharpe AH (1999) The role of CTLA-4 in regulating Th2 differentiation. J Immunol 163:2634–2639

Parry RV et al (2005) CTLA-4 and PD-1 receptors inhibit T-cell activation by distinct mechanisms. Mol Cell Biol 25:9543–9553

Paterson AM et al (2015) Deletion of CTLA-4 on regulatory T cells during adulthood leads to resistance to autoimmunity. J Exp Med 212:1603–1621

Pawlak-Adamska E et al (2017) PD-1 gene polymorphic variation is linked with first symptom of disease and severity of relapsing-remitting form of MS. J Neuroimmunol 305:115–127

Perrin PJ et al (1995) Role of B7:CD28/CTLA-4 in the induction of chronic relapsing experimental allergic encephalomyelitis. J Immunol 154:1481–1490

Phan GQ et al (2003) Cancer regression and autoimmunity induced by cytotoxic T lymphocyte-associated antigen 4 blockade in patients with metastatic melanoma. Proc Natl Acad Sci U S A 100:8372–8377

Pizarro C, Garcia-Diaz DF, Codner E, Salas-Perez F, Carrasco E, Perez-Bravo F (2014) PD-L1 gene polymorphisms and low serum level of PD-L1 protein are associated to type 1 diabetes in Chile. Diabetes Metab Res Rev 30:761–766

Prokunina L et al (2002) A regulatory polymorphism in PDCD1 is associated with susceptibility to systemic lupus erythematosus in humans. Nat Genet 32:666–669

Rajasalu T et al (2010) Deficiency in B7-H1 (PD-L1)/PD-1 coinhibition triggers pancreatic beta-cell destruction by insulin-specific, murine CD8 T-cells. Diabetes 59:1966–1973

Raptopoulou AP et al (2010) The programmed death 1/programmed death ligand 1 inhibitory pathway is up-regulated in rheumatoid synovium and regulates peripheral T cell responses in human and murine arthritis. Arthritis Rheum 62:1870–1880

Robert C et al (2015) Pembrolizumab versus ipilimumab in advanced melanoma. N Engl J Med 372:2521–2532

Romo-Tena J, Gomez-Martin D, Alcocer-Varela J (2013) CTLA-4 and autoimmunity: new insights into the dual regulator of tolerance. Autoimmun Rev 12:1171–1176

Salama AD et al (2003) Critical role of the programmed death-1 (PD-1) pathway in regulation of experimental autoimmune encephalomyelitis. J Exp Med 198:71–78

Salomon B, Lenschow DJ, Rhee L, Ashourian N, Singh B, Sharpe A, Bluestone JA (2000) B7/CD28 costimulation is essential for the homeostasis of the CD4+CD25+ immunoregulatory T cells that control autoimmune diabetes. Immunity 12:431–440

Salomon B et al (2001) Development of spontaneous autoimmune peripheral polyneuropathy in B7-2-deficient NOD mice. J Exp Med 194:677–684

Schildberg FA, Klein SR, Freeman GJ, Sharpe AH (2016) Coinhibitory pathways in the B7-CD28 ligand-receptor family. Immunity 44:955–972

Schubert D et al (2014) Autosomal dominant immune dysregulation syndrome in humans with CTLA4 mutations. Nat Med 20:1410–1416

Shahinian A et al (1993) Differential T cell costimulatory requirements in CD28-deficient mice. Science 261:609–612

Shimatani K, Yoshimoto T, Doi Y, Sonoda T, Yamamoto S, Kanematsu A (2018) Two cases of nonbacterial cystitis associated with nivolumab, the anti-programmed-death-receptor-1 inhibitor. Urol Case Rep 17:97–99

Stumpf M, Zhou X, Bluestone JA (2013) The B7-independent isoform of CTLA-4 functions to regulate autoimmune diabetes. J Immunol 190:961–969

Suchard SJ et al (2013) A monovalent anti-human CD28 domain antibody antagonist: preclinical efficacy and safety. J Immunol 191:4599–4610

Sugino Y et al (2012) BALB/c-Fcgr2bPdcd1 mouse expressing anti-urothelial antibody is a novel model of autoimmune cystitis. Sci Rep 2:317

Tabares P et al (2014) Human regulatory T cells are selectively activated by low-dose application of the CD28 superagonist TGN1412/TAB08. Eur J Immunol 44:1225–1236

Tada Y et al (1999) Role of the costimulatory molecule CD28 in the development of lupus in MRL/lpr mice. J Immunol 163:3153–3159

Takahashi S et al (2005) In vivo overexpression of CTLA-4 suppresses lymphoproliferative diseases and thymic negative selection. Eur J Immunol 35:399–407

Takahashi Y et al (2013) Genetic variations of immunoregulatory genes associated with Rasmussen syndrome. Epilepsy Res 107:238–243

Tanasilovic S, Popadic S, Medenica L, Popadic D (2017) Pemphigus vulgaris and pemphigus foliaceus determined by CD86 and CTLA4 polymorphisms. Clin Dermatol 35:236–241

Tang Q et al (2003) Cutting edge: CD28 controls peripheral homeostasis of CD4+CD25+ regulatory T cells. J Immunol 171:3348–3352

Tarrio ML, Grabie N, Bu DX, Sharpe AH, Lichtman AH (2012) PD-1 protects against inflammation and myocyte damage in T cell-mediated myocarditis. J Immunol 188:4876–4884

Tivol EA, Gorski J (2002) Re-establishing peripheral tolerance in the absence of CTLA-4: complementation by wild-type T cells points to an indirect role for CTLA-4. J Immunol 169:1852–1858

Tivol EA, Borriello F, Schweitzer AN, Lynch WP, Bluestone JA, Sharpe AH (1995) Loss of CTLA-4 leads to massive lymphoproliferation and fatal multiorgan tissue destruction, revealing a critical negative regulatory role of CTLA-4. Immunity 3:541–547

Tjarnlund A et al (2018) Abatacept in the treatment of adult dermatomyositis and polymyositis: a randomised, phase IIb treatment delayed-start trial. Ann Rheum Dis 77:55–62

Topalian SL et al (2012) Safety, activity, and immune correlates of anti-PD-1 antibody in cancer. N Engl J Med 366:2443–2454

Tyrsin D, Chuvpilo S, Matskevich A, Nemenov D, Romer PS, Tabares P, Hunig T (2016) From TGN1412 to TAB08: the return of CD28 superagonist therapy to clinical development for the treatment of rheumatoid arthritis. Clin Exp Rheumatol 34:45–48

Ueda H et al (2003) Association of the T-cell regulatory gene CTLA4 with susceptibility to autoimmune disease. Nature 423:506–511

Varricchi G et al (2017) Cardiotoxicity of immune checkpoint inhibitors. ESMO Open 2:e000247

Vijayakrishnan L et al (2004) An autoimmune disease-associated CTLA-4 splice variant lacking the B7 binding domain signals negatively in T cells. Immunity 20:563–575

Vincenti F et al (2016) Belatacept and long-term outcomes in kidney transplantation. N Engl J Med 374:333–343

Wagner M et al (2015) Polymorphisms in CD28, CTLA-4, CD80 and CD86 genes may influence the risk of multiple sclerosis and its age of onset. J Neuroimmunol 288:79–86

Walker LS, Sansom DM (2015) Confusing signals: recent progress in CTLA-4 biology. Trends Immunol 36:63–70

Wang J, Yoshida T, Nakaki F, Hiai H, Okazaki T, Honjo T (2005) Establishment of NOD-Pdcd1−/− mice as an efficient animal model of type I diabetes. Proc Natl Acad Sci U S A 102:11823–11828

Wang J et al (2010) PD-1 deficiency results in the development of fatal myocarditis in MRL mice. Int Immunol 22:443–452

Wang G, Hu P, Yang J, Shen G, Wu X (2011) The effects of PDL-Ig on collagen-induced arthritis. Rheumatol Int 31:513–519

Waterhouse P et al (1995) Lymphoproliferative disorders with early lethality in mice deficient in Ctla-4. Science 270:985–988

Wing K et al (2008) CTLA-4 control over Foxp3+ regulatory T cell function. Science 322:271–275

Wing K, Yamaguchi T, Sakaguchi S (2011) Cell-autonomous and -non-autonomous roles of CTLA-4 in immune regulation. Trends Immunol 32:428–433

Woo SR et al (2012) Immune inhibitory molecules LAG-3 and PD-1 synergistically regulate T-cell function to promote tumoral immune escape. Cancer Res 72:917–927

Yanagawa T, Hidaka Y, Guimaraes V, Soliman M, DeGroot LJ (1995) CTLA-4 gene polymorphism associated with Graves' disease in a Caucasian population. J Clin Endocrinol Metab 80:41–45

Yang Q, Liu Y, Liu D, Zhang Y, Mu K (2011) Association of polymorphisms in the programmed cell death 1 (PD-1) and PD-1 ligand genes with ankylosing spondylitis in a Chinese population. Clin Exp Rheumatol 29:13–18

Yang Z et al (2015) Integrated pharmacokinetic/pharmacodynamic analysis for determining the minimal anticipated biological effect level of a novel anti-CD28 receptor antagonist BMS-931699. J Pharmacol Exp Ther 355:506–515

Yokosuka T, Takamatsu M, Kobayashi-Imanishi W, Hashimoto-Tane A, Azuma M, Saito T (2012) Programmed cell death 1 forms negative costimulatory microclusters that directly inhibit T cell receptor signaling by recruiting phosphatase SHP2. J Exp Med 209:1201–1217

Yoshida T, Jiang F, Honjo T, Okazaki T (2008) PD-1 deficiency reveals various tissue-specific autoimmunity by H-2b and dose-dependent requirement of H-2g7 for diabetes in NOD mice. Proc Natl Acad Sci U S A 105:3533–3538

Yu Y et al (2016) Single-cell RNA-seq identifies a PD-1(hi) ILC progenitor and defines its development pathway. Nature 539:102–106

Zamani MR, Asbagh FA, Massoud AH, Salmaninejad A, Massoud A, Rezaei N (2015) Association between a PD-1 gene polymorphism and antisperm antibody-related infertility in Iranian men. J Assist Reprod Genet 32:103–106

Zhang Q, Vignali DA (2016) Co-stimulatory and co-inhibitory pathways in autoimmunity. Immunity 44:1034–1051

Zhong X, Tumang JR, Gao W, Bai C, Rothstein TL (2007) PD-L2 expression extends beyond dendritic cells/macrophages to B1 cells enriched for V(H)11/V(H)12 and phosphatidylcholine binding. Eur J Immunol 37:2405–2410

Zhu B et al (2006) Differential role of programmed death-ligand 1 [corrected] and programmed death-ligand 2 [corrected] in regulating the susceptibility and chronic progression of experimental autoimmune encephalomyelitis. J Immunol 176:3480–3489

Chapter 9
Co-signaling Molecules in Neurological Diseases

Pia Kivisäkk and Samia J. Khoury

Abstract Inflammation plays an important role in the onset and progression of many neurological diseases. As the central nervous system (CNS) constitutes a highly specialized environment where immune activation can be detrimental, it is crucial to understand mechanisms by which the immune system is regulated during neurological diseases. The system of co-signaling pathways provides the immune system with the means to fine-tune immune responses by turning on and off immune cell activation. Studies of co-signaling molecules in neurological diseases and their animal models have highlighted the complexities of immune regulation within the CNS and the intricacies of the interplay between the different cells of the immune system and how they interact with the resident cells of the CNS. This complexity poses challenges when targeting co-signaling pathway to treat neurological diseases and may explain why no drugs targeting these pathways have been successfully developed this far. Here, we will review the current literature on some important co-signaling pathways in multiple sclerosis (MS), Alzheimer's disease, amyotrophic lateral sclerosis (ALS), Parkinson's disease, and ischemic stroke to understand these pathways in mediating and controlling neuroinflammation.

Keywords Costimulatory molecules · Neurological diseases · Multiple sclerosis · Alzheimer's disease · Amyotrophic lateral sclerosis · Parkinson's disease · Ischemic stroke

---

P. Kivisäkk
Ann Romney Center for Neurologic Diseases, Brigham and Women's Hospital, Harvard Medical School, Boston, MA, USA
e-mail: pkivisakk@mgh.harvard.edu

S. J. Khoury (✉)
Abou Haidar Neuroscience Institute and Nehme and Therese Tohme Multiple Sclerosis Center, Faculty of Medicine, American University of Beirut Medical Center, Beirut, Lebanon
e-mail: sk88@aub.edu.lb

© Springer Nature Singapore Pte Ltd. 2019
M. Azuma, H. Yagita (eds.), *Co-signal Molecules in T Cell Activation*,
Advances in Experimental Medicine and Biology 1189,
https://doi.org/10.1007/978-981-32-9717-3_9

9.1 Introduction

The central nervous system (CNS) constitutes a highly specialized environment where immune activation can be detrimental. Traditionally, it was believed that the CNS is immunologically privileged and shielded from the peripheral immune system by the blood–brain barrier (BBB), but it is clear that peripheral immune cells can enter the CNS as part of physiological immune surveillance, recognize cognate antigens, and elicit an adaptive inflammatory response (Korn and Kallies 2017). Resident CNS cells, in particular, activated microglia, play an important role in CNS inflammation as professional antigen-presenting cells (APCs) that secrete a vast array of inflammatory mediators, which modulate both innate and adaptive immune responses (Almolda et al. 2015). Many neurological diseases are associated with CNS inflammation, not only the classical inflammatory demyelinating diseases exemplified by multiple sclerosis (MS), but also neurodegenerative disorders such as Alzheimer's disease (AD), amyotrophic lateral sclerosis (ALS), Parkinson's disease (PD), and ischemic stroke (Puentes et al. 2016; Gendelman and Mosley 2015; Cebrian et al. 2015; Famakin 2014). As neurons are unable to regenerate and often are integrated into highly complex networks, immune responses in the CNS need to be tightly controlled, balancing the need to protect the organism from foreign threats while minimizing immune-mediated bystander damage (Korn and Kallies 2017).

The system of co-signaling pathways provides the immune system with the means to fine-tune immune responses by turning on and off immune cell activation. It has long been known that activation of T cells requires two signals: The first consists of the interaction of the T-cell receptor (TCR) with its cognate antigen presented in the context of major histocompatibility complex (MHC) molecules on the surface of APCs, and the second consists of the interaction of co-signaling receptors on the T cell with ligands expressed by the APCs (Bretscher and Cohn 1970). As co-signaling receptors can be both stimulatory, promoting T-cell activation, differentiation, and survival, or inhibitory, dampening T-cell activation, the net outcome of TCR stimulation is decided by the combination of the different stimulatory and inhibitory signals (Zhang and Vignali 2016). Similarly, B cells and other immune cells also require two signals for their activation, maturation, and function (Bretscher and Cohn 1970). In addition to microglia, other resident cells of the CNS including astrocytes, neurons, and neural stem and progenitor cells may also express co-signaling molecules under various conditions providing a mechanism by which CNS cells can interact with the immune system and modulate its effects. In this chapter, we will review the literature on some important co-signaling pathways and discuss their role in mediating and controlling neuroinflammation.

9.2 Resident CNS Cells

Microglia are the main immunocompetent cells in the CNS and function as the resident macrophages of the CNS parenchyma. They are constantly surveying the CNS parenchyma and are ready to rapidly respond to disturbances in the microenvironment, serving as a first line of defense against infection or injury (Ransohoff and El Khoury 2015). Under normal conditions, microglia display a quiescent phenotype characterized by the lack or low expression of many molecules normally expressed by other tissue macrophages to prevent the CNS from unwanted immune-mediated inflammation (Perry 2016). Consistent with this quiescent phenotype, unstimulated microglia express only low or undetectable levels of costimulatory molecules (Aloisi et al. 1998; Almolda et al. 2015). An exception is Tim-3, an inhibitory co-signaling receptor regulating peripheral tolerance and the expansion of effector Th1 cells, preventing uncontrolled inflammation, which is constitutively expressed by microglia isolated from autopsy tissue from subjects with no evident inflammatory disease (Anderson et al. 2007).

Neurons in the local microenvironment control microglial activation and contribute to their quiescent state by secreting soluble factors and through cell–cell interactions (Chavarria and Cardenas 2013). The expression of the costimulatory molecules CD40 and CD86 is downregulated in cultured microglia by nerve growth factor (NGF) released by neurons (Wei and Jonakait 1999). Neurons also express CD200 (Koning et al. 2009), a nonsignaling molecule that triggers anti-inflammatory signaling in CD200R-expressing cells including microglia (Walker and Lue 2013). Microglia from CD200-deficient mice exhibited an activated phenotype, while IL-4-mediated neuronal CD200 expression is protected against lipopolysaccharide (LPS)-induced microglial activation (Hoek et al. 2000; Lyons et al. 2009).

Consistent with their role as sentinels of the CNS, microglia rapidly become highly activated upon insults to the brain. Depending on the specific stimuli and the condition of the microenvironment, microglia can exert neuroprotective functions or upregulate factors involved in phagocytosis, antigen presentation, and secretion of neurotoxic factors, showing a high degree of plasticity (Ransohoff and Perry 2009). In vitro experiments have consistently shown that activated microglia can be induced to express costimulatory molecules. The expression of CD40 is upregulated on microglia by proinflammatory cytokines such as IFN-γ and GM-CSF, while anti-inflammatory cytokines such as TGF-β and IL-4 downregulate its expression (Almolda et al. 2015). Activated microglia isolated from the CNS during demyelinating diseases such as MS and experimental autoimmune encephalomyelitis (EAE), its animal model, have been shown to express CD40 (Vogel et al. 2013; Becher et al. 2001; Ponomarev et al. 2006), CD80/CD86 (Issazadeh et al. 1998), and PD-L1 (Schreiner et al. 2008; Pittet et al. 2011; Ortler et al. 2008). CD40-positive microglia can also be detected in the CNS during neurodegenerative disorders such as AD and the SOD1 mouse model of ALS (Okuno et al. 2004; Togo et al. 2000), while CD40 and PD-1 are upregulated in microglia during reperfusion after middle cerebral artery occlusion (MCAO), an animal model of ischemic stroke in mice (Klohs et al. 2008; Ren et al. 2011).

The role of astrocytes in regulating the immune system is less well understood. Astrocytes have a range of functions most importantly maintaining neuronal health (Sofroniew and Vinters 2010). Reactive astrogliosis, a defensive reaction of astrocytes aimed at limiting tissue damage and restoring homeostasis, is observed in many neurological disorders. Reactive astroglia signal to surrounding cells both by cell–cell interactions and by secreting numerous growth factors, neurotransmitters, cytokines, and chemokines (Pekny et al. 2016). Astrocytes protect the CNS from unwanted adaptive immune responses by the expression of inhibitory co-signaling receptors. In vitro experiments have shown that astrocytes can suppress T-cell proliferation and effector functions by upregulation of the inhibitory receptor CTLA-4 (Gimsa et al. 2004). Astrocytes can also be induced in vitro to express PD-L1 and galectin-9 (Gal-9) that bind to the coinhibitory receptors PD-1 and Tim-3, respectively (Yoshida et al. 2001; Magnus et al. 2005; Pittet et al. 2011). Furthermore, PD-L1 and Gal-9 immunoreactivity has been reported in astrocytes in a mouse model of axonal injury and in MS brain lesions (Anderson et al. 2007; Lipp et al. 2007; Pittet et al. 2011).

Astrocytes may also express CD40L, a ligand for the stimulatory receptor CD40, during physiologic aging as well as in AD (Calingasan et al. 2002), highlighting the complexity of astrocyte responses. In vitro studies have shown inconsistent results with regard to the expression of CD80 and CD86 on astrocytes (Chastain et al. 2011), but it should be noted that both astrocytes and microglia are known to rapidly change their phenotype and gene expression profile when removed from the complex support structure in the brain rendering them difficult to study in vitro (Butovsky et al. 2014). CD80 and CD86 expression was reported in astrocytes during EAE in some models but not others (Issazadeh et al. 1998; Cross and Ku 2000) and could be observed on astrocytes in chronic active MS lesions (Togo et al. 2000; Zeinstra et al. 2003).

Neurons can directly interact with autoreactive encephalitogenic T cells and convert them to T_{regs} of the traditional Foxp3+ phenotype or a recently described FoxA1+ phenotype (Liu et al. 2006, 2014). FoxA1+ T_{regs} were originally identified in IFN-β-deficient mice and can be induced by IFN-β both in vivo and in vitro (Liu et al. 2014). These cells are characterized by high expression of PD-L1 and can suppress autoreactive T cells in the CNS during EAE in a PD-L1-dependent manner (Liu et al. 2014). PD-L1 expression on neurons is essential for their ability to interact with encephalitogenic T cells and convert them to FoxA1+ T_{regs} (Liu et al. 2017b). Mechanistic studies showed that endogenous neuronal IFN-β triggers the PI3K/Akt pathway through autocrine signaling resulting in translocation of the transcription factor FoxA1 to the nucleus, inducing PD-L1 expression (Liu et al. 2017b).

9.3 Multiple Sclerosis and Experimental Autoimmune Encephalomyelitis

MS is an immune-mediated disease characterized by immune cell infiltration in the CNS and associated inflammation, demyelination, and neuronal degeneration (Dendrou et al. 2015). The initiating factor is still unknown, but evidence suggests that MS, especially in the earlier stages of the disease, is a T-cell-driven disease where autoreactive T cells are activated and migrate to the CNS, where they trigger an inflammatory response with accumulation of macrophages, T cells, B cells, and plasma cells (Dendrou et al. 2015; Ransohoff et al. 2015). This inflammatory response is accompanied by activation of microglia and astrocytes, as well as damage to myelin and neurons. As the disease progresses, the inflammation becomes more diffuse and sequestered within the CNS with fewer infiltrating cells and more pronounced neuro-degeneration (Dendrou et al. 2015). Much insight into the pathogenesis of MS has been gained from its animal model, experimental autoimmune encephalomyelitis (EAE) that is typically initiated by peripheral immunization with myelin proteins/peptides or by adoptive transfer of autoreactive T cells. Peripherally generated pathogenic CD4+ T helper (Th) cells expressing Th1 and Th17 cytokine profiles cross the BBB and trigger an inflammatory response in the CNS upon encountering their cognate antigens resulting in a model primarily resembling aspects of the early inflammatory phase of MS (Lassmann and Brad, Acta Neuropath, 2017).

All current FDA-approved disease-modifying drugs in MS target the immune system, confirming that modulation of inflammation can reduce disease activity in MS. Several co-signaling pathways have been targeted in EAE with positive effects, but none of the molecules tested in clinical trials this far have shown efficacy in MS. Studies of co-signaling molecules in MS and EAE have, however, provided much insight into the role of the immune system in CNS inflammatory diseases and how these diseases are regulated.

9.3.1 CD28/CTLA-4

The CD28 costimulatory pathway plays a central role in modulating T-cell functions, and there is an extensive literature showing that CD28 and CTLA-4 (cytotoxic T-lymphocyte-associated protein 4) are critical regulators of autoimmune diseases (Esensten et al. 2016). CD28 and CTLA-4 are highly homologous and compete for the same two ligands, CD80 and CD86, but have opposing effects on T-cell activation. CD28 is constitutively expressed on T cells and is involved in TCR signaling and IL-2 production, providing an activating signal that promotes T-cell proliferation and survival. In contrast, the expression of CTLA-4 is upregulated upon T-cell activation and competes with CD28 due to its higher affinity for CD80 and CD86, triggering a negative signal that downregulates T-cell activation.

CD28-deficient mice are resistant to EAE (Oliveira-dos-Santos et al. 1999), and blockade of CD28-CD80/86 signaling ameliorates EAE both when administered during antigen priming and after disease onset (Perrin et al. 1999; Schaub et al. 1999). CTLA-4 plays a critical role in maintaining tolerance to peripheral self-antigens, as evidenced by lethal, multiorgan autoimmunity in CTLA-4-deficient mice (Waterhouse et al. 1995). Anti-CTLA-4 treatment of mice exacerbates EAE both in adoptive transfer and active immunization models of EAE (Karandikar et al. 2000; Perrin et al. 1996; Hurwitz et al. 1997), and anti-CTLA-4 treatment during EAE remission resulted in the exacerbation of relapses (Karandikar et al. 1996). Blockade of CTLA-4 completely reversed peripheral tolerance to EAE induced by intravenous (i.v.) administration of antigen-coupled splenocytes indicating that peripheral tolerance is dependent on CTLA-4 (Eagar et al. 2002).

Conditional deletion of CTLA-4 in adult mice also resulted in spontaneous lymphoproliferation and multiorgan inflammation, but was not lethal (Klocke et al. 2016). In contrast to mice deficient of CTLA-4 from birth, mice depleted of CTLA-4 in adulthood were protected against MOG peptide-induced EAE and displayed delayed onset of protein-induced EAE (Klocke et al. 2016; Paterson et al. 2015). CD4+ T cells in draining lymph nodes from adult CTLA-4-deficient mice did not differ from littermate controls in their production of IFN-γ, IL-17, or GM-CSF, and these mice had similar numbers of T cells infiltrating into the CNS (Paterson et al. 2015; Klocke et al. 2016). However, adult CTLA-4-deficient mice had a preferential expansion of T_{regs} with more than twofold increase in the T_{reg}/$T_{conventional}$ cell ratio in the CNS. It was previously shown that expansion of T_{reg} numbers prevents spontaneous EAE in CTLA-4-deficient MBP-peptide TCR transgenic mice (Verhagen et al. 2009), and loss of CTLA-4 on T_{regs} alone is sufficient to confer EAE resistance (Paterson et al. 2015). CTLA-4-deficient T_{regs} are functionally suppressive but use non-CTLA-4-dependent mechanisms to suppress immune responses (Wing et al. 2008; Paterson et al. 2015). Interestingly, the protective effects of T_{regs} were not as pronounced in protein-induced EAE, where disease incidence and severity in mice depleted of CTLA-4 during adulthood were similar to that in control mice (Klocke et al. 2016). An explanation for this may be that protein-induced EAE is more dependent on B cells (Lyons et al. 1999), and as CTLA-4 inhibits stimulatory function of T follicular helper (Tfh) cells, deletion of CTLA-4 on Tfh may lead to increased antibody production (Sage et al. 2014; Wing et al. 2014; Klocke et al. 2016).

CTLA-4Ig is a fusion protein linking a soluble CTLA-4-binding domain to an Ig constant region, which binds to CD80/CD86 and blocks their interaction with CD28 (Perrin et al. 1996). CTLA-4Ig has been shown to profoundly suppress EAE, even when distributed after the onset of clinical disease (Arima et al. 1996; Khoury et al.

1995; Cross et al. 1999). Two CTLA-4Ig drugs are currently approved by the FDA, abatacept and belatacept (a higher affinity version). They have shown therapeutic effectiveness in rheumatoid arthritis, juvenile idiopathic arthritis, and prevention of acute rejection of renal transplants (Genovese et al. 2005; Ruperto et al. 2008; Vincenti et al. 2005). CTLA-4Ig has been tested in MS with less encouraging results. An open-label phase I trial of CTLA-4Ig in relapsing–remitting MS (RRMS) showed that CTLA-4Ig was well tolerated and that it reduced T-cell proliferation and production of IFN-γ by peripheral blood mononuclear cells (PBMCs) in response to myelin peptide stimulation in vitro (Viglietta et al. 2008). A phase II randomized double-blind placebo-controlled study of abatacept in RRMS was terminated prematurely by the sponsor due to treatment group imbalance but hinted toward a clinical efficacy in the higher-dose group (10 mg/kg; SYNOPSIS. Clinical study report IM101200, http://ctr.bms.com/pdf/IM101200.pdf). This was followed by a second phase II randomized double-blind placebo-controlled study of abatacept in RRMS (Khoury et al. 2017). The study did not find any statistically significant effects on the number of new gadolinium-enhancing (Gd+) lesions on brain MRI or clinical measures including no evidence of disease activity (NEDA). The study had some limitations, most notably low enrollment and a predominance for stable patients with low numbers of new Gd+ lesions reflecting a reluctance of treating physicians to enroll more active patients in placebo-controlled studies when several disease-modifying mediations are available for the treatment of RRMS.

CTLA-4-blocking agents are currently in use to treat patients with malignancies, utilizing the ability of CTLA-4 to serve as an immune checkpoint inhibitor, shifting the immune status from T-cell exhaustion to a functional antitumor response. Treatment with ipilimumab, the first immunomodulatory checkpoint inhibitor approved by the FDA (Hodi et al. 2010), was associated with inflammatory side effects, termed "immune-related adverse events" (Kong and Flynn 2014; Weber et al. 2012). Interestingly, a few case reports have shown transition from a subclinical radiologically isolated syndrome (RIS) to clinically overt MS, clinical exacerbations, and increased MRI activity in patients with preexisting MS, or apparent de novo development of MS in individual patients treated with ipilimumab (Gettings et al. 2015; Gerdes et al. 2016; Cao et al. 2016), while others reported no worsening of MS (Johnson et al. 2016; Kyi et al. 2014). A more thorough follow-up of patients with underlying autoimmune conditions treated with ipilimumab is needed to increase our understanding of immunotherapies in this patient population.

9.3.2 PD-1

Programmed cell death protein-1 (PD-1) is a member of the B7–CD28 family that was proposed to serve as a first-tier coinhibitory receptor together with CTLA-4, playing an important role in maintaining peripheral tolerance (Fife and Bluestone

2008; Anderson et al. 2016). In contrast to CTLA-4 that inhibits the initial stage of activation of naïve T cells typically within lymphoid tissues, PD-1 downregulates previously activated T cells during the effector phase of an immune response primarily in peripheral tissues and may serve to maintain tolerance within locally infiltrated tissues, reducing organ damage (Keir et al. 2006). PD-1 signaling results in the inhibition of TCR-mediated responses including T-cell proliferation, cytokine production, cytotoxicity, and reduced T-cell survival (Buchbinder and Desai 2016).

PD-1 is broadly expressed on T cells, B cells, and myeloid cells upon activation, and its expression is maintained in settings of persistent antigenic stimulation (Yamazaki et al. 2002; Liang et al. 2003). The expression of its two ligands PD-L1 and PL-L2 is regulated by inflammatory stimuli, especially cytokines, with the expression of PD-L2 restricted to APCs, while PD-L1 is expressed by a wide range of cells including leukocytes, nonhematopoietic cells, and parenchymal cells (Chen 2004). PD-L1 and PD-L2 are not expressed by resting human CNS cells, but inflammatory cytokines including IFN-γ and TNF-α upregulate PD-L1 expression on human astrocytes and microglia in vitro (Pittet et al. 2011), and PD-L1 expression is detected on glial cells in MS lesions (Pittet et al. 2011; Ortler et al. 2008). PD-1 and PD-L1 are expressed on CNS infiltrating cells in EAE with a temporal pattern following the clinical course of the disease (Salama et al. 2003; Schreiner et al. 2008), and PD-L1 is also upregulated on vascular endothelial cells and microglia in mice with EAE (Liang et al. 2003; Magnus et al. 2005; Schreiner et al. 2008).

Several studies have shown that blockade of PD-L1 and/or PD-L2 increases the susceptibility to EAE and enhances disease severity (Zhu et al. 2006; Salama et al. 2003). While initial studies indicated that interactions between PD-1 and PD-L2 constitute the dominant pathway in regulating EAE, later studies showed that the relative importance of the two ligands is strain specific and dependent on the genetic background (Zhu et al. 2006). Experiments in knockout (KO) mice showed that PD-1- and PD-L1-deficient, but not PD-L2-deficient, mice developed more severe EAE (Latchman et al. 2004; Carter et al. 2007; Wang et al. 2010) and that genetic disruption of PD-L1 alone is sufficient to convert an EAE-resistant strain into a fully permissive one (Latchman et al. 2004). It is believed that increased CNS expression of PD-L1 during EAE serves as a negative feedback mechanism limiting encephalitogenic T-cell responses and inflammatory tissue damage, and it is likely that these effects are mediated at least in part by T_{regs} that constitutively express PD-L1 and upregulate PD-1 expression following TCR stimulation (Keir et al. 2007; Taylor et al. 2004). PD-1-deficient mice have reduced frequencies of T_{regs} in vivo, lowering the threshold for disease induction, and PD-1 expression contributes to the conversion of naïve myelin-specific CD4+ T cells into T_{regs} in vitro, correlating with their suppressive activity (Wang et al. 2010).

Single-nucleotide polymorphisms (SNPs) in the Pdcd-1 gene that encodes PD-1 have been associated with several autoimmune diseases including MS (Kasagi et al. 2011). The only SNP associated with MS is the regulatory SNP PD1.3A that increases the probability of disease progression in MS (Kroner et al. 2005). This SNP is also associated with increased susceptibility to diseases such as systemic lupus erythematosus (SLE), diabetes, and rheumatoid arthritis (Kasagi et al. 2011).

The PD1.3A polymorphism is not associated with a measurable change in expression of PD-1 on T cells, but functional experiments showed that PD-1-mediated inhibition of IFN-γ secretion is impaired in patients carrying the mutated allele, which could result in continuous activation of self-reactive T-cells perpetuating CNS inflammation (Kroner et al. 2005).

A few studies have analyzed the expression of PD-1 and its ligands in patients with MS, suggesting that PD-1 and PD-L1 may be involved in controlling disease activity. Relative expression of PD-1 and PD-L1 was lower in total PBMCs from MS patients compared to healthy controls (Javan et al. 2016). The expression of PD-1 was significantly increased in MBP-stimulated T cells from MS patients with stable disease compared to patients with active disease, and the expression of PD-L1 was increased in B cells and monocytes from the same patients (Trabattoni et al. 2009). Interestingly, a large proportion of CD8+ T cells identified within MS lesions did not express PD-1 and are hence resistant to regulation through PD-L1 (Pittet et al. 2011). Treatment with IFN-β resulted in increased expression of PD-L1 and PD-L2 on monocytes as well as PD-L1 on CD4+ T cells both in vivo and in vitro (Schreiner et al. 2008; Wiesemann et al. 2008), and an upregulation of PD-L2 was associated with treatment response to IFN-β in a small cohort of MS patients (Wiesemann et al. 2008).

9.3.3 TIGIT/CD226

A more recently defined network of costimulatory molecules with similarities to the CD28/CTLA-4/CD80/CD86 family is the TIGIT (T-cell immunoreceptor with Ig and ITIM domains)/CD226/CD112/CD155 network (Anderson et al. 2016). Both TIGIT and CD226 are expressed on NK cells, effector and memory T cells, and T_{regs} and share the two ligands CD112 and CD155 that are expressed by APCs, T cells, and a variety of non-hematopoietic cells including tumor cells. In analogy with CTLA-4, TIGIT binds to its ligands with higher affinity than CD226 and provides an inhibitory signal, while CD226 acts as a costimulatory molecule for T cells.

Transgenic mice expressing TIGIT on T and B cells and mice treated with a TIGIT agonist are protected from EAE (Levin et al. 2011), while TIGIT-deficient mice are susceptible to EAE and display higher frequencies of encephalitogenic T cells and higher levels of proinflammatory cytokines (Joller et al. 2011; Levin et al. 2011). TIGIT-deficient mice developed spontaneous atypical EAE, characterized by neurological symptoms similar to those associated with Th17-driven EAE (Jäger et al. 2009) when crossed with MOG35-55-specific TCR transgenic 2D2 mice, suggesting that TIGIT is involved in regulating the threshold of T-cell activation and is important in maintaining peripheral tolerance (Joller et al. 2011). In addition to a direct inhibitory effect on T-cell activation and expansion (Joller et al. 2011; Levin et al. 2011; Lozano et al. 2012), TIGIT also inhibits immune responses by inducing tolerogenic DCs that secrete more IL-10 and less IL-12p40, by inhibiting cytotoxicity in NK cells, and by promoting T_{reg}-mediated suppression through the induction of IL-10 and Fgl2 that selectively suppresses Th1 and Th17 responses (Stanietsky et al. 2009; Anderson et al. 2016).

Little is known about the role of TIGIT in MS, but preliminary data indicate that TIGIT is present in mononuclear cell infiltrates in glioblastoma multiforme while it is nearly absent from inflammatory MS lesions (Lowther et al. 2015). In contrast, CD226 and CD155 were detected in glioblastoma infiltrates and in MS lesions suggesting that TIGIT may be a checkpoint inhibitor for tumor evasion in the CNS, while lack of TIGIT may aggravate MS.

Genome-wide association studies have shown an association of the Gly307Ser SNP in the CD226 gene with MS susceptibility (Hafler et al. 2009). Using several large-scale expression quantitative trait loci (eQTL) datasets, a correlation between the MS risk haplotype rs763361[T] and reduced CD226 expression was observed in PBMCs and brain tissue (Liu et al. 2017a). Interestingly, more in-depth characterization of the CD226 genetic variant showed that healthy subjects carrying the MS risk haplotype had reduced CD226 expression on T cells, while MS patients had a CD226 expression level comparable to the risk haplotype and showed no haplotype-dependent differences (Piedavent-Salomon et al. 2015). CD226 promotes Th1 and Th17 responses and suppresses Th2 function, and blockade of CD226 delayed the onset and reduced the reduced severity of EAE (Dardalhon et al. 2005; Lozano et al. 2013; Zhang et al. 2016), raising the question how reduced expression of CD226 is associated with increased risk of MS. The answer to this apparent contradiction may be related to CD226 expression on T_{regs}, as CD226 is highly expressed in IL10-producing Tr1 cells as well as in classical Foxp3+ T_{regs} (Gagliani et al. 2013; Koyama et al. 2013). CD226-deficient T_{regs} showed reduced inhibitory activity, which was associated with an exacerbated course of EAE in CD226-deficient mice (Piedavent-Salomon et al. 2015). Similar to the situation with CTLA-4, treatment with anti-CD226 antibodies may predominantly affect effector T cells with high CD226 expression, while CD226-deficient mice may more accurately reflect the genetically encoded reduced CD226 expression observed in humans (Piedavent-Salomon et al. 2015).

CD226 and its two ligands also play an important role in NK cell-mediated lysis of activated T cells (de Andrade et al. 2014). Antigen-activated T cells induce cytolytic activity in NK cells, a process that is dependent on CD155 (Gross et al. 2016). NK cells derived from MS patients exhibited reduced cytolytic activity in response to antigen-activated T cells due to reduced expression of CD226 on NK cells, which increases the threshold for NK cell activation, at the same time as their CD4+ T cells failed to upregulate CD155 upon antigen activation (Gross et al. 2016). Treatment with daclizumab, a humanized anti-CD25 antibody previously used for the treatment of MS but now removed from the market because of unexpected complications, resulted in increased expression of CD155 on CD4+ T cells and restored cytolytic activity of NK cells (Gross et al. 2016).

9.3.4 LAG-3

Lymphocyte activation gene-3 (LAG-3) is a coinhibitory receptor that is expressed by activated T cells, NK cells, B cells, and plasmacytoid DCs (Sierro et al. 2011; Anderson et al. 2016). LAG-3 negatively regulates proliferation and activation of T cells, while being crucial for T_{reg} suppression. LAG-3-deficient mice do not spontaneously develop autoimmunity but display augmented disease in susceptible strains.

A recent study showed that CD4+ intraepithelial lymphocytes (IELs) isolated from the gut epithelium of MOG35-55 TCR transgenic mice can inhibit EAE on transfer (Kadowaki et al. 2016). These cells express immune regulatory molecules such as LAG-3, CTLA-4, and TGF-β and can inhibit T-cell proliferation in vitro by a mechanism dependent on these molecules. LAG-3-blocking antibodies increased the severity of EAE induced by MOG35-55 TCR transgenic IELs. Interestingly, these regulatory IELs were influenced by stimuli from the gut environment, such as the microbiota and aryl hydrocarbon receptor (AHR) ligands in the diet providing a mechanism for how the gut microbiome can control extraintestinal autoimmune diseases such as MS.

9.3.5 Tim-3

T-cell immunoglobulin and mucin domain 3 (Tim-3) is an inhibitory receptor that triggers apoptosis upon interaction with its ligand, galectin-9 (Gal-9) (Anderson et al. 2016). Tim-3 is highly expressed by terminally activated Th1 cells, expressed at lower levels on Th17 cells, and is absent on naïve T cells and Th2 cells (Hastings et al. 2009). In addition, Tim-3 is constitutively expressed by DCs and microglia (Anderson et al. 2007). Tim-3 is an inhibitory molecule regulating peripheral tolerance and the expansion of effector Th1 cells, preventing uncontrolled inflammation. It can be protective in autoimmunity, but has been more extensively studied in cancer and chronic viral infections, where it contributes to the dampening of protective immunity (Anderson et al. 2016).

Tim-3-positive cells accumulate in the CNS of mice with EAE and peak at the onset of clinical symptoms (Monney et al. 2002; Anderson et al. 2007). Administration of an anti-Tim-3 antibody during EAE induction resulted in hyperacute disease with high numbers of activated macrophages, increased numbers of inflammatory foci in the CNS, and increased mortality (Monney et al. 2002), and blockade of Tim-3 signaling resulted in hyperproliferation of Th1 cells, increased release of IFN-γ and IL-2, and lack of antigen-specific tolerance (Sabatos et al. 2003). Along the same line, silencing of Gal-9 with siRNA exacerbated EAE, while in vivo administration of Gal-9 resulted in selective loss of IFN-γ-producing cells, attenuated Th1 responses, and ameliorated EAE (Zhu et al. 2005). More recent data suggest that interfering with the Tim-3–Gal-9 axis in CD4+ T cells changes the pattern of inflammation in the brain and spinal cord due to differential effects on Th1 versus Th17 cells (Lee and Goverman 2013). As Tim-3 signaling predominantly controls the expansion of pathogenic IFN-γ-secreting Th1 cells, blockade of Tim-3 in Th1-mediated EAE exacerbates disease severity, while blockade in Th17-mediated EAE selectively increases the survival of Th1 cells, changing the ratio of Th1/Th17 cells and resulting in decreased inflammation in the brain, but not in the spinal cord.

Evidence suggests that CD4+ T cells from MS patients have a reduced ability to upregulate Tim-3 upon stimulation (Koguchi et al. 2006; Yang et al. 2008). CD4+ T-cell clones generated from the cerebrospinal fluid (CSF) of MS patients expressed less Tim-3 than clones from controls, and this was associated with higher levels of IFN-γ production (Koguchi et al. 2006). Th1 polarization increased IFN-γ secretion in clones from MS patients, but this was associated with a relative inability to upregulate Tim-3. Similarly, Tim-3 blockade during ex vivo activation of CD4+ T cells from peripheral blood of controls enhanced IFN-γ secretion, but had no effect on CD4+ T cells from untreated MS patients (Yang et al. 2008). Interestingly, treatment of MS patients with the disease-modifying drugs IFN-β and glatiramer acetate restored the expression and function of Tim-3 (Yang et al. 2008).

MS patients with a benign course have increased expression of Tim-3 and Gal-9 in MBP-stimulated CD4+ T cells isolated from peripheral blood compared to other forms of MS, resulting in an augmented death rate of MBP-specific CD4+ T cells, while PPMS patients had reduced expression of the same two molecules (Saresella et al. 2014). Furthermore, patients with benign MS had decreased expression of Bat3 (HLA-B-associated transcript 3), a repressor of Tim-3 that protects Th1 cells from Gal-9-mediated cell death and facilitates the development of EAE (Rangachari et al. 2012), in MBP-stimulated CD4+ T cells, while Bat3 expression was increased in PPMS (Saresella et al. 2014).

High CSF levels of Gal-9 have been observed in two independent cohorts of SPMS patients when compared to RRMS patients (Burman and Svenningsson 2016). Gal-9 levels did not correlate with markers of adaptive immunity, and it was suggested that they were driven by cells of the innate immune system within the CNS such as activated astrocytes in chronically active white matter lesions (Anderson et al. 2007).

9.3.6 ICOS

Inducible T-cell costimulator (ICOS) is a costimulatory molecule structurally and genetically related to CD28 and CTLA-4 (Wikenheiser and Stumhofer 2016). It is not constitutively expressed on resting T cells, but is rapidly induced on CD4+ and CD8+ T cells following TCR cross-linking or CD28 activation. ICOS binds to the ICOS ligand (ICOSL) that is expressed on APCs and also on non-lymphoid cells such as fibroblasts, endothelial cells, and some epithelial cells. Like CD28, ICOS has positive costimulatory activities, including enhanced cytokine production, upregulation of CD40L expression, and providing help for Ig isotype class switching by B cells.

The role for ICOS signaling in EAE is complex. ICOS-deficient mice develop a severe form of EAE, characterized by massive CNS infiltrates even when induced on a genetically resistant background (Dong et al. 2001). Blockade of the ICOS–ICOSL interaction during the priming phase (1–10 days p.i.) exacerbated EAE, while blockade during the effector phase (9–20 days p.i.) attenuated the disease (Rottman et al. 2001). Effector and memory T cells have different costimulatory requirements, and blockade of ICOSL reduced memory cell-induced EAE but worsened effector cell-mediated disease (Elyaman et al. 2008). ICOS plays an important role in inducing the production of IL-10, a key immunoregulatory cytokine involved in the induction of regulatory T type 1 (Tr1) cells, and it is likely that the effects of ICOS blockade in EAE are related to impairment of the generation or function of IL-10-producing regulatory cells (Sporici et al. 2001; Greve et al. 2004; Rojo et al. 2008). ICOSL is upregulated in tissues in response to inflammatory cytokines, and the ICOS/ICOSL system may dampen immune activation in EAE and contribute to terminating the inflammation. This was further supported in studies of mucosal tolerance in EAE, where ICOS-deficient mice were resistant to the induction of mucosal tolerance to myelin peptides (Miyamoto et al. 2005), a process where IL-10-producing Tr1 cells are of crucial importance (Weiner et al. 2011).

It is also possible that other cell types are affected by ICOS/ICOSL signaling. Evidence suggest that helminth-infected MS patients have reduced disease activity (Correale and Farez 2007), which has been linked to the induction of IL-10-producing regulatory B cells through a mechanism mediated at least in part by the ICOS/ICOSL pathway (Correale et al. 2008). T cells expressing the invariant $V\alpha19i$ chain inhibited both the induction and progression of EAE through reduced production of inflammatory cytokines and increased secretion of IL-10 by B cells, a process that could be blocked by anti-ICOSL antibodies (Croxford et al. 2006).

Recent studies in patients with MS have focused on ICOS+ Tfh cells. Tfh cells play a fundamental role in humoral immunity by providing help for germinal center (GC) formation, B-cell differentiation into plasma cells, and antibody production in secondary lymphoid tissues (Fan et al. 2015b). RR and SPMS patients have increased frequencies of activated ICOS+ Tfh cells in peripheral blood compared to healthy controls (Romme Christensen et al. 2013), and the frequencies of ICOS+CCR7+ memory Tfh cells were further increased in MS patients examined during exacerbation (Fan et al. 2015a). The frequency of ICOS+ Tfh cells correlated with disease progression in progressive patients and with number of plasmablasts, suggesting that ICOS+ Tfh cells may play a role in B-cell activation (Romme Christensen et al. 2013).

9.3.7 CD40

CD40 is a member of the tumor necrosis factor (TNF) receptor family that is constitutively expressed by APCs, including DCs, B cells, and macrophages, and that can be expressed by endothelial cells, smooth muscle cells, fibroblasts, and epithelial cells (Chatzigeorgiou et al. 2009). CD40 binds to one ligand, CD40L (CD154) that is mainly expressed on activated T cells, but other cells such as endothelial cells, microglia, and astrocytes can be induced to express CD40L. CD40 was originally identified as a costimulatory molecule important in T-cell-mediated B-cell activation and differentiation, but signaling through CD40 also stimulates cells to produce cytokines and chemokines and express adhesion molecules, costimulatory molecules, and various enzymes, all of which are involved in the local inflammatory processes taking place during chronic inflammation (reviewed by (Chatzigeorgiou et al. 2009)).

Both CD40 and CD40L can be detected in the CNS of mice with EAE, and their expression correlates with disease activity and production of IFN-γ (Issazadeh et al. 1998). Mice without functional CD40/CD40L signaling due to genetic deletion of CD40L or treatment with antagonistic anti-CD40L antibodies during the priming stage are resistant to EAE, while treatment during the peak of disease or during remission reduces the severity of EAE (Grewal et al. 1996; Gerritse et al. 1996; Howard et al. 1999; Howard and Miller 2001; Becher et al. 2001). This was initially believed to be due to an inability of APCs to upregulate the expression of CD80/CD86 and produce IL-12, which is necessary for Th1 differentiation during the priming phase (Grewal et al. 1996; Constantinescu et al. 1999). Later studies revealed that even though encephalitogenic T cells were generated in CD40L-treated mice and were able to enter the CNS, the expansion and retention of these cells were impaired (Howard and Miller 2001). Using bone-marrow chimeras, it was demonstrated that mice lacking CD40 expression on CNS-resident microglia developed less severe EAE with reduced number of inflammatory cell infiltrates in the CNS (Becher et al. 2001; Ponomarev et al. 2006). This was associated with an inability of encephalitogenic T cells to fully activate microglia, blocking their ability to upregulate CD80/CD86 expression and to present CNS antigens to T cells (Ponomarev et al. 2006). Interestingly, CD40-deficient microglia were able to achieve an intermediary stage of activation with increased MHC class II expression, but in the absence of CD80/CD86 co-stimulation, these cells may trigger a tolerogenic signal resulting in downmodulation of CNS infiltration. A more recent study showed that MHC class II+CD40^{dim}CD86^{dim}IL-10+ microglia are potent inducers of antigen-specific CD4+Foxp3+ T_{regs} in vitro and that blocking CD40/CD40L signaling resulted in reduced numbers of CD25+Foxp3- effector cells, but did not affect the number of CD25+Foxp3+ T_{regs} (Ebner et al. 2013).

CD40 and CD40L immunoreactivity has been detected in close proximity to each other in perivascular infiltrates in active MS lesions (Gerritse et al. 1996). MS patients have higher frequencies of CD40L+ T cells in blood compared to controls, with levels decreasing during IFN-β treatment (Teleshova et al. 2000; Jensen et al. 2001; Filion et al. 2003). MS patients also have an increased frequency of a subset of CD4+ T cells expressing CD40 compared to healthy subjects and controls with non-autoimmune diseases (Waid et al. 2014). These cells displayed a CD45RO[hi] phenotype, recognized myelin peptides, and produced both IFN-γ and IL-17 consistent with an autoaggressive effector phenotype. PBMCs from SPMS, but not RRMS, patients produced more IL-12 and IFN-γ when restimulated in vitro, a process which was dependent on CD40/CD40L signaling (Balashov et al. 1997).

Although CD40 is of vital importance for B-cell development, little is known about effects of CD40/CD40L blockade on the B-cell compartment in EAE. B10 cells constitute a small subset of regulatory B cells that inhibit antigen-specific inflammatory reactions through IL-10 secretion (Yanaba et al. 2008). These cells are dependent on IL-21 and CD40 for their development and expansion and can inhibit EAE when transferred into mice with established autoimmune disease (Yoshizaki et al. 2012). Memory B cells from MS patients respond with enhanced proliferation when stimulated with low-dose CD40L compared to healthy subjects (Ireland et al. 2014). This hyperresponsiveness to CD40 signaling in B cells was associated with dysregulation of the canonical NF-kB pathway in MS patients (Chen et al. 2016) and was normalized in patients treated with glatiramer acetate (Ireland et al. 2014). One study reported increased frequencies of CD40+ B cells in RRMS and patients with a clinically isolated syndrome representing very early MS, especially around the time of a relapse (Mathias et al. 2017), but another study reported decreased frequencies of CD40+ B cells in RRMS patients (Field et al. 2015).

CD40–1C>T (rs1883832) is a functional SNP, which has been studied extensively in different MS populations. A recent meta-analysis indicated that the rs1883832 SNP is associated with increased risk of MS (Qin et al. 2017). Intriguingly, the risk allele for MS at rs1883832 is associated with reduced expression of CD40 (Jacobson et al. 2005) suggesting a protective effect of CD40 in MS and highlighting the complexity of costimulatory pathways that can affect regulatory as well as effector cells.

9.4   Alzheimer's Disease

Alzheimer's disease (AD) is a neurodegenerative disorder distinguished from other forms of dementia by the deposition of extracellular amyloid-beta protein (Aβ) and the formation of neurofibrillary tangles. This is associated with neuronal injury and low-level inflammation characterized by chronic activation of microglia and astrocytes (Heneka et al. 2015). Aβ peptides play a central role in this process by promoting microglial activation and perpetuating the inflammatory response. Evidence suggests that signaling through CD40 is essential for Aβ-induced microglial activation in AD and that this is an early event in the disease pathogenesis. Resting microglia express only low levels of CD40 and its expression is tightly regulated under physiological conditions in the CNS (Tan et al. 1999b). Aβ treatment activates cultured microglia, and this is enhanced in the presence of inflammatory mediators (Meda et al. 1995). Aβ-induced microglial activation upregulated the expression of CD40 in vitro (Tan et al. 1999a), and abundant CD40 immunoreactivity has been detected on activated microglia adjacent to Aβ-containing senile plaques within AD brains (Togo et al. 2000). CD40L-positive astrocytes within AD plaques are able to trigger CD40 signaling (Calingasan et al. 2002), which is functionally relevant since CD40L treatment of Aβ-stimulated microglia led to decreased phagocytosis of exogenous Aβ and increased production of proinflammatory cytokines (Townsend et al. 2005), as well as enhanced neuronal cell injury in coculture experiments (Tan et al. 1999a). In APPSw or PSAPP mice characterized by deposition of Aβ in the brain mimicking the pathology in AD, interference with CD40/CD40L signaling through genetic manipulation or by treatment with blocking antibodies decreases microglial activation and amyloid burden (Tan et al. 1999a; Ait-Ghezala et al. 2005). Furthermore, CD40 ligation has a direct effect on tau phosphorylation, a process contributing to the formation of neurofibrillary tangles, which is independent of Aβ pathology (Laporte et al. 2008). Taken together, the data suggests that CD40/CD40L-mediated microgliosis is pathogenic in AD and that interfering with this pathway reduces Aβ accumulation in animal models of the disease.

Aβ is also deposited in the walls of cerebral vessels resulting in degeneration of the vessel wall. Release of soluble CD40L (sCD40L) from activated platelets in damaged microvessels and its subsequent binding to CD40 expressed on the endothelial surface lead to upregulation of adhesion molecules and stimulation of endothelial release of proinflammatory cytokines (Zhang et al. 2013). sCD40L can also negatively affect endothelial regeneration (Hristov et al. 2010) further augmenting vessel damage and contributing to a potentially self-perpetuating inflammatory process.

Clinical studies have shown an association between increased levels of soluble CD40 (sCD40) or sCD40L in serum or plasma from AD patients compared to healthy subjects or controls with Parkinson's or non-AD dementia (Mocali et al. 2004; Ait-ghezala et al. 2008; Desideri et al. 2008; Buchhave et al. 2009; Yu et al. 2016). Circulating sCD40L levels correlated with disease severity and predicted disease progression using the Clinical Dementia Rating (CDR) or the Mini-Mental State Examination (MMSE) during a 2-year follow-up (Desideri et al. 2008). Baseline levels of sCD40 were elevated in patients with mild cognitive impairment (MCI), who subsequently developed AD during a follow-up period of 4–7 years, while MCI patients who had vascular dementia or remained cognitively stable did not differ from controls (Buchhave et al. 2009). Combinations of sCD40 and sCD40L together with other markers such as Aβ, apoE, and VEGF have been suggested as biomarkers in AD (Ait-ghezala et al. 2008; Yu et al. 2016).

Changes in immune cell phenotype and function in peripheral blood have also been reported in patients with AD, although it is not clear if peripheral immune cell activation is detrimental to the disease or an attempt of the immune system to reduce the effects of Aβ deposition in the brain (Gendelman and Mosley 2015). Little has been done to determine which costimulatory pathways are involved in the peripheral immune activation in AD, but two papers suggested dysregulation of PD-1 and PD-L1 (Saresella et al. 2010, 2012). Patients with AD or MCI had lower numbers of PD-1-positive CD4+ T cells and reduced PD-L1 expression on CD14+ monocytes after Aβ-stimulation of PBMCs compared to healthy controls (Saresella et al. 2012). This was associated with increased proliferation of Aβ-specific CD4+ T cells and lower number of IL-10-producing monocytes. The expression of PD-1 on T_{regs} was also changed in AD (Saresella et al. 2010). Both AD patients and patients with MCI had increased frequency of T_{regs} compared to healthy controls, but AD patients had decreased frequency of PD-1-negative T_{regs}, and functionally, T_{regs} from AD patients displayed reduced suppressive ability compared to MCI patients. Taken together, these findings suggest that AD patients have increased activation of antigen-specific T cells in the periphery, but further studies are needed to determine the functional significance of these cells and if the abnormalities of the PD-1/PD-L1 pathway are of significance.

9.5 Amyotrophic Lateral Sclerosis (ALS)

Amyotrophic lateral sclerosis (ALS) is a progressive, paralytic disorder character-ized by degeneration of motor neurons in the brain and spinal cord associated with aggregation of cytoplasmic proteins predominantly, but not exclusively, within neu-rons (Sreedharan and Brown 2013). Genetic analysis of familiar ALS cases identi-fied a large number of mutations associated with ALS and provided insights into disease pathogenesis. A significant proportion of the familial cases has mutations in the enzyme superoxide dismutase type 1 (SOD1) that causes protein misfolding and gain of toxic functions (Sau et al. 2007). This discovery has led to the development of transgenic mice expressing the mutant SOD-1, which display an ALS-like phe-notype (Gurney et al. 1994). Endogenous factors such as aggregated and misfolded proteins result in robust activation of microglia both in patients with ALS and SOD-1 mutant mice triggering an innate immune response (Puentes et al. 2016). Microglia isolated from SOD-1 mice express both potentially neuroprotective and toxic factors (Chiu et al. 2013) and can produce both pro- and anti-inflammatory cytokines (Puentes et al. 2016) showing that microglia plays a complex role in ALS.

Differential regulation of the CD40–CD40L pathway was found in SOD-1 mice during the presymptomatic stage and at symptom onset using unbiased transcrip-tome profiling (Lincecum et al. 2010). Treatment with a blocking anti-CD40L anti-body delayed paralysis onset, extended survival, and increased the number of motor neuron bodies in the spinal cord when administered before symptom onset. The mechanisms of anti-CD40L treatment remain unclear, but it was suggested that its therapeutic effects were mediated through immune modulation as anti-CD40L-treated mice had reduced numbers of infiltrating CD68+ macrophages in peripheral nerves and lower frequencies of CD8+ cytotoxic T cells in draining lymph nodes (Lincecum et al. 2010). CD40 may also have direct neurotoxic effects, as CD40 stimulation of primary spinal cord cultures caused motor neuron loss by inducing cyclooxygenase-2 (COX-2) (Okuno et al. 2004). CD40 expression is increased in reactive microglia and astrocytes in the spinal cord of SOD-1 mice (Okuno et al. 2004), and CD40 immunoreactivity is present in the spinal cord of patients with ALS (Graves et al. 2004). Further studies are needed to understand the role of costimulatory signals in ALS and whether manipulation of these pathways may be used to control neuronal loss in ALS (Puentes et al. 2016).

9.6 Parkinson's Disease

Parkinson's disease (PD) is a neurodegenerative disease where death of dopaminergic neurons in the substantia nigra leads to a movement disorder characterized by tremor, rigidity, and slowness of movement, accompanied by non-motor symptoms including dementia. PD is pathologically characterized by intracellular Lewy bodies within neurons containing aggregates of misfolded and insoluble α-synuclein (α-syn) (Kalia and Lang 2015). In addition to being toxic to neurons, misfolded α-syn can also activate microglia either through factors from stressed neurons or by direct interactions with extracellular α-syn aggregates. Secretion of proinflammatory and neurotoxic mediators by activated microglia further damage neurons causing a vicious cycle of neuroinflammation and neurodegeneration, although it is also possible that the inflammatory response triggered by microglia in some instances may provide neuroprotection (Cebrian et al. 2015). There is increasing evidence that the adaptive immune system plays an important role in PD. T cells from PD patients can respond to α-syn peptides in vitro (Sulzer et al. 2017), and microglia activated by α-syn can induce MHC class I expression on neurons rendering them susceptible to killing by CD8+ cytotoxic T cells (Cebrian et al. 2014).

CD200 and its receptor CD200R are considered key regulators of CNS inflammation through modulation of microglial activation. CD200 is highly expressed by neurons, but is also expressed by endothelial cells, astrocytes, and activated T and B cells, whereas CD200R is selectively expressed by myeloid cells (Walker and Lue 2013). CD200-deficient mice are characterized by spontaneously activated microglia and an increased susceptibility to EAE (Hoek et al. 2000), whereas mice with increased CD200 expression were protected against EAE (Chitnis et al. 2007). Taken together, it is believed that neuronal CD200 expression is actively maintaining microglia in a quiescent state through CD200R signaling (Walker and Lue 2013). Decreased expression of CD200 was observed in chronic MS lesions, which has been attributed either to neuronal damage or downregulation of CD200 due to reduced levels of anti-inflammatory cytokines such as IL-4 (Lyons et al. 2009; Koning et al. 2007). Decreased expression of CD200 and CD200R was also observed in brain regions affected by neurodegeneration in patients with AD (Walker et al. 2009).

It has been suggested that dysregulation of the CD200–CD200R axis contributes to the pathology in PD. CD200 expression is decreased with aging in the human brain (Frank et al. 2006), and monocyte-derived macrophages from older subjects including patients with PD responded to stimulation in vitro by reduced CD200R upregulation (Luo et al. 2010). Blockade of CD200R after injection with 6-hydroxydopamine into the substantia nigra in rats resulted in microglial activation associated with significantly increased loss of dopaminergic neurons and more Parkinson-like movement disorder (Zhang et al. 2011). Furthermore, CD200R blockade enhanced the susceptibility of dopaminergic neurons to rotenone-induced neurotoxicity in vitro. Microglial activation after peripheral injection of LPS in rats was associated with a reduction in the numbers of dopaminergic neurons and increased expression of CD200 and CD200R in the substantia nigra (Xie et al.

2017). Injection of a CD200 agonist (CD200Fc) into the substantia nigra reduced the loss of dopaminergic neurons after LPS injection showing a protective role of CD200/CD200R signaling in preventing neurodegeneration induced by peripheral inflammation (Xie et al. 2017). Interestingly, treadmill exercise ameliorated the motor balance and coordination dysfunction in the 1-methyl-4-phenyl-1,2,3,6-tetrahydropyridine/probenecid (MPTP/P) model of Parkinson's disease mice. Mice in the exercise group had reduced microglial activation and reduced loss of dopaminergic neurons that were associated with increased levels of CD200 and CD200R in the CNS (Sung et al. 2012). The expression of CD200 or CD200R has not been studied in the substantia nigra of patients with PD, but a recent study showed that CD200 expression was not affected in brains from patients with Lewy body dementia, a condition with cortical deposition of modified α-syn (Walker et al. 2017). While it is well established that aggregated α-syn can activate microglia in vitro (Zhang et al. 2005), it was suggested that α-syn aggregates in Lewy body dementia are mainly localized intracellularly where they are shielded from microglia (Walker et al. 2017).

It is likely that other costimulatory pathways are of important in the regulation of PD, but few studies have addressed this issue. One recent study identified LAG-3 as a major binding site for pathological α-syn by performing an unbiased screen of binding sites (Mao et al. 2016). Deletion of LAG-3 reduced the endocytosis as well as the neuron-to-neuron transmission of pathological α-syn, and this was associated with delayed α-syn-induced neurotoxicity and behavioral deficits in vivo. LAG-3 expression has previously been detected in the CNS (Workman et al. 2002), but little is known about its functions in this organ.

9.7 Ischemic Stroke

It is clear that the immune system is activated after focal cerebral ischemia and that inflammation plays a role in the outcome of ischemic stroke (Famakin 2014). The initial response after transient ischemia consists of microglial activation and rapid infiltration of innate immune cells into the ischemic tissue. Inflammatory mediators released during this initial phase results in the influx of lymphocytes and activation of adaptive immune responses. The detrimental effect of the adaptive immune responses is shown in experimental models of stroke such as middle cerebral artery occlusion (MCAO) where mice deficient in T cells (either CD4+ or CD8+) experienced a better outcome with smaller infarct volume and less neurological deficits (Yilmaz et al. 2006). The PD-1 pathway has been shown to be of importance in regulating inflammation and minimizing damage to bystander cells after ischemic stroke (Zhao et al. 2014). PD-1 expression is strongly upregulated on activated microglia and infiltrating macrophages in the ischemic hemisphere of MCAO mice, while the expression of its two ligands PD-L1 and PD-L2 was upregulated on B cells in the same areas (Ren et al. 2011). PD-1 deficient mice had worse infarct outcome with larger infarct size, enhanced microglial activation, and increased numbers of infiltrating immune cells 96 h after MCAO, but not after 24 h, consistent with a dampening effect of PD-1 signaling during the later stages of adaptive immune responses (Ren et al. 2011; Kleinschnitz et al. 2010). Transfer of IL-10-producing regulatory B cells reduced the infarct volume after MCAO by creating a less inflammatory milieu in the postischemic brain, a process that is associated with increased expression of PD-1 on infiltrating T cells and macrophages (Bodhankar et al. 2013a). In contrast, PD-L1 or PD-L2 deficient mice or mice treated with neutralizing anti-PD-L1 antibodies had smaller infarct volumes and decreased infiltration of immune cells into the ischemic hemisphere compared to WT mice (Bodhankar et al. 2015, 2013b). This was associated with migration of CD8+CD122+ regulatory T cells, a subset of naturally occurring T_{regs} cells that produce large amounts of IL-10 (Rifa'i et al. 2004), from the spleen to the ischemic lesion. While anti-PD-L1 treatment after MCAO had a beneficial effect on stroke outcome, it was also associated with increased risk of hemorrhage after reperfusion (Bodhankar et al. 2015). Neutralization of PD-L1 inhibits the ability of CD4+CD25^{hi} T_{regs} to suppress the production of matrix metalloproteinase-9 (MMP-9) from neutrophils and mice treated with PD-L1 deficient T_{regs} had enhanced BBB damage compared to mice treated with intact T_{regs} after MCAO (Li et al. 2014). PD-L1 treatment was further shown to protect against brain injury in an experimental model of intracerebral hemorrhage by shifting the inflammatory response from a Th1- and Th17-dominated response to a response dominated by Th2 and CD4+CD25+Foxp3+ T_{regs} (Han et al. 2017). In addition to this shift in inflammatory milieu, PD-L1 treatment improved BBB integrity and protected against neuronal loss. Taken together these results show the complexity of the PD-1/PD-L1 pathway and the distinct roles of different effector and regulatory cell types in controlling CNS inflammation.

9.8 Conclusions

It is clear that inflammation plays an important role in the onset and progression of many neurological diseases and that suppression of inflammation can reduce disease burden and neuronal loss in these diseases. The co-signaling pathways provide a powerful means to manipulate the immune system as was recently shown with the breakthrough of checkpoint inhibitors in the field of tumor immunology. Early studies using blocking antibodies or genetic depletion of co-signaling pathways at a systems level have been replaced with refined methods targeting specific cellular subsets highlighting the complexities of immune regulation in neurological diseases. Seemingly contradictory findings in earlier studies appear to be related to the expression of co-signaling molecules in different subpopulations of cells, shifting the balance between effector and regulatory subsets, or different effector subsets. This highlights the intricacies of the interplay between the different cells of the immune system and how they interact with the resident cells of the CNS. This complexity poses challenges when targeting co-signaling pathway to treat neurological diseases and may explain why no drugs targeting these pathways have been successfully developed this far. More studies are needed to fully understand the regulatory network within the CNS and how to harness the co-signaling pathways to limit cytotoxicity and enhance neuroprotection once an inflammatory response has been initiated. It is also intriguing to speculate if co-signaling pathways can be used to stimulate regenerative processes within the CNS, an area that currently has not been addressed at depth.

References

Ait-Ghezala G, Mathura VS, Laporte V, Quadros A, Paris D, Patel N, Volmar CH, Kolippakkam D, Crawford F, Mullan M (2005) Genomic regulation after CD40 stimulation in microglia: relevance to Alzheimer's disease. Brain Res Mol Brain Res 140(1–2):73–85. https://doi.org/10.1016/j.molbrainres.2005.07.014

Ait-ghezala G, Abdullah L, Volmar CH, Paris D, Luis CA, Quadros A, Mouzon B, Mullan MA, Keegan AP, Parrish J, Crawford FC, Mathura VS, Mullan MJ (2008) Diagnostic utility of APOE, soluble CD40, CD40L, and Abeta1-40 levels in plasma in Alzheimer's disease. Cytokine 44(2):283–287. https://doi.org/10.1016/j.cyto.2008.08.013

Almolda B, Gonzalez B, Castellano B (2015) Are microglial cells the regulators of lymphocyte responses in the CNS? Front Cell Neurosci 9:440. https://doi.org/10.3389/fncel.2015.00440

Aloisi F, Ria F, Penna G, Adorini L (1998) Microglia are more efficient than astrocytes in antigen processing and in Th1 but not Th2 cell activation. J Immunol 160(10):4671–4680

Anderson AC, Anderson DE, Bregoli L, Hastings WD, Kassam N, Lei C, Chandwaskar R, Karman J, Su EW, Hirashima M, Bruce JN, Kane LP, Kuchroo VK, Hafler DA (2007) Promotion of tissue inflammation by the immune receptor Tim-3 expressed on innate immune cells. Science 318(5853):1141–1143. https://doi.org/10.1126/science.1148536

Anderson AC, Joller N, Kuchroo VK (2016) Lag-3, Tim-3, and TIGIT: Co-inhibitory receptors with specialized functions in immune regulation. Immunity 44(5):989–1004. https://doi.org/10.1016/j.immuni.2016.05.001

Arima T, Rehman A, Hickey WF, Flye MW (1996) Inhibition by CTLA4Ig of experimental allergic encephalomyelitis. J Immunol 156(12):4916–4924

Balashov KE, Smith DR, Khoury SJ, Hafler DA, Weiner HL (1997) Increased interleukin 12 production in progressive multiple sclerosis: induction by activated CD4+ T cells via CD40 ligand. Proc Natl Acad Sci USA 94(2):599–603

Becher B, Durell BG, Miga AV, Hickey WF, Noelle RJ (2001) The clinical course of experimental autoimmune encephalomyelitis and inflammation is controlled by the expression of CD40 within the central nervous system. J Exp Med 193(8):967–974

Bodhankar S, Chen Y, Vandenbark AA, Murphy SJ, Offner H (2013a) IL-10-producing B-cells limit CNS inflammation and infarct volume in experimental stroke. Metab Brain Dis 28(3):375–386. https://doi.org/10.1007/s11011-013-9413-3

Bodhankar S, Chen Y, Vandenbark AA, Murphy SJ, Offner H (2013b) PD-L1 enhances CNS inflammation and infarct volume following experimental stroke in mice in opposition to PD-1. J Neuroinflammation 10:111. https://doi.org/10.1186/1742-2094-10-111

Bodhankar S, Chen Y, Lapato A, Dotson AL, Wang J, Vandenbark AA, Saugstad JA, Offner H (2015) PD-L1 monoclonal antibody treats ischemic stroke by controlling central nervous system inflammation. Stroke 46(10):2926–2934. https://doi.org/10.1161/STROKEAHA.115.010592

Bretscher P, Cohn M (1970) A theory of self-nonself discrimination. Science 169(3950):1042–1049

Buchbinder EI, Desai A (2016) CTLA-4 and PD-1 pathways: similarities, differences, and implications of their inhibition. Am J Clin Oncol 39(1):98–106. https://doi.org/10.1097/COC.0000000000000239

Buchhave P, Janciauskiene S, Zetterberg H, Blennow K, Minthon L, Hansson O (2009) Elevated plasma levels of soluble CD40 in incipient Alzheimer's disease. Neurosci Lett 450(1):56–59. https://doi.org/10.1016/j.neulet.2008.10.091

Burman J, Svenningsson A (2016) Cerebrospinal fluid concentration of Galectin-9 is increased in secondary progressive multiple sclerosis. J Neuroimmunol 292:40–44. https://doi.org/10.1016/j.jneuroim.2016.01.008

Butovsky O, Jedrychowski MP, Moore CS, Cialic R, Lanser AJ, Gabriely G, Koeglsperger T, Dake B, Wu PM, Doykan CE, Fanek Z, Liu L, Chen Z, Rothstein JD, Ransohoff RM, Gygi SP, Antel JP, Weiner HL (2014) Identification of a unique TGF-beta-dependent molecular and functional signature in microglia. Nat Neurosci 17(1):131–143. https://doi.org/10.1038/nn.3599

Calingasan NY, Erdely HA, Altar CA (2002) Identification of CD40 ligand in Alzheimer's disease and in animal models of Alzheimer's disease and brain injury. Neurobiol Aging 23(1):31–39

Cao Y, Nylander A, Ramanan S, Goods BA, Ponath G, Zabad R, Chiang VL, Vortmeyer AO, Hafler DA, Pitt D (2016) CNS demyelination and enhanced myelin-reactive responses after ipilimumab treatment. Neurology 86(16):1553–1556. https://doi.org/10.1212/WNL.0000000000002594

Carter LL, Leach MW, Azoitei ML, Cui J, Pelker JW, Jussif J, Benoit S, Ireland G, Luxenberg D, Askew GR, Milarski KL, Groves C, Brown T, Carito BA, Percival K, Carreno BM, Collins M, Marusic S (2007) PD-1/PD-L1, but not PD-1/PD-L2, interactions regulate the severity of experimental autoimmune encephalomyelitis. J Neuroimmunol 182(1-2):124–134. https://doi.org/10.1016/j.jneuroim.2006.10.006

Cebrian C, Zucca FA, Mauri P, Steinbeck JA, Studer L, Scherzer CR, Kanter E, Budhu S, Mandelbaum J, Vonsattel JP, Zecca L, Loike JD, Sulzer D (2014) MHC-I expression renders catecholaminergic neurons susceptible to T-cell-mediated degeneration. Nat Commun 5:3633. https://doi.org/10.1038/ncomms4633

Cebrian C, Loike JD, Sulzer D (2015) Neuroinflammation in Parkinson's disease animal models: a cell stress response or a step in neurodegeneration? Curr Top Behav Neurosci 22:237–270. https://doi.org/10.1007/7854_2014_356

Chastain EM, Duncan DS, Rodgers JM, Miller SD (2011) The role of antigen presenting cells in multiple sclerosis. Biochim Biophys Acta 1812(2):265–274. https://doi.org/10.1016/j.bbadis.2010.07.008

Chatzigeorgiou A, Lyberi M, Chatzilymperis G, Nezos A, Kamper E (2009) CD40/CD40L signaling and its implication in health and disease. Biofactors 35(6):474–483. https://doi.org/10.1002/biof.62

Chavarria A, Cardenas G (2013) Neuronal influence behind the central nervous system regulation of the immune cells. Front Integr Neurosci 7:64. https://doi.org/10.3389/fnint.2013.00064

Chen L (2004) Co-inhibitory molecules of the B7-CD28 family in the control of T-cell immunity. Nat Rev Immunol 4(5):336–347. https://doi.org/10.1038/nri1349

Chen D, Ireland SJ, Remington G, Alvarez E, Racke MK, Greenberg B, Frohman EM, Monson NL (2016) CD40-mediated NF-kappaB activation in B cells is increased in multiple sclerosis and modulated by therapeutics. J Immunol 197(11):4257–4265. https://doi.org/10.4049/jimmunol.1600782

Chitnis T, Imitola J, Wang Y, Elyaman W, Chawla P, Sharuk M, Raddassi K, Bronson RT, Khoury SJ (2007) Elevated neuronal expression of CD200 protects Wlds mice from inflammation-mediated neurodegeneration. Am J Pathol 170(5):1695–1712. https://doi.org/10.2353/ajpath.2007.060677

Chiu AS, Gehringer MM, Braidy N, Guillemin GJ, Welch JH, Neilan BA (2013) Gliotoxicity of the cyanotoxin, beta-methyl-amino-L-alanine (BMAA). Sci Rep 3:1482. https://doi.org/10.1038/srep01482

Constantinescu CS, Hilliard B, Wysocka M, Ventura ES, Bhopale MK, Trinchieri G, Rostami AM (1999) IL-12 reverses the suppressive effect of the CD40 ligand blockade on experimental autoimmune encephalomyelitis (EAE). J Neurol Sci 171(1):60–64

Correale J, Farez M (2007) Association between parasite infection and immune responses in multiple sclerosis. Ann Neurol 61(2):97–108. https://doi.org/10.1002/ana.21067

Correale J, Farez M, Razzitte G (2008) Helminth infections associated with multiple sclerosis induce regulatory B cells. Ann Neurol 64(2):187–199. https://doi.org/10.1002/ana.21438

Cross AH, Ku G (2000) Astrocytes and central nervous system endothelial cells do not express B7-1 (CD80) or B7-2 (CD86) immunoreactivity during experimental autoimmune encephalomyelitis. J Neuroimmunol 110(1-2):76–82

Cross AH, San M, Keeling RM, Karr RW (1999) CTLA-4-Fc treatment of ongoing EAE improves recovery, but has no effect upon relapse rate. Implications for the mechanisms involved in disease perpetuation. J Neuroimmunol 96(2):144–147

Croxford JL, Miyake S, Huang YY, Shimamura M, Yamamura T (2006) Invariant V(alpha)19i T cells regulate autoimmune inflammation. Nat Immunol 7(9):987–994. https://doi.org/10.1038/ni1370

Dardalhon V, Schubart AS, Reddy J, Meyers JH, Monney L, Sabatos CA, Ahuja R, Nguyen K, Freeman GJ, Greenfield EA, Sobel RA, Kuchroo VK (2005) CD226 is specifically expressed on the surface of Th1 cells and regulates their expansion and effector functions. J Immunol 175(3):1558–1565

de Andrade LF, Smyth MJ, Martinet L (2014) DNAM-1 control of natural killer cells functions through nectin and nectin-like proteins. Immunol Cell Biol 92(3):237–244. https://doi.org/10.1038/icb.2013.95

Dendrou CA, Fugger L, Friese MA (2015) Immunopathology of multiple sclerosis. Nat Rev Immunol 15(9):545–558. https://doi.org/10.1038/nri3871

Desideri G, Cipollone F, Necozione S, Marini C, Lechiara MC, Taglieri G, Zuliani G, Fellin R, Mezzetti A, di Orio F, Ferri C (2008) Enhanced soluble CD40 ligand and Alzheimer's disease: evidence of a possible pathogenetic role. Neurobiol Aging 29(3):348–356. https://doi.org/10.1016/j.neurobiolaging.2006.10.019

Dong C, Juedes AE, Temann UA, Shresta S, Allison JP, Ruddle NH, Flavell RA (2001) ICOS co-stimulatory receptor is essential for T-cell activation and function. Nature 409(6816):97–101. https://doi.org/10.1038/35051100

Eagar TN, Karandikar NJ, Bluestone JA, Miller SD (2002) The role of CTLA-4 in induction and maintenance of peripheral T cell tolerance. Eur J Immunol 32(4):972–981. https://doi.org/10.1002/1521-4141(200204)32:4<972::AID-IMMU972>3.0.CO;2-M

Ebner F, Brandt C, Thiele P, Richter D, Schliesser U, Siffrin V, Schueler J, Stubbe T, Ellinghaus A, Meisel C, Sawitzki B, Nitsch R (2013) Microglial activation milieu controls regulatory T cell responses. J Immunol 191(11):5594–5602. https://doi.org/10.4049/jimmunol.1203331

Elyaman W, Kivisäkk P, Reddy J, Chitnis T, Raddassi K, Imitola J, Bradshaw E, Kuchroo VK, Yagita H, Sayegh MH, Khoury SJ (2008) Distinct functions of autoreactive memory and effector CD4+ T cells in experimental autoimmune encephalomyelitis. Am J Pathol 173(2):411–422. https://doi.org/10.2353/ajpath.2008.080142

Esensten JH, Helou YA, Chopra G, Weiss A, Bluestone JA (2016) CD28 costimulation: from mechanism to therapy. Immunity 44(5):973–988. https://doi.org/10.1016/j.immuni.2016.04.020

Famakin BM (2014) The immune response to acute focal cerebral ischemia and associated post-stroke immunodepression: a focused review. Aging Dis 5(5):307–326. https://doi.org/10.14336/AD.2014.0500307

Fan X, Jin T, Zhao S, Liu C, Han J, Jiang X, Jiang Y (2015a) Circulating CCR7+ICOS+ memory T follicular helper cells in patients with multiple sclerosis. PLoS One 10(7):e0134523. https://doi.org/10.1371/journal.pone.0134523

Fan X, Lin C, Han J, Jiang X, Zhu J, Jin T (2015b) Follicular helper CD4+ T cells in human neuroautoimmune diseases and their animal models. Mediators Inflamm 2015:638968. https://doi.org/10.1155/2015/638968

Field J, Shahijanian F, Schibeci S, Australia, New Zealand MSGC, Johnson L, Gresle M, Laverick L, Parnell G, Stewart G, McKay F, Kilpatrick T, Butzkueven H, Booth D (2015) The MS risk allele of CD40 is associated with reduced cell-membrane bound expression in antigen presenting cells: implications for gene function. PLoS One 10(6):e0127080. https://doi.org/10.1371/journal.pone.0127080

Fife BT, Bluestone JA (2008) Control of peripheral T-cell tolerance and autoimmunity via the CTLA-4 and PD-1 pathways. Immunol Rev 224:166–182. https://doi.org/10.1111/j.1600-065X.2008.00662.x

Filion LG, Matusevicius D, Graziani-Bowering GM, Kumar A, Freedman MS (2003) Monocyte-derived IL12, CD86 (B7-2) and CD40L expression in relapsing and progressive multiple sclerosis. Clin Immunol 106(2):127–138

Frank MG, Barrientos RM, Biedenkapp JC, Rudy JW, Watkins LR, Maier SF (2006) mRNA upregulation of MHC II and pivotal pro-inflammatory genes in normal brain aging. Neurobiol Aging 27(5):717–722. https://doi.org/10.1016/j.neurobiolaging.2005.03.013

Gagliani N, Magnani CF, Huber S, Gianolini ME, Pala M, Licona-Limon P, Guo B, Herbert DR, Bulfone A, Trentini F, Di Serio C, Bacchetta R, Andreani M, Brockmann L, Gregori S, Flavell RA, Roncarolo MG (2013) Coexpression of CD49b and LAG-3 identifies human and mouse T regulatory type 1 cells. Nat Med 19(6):739–746. https://doi.org/10.1038/nm.3179

Gendelman HE, Mosley RL (2015) A perspective on roles played by innate and adaptive immunity in the pathobiology of neurodegenerative disorders. J Neuroimmune Pharmacol 10(4):645–650. https://doi.org/10.1007/s11481-015-9639-4

Genovese MC, Becker JC, Schiff M, Luggen M, Sherrer Y, Kremer J, Birbara C, Box J, Natarajan K, Nuamah I, Li T, Aranda R, Hagerty DT, Dougados M (2005) Abatacept for rheumatoid arthritis refractory to tumor necrosis factor alpha inhibition. N Engl J Med 353(11):1114–1123. https://doi.org/10.1056/NEJMoa050524

Gerdes LA, Held K, Beltran E, Berking C, Prinz JC, Junker A, Tietze JK, Ertl-Wagner B, Straube A, Kumpfel T, Dornmair K, Hohlfeld R (2016) CTLA4 as immunological checkpoint in the development of multiple sclerosis. Ann Neurol 80(2):294–300. https://doi.org/10.1002/ana.24715

Gerritse K, Laman JD, Noelle RJ, Aruffo A, Ledbetter JA, Boersma WJ, Claassen E (1996) CD40-CD40 ligand interactions in experimental allergic encephalomyelitis and multiple sclerosis. Proc Natl Acad Sci USA 93(6):2499–2504

Gettings EJ, Hackett CT, Scott TF (2015) Severe relapse in a multiple sclerosis patient associated with ipilimumab treatment of melanoma. Mult Scler 21(5):670. https://doi.org/10.1177/1352458514549403

Gimsa U, ØRen A, Pandiyan P, Teichmann D, Bechmann I, Nitsch R, Brunner-Weinzierl MC (2004) Astrocytes protect the CNS: antigen-specific T helper cell responses are inhibited by astrocyte-induced upregulation of CTLA-4 (CD152). J Mol Med (Berl) 82(6):364–372. https://doi.org/10.1007/s00109-004-0531-6

Graves MC, Fiala M, Dinglasan LA, Liu NQ, Sayre J, Chiappelli F, van Kooten C, Vinters HV (2004) Inflammation in amyotrophic lateral sclerosis spinal cord and brain is mediated by activated macrophages, mast cells and T cells. Amyotroph Lateral Scler Other Motor Neuron Disord 5(4):213–219

Greve B, Vijayakrishnan L, Kubal A, Sobel RA, Peterson LB, Wicker LS, Kuchroo VK (2004) The diabetes susceptibility locus Idd5.1 on mouse chromosome 1 regulates ICOS expression and modulates murine experimental autoimmune encephalomyelitis. J Immunol 173(1):157–163

Grewal IS, Foellmer HG, Grewal KD, Xu J, Hardardottir F, Baron JL, Janeway CA Jr, Flavell RA (1996) Requirement for CD40 ligand in costimulation induction, T cell activation, and experimental allergic encephalomyelitis. Science 273(5283):1864–1867

Gross CC, Schulte-Mecklenbeck A, Runzi A, Kuhlmann T, Posevitz-Fejfar A, Schwab N, Schneider-Hohendorf T, Herich S, Held K, Konjevic M, Hartwig M, Dornmair K, Hohlfeld R, Ziemssen T, Klotz L, Meuth SG, Wiendl H (2016) Impaired NK-mediated regulation of T-cell activity in multiple sclerosis is reconstituted by IL-2 receptor modulation. Proc Natl Acad Sci USA 113(21):E2973–E2982. https://doi.org/10.1073/pnas.1524924113

Gurney ME, Pu H, Chiu AY, Dal Canto MC, Polchow CY, Alexander DD, Caliendo J, Hentati A, Kwon YW, Deng HX et al (1994) Motor neuron degeneration in mice that express a human Cu,Zn superoxide dismutase mutation. Science 264(5166):1772–1775

Hafler JP, Maier LM, Cooper JD, Plagnol V, Hinks A, Simmonds MJ, Stevens HE, Walker NM, Healy B, Howson JM, Maisuria M, Duley S, Coleman G, Gough SC, International Multiple Sclerosis Genetics C, Worthington J, Kuchroo VK, Wicker LS, Todd JA (2009) CD226 Gly307Ser association with multiple autoimmune diseases. Genes Immun 10(1):5–10. https://doi.org/10.1038/gene.2008.82

Han R, Luo J, Shi Y, Yao Y, Hao J (2017) PD-L1 (Programmed Death Ligand 1) protects against experimental intracerebral hemorrhage-induced brain injury. Stroke 48(8):2255–2262. https://doi.org/10.1161/STROKEAHA.117.016705

Hastings WD, Anderson DE, Kassam N, Koguchi K, Greenfield EA, Kent SC, Zheng XX, Strom TB, Hafler DA, Kuchroo VK (2009) TIM-3 is expressed on activated human CD4+ T cells and regulates Th1 and Th17 cytokines. Eur J Immunol 39(9):2492–2501. https://doi.org/10.1002/eji.200939274

Heneka MT, Carson MJ, El Khoury J, Landreth GE, Brosseron F, Feinstein DL, Jacobs AH, Wyss-Coray T, Vitorica J, Ransohoff RM, Herrup K, Frautschy SA, Finsen B, Brown GC, Verkhratsky A, Yamanaka K, Koistinaho J, Latz E, Halle A, Petzold GC, Town T, Morgan D, Shinohara ML, Perry VH, Holmes C, Bazan NG, Brooks DJ, Hunot S, Joseph B, Deigendesch N, Garaschuk O, Boddeke E, Dinarello CA, Breitner JC, Cole GM, Golenbock DT, Kummer MP (2015) Neuroinflammation in Alzheimer's disease. Lancet Neurol 14(4):388–405. https://doi.org/10.1016/S1474-4422(15)70016-5

Hodi FS, O'Day SJ, McDermott DF, Weber RW, Sosman JA, Haanen JB, Gonzalez R, Robert C, Schadendorf D, Hassel JC, Akerley W, van den Eertwegh AJ, Lutzky J, Lorigan P, Vaubel JM, Linette GP, Hogg D, Ottensmeier CH, Lebbe C, Peschel C, Quirt I, Clark JI, Wolchok JD, Weber JS, Tian J, Yellin MJ, Nichol GM, Hoos A, Urba WJ (2010) Improved survival with ipilimumab in patients with metastatic melanoma. N Engl J Med 363(8):711–723. https://doi.org/10.1056/NEJMoa1003466

Hoek RM, Ruuls SR, Murphy CA, Wright GJ, Goddard R, Zurawski SM, Blom B, Homola ME, Streit WJ, Brown MH, Barclay AN, Sedgwick JD (2000) Down-regulation of the macrophage lineage through interaction with OX2 (CD200). Science 290(5497):1768–1771

Howard LM, Miller SD (2001) Autoimmune intervention by CD154 blockade prevents T cell retention and effector function in the target organ. J Immunol 166(3):1547–1553

Howard LM, Miga AJ, Vanderlugt CL, Dal Canto MC, Laman JD, Noelle RJ, Miller SD (1999) Mechanisms of immunotherapeutic intervention by anti-CD40L (CD154) antibody in an animal model of multiple sclerosis. J Clin Invest 103(2):281–290. https://doi.org/10.1172/JCI5388

Hristov M, Gumbel D, Lutgens E, Zernecke A, Weber C (2010) Soluble CD40 ligand impairs the function of peripheral blood angiogenic outgrowth cells and increases neointimal formation after arterial injury. Circulation 121(2):315–324. https://doi.org/10.1161/CIRCULATIONAHA.109.862771

Hurwitz AA, Sullivan TJ, Krummel MF, Sobel RA, Allison JP (1997) Specific blockade of CTLA-4/B7 interactions results in exacerbated clinical and histologic disease in an actively-induced model of experimental allergic encephalomyelitis. J Neuroimmunol 73(1-2):57–62

Ireland SJ, Guzman AA, O'Brien DE, Hughes S, Greenberg B, Flores A, Graves D, Remington G, Frohman EM, Davis LS, Monson NL (2014) The effect of glatiramer acetate therapy on functional properties of B cells from patients with relapsing-remitting multiple sclerosis. JAMA Neurol 71(11):1421–1428. https://doi.org/10.1001/jamaneurol.2014.1472

Issazadeh S, Navikas V, Schaub M, Sayegh M, Khoury S (1998) Kinetics of expression of costimulatory molecules and their ligands in murine relapsing experimental autoimmune encephalomyelitis in vivo. J Immunol 161(3):1104–1112

Jacobson EM, Concepcion E, Oashi T, Tomer Y (2005) A Graves' disease-associated Kozak sequence single-nucleotide polymorphism enhances the efficiency of CD40 gene translation: a case for translational pathophysiology. Endocrinology 146(6):2684–2691. https://doi.org/10.1210/en.2004-1617

Jäger A, Dardalhon V, Sobel RA, Bettelli E, Kuchroo VK (2009) Th1, Th17, and Th9 effector cells induce experimental autoimmune encephalomyelitis with different pathological phenotypes. J Immunol 183(11):7169–7177. https://doi.org/10.4049/jimmunol.0901906

Javan MR, Aslani S, Zamani MR, Rostamnejad J, Asadi M, Farhoodi M, Nicknam MH (2016) Downregulation of immunosuppressive molecules, PD-1 and PD-L1 but not PD-L2, in the patients with multiple sclerosis. Iran J Allergy Asthma Immunol 15(4):296–302

Jensen J, Krakauer M, Sellebjerg F (2001) Increased T cell expression of CD154 (CD40-ligand) in multiple sclerosis. Eur J Neurol 8(4):321–328

Johnson DB, Sullivan RJ, Ott PA, Carlino MS, Khushalani NI, Ye F, Guminski A, Puzanov I, Lawrence DP, Buchbinder EI, Mudigonda T, Spencer K, Bender C, Lee J, Kaufman HL,

Menzies AM, Hassel JC, Mehnert JM, Sosman JA, Long GV, Clark JI (2016) Ipilimumab therapy in patients with advanced melanoma and preexisting autoimmune disorders. JAMA Oncol 2(2):234–240. https://doi.org/10.1001/jamaoncol.2015.4368

Joller N, Hafler JP, Brynedal B, Kassam N, Spoerl S, Levin SD, Sharpe AH, Kuchroo VK (2011) Cutting edge: TIGIT has T cell-intrinsic inhibitory functions. J Immunol 186(3):1338–1342. https://doi.org/10.4049/jimmunol.1003081

Kadowaki A, Miyake S, Saga R, Chiba A, Mochizuki H, Yamamura T (2016) Gut environment-induced intraepithelial autoreactive CD4(+) T cells suppress central nervous system autoimmunity via LAG-3. Nat Commun 7:11639. https://doi.org/10.1038/ncomms11639

Kalia LV, Lang AE (2015) Parkinson's disease. Lancet 386(9996):896–912. https://doi.org/10.1016/S0140-6736(14)61393-3

Karandikar NJ, Vanderlugt CL, Walunas TL, Miller SD, Bluestone JA (1996) CTLA-4: a negative regulator of autoimmune disease. J Exp Med 184(2):783–788

Karandikar NJ, Eagar TN, Vanderlugt CL, Bluestone JA, Miller SD (2000) CTLA-4 downregulates epitope spreading and mediates remission in relapsing experimental autoimmune encephalomyelitis. J Neuroimmunol 109(2):173–180

Kasagi S, Kawano S, Kumagai S (2011) PD-1 and autoimmunity. Crit Rev Immunol 31(4):265–295

Keir ME, Liang SC, Guleria I, Latchman YE, Qipo A, Albacker LA, Koulmanda M, Freeman GJ, Sayegh MH, Sharpe AH (2006) Tissue expression of PD-L1 mediates peripheral T cell tolerance. J Exp Med 203(4):883–895. https://doi.org/10.1084/jem.20051776

Keir ME, Francisco LM, Sharpe AH (2007) PD-1 and its ligands in T-cell immunity. Curr Opin Immunol 19(3):309–314. https://doi.org/10.1016/j.coi.2007.04.012

Khoury SJ, Gallon L, Chen W, Betres K, Russell ME, Hancock WW, Carpenter CB, Sayegh MH, Weiner HL (1995) Mechanisms of acquired thymic tolerance in experimental autoimmune encephalomyelitis: thymic dendritic-enriched cells induce specific peripheral T cell unresponsiveness in vivo. J Exp Med 182(2):357–366

Khoury SJ, Rochon J, Ding L, Byron M, Ryker K, Tosta P, Gao W, Freedman MS, Arnold DL, Sayre PH, Smilek DE, Group AS (2017) ACCLAIM: a randomized trial of abatacept (CTLA4-Ig) for relapsing-remitting multiple sclerosis. Mult Scler 23(5):686–695. https://doi.org/10.1177/1352458516662727

Kleinschnitz C, Schwab N, Kraft P, Hagedorn I, Dreykluft A, Schwarz T, Austinat M, Nieswandt B, Wiendl H, Stoll G (2010) Early detrimental T-cell effects in experimental cerebral ischemia are neither related to adaptive immunity nor thrombus formation. Blood 115(18):3835–3842. https://doi.org/10.1182/blood-2009-10-249078

Klocke K, Sakaguchi S, Holmdahl R, Wing K (2016) Induction of autoimmune disease by deletion of CTLA-4 in mice in adulthood. Proc Natl Acad Sci USA 113(17):E2383–E2392. https://doi.org/10.1073/pnas.1603892113

Klohs J, Grafe M, Graf K, Steinbrink J, Dietrich T, Stibenz D, Bahmani P, Kronenberg G, Harms C, Endres M, Lindauer U, Greger K, Stelzer EH, Dirnagl U, Wunder A (2008) In vivo imaging of the inflammatory receptor CD40 after cerebral ischemia using a fluorescent antibody. Stroke 39(10):2845–2852. https://doi.org/10.1161/STROKEAHA.107.509844

Koguchi K, Anderson DE, Yang L, O'Connor KC, Kuchroo VK, Hafler DA (2006) Dysregulated T cell expression of TIM3 in multiple sclerosis. J Exp Med 203(6):1413–1418. https://doi.org/10.1084/jem.20060210

Kong YC, Flynn JC (2014) Opportunistic autoimmune disorders potentiated by immune-checkpoint inhibitors anti-CTLA-4 and anti-PD-1. Front Immunol 5:206. https://doi.org/10.3389/fimmu.2014.00206

Koning N, Bo L, Hoek RM, Huitinga I (2007) Downregulation of macrophage inhibitory molecules in multiple sclerosis lesions. Ann Neurol 62(5):504–514. https://doi.org/10.1002/ana.21220

Koning N, Swaab DF, Hoek RM, Huitinga I (2009) Distribution of the immune inhibitory molecules CD200 and CD200R in the normal central nervous system and multiple sclerosis lesions suggests neuron-glia and glia-glia interactions. J Neuropathol Exp Neurol 68(2):159–167. https://doi.org/10.1097/NEN.0b013e3181964113

Korn T, Kallies A (2017) T cell responses in the central nervous system. Nat Rev Immunol 17(3):179–194. https://doi.org/10.1038/nri.2016.144

Koyama M, Kuns RD, Olver SD, Lineburg KE, Lor M, Teal BE, Raffelt NC, Leveque L, Chan CJ, Robb RJ, Markey KA, Alexander KA, Varelias A, Clouston AD, Smyth MJ, MacDonald KP, Hill GR (2013) Promoting regulation via the inhibition of DNAM-1 after transplantation. Blood 121(17):3511–3520. https://doi.org/10.1182/blood-2012-07-444026

Kroner A, Mehling M, Hemmer B, Rieckmann P, Toyka KV, Maurer M, Wiendl H (2005) A PD-1 polymorphism is associated with disease progression in multiple sclerosis. Ann Neurol 58(1):50–57. https://doi.org/10.1002/ana.20514

Kyi C, Carvajal RD, Wolchok JD, Postow MA (2014) Ipilimumab in patients with melanoma and autoimmune disease. J Immunother Cancer 2(1):35. https://doi.org/10.1186/s40425-014-0035-z

Laporte V, Ait-Ghezala G, Volmar CH, Ganey C, Ganey N, Wood M, Mullan M (2008) CD40 ligation mediates plaque-associated tau phosphorylation in beta-amyloid overproducing mice. Brain Res 1231:132–142. https://doi.org/10.1016/j.brainres.2008.06.032

Latchman YE, Liang SC, Wu Y, Chernova T, Sobel RA, Klemm M, Kuchroo VK, Freeman GJ, Sharpe AH (2004) PD-L1-deficient mice show that PD-L1 on T cells, antigen-presenting cells, and host tissues negatively regulates T cells. Proc Natl Acad Sci USA 101(29):10691–10696. https://doi.org/10.1073/pnas.0307252101

Lee SY, Goverman JM (2013) The influence of T cell Ig mucin-3 signaling on central nervous system autoimmune disease is determined by the effector function of the pathogenic T cells. J Immunol 190(10):4991–4999. https://doi.org/10.4049/jimmunol.1300083

Levin SD, Taft DW, Brandt CS, Bucher C, Howard ED, Chadwick EM, Johnston J, Hammond A, Bontadelli K, Ardourel D, Hebb L, Wolf A, Bukowski TR, Rixon MW, Kuijper JL, Ostrander CD, West JW, Bilsborough J, Fox B, Gao Z, Xu W, Ramsdell F, Blazar BR, Lewis KE (2011) Vstm3 is a member of the CD28 family and an important modulator of T-cell function. Eur J Immunol 41(4):902–915. https://doi.org/10.1002/eji.201041136

Li P, Mao L, Liu X, Gan Y, Zheng J, Thomson AW, Gao Y, Chen J, Hu X (2014) Essential role of program death 1-ligand 1 in regulatory T-cell-afforded protection against blood-brain barrier damage after stroke. Stroke 45(3):857–864. https://doi.org/10.1161/STROKEAHA.113.004100

Liang SC, Latchman YE, Buhlmann JE, Tomczak MF, Horwitz BH, Freeman GJ, Sharpe AH (2003) Regulation of PD-1, PD-L1, and PD-L2 expression during normal and autoimmune responses. Eur J Immunol 33(10):2706–2716. https://doi.org/10.1002/eji.200324228

Lincecum JM, Vieira FG, Wang MZ, Thompson K, De Zutter GS, Kidd J, Moreno A, Sanchez R, Carrion IJ, Levine BA, Al-Nakhala BM, Sullivan SM, Gill A, Perrin S (2010) From transcriptome analysis to therapeutic anti-CD40L treatment in the SOD1 model of amyotrophic lateral sclerosis. Nat Genet 42(5):392–399. https://doi.org/10.1038/ng.557

Lipp M, Brandt C, Dehghani F, Kwidzinski E, Bechmann I (2007) PD-L1 (B7-H1) regulation in zones of axonal degeneration. Neurosci Lett 425(3):156–161. https://doi.org/10.1016/j.neulet.2007.07.053

Liu Y, Teige I, Birnir B, Issazadeh-Navikas S (2006) Neuron-mediated generation of regulatory T cells from encephalitogenic T cells suppresses EAE. Nat Med 12(5):518–525. https://doi.org/10.1038/nm1402

Liu Y, Carlsson R, Comabella M, Wang J, Kosicki M, Carrion B, Hasan M, Wu X, Montalban X, Dziegiel MH, Sellebjerg F, Sorensen PS, Helin K, Issazadeh-Navikas S (2014) FoxA1 directs the lineage and immunosuppressive properties of a novel regulatory T cell population in EAE and MS. Nat Med 20(3):272–282. https://doi.org/10.1038/nm.3485

Liu G, Hu Y, Jin S, Jiang Q (2017a) Genetic variant rs763361 regulates multiple sclerosis CD226 gene expression. Proc Natl Acad Sci USA 114(6):E906–E907. https://doi.org/10.1073/pnas.1618520114

Liu Y, Marin A, Ejlerskov P, Rasmussen LM, Prinz M, Issazadeh-Navikas S (2017b) Neuronal IFN-beta-induced PI3K/Akt-FoxA1 signalling is essential for generation of FoxA1+Treg cells. Nat Commun 8:14709. https://doi.org/10.1038/ncomms14709

Lowther D, Ramanan S, DeBartolo D, Park C, Duan X, Hafler D, Pitt D (2015) The TIGIT/CD226/CD155 axis is differentially expressed in MS and glioblastoma: implications for autoimmunity and tumor immune escape. Neurology 84(14):Supplement P4.043

Lozano E, Dominguez-Villar M, Kuchroo V, Hafler DA (2012) The TIGIT/CD226 axis regulates human T cell function. J Immunol 188(8):3869–3875. https://doi.org/10.4049/jimmunol.1103627

Lozano E, Joller N, Cao Y, Kuchroo VK, Hafler DA (2013) The CD226/CD155 interaction regulates the proinflammatory (Th1/Th17)/anti-inflammatory (Th2) balance in humans. J Immunol 191(7):3673–3680. https://doi.org/10.4049/jimmunol.1300945

Luo XG, Zhang JJ, Zhang CD, Liu R, Zheng L, Wang XJ, Chen SD, Ding JQ (2010) Altered regulation of CD200 receptor in monocyte-derived macrophages from individuals with Parkinson's disease. Neurochem Res 35(4):540–547. https://doi.org/10.1007/s11064-009-0094-6

Lyons JA, Zhao ML, Fritz RB (1999) Pathogenesis of acute passive murine encephalomyelitis II. Th1 phenotype of the inducing population is not sufficient to cause disease. J Neuroimmunol 93(1–2):26–36

Lyons A, McQuillan K, Deighan BF, O'Reilly JA, Downer EJ, Murphy AC, Watson M, Piazza A, O'Connell F, Griffin R, Mills KH, Lynch MA (2009) Decreased neuronal CD200 expression in IL-4-deficient mice results in increased neuroinflammation in response to lipopolysaccharide. Brain Behav Immun 23(7):1020–1027. https://doi.org/10.1016/j.bbi.2009.05.060

Magnus T, Schreiner B, Korn T, Jack C, Guo H, Antel J, Ifergan I, Chen L, Bischof F, Bar-Or A, Wiendl H (2005) Microglial expression of the B7 family member B7 homolog 1 confers strong immune inhibition: implications for immune responses and autoimmunity in the CNS. J Neurosci 25(10):2537–2546. https://doi.org/10.1523/JNEUROSCI.4794-04.2005

Mao X, Ou MT, Karuppagounder SS, Kam TI, Yin X, Xiong Y, Ge P, Umanah GE, Brahmachari S, Shin JH, Kang HC, Zhang J, Xu J, Chen R, Park H, Andrabi SA, Kang SU, Goncalves RA, Liang Y, Zhang S, Qi C, Lam S, Keiler JA, Tyson J, Kim D, Panicker N, Yun SP, Workman CJ, Vignali DA, Dawson VL, Ko HS, Dawson TM (2016) Pathological alpha-synuclein transmission initiated by binding lymphocyte-activation gene 3. Science 353(6307). https://doi.org/10.1126/science.aah3374

Mathias A, Perriard G, Canales M, Soneson C, Delorenzi M, Schluep M, Du Pasquier RA (2017) Increased ex vivo antigen presentation profile of B cells in multiple sclerosis. Mult Scler 23(6):802–809. https://doi.org/10.1177/1352458516664210

Meda L, Cassatella MA, Szendrei GI, Otvos L Jr, Baron P, Villalba M, Ferrari D, Rossi F (1995) Activation of microglial cells by beta-amyloid protein and interferon-gamma. Nature 374(6523):647–650. https://doi.org/10.1038/374647a0

Miyamoto K, Kingsley CI, Zhang X, Jabs C, Izikson L, Sobel RA, Weiner HL, Kuchroo VK, Sharpe AH (2005) The ICOS molecule plays a crucial role in the development of mucosal tolerance. J Immunol 175(11):7341–7347

Mocali A, Cedrola S, Della Malva N, Bontempelli M, Mitidieri VA, Bavazzano A, Comolli R, Paoletti F, La Porta CA (2004) Increased plasma levels of soluble CD40, together with the decrease of TGF beta 1, as possible differential markers of Alzheimer disease. Exp Gerontol 39(10):1555–1561. https://doi.org/10.1016/j.exger.2004.07.007

Monney L, Sabatos CA, Gaglia JL, Ryu A, Waldner H, Chernova T, Manning S, Greenfield EA, Coyle AJ, Sobel RA, Freeman GJ, Kuchroo VK (2002) Th1-specific cell surface protein Tim-3 regulates macrophage activation and severity of an autoimmune disease. Nature 415(6871):536–541. https://doi.org/10.1038/415536a

Okuno T, Nakatsuji Y, Kumanogoh A, Koguchi K, Moriya M, Fujimura H, Kikutani H, Sakoda S (2004) Induction of cyclooxygenase-2 in reactive glial cells by the CD40 pathway: relevance to amyotrophic lateral sclerosis. J Neurochem 91(2):404–412. https://doi.org/10.1111/j.1471-4159.2004.02727.x

Oliveira-dos-Santos AJ, Ho A, Tada Y, Lafaille JJ, Tonegawa S, Mak TW, Penninger JM (1999) CD28 costimulation is crucial for the development of spontaneous autoimmune encephalomyelitis. J Immunol 162(8):4490–4495

9 Co-signaling Molecules in Neurological Diseases

Ortler S, Leder C, Mittelbronn M, Zozulya AL, Knolle PA, Chen L, Kroner A, Wiendl H (2008) B7-H1 restricts neuroantigen-specific T cell responses and confines inflammatory CNS damage: implications for the lesion pathogenesis of multiple sclerosis. Eur J Immunol 38(6):1734–1744. https://doi.org/10.1002/eji.200738071

Paterson AM, Lovitch SB, Sage PT, Juneja VR, Lee Y, Trombley JD, Arancibia-Carcamo CV, Sobel RA, Rudensky AY, Kuchroo VK, Freeman GJ, Sharpe AH (2015) Deletion of CTLA-4 on regulatory T cells during adulthood leads to resistance to autoimmunity. J Exp Med 212(10):1603–1621. https://doi.org/10.1084/jem.20141030

Pekny M, Pekna M, Messing A, Steinhauser C, Lee JM, Parpura V, Hol EM, Sofroniew MV, Verkhratsky A (2016) Astrocytes: a central element in neurological diseases. Acta Neuropathol 131(3):323–345. https://doi.org/10.1007/s00401-015-1513-1

Perrin PJ, Maldonado JH, Davis TA, June CH, Racke MK (1996) CTLA-4 blockade enhances clinical disease and cytokine production during experimental allergic encephalomyelitis. J Immunol 157(4):1333–1336

Perrin PJ, June CH, Maldonado JH, Ratts RB, Racke MK (1999) Blockade of CD28 during in vitro activation of encephalitogenic T cells or after disease onset ameliorates experimental autoimmune encephalitis. J Immunol 163(3):1704–1710

Perry VH (2016) Microglia. Microbiol Spectr 4(3). https://doi.org/10.1128/microbiolspec. MCHD-0003-2015

Piedavent-Salomon M, Willing A, Engler JB, Steinbach K, Bauer S, Eggert B, Ufer F, Kursawe N, Wehrmann S, Jager J, Reinhardt S, Friese MA (2015) Multiple sclerosis associated genetic variants of CD226 impair regulatory T cell function. Brain 138(Pt 11):3263–3274. https://doi. org/10.1093/brain/awv256

Pittet CL, Newcombe J, Antel JP, Arbour N (2011) The majority of infiltrating CD8 T lymphocytes in multiple sclerosis lesions is insensitive to enhanced PD-L1 levels on CNS cells. Glia 59(5):841–856. https://doi.org/10.1002/glia.21158

Ponomarev ED, Shriver LP, Dittel BN (2006) CD40 expression by microglial cells is required for their completion of a two-step activation process during central nervous system autoimmune inflammation. J Immunol 176(3):1402–1410

Puentes F, Malaspina A, van Noort JM, Amor S (2016) Non-neuronal cells in ALS: role of glial, immune cells and blood-CNS barriers. Brain Pathol 26(2):248–257. https://doi.org/10.1111/bpa.12352

Qin J, Xing J, Liu R, Chen B, Chen Y, Zhuang X (2017) Association between CD40 rs1883832 and immune-related diseases susceptibility: a meta-analysis. Oncotarget. https://doi.org/10.18632/oncotarget.18704

Rangachari M, Zhu C, Sakuishi K, Xiao S, Karman J, Chen A, Angin M, Wakeham A, Greenfield EA, Sobel RA, Okada H, McKinnon PJ, Mak TW, Addo MM, Anderson AC, Kuchroo VK (2012) Bat3 promotes T cell responses and autoimmunity by repressing Tim-3-mediated cell death and exhaustion. Nat Med 18(9):1394–1400. https://doi.org/10.1038/nm.2871

Ransohoff RM, El Khoury J (2015) Microglia in health and disease. Cold Spring Harb Perspect Biol 8(1):a020560. https://doi.org/10.1101/cshperspect.a020560

Ransohoff RM, Perry VH (2009) Microglial physiology: unique stimuli, specialized responses. Annu Rev Immunol 27:119–145. https://doi.org/10.1146/annurev.immunol.021908.132528

Ransohoff RM, Hafler DA, Lucchinetti CF (2015) Multiple sclerosis-a quiet revolution. Nat Rev Neurol 11(3):134–142. https://doi.org/10.1038/nrneurol.2015.14

Ren X, Akiyoshi K, Vandenbark AA, Hurn PD, Offner H (2011) Programmed death-1 pathway limits central nervous system inflammation and neurologic deficits in murine experimental stroke. Stroke 42(9):2578–2583. https://doi.org/10.1161/STROKEAHA.111.613182

Rifa'i M, Kawamoto Y, Nakashima I, Suzuki H (2004) Essential roles of CD8+CD122+ regulatory T cells in the maintenance of T cell homeostasis. J Exp Med 200(9):1123–1134. https://doi. org/10.1084/jem.20040395

Rojo JM, Pini E, Ojeda G, Bello R, Dong C, Flavell RA, Dianzani U, Portoles P (2008) CD4+ICOS+ T lymphocytes inhibit T cell activation 'in vitro' and attenuate autoimmune encephalitis 'in vivo'. Int Immunol 20(4):577–589. https://doi.org/10.1093/intimm/dxn016

Romme Christensen J, Bornsen L, Ratzer R, Piehl F, Khademi M, Olsson T, Sorensen PS, Sellebjerg F (2013) Systemic inflammation in progressive multiple sclerosis involves follicular T-helper, Th17- and activated B-cells and correlates with progression. PLoS One 8(3):e57820. https://doi.org/10.1371/journal.pone.0057820

Rottman JB, Smith T, Tonra JR, Ganley K, Bloom T, Silva R, Pierce B, Gutierrez-Ramos JC, Ozkaynak E, Coyle AJ (2001) The costimulatory molecule ICOS plays an important role in the immunopathogenesis of EAE. Nat Immunol 2(7):605–611. https://doi.org/10.1038/89750

Ruperto N, Lovell DJ, Quartier P, Paz E, Rubio-Perez N, Silva CA, Abud-Mendoza C, Burgos-Vargas R, Gerloni V, Melo-Gomes JA, Saad-Magalhaes C, Sztajnbok F, Goldenstein-Schainberg C, Scheinberg M, Penades IC, Fischbach M, Orozco J, Hashkes PJ, Hom C, Jung L, Lepore L, Oliveira S, Wallace CA, Sigal LH, Block AJ, Covucci A, Martini A, Giannini EH, Paediatric Rheumatology ITO, Pediatric Rheumatology Collaborative Study G (2008) Abatacept in children with juvenile idiopathic arthritis: a randomised, double-blind, placebo-controlled withdrawal trial. Lancet 372(9636):383–391. https://doi.org/10.1016/S0140-6736(08)60998-8

Sabatos CA, Chakravarti S, Cha E, Schubart A, Sanchez-Fueyo A, Zheng XX, Coyle AJ, Strom TB, Freeman GJ, Kuchroo VK (2003) Interaction of Tim-3 and Tim-3 ligand regulates T helper type 1 responses and induction of peripheral tolerance. Nat Immunol 4(11):1102–1110. https://doi.org/10.1038/ni988

Sage PT, Paterson AM, Lovitch SB, Sharpe AH (2014) The coinhibitory receptor CTLA-4 controls B cell responses by modulating T follicular helper, T follicular regulatory, and T regulatory cells. Immunity 41(6):1026–1039. https://doi.org/10.1016/j.immuni.2014.12.005

Salama AD, Chitnis T, Imitola J, Ansari MJ, Akiba H, Tushima F, Azuma M, Yagita H, Sayegh MH, Khoury SJ (2003) Critical role of the programmed death-1 (PD-1) pathway in regulation of experimental autoimmune encephalomyelitis. J Exp Med 198(1):71–78. https://doi.org/10.1084/jem.20022119

Saresella M, Calabrese E, Marventano I, Piancone F, Gatti A, Calvo MG, Nemni R, Clerici M (2010) PD1 negative and PD1 positive CD4+ T regulatory cells in mild cognitive impairment and Alzheimer's disease. J Alzheimers Dis 21(3):927–938. https://doi.org/10.3233/JAD-2010-091696

Saresella M, Calabrese E, Marventano I, Piancone F, Gatti A, Farina E, Alberoni M, Clerici M (2012) A potential role for the PD1/PD-L1 pathway in the neuroinflammation of Alzheimer's disease. Neurobiol Aging 33(3):624 e611–622. doi:https://doi.org/10.1016/j.neurobiolaging.2011.03.004

Saresella M, Piancone F, Marventano I, La Rosa F, Tortorella P, Caputo D, Rovaris M, Clerici M (2014) A role for the TIM-3/GAL-9/BAT3 pathway in determining the clinical phenotype of multiple sclerosis. FASEB J 28(11):5000–5009. https://doi.org/10.1096/fj.14-258194

Sau D, De Biasi S, Vitellaro-Zuccarello L, Riso P, Guarnieri S, Porrini M, Simeoni S, Crippa V, Onesto E, Palazzolo I, Rusmini P, Bolzoni E, Bendotti C, Poletti A (2007) Mutation of SOD1 in ALS: a gain of a loss of function. Hum Mol Genet 16(13):1604–1618. https://doi.org/10.1093/hmg/ddm110

Schaub M, Issazadeh S, Stadlbauer TH, Peach R, Sayegh MH, Khoury SJ (1999) Costimulatory signal blockade in murine relapsing experimental autoimmune encephalomyelitis. J Neuroimmunol 96(2):158–166

Schreiner B, Bailey SL, Shin T, Chen L, Miller SD (2008) PD-1 ligands expressed on myeloid-derived APC in the CNS regulate T-cell responses in EAE. Eur J Immunol 38(10):2706–2717. https://doi.org/10.1002/eji.200838137

Sierro S, Romero P, Speiser DE (2011) The CD4-like molecule LAG-3, biology and therapeutic applications. Expert Opin Ther Targets 15(1):91–101. https://doi.org/10.1517/14712598.2011.540563

Sofroniew MV, Vinters HV (2010) Astrocytes: biology and pathology. Acta Neuropathol 119(1):7–35. https://doi.org/10.1007/s00401-009-0619-8

Sporici RA, Beswick RL, von Allmen C, Rumbley CA, Hayden-Ledbetter M, Ledbetter JA, Perrin PJ (2001) ICOS ligand costimulation is required for T-cell encephalitogenicity. Clin Immunol 100(3):277–288. https://doi.org/10.1006/clim.2001.5074

Sreedharan J, Brown RH Jr (2013) Amyotrophic lateral sclerosis: problems and prospects. Ann Neurol 74(3):309–316. https://doi.org/10.1002/ana.24012

Stanietsky N, Simic H, Arapovic J, Toporik A, Levy O, Novik A, Levine Z, Beiman M, Dassa L, Achdout H, Stern-Ginossar N, Tsukerman P, Jonjic S, Mandelboim O (2009) The interaction of TIGIT with PVR and PVRL2 inhibits human NK cell cytotoxicity. Proc Natl Acad Sci USA 106(42):17858–17863. https://doi.org/10.1073/pnas.0903474106

Sulzer D, Alcalay RN, Garretti F, Cote L, Kanter E, Agin-Liebes J, Liong C, McMurtrey C, Hildebrand WH, Mao X, Dawson VL, Dawson TM, Oseroff C, Pham J, Sidney J, Dillon MB, Carpenter C, Weiskopf D, Phillips E, Mallal S, Peters B, Frazier A, Lindestam Arlehamn CS, Sette A (2017) T cells from patients with Parkinson's disease recognize alpha-synuclein peptides. Nature 546(7660):656–661. https://doi.org/10.1038/nature22815

Sung YH, Kim SC, Hong HP, Park CY, Shin MS, Kim CJ, Seo JH, Kim DY, Kim DJ, Cho HJ (2012) Treadmill exercise ameliorates dopaminergic neuronal loss through suppressing microglial activation in Parkinson's disease mice. Life Sci 91(25-26):1309–1316. https://doi.org/10.1016/j.lfs.2012.10.003

Tan J, Town T, Paris D, Mori T, Suo Z, Crawford F, Mattson MP, Flavell RA, Mullan M (1999a) Microglial activation resulting from CD40-CD40L interaction after beta-amyloid stimulation. Science 286(5448):2352–2355

Tan J, Town T, Paris D, Placzek A, Parker T, Crawford F, Yu H, Humphrey J, Mullan M (1999b) Activation of microglial cells by the CD40 pathway: relevance to multiple sclerosis. J Neuroimmunol 97(1–2):77–85

Taylor A, Verhagen J, Akdis CA, Akdis M (2004) T regulatory cells in allergy and health: a question of allergen specificity and balance. Int Arch Allergy Immunol 135(1):73–82. https://doi.org/10.1159/000080523

Teleshova N, Bao W, Kivisäkk P, Özenci V, Mustafa M, Link H (2000) Elevated CD40 ligand expressing blood T-cell levels in multiple sclerosis are reversed by interferon-beta treatment. Scand J Immunol 51(3):312–320

Togo T, Akiyama H, Kondo H, Ikeda K, Kato M, Iseki E, Kosaka K (2000) Expression of CD40 in the brain of Alzheimer's disease and other neurological diseases. Brain Res 885(1):117–121

Townsend KP, Town T, Mori T, Lue LF, Shytle D, Sanberg PR, Morgan D, Fernandez F, Flavell RA, Tan J (2005) CD40 signaling regulates innate and adaptive activation of microglia in response to amyloid beta-peptide. Eur J Immunol 35(3):901–910. https://doi.org/10.1002/eji.200425585

Trabattoni D, Saresella M, Pacei M, Marventano I, Mendozzi L, Rovaris M, Caputo D, Borelli M, Clerici M (2009) Costimulatory pathways in multiple sclerosis: distinctive expression of PD-1 and PD-L1 in patients with different patterns of disease. J Immunol 183(8):4984–4993. https://doi.org/10.4049/jimmunol.0901038

Verhagen J, Gabrysova L, Minaee S, Sabatos CA, Anderson G, Sharpe AH, Wraith DC (2009) Enhanced selection of FoxP3+ T-regulatory cells protects CTLA-4-deficient mice from CNS autoimmune disease. Proc Natl Acad Sci USA 106(9):3306–3311. https://doi.org/10.1073/pnas.0803186106

Viglietta V, Bourcier K, Buckle GJ, Healy B, Weiner HL, Hafler DA, Egorova S, Guttmann CR, Rusche JR, Khoury SJ (2008) CTLA4Ig treatment in patients with multiple sclerosis: an open-label, phase 1 clinical trial. Neurology 71(12):917–924. https://doi.org/10.1212/01.wnl.0000325915.00112.61

Vincenti F, Larsen C, Durrbach A, Wekerle T, Nashan B, Blancho G, Lang P, Grinyo J, Halloran PF, Solez K, Hagerty D, Levy E, Zhou W, Natarajan K, Charpentier B, Belatacept Study G (2005) Costimulation blockade with belatacept in renal transplantation. N Engl J Med 353(8):770–781. https://doi.org/10.1056/NEJMoa050085

Vogel DY, Vereyken EJ, Glim JE, Heijnen PD, Moeton M, van der Valk P, Amor S, Teunissen CE, van Horssen J, Dijkstra CD (2013) Macrophages in inflammatory multiple sclerosis lesions have an intermediate activation status. J Neuroinflammation 10:35. https://doi.org/10.1186/1742-2094-10-35

Waid DM, Schreiner T, Vaitaitis G, Carter JR, Corboy JR, Wagner DH Jr (2014) Defining a new biomarker for the autoimmune component of Multiple Sclerosis: Th40 cells. J Neuroimmunol 270(1-2):75–85. https://doi.org/10.1016/j.jneuroim.2014.03.009

Walker DG, Lue LF (2013) Understanding the neurobiology of CD200 and the CD200 receptor: a therapeutic target for controlling inflammation in human brains? Future Neurol 8(3). https://doi.org/10.2217/fnl.13.14

Walker DG, Dalsing-Hernandez JE, Campbell NA, Lue LF (2009) Decreased expression of CD200 and CD200 receptor in Alzheimer's disease: a potential mechanism leading to chronic inflammation. Exp Neurol 215(1):5–19. https://doi.org/10.1016/j.expneurol.2008.09.003

Walker DG, Lue LF, Tang TM, Adler CH, Caviness JN, Sabbagh MN, Serrano GE, Sue LI, Beach TG (2017) Changes in CD200 and intercellular adhesion molecule-1 (ICAM-1) levels in brains of Lewy body disorder cases are associated with amounts of Alzheimer's pathology not alpha-synuclein pathology. Neurobiol Aging 54:175–186. https://doi.org/10.1016/j.neurobiolaging.2017.03.007

Wang C, Li Y, Proctor TM, Vandenbark AA, Offner H (2010) Down-modulation of programmed death 1 alters regulatory T cells and promotes experimental autoimmune encephalomyelitis. J Neurosci Res 88(1):7–15. https://doi.org/10.1002/jnr.22181

Waterhouse P, Penninger JM, Timms E, Wakeham A, Shahinian A, Lee KP, Thompson CB, Griesser H, Mak TW (1995) Lymphoproliferative disorders with early lethality in mice deficient in Ctla-4. Science 270(5238):985–988

Weber JS, Kahler KC, Hauschild A (2012) Management of immune-related adverse events and kinetics of response with ipilimumab. J Clin Oncol 30(21):2691–2697. https://doi.org/10.1200/JCO.2012.41.6750

Wei R, Jonakait GM (1999) Neurotrophins and the anti-inflammatory agents interleukin-4 (IL-4), IL-10, IL-11 and transforming growth factor-beta1 (TGF-beta1) down-regulate T cell costimulatory molecules B7 and CD40 on cultured rat microglia. J Neuroimmunol 95(1-2):8–18

Weiner HL, da Cunha AP, Quintana F, Wu H (2011) Oral tolerance. Immunol Rev 241(1):241–259. https://doi.org/10.1111/j.1600-065X.2011.01017.x

Wiesemann E, Deb M, Trebst C, Hemmer B, Stangel M, Windhagen A (2008) Effects of interferon-beta on co-signaling molecules: upregulation of CD40, CD86 and PD-L2 on monocytes in relation to clinical response to interferon-beta treatment in patients with multiple sclerosis. Mult Scler 14(2):166–176. https://doi.org/10.1177/1352458507081342

Wikenheiser DJ, Stumhofer JS (2016) ICOS Co-Stimulation: Friend or Foe? Front Immunol 7:304. https://doi.org/10.3389/fimmu.2016.00304

Wing K, Onishi Y, Prieto-Martin P, Yamaguchi T, Miyara M, Fehervari Z, Nomura T, Sakaguchi S (2008) CTLA-4 control over Foxp3+ regulatory T cell function. Science 322(5899):271–275. https://doi.org/10.1126/science.1160062

Wing JB, Ise W, Kurosaki T, Sakaguchi S (2014) Regulatory T cells control antigen-specific expansion of Tfh cell number and humoral immune responses via the coreceptor CTLA-4. Immunity 41(6):1013–1025. https://doi.org/10.1016/j.immuni.2014.12.006

Workman CJ, Rice DS, Dugger KJ, Kurschner C, Vignali DA (2002) Phenotypic analysis of the murine CD4-related glycoprotein, CD223 (LAG-3). Eur J Immunol 32(8):2255–2263. https://doi.org/10.1002/1521-4141(200208)32:8<2255::AID-IMMU2255>3.0.CO;2-A

Xie X, Luo X, Liu N, Li X, Lou F, Zheng Y, Ren Y (2017) Monocytes, microglia, and CD200-CD200R1 signaling are essential in the transmission of inflammation from the periphery to the central nervous system. J Neurochem 141(2):222–235. https://doi.org/10.1111/jnc.13972

Yamazaki T, Akiba H, Iwai H, Matsuda H, Aoki M, Tanno Y, Shin T, Tsuchiya H, Pardoll DM, Okumura K, Azuma M, Yagita H (2002) Expression of programmed death 1 ligands by murine T cells and APC. J Immunol 169(10):5538–5545

Yanaba K, Bouaziz JD, Haas KM, Poe JC, Fujimoto M, Tedder TF (2008) A regulatory B cell subset with a unique CD1dhiCD5+ phenotype controls T cell-dependent inflammatory responses. Immunity 28(5):639–650. https://doi.org/10.1016/j.immuni.2008.03.017

Yang L, Anderson DE, Kuchroo J, Hafler DA (2008) Lack of TIM-3 immunoregulation in multiple sclerosis. J Immunol 180(7):4409–4414

Yilmaz G, Arumugam TV, Stokes KY, Granger DN (2006) Role of T lymphocytes and interferon-gamma in ischemic stroke. Circulation 113(17):2105–2112. https://doi.org/10.1161/CIRCULATIONAHA.105.593046

Yoshida H, Imaizumi T, Kumagai M, Kimura K, Satoh C, Hanada N, Fujimoto K, Nishi N, Tanji K, Matsumiya T, Mori F, Cui XF, Tamo W, Shibata T, Takanashi S, Okumura K, Nakamura T, Wakabayashi K, Hirashima M, Sato Y, Satoh K (2001) Interleukin-1beta stimulates galectin-9 expression in human astrocytes. Neuroreport 12(17):3755–3758

Yoshizaki A, Miyagaki T, DiLillo DJ, Matsushita T, Horikawa M, Kountikov EI, Spolski R, Poe JC, Leonard WJ, Tedder TF (2012) Regulatory B cells control T-cell autoimmunity through IL-21-dependent cognate interactions. Nature 491(7423):264–268. https://doi.org/10.1038/nature11501

Yu S, Liu YP, Liu YH, Jiao SS, Liu L, Wang YJ, Fu WL (2016) Diagnostic utility of VEGF and soluble CD40L levels in serum of Alzheimer's patients. Clin Chim Acta 453:154–159. https://doi.org/10.1016/j.cca.2015.12.018

Zeinstra E, Wilczak N, De Keyser J (2003) Reactive astrocytes in chronic active lesions of multiple sclerosis express co-stimulatory molecules B7-1 and B7-2. J Neuroimmunol 135(1–2):166–171

Zhang Q, Vignali DA (2016) Co-stimulatory and co-inhibitory pathways in autoimmunity. Immunity 44(5):1034–1051. https://doi.org/10.1016/j.immuni.2016.04.017

Zhang W, Wang T, Pei Z, Miller DS, Wu X, Block ML, Wilson B, Zhang W, Zhou Y, Hong JS, Zhang J (2005) Aggregated alpha-synuclein activates microglia: a process leading to disease progression in Parkinson's disease. FASEB J 19(6):533–542. https://doi.org/10.1096/fj.04-2751com

Zhang S, Wang XJ, Tian LP, Pan J, Lu GQ, Zhang YJ, Ding JQ, Chen SD (2011) CD200-CD200R dysfunction exacerbates microglial activation and dopaminergic neurodegeneration in a rat model of Parkinson's disease. J Neuroinflammation 8:154. https://doi.org/10.1186/1742-2094-8-154

Zhang W, Huang W, Jing F (2013) Contribution of blood platelets to vascular pathology in Alzheimer's disease. J Blood Med 4:141–147. https://doi.org/10.2147/JBM.S45071

Zhang R, Zeng H, Zhang Y, Chen K, Zhang C, Song C, Fang L, Xu Z, Yang K, Jin B, Wang Q, Chen L (2016) CD226 ligation protects against EAE by promoting IL-10 expression via regulation of CD4+ T cell differentiation. Oncotarget 7(15):19251–19264. https://doi.org/10.18632/oncotarget.7834

Zhao S, Li F, Leak RK, Chen J, Hu X (2014) Regulation of neuroinflammation through programed death-1/programed death ligand signaling in neurological disorders. Front Cell Neurosci 8:271. https://doi.org/10.3389/fncel.2014.00271

Zhu C, Anderson AC, Schubart A, Xiong H, Imitola J, Khoury SJ, Zheng XX, Strom TB, Kuchroo VK (2005) The Tim-3 ligand galectin-9 negatively regulates T helper type 1 immunity. Nat Immunol 6(12):1245–1252. https://doi.org/10.1038/ni1271

Zhu B, Guleria I, Khosroshahi A, Chitnis T, Imitola J, Azuma M, Yagita H, Sayegh MH, Khoury SJ (2006) Differential role of programmed death-ligand 1 [corrected] and programmed death-ligand 2 [corrected] in regulating the susceptibility and chronic progression of experimental autoimmune encephalomyelitis. J Immunol 176(6):3480–3489

Chapter 10
Costimulation Blockade in Transplantation

Melissa Y. Yeung, Tanja Grimmig, and Mohamed H. Sayegh

Abstract T cells play a pivotal role in orchestrating immune responses directed against a foreign (allogeneic) graft. For T cells to become fully activated, the T-cell receptor (TCR) must interact with the major histocompatibility complex (MHC) plus peptide complex on antigen-presenting cells (APCs), followed by a second "positive" costimulatory signal. In the absence of this second signal, T cells become anergic or undergo deletion. By blocking positive costimulatory signaling, T-cell allo-responses can be aborted, thus preventing graft rejection and promoting long-term allograft survival and possibly tolerance (Alegre ML, Najafian N, Curr Mol Med 6:843–857, 2006; Li XC, Rothstein DM, Sayegh MH, Immunol Rev 229:271–293, 2009). In addition, costimulatory molecules can provide negative "coinhibitory" signals that inhibit T-cell activation and terminate immune responses; strategies to promote these pathways can also lead to graft tolerance (Boenisch O, Sayegh MH, Najafian N, Curr Opin Organ Transplant 13:373–378, 2008). However, T-cell costimulation involves an incredibly complex array of interactions that may act simultaneously or at different times in the immune response and whose relative importance varies depending on the different T-cell subsets and activation status. In transplantation, the presence of foreign alloantigen incites not only destructive T effector cells but also protective regulatory T cells, the balance of which ultimately determines the fate of the allograft (Lechler RI, Garden OA, Turka LA, Nat Rev

---

M. Y. Yeung (✉)
Department of Medicine, Renal Division, Brigham and Women's Hospital, Boston, MA, USA

Harvard Medical School, Boston, MA, USA
e-mail: myeung@rics.bwh.harvard.edu

T. Grimmig
Department of Surgery, Molecular Oncology and Immunology, University of Wuerzburg, Wuerzburg, Germany

M. H. Sayegh
Department of Medicine, Renal Division, Brigham and Women's Hospital, Boston, MA, USA

Harvard Medical School, Boston, MA, USA

Department of Medicine and Immunology, American University of Beirut, Beirut, Lebanon

© Springer Nature Singapore Pte Ltd. 2019
M. Azuma, H. Yagita (eds.), *Co-signal Molecules in T Cell Activation*,
Advances in Experimental Medicine and Biology 1189,
https://doi.org/10.1007/978-981-32-9717-3_10

Immunol 3:147–158, 2003). Since the processes of alloantigen-specific rejection and regulation both require activation of T cells, costimulatory interactions may have opposing or synergistic roles depending on the cell being targeted. Such complexities present both challenges and opportunities in targeting T-cell costimulatory pathways for therapeutic purposes. In this chapter, we summarize our current knowledge of the various costimulatory pathways in transplantation and review the current state and challenges of harnessing these pathways to promote graft tolerance (summarized in Table 10.1).

Keywords Transplant · Allograft · Alloimmune · Costimulation blockade · Tolerance · Belatacept

10.1 Introduction

T cells play a pivotal role in orchestrating immune responses directed against a foreign (allogeneic) graft. For T cells to become fully activated, the T-cell receptor (TCR) must interact with the major histocompatibility complex (MHC) plus peptide complex on antigen-presenting cells (APCs), followed by a second "positive" costimulatory signal. In the absence of this second signal, T cells become anergic or undergo deletion. By blocking positive costimulatory signaling, T-cell allo-responses can be aborted, thus preventing graft rejection and promoting long-term allograft survival and possibly tolerance (Alegre and Najafian 2006; Li et al. 2009). In addition, costimulatory molecules can provide negative "coinhibitory" signals that inhibit T-cell activation and terminate immune responses; strategies to promote these pathways can also lead to graft tolerance (Boenisch et al. 2008). However, T-cell costimulation involves an incredibly complex array of interactions that may act simultaneously or at different times in the immune response and whose relative importance varies depending on the different T-cell subsets and activation status. In transplantation, the presence of foreign alloantigen incites not only destructive T effector cells but also protective regulatory T cells, the balance of which ultimately determines the fate of the allograft (Lechler et al. 2003). Since the processes of alloantigen-specific rejection and regulation both require activation of T cells, costimulatory interactions may have opposing or synergistic roles depending on the cell being targeted. Such complexities present both challenges and opportunities in targeting T-cell costimulatory pathways for therapeutic purposes. In this chapter, we summarize our current knowledge of the various costimulatory pathways in transplantation and review the current state and challenges of harnessing these pathways to promote graft tolerance (summarized in Table 10.1).

Table 10.1 Role of costimulatory pathways in transplantation

Pathway	Effect on Tconv	Effect on Tregs	Strategies to target	Clinical trials	Important considerations
CD28/B7	Positive costimulatory signal	Important for thymic development, peripheral homeostasis, self-tolerance	CTLA-4-Ig (belatacept); blockade of B7	BENEFIT, BENEFIT-EXT trials showing superior efficacy over CNI-based regimens	Also inhibits CTLA-4/B7 and PD-1/B7 coinhibition, impairs Treg homeostasis and function, ineffective against memory responses
			Antagonistic anti-B7-1/B7-2 mAbs	Phase I trials showed safety, phase II never pursued	Blockade of both ligands required to prevent rejection, also blocks CTLA-4/B7 and PD-1/B7 coinhibition, impairs Tregs
			Antagonistic anti-CD28 mAb	Phase I trial with TGN1412 led to multisystem organ failure and death	Allows for CTLA-4 signaling, but CD28 mAbs can be superagonistic and trigger CD28 signaling
			Modified anti-CD28 mAb (sc28AT, FR104, lulizumab)	Phase I trials with FR104, lulizumab: safe, no superagonistic activity	Allows for CTLA-4 signaling but still impairs CD28 on Tregs
CTLA-4/ B7	Negative costimulatory signal	Critical to suppressive ability, maintenance of self-tolerance			CTLA-4 binds with much higher affinity to B7, interrupts CD28 signaling
PD-1/ PD-L	Negative costimulatory signal				PD-L1 expression on donor tissue also promotes graft tolerance
ICOS/ ICOS-L	Positive costimulatory signal, role in memory T-cell and germinal center responses	Promotes induction of potent Tregs	Blockade with ICOS-Ig, anti-ICOS mAb, anti-ICOS-L mAb	Phase I trial with MEDI-570 (anti-ICOS mAb) as an immune checkpoint inhibitor for treatment of lymphoma currently underway; trial for treatment of lupus was terminated for business reasons	Blockade shows only modest improvement in graft survival; mixed results, when combined with CD28 blockade, may be dependent on timing of treatment; ICOS-L can also interact with CD28 and CTLA-4 and/ or the effects on ICOS signaling in Tregs

(continued)

Table 10.1 (continued)

Pathway	Effect on Tconv	Effect on Tregs	Strategies to target	Clinical trials	Important considerations
B7-H3/ unknown	Unclear				Both costimulatory and coinhibitory functions reported, conflicting roles in graft outcomes
B7-H4/ unknown	Negative costimulatory signal				Overexpression of B7-H4 on donor islet cells also promotes graft survival
CD40/ CD40L	Positive costimulatory signal	Involved in Treg development and homeostasis	Antagonistic anti-CD40L mAbs (hu5C8, IDEC-131, ABI793)	Discontinued because of thromboembolic complications	Blockade can prevent acute rejection but not CAV, associated with thromboembolic side effects because of CD40L expression on platelets
			Modified anti-CD40L mAbs (aglycosylated mAb, Fc-silent domain Ab)		
			Antagonistic anti-CD40 mAbs (ASKP1240, CFZ533, 3A8, 2C10R4)	Phase I trial with ASP1240 showed safety, phase II trial underway; proof-of-concept clinical trial with CFZ533 underway	
OX40/ OX40L	Positive costimulatory signal, promotes transition from effector to memory phenotype	OX40 signaling *inhibits* Treg suppressive function and prevents their induction	Antagonistic anti-OX40 mAbs (GBR 830)	Phase I trial with GBR 830 showed safety	Blockade alone is insufficient in preventing rejection but shows efficacy in combination with CD28 or CD40 blockade, unique in that inhibition can restrain T effector responses while promoting Tregs
CD27/ CD70	Positive costimulatory signal	Increases frequency of Tregs, reduces their apoptosis			

GITR/ GITRL	Positive costimulatory signal	GITR signaling *disarms* Tregs and breaks self-tolerance	May show opposing roles in T effector/Treg, but yet to be explored in transplant
CD137/ CD137L	Positive costimulatory signal	CD137 signaling *reprograms* Tregs into cytotoxic CD4 T cells	May show opposing roles in T effector/Treg, but yet to be explored in transplant
TIM-1/ unknown	Positive costimulatory signal	Hinders development of Tregs	May have a more dominant role in tolerance mediated by regulatory B cells
unknown/ TIM-4	Positive costimulatory signal in transplant		Also involved in apoptotic cell uptake, rendering it difficult to dissect T-cell costimulatory roles in vivo
TIM-3/ galectin-9	Promotes T effector cell death	Enhances immunosuppressive function	Also involved in apoptotic cell uptake and mediates cross-presentation of antigens associated with dying cells

10.2 B7/CD28 Family

10.2.1 CD28/CTLA-4/B7 Pathway

Since the discovery of CD28 as a key T-cell costimulatory receptor, its blockade has become a major goal in the development of therapeutic strategies to promote transplant tolerance (reviewed in Yeung et al. (2014)). CD28 is a transmembrane protein that is constitutively expressed on nearly all CD4+ T cells and 50% of CD8+ T cells in humans (Hamann et al. 1997). Engagement of CD28 with its ligands B7-1 (CD80) and B7-2 (CD86) on APCs results in T-cell activation. Following TCR ligation/ CD28 costimulation, CTLA-4, a homolog of CD28, becomes highly upregulated on the T-cell surface (Alegre et al. 1996). It competitively inhibits CD28 signaling by binding with much higher affinity to B7-1 and B7-2, and delivers a negative costimulatory signal (Walunas et al. 1996). This results in attenuation of the T-cell response and acts as a counter-regulatory feedback mechanism to dampen the immune response following resolution of the threat (Perez 1997). Therapeutic attempts to directly block the CD28 receptor itself have been challenging because of the potential for anti-CD28 monoclonal antibodies (mAbs) to elicit a stimulating response. Thus strategies to block its ligands, such as the use of mAbs directed against B7 and CTLA-4-Ig fusion proteins, have been developed as alternatives.

10.2.1.1 Use of CTLA-4 Recombinant Fusion Proteins

CTLA-4 fusion proteins (CTLA-4-Ig), consisting of the extracellular domain of CTLA-4 fused to the Fc region of human IgG1 (Vincenti et al. 2011), were developed to capitalize on the finding that CTLA-4 has a much higher binding affinity to B7 molecules than CD28. As such, they act as a competitive inhibitor of CD28/B7 interactions. Abatacept (Orencia®, Bristol-Myers Squibb) was the first to be approved by the US Food and Drug Administration for the treatment of rheumatoid arthritis and psoriasis (Kremer et al. 2003) (Mease et al. 2011). However, in nonhuman primate studies of transplantation, it proved ineffective in prolonging allograft survival (Kirk et al. 1997; Levisetti et al. 1997), largely because it was 100-fold less potent than endogenous CTLA-4 at inhibiting B7-2 (CD86) costimulation (Linsley et al. 1994), resulting in incomplete blockade of B7-mediated T-cell activation in vivo (Sayegh et al. 1995; Ronchese et al. 1994; Khoury et al. 1995). This led to the re-engineered CTLA-4-Ig belatacept (Nulojix®, Bristol-Myers Squibb) which differs from abatacept by two amino acid substitutions at the ligand-binding domain and binds to B7-1 (CD80) and B7-2 (CD86) with greater avidity, thereby producing greater immunosuppressive effects (Larsen et al. 2005; Vincenti et al. 2011).

In mixed lymphocyte cultures, CTLA-4-Ig can completely block T-cell proliferation and effector functions in response to alloantigen stimulation (Tan et al. 1993; Zheng et al. 1999) and induce T-cell anergy (Judge et al. 1999). In rodent transplant models, a brief course of CTLA-4-Ig, especially when combined with a single donor-specific transfusion, consistently prevents rejection of fully MHC-mismatched heart, kidney, liver, and pancreatic islet allografts (Turka 1992; Li 2001; Lenschow et al. 1992) and, in some cases, induces donor-specific tolerance (Zheng et al. 1999; Pearson et al. 1996). However, in more stringent rodent models, such as skin transplantation, or in nonhuman primate models, short-term blockade of the CD28/B7 pathway fails to prevent transplant rejection (Williams et al. 2000; Kirk et al. 1997; Zheng et al. 2003). The failure of CD28/B7 costimulatory blockade to uniformly induce tolerance likely relates to a number of factors and will be discussed further below. Focus has now shifted away from utilizing CTLA-4-Ig as a tolerogenic agent to pairing it with other maintenance immunosuppression regimens to minimize calcineurin inhibitor (CNI) exposure and reduce nephrotoxic and cardiovascular side effects associated with CNI-based regimens.

In general, disruption of the CD28/B7 pathway with CTLA-4-Ig can be successfully combined with blockade of other positive costimulatory pathways or current immunosuppressive drugs to enhance survival of fully MHC-mismatched transplants (Li et al. 2009). The combination of CTLA-4-Ig and sirolimus, a mammalian target of rapamycin (mTOR) inhibitor, has been shown to induce tolerance in naive animal models (Li et al. 1999; Xu et al. 2003; D'Addio et al. 2010). However, not all immunosuppressive agents are additive when combined with costimulatory blockade. Calcineurin inhibitors (CNIs), such as cyclosporine and tacrolimus, appear to be capable of antagonizing the therapeutic effects of CTLA-4-Ig, particularly in fully MHC-mismatched transplant models (Li et al. 1999; Kirk et al. 1999).

Currently, belatacept (Nulojix®, Bristol-Myers Squibb) is the only clinically approved costimulatory blockade agent in transplantation (approved by the US Food and Drug Administration in June 2011 and by European Medicines Agency in April 2011) and is indicated as an alternative to the use of calcineurin inhibitors in renal transplantation (Archdeacon et al. 2012). In the Belatacept Evaluation of Nephroprotection and Efficacy as First-line Immunosuppression Trial (BENEFIT), 686 recipients of a living or standard criteria deceased donor kidney transplant were randomly assigned to receive more intensive (MI) belatacept, less intensive (LI) belatacept, or cyclosporine, in addition to receiving mycophenolate and steroids (Vincenti et al. 2010). At 7 years post-transplantation, patients treated with belatacept had a 43% lower risk of death or graft loss compared with those receiving an immunosuppressive regimen containing cyclosporine (Vincenti et al. 2016). Additionally, these patients showed superior renal function with 1.5-fold higher estimated glomerular filtration rates (eGFR of ~70 vs 45 ml/min/m2). These longterm benefits of belatacept were despite a significant increase in incidence and higher grade of acute rejection within the first year (22 and 17 versus 7 percent in the MI, LI, and cyclosporine arms, respectively). Similar results demonstrating the superior efficacy of belatacept was seen in the BENEFIT-EXT trial, which enrolled recipients who received kidney transplants from extended criteria donors (Durrbach et al. 2010, 2016). A major limitation of these two seminal studies was the concern that belatacept was not compared with modern-day practice of using a tacrolimus-based maintenance immunosuppression regimen. However, a subsequent randomized control trial comparing belatacept with a tacrolimus-based, steroid-avoiding maintenance regimen has confirmed belatacept's superiority in preserving renal function (Ferguson et al. 2011).

10.2.1.2 Challenges Encountered in Use of CTLA-4-Ig

Despite belatacept's superior ability to preserve long-term graft function, the increased rates of acute rejection remain of concern and point to important biological complexities of targeting T-cell costimulation. Results from studies in preclinical (mouse and nonhuman primate) models, as well as ex vivo analyses of human cells, have suggested this higher rate of rejection may be mediated by belatacept's interruption of inhibitory pathways (Perez 1997; Butte et al. 2007), its negative effects on regulatory T cells (Tang et al. 2003; Vasu et al. 2004; Greenwald et al. 2005), and/or its inability to target memory T cells (Adams et al. 2003; Ford et al. 2007; Nadazdin et al. 2011) or CD4+ Th17 cells (Yuan et al. 2008; Burrell et al. 2008).

Negative Impact on CTLA-4 Inhibitory Pathway

Because belatacept binds to B7-1 and B7-2 on APCs, it is capable of also inhibiting tolerance-promoting CTLA-4 signals, through both cell-intrinsic and cell-extrinsic mechanisms (reviewed in Salomon and Bluestone 2001; Rudd 2008; Rudd et al. 2009). B7 engagement with CTLA-4 is required for the induction of peripheral tolerance and the prevention of autoimmunity. CTLA-4-deficient mice die within 3 weeks of birth from massive tissue destruction caused by unrestrained T-cell activation (Tivol et al. 1995; Waterhouse et al. 1995), and in humans, polymorphisms in the *ctla-4* gene have been linked to susceptibility to autoimmune diseases such as type 1 diabetes, rheumatoid arthritis, and systemic lupus erythematosus (Ueda 2003). Similarly, B7 interactions with CTLA-4 have been shown to be crucial in maintaining transplant tolerance (Zheng et al. 1999; Tsai et al. 2004). Additionally, CTLA-4-Ig is capable of blocking CD80 binding to PD-L1 (programmed cell death 1 ligand 1, discussed further below), another key coinhibitory signal (Butte et al. 2007).

Because CD28 is a highly expressed but low-affinity receptor, whereas CTLA-4 is a low abundance but higher-affinity receptor, experts have postulated that a high concentration of belatacept would block both pathways, whereas at lower in vivo concentrations, it would preferentially block CD28 signaling (Kean et al. 2017). This theory could explain why the lower-intensity regimen of belatacept was associated with less episodes of rejection. Conceptually, selective blockade of CD28 would allow for specific targeting of the positive costimulatory signal while still allowing for CTLA-4-mediated coinhibitory signaling. Development of therapeutics to achieve such a goal is discussed further below (Section "Targeting CD28").

Impact on Regulatory T Cells

Transplantation incites not only destructive T effector cells but also protective regulatory T cells; this balance between T effector cells and Tregs ultimately determines the fate of the allograft (Lechler et al. 2003; Yeung and Sayegh 2009). Regulatory T cells appear critical in regulating allospecific tolerance and achieving long-term graft survival (Wood et al. 2012). The discovery that many of the same costimulatory molecules found on effector T cells also control Treg homeostasis and function has redefined the field of costimulation and tolerance; therapeutics that modulate costimulatory signaling may have detrimental effects if they coincidentally affect Tregs. Such is the case with belatacept.

CD28 signaling appears crucial for the maintenance of Treg homeostasis and function. Both thymic development and peripheral homeostasis of Tregs require CD28-mediated production of IL-2 (Tang et al. 2003; Greenwald et al. 2005); treatment with CTLA-4-Ig leads to a decrease in Tregs (Tang et al. 2003) and disruption of self-tolerance (Lenschow et al. 1996). In certain experimental models of transplantation, interruption of CD28 signaling breaks tolerance, rather than prevents rejection (Yang et al. 2009; Riella et al. 2012a). While deficiency of CD28 or B7 in transplanted mice leads to prolonged graft survival in full MHC-mismatched models, these recipients paradoxically reject their allografts at a faster tempo when there is only a single MHC class II mismatch (Yang et al. 2009). Similar findings were observed when wild-type recipients were treated with CTLA-4-Ig (Riella et al. 2012a). In an MHC class II-mismatched model, acute rejection of the graft is inhibited by the emergence of Tregs that then restrict the clonal expansion of alloreactive T cells (Schenk et al. 2005). The absence/interruption of CD28 signaling in this situation thus negatively impacts the regulatory T-cell population. Recipients demonstrated far fewer numbers of peripheral Tregs, and in both instances, restoration of the Foxp3+ Treg population, through adoptive transfer, rescued these grafts from rejection. Similarly, in a nonhuman primate model of kidney transplantation, treatment with CTLA-4-Ig (belatacept) in combination with sirolimus, an mTOR inhibitor, successfully prevented rejection but was found to be associated with a twofold decrease in the absolute number of Tregs, with the population reemerging after belatacept was discontinued (Lo et al. 2013).

Constitutive expression of CTLA-4 on Tregs is also critical to their suppressive ability (Takahashi et al. 2000; Wing et al. 2008). As mentioned, mice completely deficient of CTLA-4 die within a few weeks of birth from massive lymphoproliferation. When CTLA-4 was specifically deleted in Tregs using a conditional knockout approach, spontaneous development of lymphoproliferation and fatal autoimmune disease still developed, albeit at a slower tempo (Wing et al. 2008). Thus CTLA-4 deficiency in Tregs alone is sufficient to cause fatal disease. Several models have been proposed to explain the role of CTLA-4 on Tregs. Firstly, engagement of CTLA-4 may lead to the development of antigen-specific Tregs, leading to inhibition of T-cell responses (Vasu et al. 2004). In a cell-extrinsic manner, engagement of B7 on DCs by CTLA-4 initially leads to increased IFN-γ, which acts in a paracrine fashion to increase indoleamine 2,3-dioxygenase (IDO), thereby inhibiting

T-cell proliferation (Fallarino et al. 2003; Grohmann et al. 2002). As Tregs highly express CTLA-4, a mechanism of Treg suppression has been proposed where IDO production by B7 expressing DCs appears to act as an important bridge between regulatory T cells and naïve responder cells (Mellor and Munn 2004). The importance of this pathway in vivo was shown in a murine model of islet transplantation, where inhibition of IDO abrogated the graft-prolonging effects of CTLA-4-Ig (Grohmann et al. 2002). Activation further augments CTLA-4 expression on Tregs (Wing et al. 2008), and this upregulation may allow Tregs to outcompete CD28 expressed on conventional T cells for their B7 ligands (Tivol et al. 1995; Waterhouse et al. 1995).

Despite the data in animal models showing the detrimental effects of CTLA-4-Ig on Tregs, it is unclear to what extent this may hold true in humans. A study retrospectively examining data from the Phase II clinical trial using a belatacept-based immunosuppressive regimen found no long-term deleterious effects on circulating Tregs, both in numbers and in in vitro functional assays, when compared to the calcineurin-treated group (Bluestone et al. 2008). Further, they observed a significant increase in Foxp3+ Tregs in rejecting kidney allograft biopsies in the belatacept-treated group. The authors postulated that the differences seen in their study, compared to experimental models, may be due to the sub-saturating dose of belatacept used in humans which could allow for residual B7 interactions. Although CD80/CD86 knockout mice were shown to be Treg deficient, CD80/CD86$^{+/-}$ heterozygotes had significant levels of Tregs, despite a 50% reduction in CD80 and CD86 expression (Bluestone et al. 2008). If this tenet is correct, then there may be an optimal dose of belatacept that could preferentially inhibit graft-destructive effector T-cell responses while preserving the regulatory T-cell compartment.

Inability to Modulate Memory T-Cell Responses

Many studies, but not all, have shown memory T cells to be less dependent on CD28/B7 costimulation for activation and thus resistant to the immunomodulatory effects of belatacept. Animal models have demonstrated the relative ineffectiveness of CTLA-4-Ig in prolonging graft survival when the recipient possessed donor-specific memory T cells (Valujskikh et al. 2002). This presents a problematic clinical situation since in humans, memory T cells comprise of 1–10% of our T-cell repertoire and alloreactive memory T cell exist at a frequency of 1/200,000 T cells (Blattman et al. 2002; Suchin et al. 2001), even in the absence of prior alloantigen exposure such as pregnancy, blood transfusion, and previous transplants. These memory cells that are cross-reactive to transplant antigens, including recognition of foreign MHC, are thought to have arisen through prior encounter with pathogens (heterologous immunity) (Pantenburg et al. 2002; Adams et al. 2003). Additionally, following the use of lymphodepleting agents at the time of transplant, this memory T-cell pool can expand through homeostatic proliferation, when naïve T cells can convert into effector memory cells even in the absence of antigen (Goldrath et al. 2000; Wu et al. 2004; Moxham et al. 2008; Valujskikh et al. 2002).

The contribution of the memory T-cell pool in mediating belatacept resistance is highlighted by the finding that kidney transplant recipients treated with belatacept who experienced rejection appear to possess a population of CD57[+]PD1[-]CD4[+] memory T cells (Espinosa et al. 2016). These cells appear to infiltrate rejecting kidneys, are cytolytic, and do not express CD28, thus rendering them resistant to belatacept therapy. Importantly, this population of cells can be identified in the peripheral blood of these patients prior to transplant and may help to identify patients who are at higher risk of rejection when receiving belatacept-based immunosuppression regimens.

It is important to note that memory T-cell populations, though resistant to CD28/B7 costimulation, can be susceptible to modulation via other costimulatory pathways. Pre-clinical studies have shown these pre-existing, donor-specific responses can be overcome by targeting pathways such as OX40 (Vu et al. 2006) or ICOS (Khayyamian et al. 2002; Schenk et al. 2009), discussed further below. Additionally, certain subsets within the memory T-cell pool can be more susceptible to CD28 blockade than others. In full MHC-mismatched transplant models where memory responses were generated through prior alloantigen exposure, CD8 memory T cells were more impervious than CD4 memory cells (Pearson et al. 1997). Within the CD8 T-cell population, central memory cells (CD62L[hi]CCR7[+]) posed a greater barrier to transplant tolerance induction than effector memory cells (CD62L[low]CCR7[-]). However, even this may depend on the nature and duration of the prior antigenic exposure; in a model of heterologous immunity, where donor-reactive memory T cells were generated via exposure to latent Epstein-Barr virus, it was the effector memory cells that posed the greater barrier to tolerance induced through costimulatory blockade (Stapler et al. 2008).

Immune Redundancy

Finally, a plethora of mechanisms and pathways, including many other T-cell costimulatory molecules (discussed below), are involved in the rejection response. In fact, CD28 knockout mice are capable of mounting effective alloimmune responses and can promptly reject MHC-mismatched transplants (Yamada et al. 2001). Although the tempo of rejection is delayed in some models, CD28 knockout mice do not consistently exhibit the markedly prolonged graft survival, likely because alternative costimulatory pathways compensate for the absence of CD28 and play a more dominant role in the rejection response (Demirci et al. 2004; Yamada et al. 2005; Li et al. 2009). These compensatory mechanisms appear less prominent during CD28/B7 blockade with CTLA-4-Ig.

10.2.1.3 Other Strategies to Target B7-1/B7-2

Apart from the use of CTLA-4 fusion proteins, other strategies have been explored to block CD28/B7 costimulation. While B7-1 (CD80) and B7-2 (CD86) are thought to have overlapping functions, the differential expression patterns of these receptors on various cell types during immune responses suggested the potential for distinct roles in vivo. In experimental models of autoimmune diseases, selective blockade of B7-1 or B7-2 has resulted in strikingly different outcomes (Kuchroo et al. 1995; Lenschow et al. 1995a). In transplant models, however, blockade of both ligands appears to be required for optimal inhibition of rejection (Lenschow et al. 1995b; Pearson et al. 1997; Kirk et al. 2001). A Phase I study using a monoclonal antibody directed against both ligands in renal transplant recipients receiving maintenance therapy consisting of cyclosporine, mycophenolate mofetil, and steroids proved the regimen to be safe and effective. However, Phase II clinical trials to evaluate efficacy were never pursued. A soluble CD28 fusion protein, CD28-Ig (Peach et al. 1994), which also blocks CD28 signaling by binding B7, was also generated but proved largely ineffective because of its low binding affinity. As with the use of CTLA-4-Ig, each of these strategies also has the undesired effect of blocking B7 interactions with CTLA-4 and the potential to impair Treg responses.

10.2.1.4 Strategies to Selectively Target CD28

Another strategy to inhibit CD28-mediated signals involved the development of antagonistic anti-CD28 monoclonal antibody agents to directly target CD28 itself, which would allow B7/CTLA-4 signaling to remain intact. A number of blocking anti-CD28 mAbs have been shown to delay acute rejection (Dengler et al. 1999) and prevent chronic graft rejection (Dong et al. 2002) in rodent models. However, upon ligation, monoclonal antibodies can also lead to signaling through the receptor, rather than block physiologic receptor/ligand interactions, rendering it difficult to design purely antagonistic antibodies. This potential for anti-CD28 antibodies to trigger CD28 signaling in the presence of antigen (an agonistic antibody), or, for it to be superagonistic (leading to effector T-cell activation without the requirement of TCR ligation to MHC/peptide complexes) remains a major concern in the development of CD28 mAbs for therapeutic purposes (Hunig and Dennehy 2005). This latter phenomenon was seen in the case of the first-in-class, genetically engineered humanized anti-CD28 superagonistic antibody TGN1412 (TeGenero). Tragically, an unexpected and severe cytokine storm leading to end-organ damage developed in all six healthy volunteers enrolled in the Phase I clinical trial (Suntharalingam et al. 2006).

Recent advances in the generation of therapeutic mAbs have made it possible for us to modulate these reagents and create custom molecules that may overcome these limitations. For example, mAbs stripped of their Fc portion are incapable of cross-linking and delivering a stimulatory signal. Thus these novel mAbs can safely and specifically block CD28 costimulatory signals while leaving CTLA-4 coinhibitory signals intact. sc28AT (Debiopharm, Lausanne, Switzerland/TcLand, Nantes, France) is a novel monovalent anti-human CD28 antagonist generated by linking a CD28-specific single-chain Fv Ab fragment to human $\alpha 1$-antitrypsin. It has shown to selectively block CD28 interactions with its ligands without superagonistic activity (Vanhove et al. 2003). In vitro, it is incapable of stimulating human T effector cells and, when administered to nonhuman primates, does not activate or deplete T cells. Importantly, it cannot induce CD28 receptor cross-linking (Vanhove et al. 2003) and does not bind the target epitope on CD28 that is essential for inducing the TCR-independent superagonistic signal (Luhder et al. 2003). In nonhuman primates, treatment with sc28AT synergized with calcineurin inhibitors to promote acceptance of both kidney and heart allografts and reduced the severity of chronic allograft vasculopathy (Poirier et al. 2010). Treatment was associated with an increase in intragraft and peripheral blood Tregs, suggesting that its selective targeting of CD28 preserves CTLA-4-dependent Treg populations. Indeed, the graft-prolonging effects of selective CD28 blockade with sc28AT have been shown to be dependent on CTLA-4 signaling (Zhang et al. 2011), providing evidence that direct targeting of CD28 may be superior to use of CTLA-4-Ig (belatacept). Similarly, treatment of mice receiving cardiac allografts with a monovalent mouse anti-CD28 scFv (α28scFv) combined with either an anti-CD40L mAb or cyclosporine significantly increases the proportion of intragraft Tregs compared with recipients that received either treatment alone (Zhang et al. 2011). In these studies, intragraft PD-1 expression was also found to be increased, suggesting that the PD-1 coinhibitory signals remain intact and may even be enhanced in the presence of a CD28 antagonist, either through its interactions with PD-L1 or B7.

This same group has also generated a humanized PEGylated anti-CD28 Fab Ab fragment (FR104, Janssen Biotech) derived from the same high-affinity anti-human CD28 Ab (CD28.3) used in the generation of sc28AT (Vanhove et al. 2003). FR104 has been shown to prolong renal allograft survival in nonhuman primates (Ville et al. 2016). Importantly, it appears to be superior to belatacept because of its ability to preserve CTLA-4- and Treg-mediated mechanisms (Ville et al. 2016; Zaitsu et al. 2017). A Phase I clinical trial demonstrated it to be safe and well tolerated, without evidence of cytokine release syndrome (Poirier et al. 2016). Future clinical studies are planned to study its efficacy in rheumatoid arthritis and transplantation.

CD28 "domain-specific" antibodies (lulizumab, Bristol-Myers Squibb), that have been pegylated to prolong their half-life, have also been developed (Suchard et al. 2013). These dAbs inhibit both CD80- and CD86-driven T-cell proliferation and cytokine production and appear more potent and less variable than CTLA-4-Ig in inhibiting dendritic cell-driven MLRs. Importantly, they have also been shown to be devoid of agonistic activity and do not interfere with Treg function (Suchard et al. 2013). Phase I studies have been completed (Yang et al. 2015; Shi et al. 2017), and there is currently an ongoing Phase II trial to study its safety and efficacy in the treatment of lupus (NCT02265744). A second Phase II proof-of-concept study in Sjögren's syndrome (NCT02843659) was recently terminated because of inability to meet protocol objectives.

10.2.2 PD-1/PD-L Pathway

The inhibitory receptor PD-1 (CD279) is inducibly expressed on T cells and B cells upon TCR or BCR engagement, as well as on NKT cells, NK cells, activated monocytes, and some subsets of DC. PD-1 has two natural ligands, PD-L1 (B7-H1, CD274) and PD-L2 (B7-DC, CD273). PD-L1 is mainly an inducible molecule, found predominantly on APC but also on some non-hematopoietic cells. PD-L2 is expressed by DC, macrophages, some B-cell subsets, and, in humans, vascular endothelial cells (Riella et al. 2012b). Like CTLA-4, PD-1 signaling provides a coinhibitory signal in T-cell activation, and therapeutics enhancing its function may have benefit in promoting graft acceptance.

The relevance of this coinhibitory pathway in transplantation was first observed in 2002 by Ozkaynak et al. Using a murine model, they discovered that mRNA of PD-1 and both of its ligands, PD-L1 and PD-L2, was significantly induced during development of cardiac allograft rejection. Treatment with a PD-L1 fusion protein (PD-L1-Ig) promoted allograft survival when used in combination with cyclosporine or rapamycin (Ozkaynak et al. 2002). PD-L1-Ig in combination with anti-CD40L also induced long-term islet allograft survival by inhibiting both CD4 and CD8 T-cell activations (Gao et al. 2003). Conversely, mice deficient of PD-1 show accelerated cardiac allograft, and alloreactive PD-1$^{-/-}$ CD4 and CD8 T cells have enhanced proliferation and cytokine production (Wang et al. 2007b). Blockade of PD-1 by an antagonistic mAb in a non-vascularized concordant rat to mouse islet xenograft model even reversed the protective effect provided by anti-CD40L treatment, indicating that the PD-1 engagement is required for the achievement of prolonged graft survival (Mai et al. 2007). Additionally, in a weakly mismatched model using male islet grafts transplanted into female H-2(b) (C57BL/6) recipient mice, treatment with an antagonistic anti-PD-1 antibody was capable of reversing spontaneous graft tolerance (Thangavelu et al. 2011).

Studies performed in transgenic mice expressing T-cell-restricted PD-1 confirmed prolonged cardiac allograft survival in a minor MHC mismatch model is due in part to enhanced PD-1 signaling in T cells (Chen et al. 2008a). PD-1-Tg T cells demonstrated reduced proliferative and cytokine secretion capacity upon TCR stimulation. Besides its role in effector T-cell activation, several studies have focused on the role of PD-1/PD-L signaling in Tregs. Blockade of PD-L1 using an antagonistic antibody has been shown to reverse graft-protective effects of regulatory T cells in a murine skin transplantation model adoptively transferred with syngeneic conventional CD4 T cells and Treg. Similar observations were made in heart allograft experiments when PD-L1 blockade combined with CTLA-4-Ig treatment led to a significant decrease in the proportion of Foxp3-expressing cells in heart allografts compared to mice treated only with CTLA-4-Ig (del Rio et al. 2008).

10.2.2.1 Role of Donor Tissue Expression of PD-L1

PD-L1 is also expressed by a variety of parenchymal cells, including heart, lung, kidney, pancreas, endothelium, and placenta. Engagement of PD-1 by donor tissue expressing PD-L1 has also been shown to influence PD-1/PD-L1-mediated immunosuppression in transplantation (Riella et al. 2012b). Liver allografts in mice are known to be accepted across MHC barriers without the need for immunosuppression. Elevated PD-L1 expression can be detected in these allografts and is associated with apoptosis of graft-infiltrating T cells. When recipients were treated with an antagonistic anti-PD-L1 mAb or transplanted with a graft from a PD-L1-deficient donor, liver allografts were rapidly rejected and showed severe lymphocyte infiltration (Morita et al. 2010). Similar findings of accelerated rejection, increased inflammatory cell infiltration, and T-cell alloreactivity were also observed in models of islet (Ma et al. 2016) and cardiac transplantation (Yang et al. 2008) using grafts devoid of PD-L1. Tolerance induction of cardiac allografts from PD-L1 chimeric donors treated with CTLA-4-Ig appears to be dependent on both donor expression of PD-L1 on hematopoietic and non-hematopoietic cells (mainly endothelium). PD-L1 deficiency specifically on donor tissue cells results in accelerated and more aggressive rejection (Riella et al. 2011).

10.2.2.2 PD-L1/B7 Interaction

Interestingly, several studies in alloimmunity reveal a significant superior effect of blocking PD-L1 compared to blocking PD-1 using mAbs. Initially, this observation was hypothesized either to be related to the varying expression patterns of PD-1 and PD-L1 or to the half-lives and/or affinity of the used antagonistic antibodies. However, when B7-1 was subsequently identified as an additional binding partner for PD-L1, this interaction was also suspected to be a potential explanation. By using an anti-PD-L1 antibody that selectively blocks the PD-L1/B7-1 interaction (10F.2H11), blockade of the PD-L1/B7-1 pathway was demonstrated to result in significantly worse CAV together with an increase in alloreactivity and a decrease in Treg populations (Yang et al. 2011). This suggests that mechanisms that block B7 to inhibit CD28 signaling may also have the unintended consequence of also blocking pro-tolerogenic B7/PD-1 interactions.

10.2.2.3 Other Strategies to Modulate PD-1/PD-L1

Apart from the use of PD-L1-Ig, an alternative approach to enhance PD-1/PD-L1 signaling is the administration of adenoviral vectors expressing a PD-L1-Ig fusion protein. In a rat cardiac transplant model, transgenic PD-L1 expression on grafts resulted in prolonged graft survival (Dudler et al. 2006). Similarly, in mouse pancreatic islet transplantation, recombinant adenovirus-mediated expression of

PD-L1 in recipient mouse lead to significantly prolonged graft survival, even without additional immunosuppressive therapy (Li et al. 2015).

10.2.3 ICOS/ICOS-L Pathway

ICOS (Inducible T-cell COStimulator; CD278) is another member of the CD28 superfamily. However, unlike CD28, ICOS is not expressed by naïve T cells but is rapidly upregulated upon T-cell activation and is constitutively expressed by some resting memory cells (Hutloff et al. 1999; Yoshinaga et al. 1999). ICOS binds exclusively to ICOS-L (CD275, B7h, B7RP-1), which is expressed on dendritic cells, B cells, and macrophages, and can be induced under inflammatory conditions on non-lymphoid cells (Swallow et al. 1999). ICOS costimulation enhances T-cell activation, differentiation, proliferation, and effector functions. ICOS has also been directly implicated in the induction of T follicular helper cells, which play a crucial role in T-cell-dependent humoral responses (Akiba et al. 2005). Lack of ICOS signaling also results in severely deficient T-cell-dependent B-cell responses, with impairment in germinal center formation and defective immunoglobulin class switching (McAdam et al. 2001; Tafuri et al. 2001).

The finding that the ICOS/ICOS-L pathway affects not only naïve T-cell activation but also memory T cell and T-cell-dependent humoral responses such as germinal center formation and isotype switching makes it an attractive therapeutic target for use in prevention of cell-mediated and antibody-mediated rejection. In fact, graft-infiltrating CD8+ memory T cells, which are critical mediators of belatacept-resistant rejection, upregulate ICOS both in pre-clinical models (rodents and nonhuman primates) (Nanji et al. 2004; Azimzadeh et al. 2006) and in human renal allograft biopsies (Akalin et al. 2003). Although ICOS-mediated signals appear crucial for the development of both acute and chronic rejections (Ozkaynak et al. 2001), ICOS blockade alone has yielded only modest improvement in graft survival (Ozkaynak et al. 2001; Kosuge et al. 2003). This may be due, in part, to the fact that some of its actions, such as modulation of class switching, can be overcome by CD40 stimulation (McAdam et al. 2001). Indeed, combining ICOS and CD40/CD40L blockade results in prolonged graft survival in rodent islet allograft models (Nanji et al. 2006). Synergistic activity was also seen when ICOS blockade was combined with cyclosporine, leading to long-term (>100-day) cardiac allograft survival (Ozkaynak et al. 2001).

ICOS appears to function independently of CD28, suggesting that combined ICOS and CD28 blockade may also be of benefit. Following TCR engagement, ICOS becomes upregulated on T cells, even in the absence of CD28/B7 signaling (Schenk et al. 2009). Furthermore, ICOS is able to induce proliferation in T cells from mice deficient in CD28 (Yoshinaga et al. 1999). However, whereas ICOS blockade in CD28-deficient mice prolongs cardiac allograft survival, the combined use of CD28 and ICOS blockade shows mixed results. While, in mouse cardiac and islet transplant models, combined CTLA-4-Ig and ICOS blockade resulted in

10 Costimulation Blockade in Transplantation

long-term allograft survival (Nanji et al. 2004; Kosuge et al. 2003), in a rat cardiac allograft model, ICOS-Ig abrogated the graft-prolonging effect of CTLA-4-Ig when used in combination (Salama et al. 2003). In this latter study, ICOS-Ig ligation with B7RP-1 resulted in downregulation of B7 expression on APCs, providing a plausible explanation as to why CD28 blockade was rendered ineffective. In a nonhuman primate (NHP) kidney transplant model, neither ICOS-Ig therapy alone or in combination with belatacept prolonged rejection-free graft survival (Lo et al. 2015). Some studies have further suggested that the efficacy of ICOS blockade may depend on the timing of its administration, with results favoring delayed ICOS blockade (Salama et al. 2003; Harada et al. 2003; Kashizuka et al. 2005). Although targeting ICOS may be fruitful in controlling memory T-cell responses that are resistant to the effects of CD28 blockade (Khayyamian et al. 2002; Schenk et al. 2009), further studies are required to resolve these discrepant findings. One explanation may be that ICOS-L also appears to interact with both CD28 and CTLA-4; interaction between ICOS-L and CD28 helps drive primary and memory T-cell allo-responses (Pentcheva-Hoang et al. 2004), creating an intricate and intertwined relationship between these two costimulatory pathways. Additionally, ICOS has the highest expression on IL-10 producing CD4+ T cells (Lohning et al. 2003), and its signaling is linked to the induction of Tregs with potent inhibitory activity (Akbari et al. 2002). Thus, inadvertent blockade of this pro-tolerogenic function may be the cause of these disparate observations. In fact, the anti-ICOS mAb MEDI-570 is currently being evaluated as an immune checkpoint inhibitor targeting ICOS+ Tregs in a Phase I clinical trial sponsored by the National Cancer Institute for treatment of T-cell lymphoma (NCT02520791).

10.2.4 B7-H3

B7-H3 (CD276) is a member of the B7 superfamily of costimulatory molecules. It is a type 1 transmembrane protein with a short cytoplasmic tail and no known signaling domain. As such, it is thought to likely act as a ligand, rather than as a receptor. B7-H3 is broadly expressed in human tissues, and, in the immune system, its expression is induced on monocytes, DCs, and T cells upon activation (Chapoval et al. 2001). This wide pattern of expression suggests B7-H3 may have diverse immunological and non-immunological functions. Its function in T-cell activation remains unclear, with both costimulatory (Chapoval et al. 2001; Luo et al. 2004; Hashiguchi et al. 2008; Wang et al. 2005b) and coinhibitory (Suh et al. 2003; Prasad et al. 2004; Leitner et al. 2009) functions being reported.

Just as in autoimmunity and tumor immunity, the role of B7-H3 in transplantation remains controversial; it has been shown to contribute to both transplant rejection (Wang et al. 2005b) and tolerance (Ueno et al. 2012). In the study by Wang et al., hearts from BALB/c donors transplanted into B7-H3KO or control C57BL/6 mice (full MHC mismatch) were rejected at the same tempo and with the same histological features (Wang et al. 2005b). However, when recipient T-cell responses were dampened by the concomitant use of immunosuppression, it became evident that B7-H3 signaling contributes to the alloimmune response. Using a subtherapeutic regimen of cyclosporine or rapamycin, graft survival was significantly prolonged in B7-H3KO recipients. These allografts from KO recipients showed decreased expression of IL-2 and IFN-γ, and chemokines MCP-1 (monocyte chemoattractant protein) and IP-10 (IFN-inducible protein). Similar findings of graft prolongation in B7-H3-deficient recipients were seen in an islet allograft model where recipients also received rapamycin therapy and in two models of chronic rejection.

In stark contrast, results from our group support the theory that B7-H3 signaling acts as a negative costimulatory pathway (Ueno et al. 2012). Administration of two different B7-H3 fusion proteins (B7-H3-Ig), which signal through a putative B7-H3 receptor, prolonged allograft survival in a fully MHC-mismatched cardiac model by preferentially down-modulating IFN-γ production and promoting a shift toward a graft-protective Th2 milieu. To ensure that the prolongation of graft survival achieved by our fusion proteins was due to the delivery of a negative signal, rather than the blockade of positive costimulatory signals between B7-H3 and its receptor, allografts were transplanted into B7-H3-deficient recipients and treated with B7-H3-Ig or control Ig. Control-treated B7-H3-deficient mice promptly rejected their allografts at a rate comparable to that of wild-type recipients. However, the administration of B7-H3-Ig to B7-H3KO recipients significantly prolonged allograft survival in comparison to control B7-H3KO recipients, suggesting that B7-H3-Ig indeed provides a negative costimulatory signal through a putative B7-H3 receptor. Furthermore, combined treatment with B7-H3-Ig and single-dose CTLA-4-Ig further augmented cardiac allograft survival, suggesting the potential approach of utilizing B7-H3 signaling agents together with strategies to block CD28/B7 in graft-prolonging protocols.

The differing effects observed between these studies may relate to specifics of the individual B7-H3 knockout mice described and/or the binding affinity/functional activity of antibodies or fusion proteins that were studied. Several members of the CD28/B7 family of costimulatory molecules have the potential to be both activators and negative regulators of the T-cell response. It is therefore possible that B7-H3 binds to different receptors, one providing a positive signal and the other a negative signal. These receptors may be expressed at different stages of immune activation or on different T-cell subsets. Additionally, it has been shown that the functions of B7-H3 extend beyond the regulation of T cells and include the ability to inhibit NK cell function (Castriconi et al. 2004), as well as participate in non-immunological processes such as embryogenesis (Suh et al. 2004). Thus, the contrasting roles of B7-H3 could be attributed to multiple receptors on different cell types. To date, only one potential receptor of mouse B7-H3 has been identified: triggering receptor expressed on myeloid cell (TREM)-like transcript (TLT-2) (Hashiguchi et al. 2008). However, others have refuted such interactions between TLT-2 and B7-H3 (Leitner et al. 2009). Finally, B7-H3 also exists in soluble form, and sB7-H3 has been shown to compete with recombinant B7-H3-Ig for binding to the B7-H3 receptor on activated T cells, thereby affecting responses to membrane-bound B7-H3 (Zhang et al. 2008). Thus the reagents used in these studies may also differ in their ability to modulate B7-H3 signaling in these varying scenarios. Further detailed studies are required to elucidate the exact role of B7-H3 in alloimmunity and its therapeutic potential.

10.2.5 B7-H4

B7-H4 is a type 1 transmembrane protein and another member of the B7 family and appears to be a coinhibitory molecule. B7-H4 mRNA is detectable in multiple tissues including spleen, lung, liver, and pancreas (Prasad et al. 2003; Sica et al. 2003). However, its cell surface and protein expression is minimal. It is not expressed on naïve T cells, B cells, or DCs but becomes upregulated on their cell surfaces upon stimulation. Its receptor is currently unknown but is thought to be expressed on activated T cells and distinct from known members of the B7 family (CD28, CTLA-4, ICOS, and PD-1) (Zang et al. 2003). In studies using an agonistic fusion protein, B7-H4 signaling was demonstrated to inhibit T-cell proliferation and cell cycle progression and dampen IL-2 and IFN-γ production (Prasad et al. 2003; Sica et al. 2003). Increased B7-H4 expression on APCs is also associated with their suppressive function and ability to promote Treg IL-10 production (Kryczek et al. 2006).

B7-H4 signaling appears important in promoting allograft survival. While inhibition of B7-H4 signals did not affect the tempo of rejection in WT recipients of fully MHC-mismatched allografts, its blockade did result in accelerated graft rejection in recipients with either CD28 deficiency or combined B7-1/B7-2 deficiency. Furthermore, B7-H4 blockade promotes allospecific IFN-γ, IL-4, and granzyme B responses, leading to abrogation of the graft-prolonging effects of CTLA-4-Ig in WT recipients (Yamaura et al. 2010). These data suggest B7-H4 to be a coinhibitory pathway, and development of B7-H4 agonistic therapies may prove useful in promoting transplant tolerance. While agonistic B7-H4 fusion proteins have been tested in mouse autoimmune models of diabetes, EAE, and nephritis (Wang et al. 2011; Podojil et al. 2013; Pawar et al. 2015), no studies to date have evaluated its efficacy in transplant.

As mentioned, B7-H4 mRNA is expressed in many peripheral tissues, but its protein expression is very tightly controlled. Its role on parenchymal cells is controversial and may have non-immune functions (Qian et al. 2013; Zhang et al. 2013a). However, in the context of transplantation, overexpression of B7-H4 on donor islet cells has been shown to promote islet allograft survival and donor-specific tolerance (Wang et al. 2009; Yuan et al. 2009a; Wang et al. 2012). In contrast, lack of B7-H4 in donor cardiac allografts did not alter the tempo or pattern of rejection (Yamaura et al. 2010). However, this may simply reflect low basal expression of B7-H4 on this tissue. Strategies to overexpress B7-H4 on donor solid organs have yet to be investigated.

10.3 TNF-TNFR Family

10.3.1 CD40/CD40L Pathway

CD40/CD40L interactions play a crucial role in T-cell-dependent humoral immune responses, as well as T-cell-mediated activation of dendritic cells and macrophages. Induction of CD40 stimulates APC-mediated release of pro-inflammatory cytokines and chemokines. In addition, it induces upregulation of B7-1 (CD80) and B7-2 (CD86), thus contributing to CD28-mediated costimulation of activated T cells. Moreover, upon ligation with CD40L (CD154) on T cells, CD40 signaling on B cells promotes their proliferation, immunoglobulin (Ig) production, isotype switching, and memory B-cell generation (Zhang et al. 2015).

10.3.1.1 CD40L Blockade

Interference in CD40/CD40L interactions using anti-CD40L antibodies can effectively prevent acute rejection in murine models of cardiac, pancreatic islet, cornea, and bone marrow transplantation (Larsen et al. 1996; Parker et al. 1995; Zhang et al. 2015). However, CD40/CD40L blockade alone has been found to be insufficient in preventing the development of chronic rejection. Consequently, combination of CD40L inhibition with different therapeutic approaches has been pursued, including use with donor-specific transfusion (DST) and simultaneous targeting of other costimulatory/coinhibitory molecules such as ICOS, PD-L1, and CD28/CTLA-4/B7 (Larsen et al. 1996; Parker et al. 1995). Among these strategies, concurrent blockade of the CD28/B7 and CD40/CD40L pathways presents a promising regimen that promotes allograft survival. In particular, selective CD28 targeting using anti-CD28 mAb (JJ319) or monovalent single-chain variable antagonist antibody fragment (α28scFv) seemed to be advantageous over the use of CTLA-4-Ig (belatacept) when combined with CD40/CD40L blockade (Guillonneau et al. 2007; Zhang et al. 2011).

The anti-CD40L mAbs hu5C8 (ruplizumab) and IDEC-131 (toralizumab) are the two most studied reagents targeting this pathway. hu5C8, a recombinant humanized anti-CD40L monoclonal antibody targeting the 5C8 complementary determining region of CD40L, was initially reported to prevent renal graft rejection in juvenile rhesus monkeys both alone and when combined with CTLA-4-Ig treatment (Kirk et al. 1997). In one regimen, long-term acceptance of renal allografts was established in some cases for more than 1 year after cessation of therapy (Kirk et al. 1999). Even after an episode of rejection, grafts in these recipients were able to regain normal function (Malvezzi et al. 2016). Beneficial effects of this combined approach have also been observed in islet and skin transplantation in rhesus monkeys and baboons, as well as in cardiac transplantation in a cynomolgus monkey model. However, CD40L inhibition with hu5C8 alone was unable to prevent CAV (Zhang et al. 2015). IDEC-131 is a humanized anti-human CD40L mAb that has

10 Costimulation Blockade in Transplantation

been shown to prolong skin allograft survival in a combined setting with rapamycin (both with and without additional DST). It can also prevent acute renal graft rejection when given with rapamycin and DST in rhesus monkeys (Zhang et al. 2015). Again, only moderate beneficial effects of IDEC-131 monotherapy were observed after cardiac transplantation (Pfeiffer et al. 2001). Besides hu5C8 and IDEC-131, two other clones of anti-CD40L mAb, ABI793 and H106, have also been investigated in NHP transplantation models. Monotherapy with the ABI793 and combined treatment with H106 and CTLA-4-Ig were demonstrated to successfully prevent renal allograft rejection in rhesus and cynomolgus monkeys, respectively (Schuler et al. 2004; Kanmaz et al. 2004; Pearson et al. 2002).

10.3.1.2   Challenges Encountered in Use of Anti-CD40L Antibodies

Despite the promising results seen with the anti-CD40L mAbs hu5C8, IDEC-131, and ABI793 in pre-clinical models, adverse effects of these reagents have led to their discontinuation. It is now known that CD40L is not only expressed on immune cells but also on activated platelets, and CD40L blockade results in thromboembolic complications. In NHP pre-clinical studies, hu5C8 and ABI793 had already been linked to thromboembolic side effects (Schuler et al. 2004; Zhang et al. 2015) but could be prevented by the use of perioperative anticoagulation (heparin) and acetyl-salicylic acid (Kawai et al. 2000; Malvezzi et al. 2016). Subsequent Phase II clinical trials of both hu5C8 for the treatment of lupus and renal graft rejection and IDEC-131 in Crohn's disease were halted after the occurrence of unacceptable thromboembolic complications (Zhang et al. 2015). It is now thought that the Fc domain of these mAbs contributes to platelet aggregation by binding to platelet Fc receptor (Robles-Carrillo et al. 2010). Novel anti-CD40L mAbs such as an Fc-disabled aglycosylated anti-CD40L mAb and an Fc-silent anti-CD40L domain antibody are now being investigated in pre-clinical settings and have shown promising results in murine transplant models (Zhang et al. 2015).

Although the CD40/CD40L pathway appears to be important in the development and homeostasis of Foxp3+ Tregs (Guiducci et al. 2005), its blockade does not seem to have any dominant effects on Treg-mediated graft acceptance as has been seen with the use of belatacept.

10.3.1.3   CD40 Blockade

In contrast to CD40L blockade, targeting CD40 on APC represents an alternate approach to disable CD40/CD40L interaction that may not induce side effects related to enhanced platelet aggregation. Current investigated strategies include the development of inhibitory anti-CD40 antibodies (e.g., ASKP1240, CFZ533, 3A8, and 2C10R4), the application of small interfering RNA (siRNA) directed against CD40 mRNA, and gene transfer of CD40-Ig fusion proteins (Malvezzi et al. 2016; Wojciechowski and Vincenti 2016).

ASKP1240 (also known as 4D11; *Astellas, Northbrook, IL*) is a fully humanized IgG4 inhibitory mAb directed against CD40. In pre-clinical nonhuman primate models of kidney and liver transplantation, ASKP1240 increased allograft survival in both settings without increased risk of thromboembolic events (Imai et al. 2007; Oura et al. 2012). Subsequent Phase I clinical trials confirmed it did not increase the risk of thromboembolism and had an overall acceptable safety profile (Goldwater et al. 2013). ASKP1240 is currently being tested in a Phase II clinical trial for the prophylaxis of organ rejection after kidney transplant (NCT01780844) (Astellas Pharma Global Development, Kyowa Hakko Kirin Company and Inc. 2013). Another anti-CD40 antibody currently under clinical investigation is CFZ533 (Novartis Pharmaceuticals). It is undergoing Phase I trials in a number of autoimmune diseases, as well as a proof-of-concept study in kidney transplantation to investigate its safety and efficacy as a replacement for calcineurin inhibitors (NCT02217410). In a pre-clinical NHP renal transplantation model using cynomolgus monkeys, CFZ533 improved graft survival in the absence of thromboembolic events (Cordoba et al. 2015). Pre-clinical studies in NHP have also been performed with 3A8 and 2C10R4. In a model of pancreatic islet transplantation, a combined regimen of 3A8 with basiliximab and sirolimus demonstrated increase graft survival. 2C10R4 was investigated in a model of renal transplantation and showed similar results regarding graft survival compared to CTLA-4-Ig treatment (Malvezzi et al. 2016).

10.3.2 OX40/OX40L Pathway

OX40 (CD134, TNFRSF4) is expressed on most CD4$^+$ and CD8$^+$ T cells and is a strong costimulatory signal for their activation, survival, and proliferation (Chen et al. 1999; Kopf et al. 1999). It is not expressed on resting memory T cells but can be rapidly upregulated following TCR stimulation. In fact, OX40 engagement has been shown to support the transition of activated T effector cells to memory T cells. OX40 is also expressed on Foxp3+ Tregs. However, unlike CD28 costimulation which supports Tregs, OX40 signaling inhibits their suppressive function and prevents their induction. Thus OX40 inhibition may be able to restrain effector T-cell responses while also promoting optimal regulatory T-cell activity. Because of this, there is much interest in targeting this pathway to achieve transplant tolerance (Demirci and Li 2008).

In a murine cardiac transplantation model, stimulation of OX40 by an agonistic anti-OX40 mAb was found to abrogate allograft acceptance induced through CD40/ CD40L blockade, by promoting a CD4+ T-cell-mediated acute rejection (Burrell et al. 2009). Treatment with an antagonistic anti-OX40 mAb was also capable of affecting CD8+ T-cell alloreactivity and preventing rejection in a CD8+ T-cell-mediated model of skin transplantation. However, tolerance could not be induced, and allografts were eventually rejected after stopping treatment (Kinnear et al. 2010). Interestingly, later experiments by the same group showed that blockade of

OX40-OX40L interaction prevented skin allograft rejection not through inhibition of T-cell activation and proliferation but rather through impaired accumulation of effector T cells in peripheral lymph nodes and reduced ability of these cells to traffic to the allograft (Kinnear et al. 2013).

10.3.2.1 Effects of OX40 Signaling on Memory T Cells

Memory T cells (Tmem) are key mediators of chronic allograft vasculopathy (CAV) and pose a significant barrier to the induction of transplant tolerance. In fact, Tmem that are generated by either homeostatic proliferation or prior donor antigen sensitization can evoke acute skin allograft rejection, even when recipient mice are treated with combined CD28 and CD40L blockade (Vu et al. 2006). These Tmem were shown to express high levels of OX40, CD137, and ICOS on their cell surface and led to interest in targeting OX40/OX40L to mitigate the effects of these cells. Indeed, when OX40 costimulation blockade was administered in combination with either CD28 or CD40L blockade, long-term skin allograft survival of >100 days could be induced in 40% of recipients. However, blockade of OX40/OX40L alone was of no benefit in this model. In a murine cardiac transplant model, treatment with an antagonistic anti-OX40L mAb led to significant reduction in Tmem populations and prevention of CAV (Wang et al. 2014). Similar findings were confirmed in an islet transplant model, in which anti-OX40L mAb prevented activation of CD4+ Tmem and significantly prolonged graft survival.

10.3.2.2 Effects of OX40 Signaling on Regulatory T Cells

Islet allograft experiments in CD40L-deficient mice using antagonistic and agonistic anti-OX40 mAbs showed that OX40 differentially regulates effector T cells and Foxp3+ Treg (Chen et al. 2008b). While OX40 signaling promoted proliferation of T effector cells, it blocked the induction and suppressive functions of Foxp3+ Tregs in this model. Interestingly, genetic depletion of OX40 had no effect on Treg development or function (Vu et al. 2007). However, costimulation of OX40 together with TCR engagement on Tregs led to reduced Foxp3 expression and suppressive activity (Vu et al. 2007). In an alloantigen-primed islet transplantation model, the use of anti-CD40L together with anti-CD154 and anti-LFA-1 not only significantly reduced the proportion of memory T cells but also resulted in an elevated proportion of Treg in the spleen (Xia et al. 2010). Similar findings were observed in a presensitized murine cardiac transplantation model where addition of anti-OX40L to the treatment regimen restored graft tolerance by targeting memory responses and promoting tolerogenic DC and Treg. Depletion of CD25+ T cells in this model prevented establishment of allograft acceptance, suggesting a Treg-mediated mechanism of tolerance (Ge et al. 2010).

10.3.2.3 Potential Therapeutic Approaches Targeting OX40/OX40L

Blockade of the OX40/OX40L pathway alone has been shown to have little effect on allograft outcomes, but the pathway does appear to have a non-redundant function when CD28 and CD40 signaling is disabled (Vu et al. 2006; Yuan et al. 2003; Demirci et al. 2004; Wang et al. 2005a). Combining OX40 inhibition with agonistic approaches to promote coinhibitory pathways also appears promising. In a mouse model for islet allograft rejection, lentiviral vectors containing OX40L siRNA sequences and an adenovirus vector containing the PD-L1 gene were injected the day before islet transplantation. The resultant reduction in OX40L protein expression together with the increased PD-L1 protein levels led to significantly prolonged allograft survival when compared to the control or single-treatment groups (Li et al. 2014). OX40 inhibition in combination with a single low dose of rapamycin was also found to be capable of improving graft survival in a rat model of allogeneic superficial inferior epigastric artery flap transplantation (Fu et al. 2010). GBR 830, an antagonistic anti-OX40 mAb (Glenmark Pharmaceuticals), was well tolerated and showed an acceptable safety profile in Phase I studies performed in the Netherlands. A Phase II trial examining its efficacy in atopic dermatitis has just recently been completed, with results pending (NCT02683928). There are yet to be any clinical trials for use in transplantation.

10.3.3 CD27/CD70

CD27 is constitutively expressed on naive and memory T cells as well as on subsets of activated B cells, NK cells, and hematopoietic progenitor cells (Tesselaar et al. 2003). Upon T-cell activation, CD27 expression transiently increases before becoming downregulated after several rounds of cell division, such that T cells with potent effector responses become devoid of CD27. In contrast, the expression of its ligand CD70 is tightly regulated. Quiescent T cells, B cells, and DC lack CD70, but its expression can be induced upon activation via TLR, CD40, and/or antigen receptor signaling. This expression pattern suggests CD27 signaling on T cells occurs through binding with CD70 on activated B cells or DCs or via T-T interactions. Furthermore, CD70 is capable of inward signaling, allowing for bidirectional effects of CD27/CD70 interactions. This coordinated interaction promotes the development of an effective T-cell response by augmenting other costimulatory signals to enhance T-cell proliferation and cytokine production (reviewed in Watts (2005)).

Early results targeting the CD27/CD70 pathway in transplantation were discouraging. Treatment with an anti-CD70 mAb had no effect on islet survival either alone or in combination with an anti-OX40L mAb nor when used in CD28$^{-/-}$ recipient mice. However, when studied in a murine full MHC-mismatched cardiac allograft model, treatment with anti-CD70 mAb did significantly prolonged heart allograft survival (Adams et al. 2002; Yamada et al. 2005), suggesting its efficacy may be dependent on the model organ. Subsequent investigations have thus focused primarily on the application of CD70 blockade in cardiac allograft models. In a pre-sensitized model, combination therapy with anti-CD70, anti-CD40L, anti-CD8, and rapamycin has been shown to promote graft acceptance by reducing T-cell infiltration and eliminating pre-existing donor-specific antibodies (Shariff et al. 2010), indicating the potential to mitigate memory recall responses. Similar studies investigating the synergistic effect of CD44/CD70 blockade and anti-CD40L/LFA-1 demonstrated limited effects of CD44/CD70 blockade alone, but in combination with anti-CD40L/LFA-1 treatment, CD44/CD70 blockade significantly prolonged cardiac allograft survival (Shao et al. 2011b). Furthermore, when combined with donor-specific transfusion (DST), CD44/CD70 blockade notably reduced the expansion of memory T cells, enhanced the proportion of CD4 + Foxp3+ regulatory T cells (Tregs), and suppressed donor-specific responses (Shao et al. 2011a). This is somewhat at odds with findings in the cancer literature demonstrating CD27 signaling reduces Treg apoptosis and increased their frequency (Claus et al. 2012). Further studies are required to fully elucidate the role of this pathway in allospecific effector versus regulatory T-cell responses.

10.3.4   GITR/GITRL

The glucocorticoid-induced TNFR-related protein (GITR) is expressed by T lymphocytes, NK cells, and APCs. Although expressed only at low levels on resting T cells, it becomes upregulated upon activation, particularly in the presence of CD28 signaling (Kwon et al. 1999). Its ligand, GITRL, is mainly expressed on APC following TLR stimulation (Tone et al. 2003). GITR activation functions as a positive costimulatory signal, promoting proliferation and enhanced survival of naïve, Th1/Th2 CD4 T cells and CD8 T cells under limited CD3 stimulation (Tone et al. 2003; Kanamaru et al. 2004). GITR is also constitutively expressed on CD4 + CD25+ Tregs, and stimulation of GITR signaling on these cells is capable of breaking self-tolerance (Shimizu et al. 2002). Thus, GITR/GITRL interaction is one pathway by which antigen-presenting cells may enhance the adaptive response to foreign antigen by simultaneously counter-regulating Tregs and costimulating effector T cells (Sonawane et al. 2009).

The potential role of Treg in transplant recipients was first explored by the addition of depleting anti-CD25 antibody to tolerance induction protocols. However, this approach deletes not only CD25+ Tregs but also T effector cells that upregulate CD25 upon activation. This led to interest in targeting GITR to characterize the central role of Treg in graft tolerance. Using a tolerizing regimen known to generate Tregs from CD25$^-$ precursors, Bushell and colleagues showed GITR engagement attenuated Treg function and led to graft rejection (Bushell and Wood 2007). Conversely, GITR inhibition with an activation-inducible TNF receptor (AITRL)-Fc construct allowed for long-term Treg-dependent graft acceptance in a model of skin transplantation (Sonawane et al. 2009). A second strategy targeting GITRL using a soluble GITR fusion protein (GITR-Fc) also further prolonged graft survival in a full MHC-mismatched skin graft model when used in combination with an anti-CD40L antibody (Kim et al. 2010).

10.3.5 CD137/CD137L

CD137 (4-1BB, TNFRSF9) is expressed on T cells, DC, and B cells. Similar to many other costimulatory molecules discussed here, CD137 is not expressed on naïve T cells but rather on activated effector cells (Kwon and Weissman 1989). Its expression peaks early following T-cell activation and is usually rapid and transient. However, in the context of chronic infections and transplantation, where foreign antigen persists, CD137 expression can be sustained (Tan et al. 2000; Seo et al. 2003). Its ligand CD137L (4-1BBL, TNFSF9) is expressed on APCs including mature DCs, macrophages, and activated B cells, but not on resting or activated T cells (Futagawa et al. 2002). CD137 signaling augments T-cell proliferation, prevents activation-induced cell death, and, under strong antigenic stimuli, can replace CD28 costimulation in CD8 T cells (Hurtado et al. 1997; Saoulli et al. 1998; Halstead et al. 2002). Engagement of CD137L has also been shown to deliver an inward signal into monocytes and B cells (Langstein et al. 1998; Pauly et al. 2002), thus allowing for bidirectional signaling and complicating the interpretation of studies manipulating this pathway in vivo.

The relevance of the CD137/CD137L pathway in transplant immunology has been investigated by several approaches: activation or inhibition by antagonistic CD137 mAbs and genetic knockout or silencing of CD137. Treatment with an agonistic anti-CD137 mAb in murine cardiac and skin transplantation models demonstrated accelerated graft rejection, giving first evidence for the therapeutic potential of targeting CD137 (Adams et al. 2002). Meanwhile, blockade of CD137 signaling using an antagonistic anti-CD137 mAb, or CD137 deficiency in recipients, extended graft survival (Cho et al. 2004). Studies using a murine model for intestinal transplantation also revealed CD137 blockade to significantly inhibited allograft rejection, interestingly mainly mediated by CD8+ but not CD4+ T cells (Wang et al. 2003). In an additional approach, effects of disabled CD137/CD137L interaction were investigated in a rat model for liver transplantation using gene silencing of CD137 by RNA interference (RNAi) (Shi et al. 2013). While CD137 signaling has been shown to reprogram Tregs into cytotoxic effector T cells and restore antitumor immunity (Akhmetzyanova et al. 2016), its role on allospecific Tregs has yet to be explored in transplantation.

10.4 TIM Family

The T-cell immunoglobulin mucin (*TIM*) family of genes encode type 1 glycoproteins, with a common immunoglobulin V-like domain, mucin-like domain, a single transmembrane domain, and a cytoplasmic region (Freeman et al.). The TIM family comprises of eight genes on mouse chromosome 11B1.1 and three genes on the human chromosome 5q33.2. The three human *tim* genes are most similar to mouse TIM-1/TIM-2, TIM-3, and TIM-4. TIM molecules were initially described as a novel family of costimulatory molecules that are critical in directing T helper cell activation and differentiation (Rodriguez-Manzanet et al. 2009). However, further studies have ascribed differing functions, including the ability to mediate phagocytosis and regulate immunity through removal of apoptotic cells (Kobayashi et al. 2007; Nakayama et al. 2009; Brooks et al. 2015) and lymphocyte trafficking (Angiari et al. 2014; Echbarthi et al. 2015) and promote B-cell tolerance (Ding et al. 2011; Xiao et al. 2012; Yeung et al. 2015). In this review, we will focus on their roles in T-cell costimulation.

10.4.1 Tim-1

In immune cells, TIM-1 is expressed on several B- and T-cell subsets, DC, and NKT cells. While absent on naive CD4 T cells, TIM-1 expression increases following TCR stimulation. TIM-1 associates with ZAP-70 and CD3, and its engagement leads to amplification of TCR signaling (Binne et al. 2007; Kane 2010). Monoclonal Abs targeting TIM-1 have been shown to elicit differing cytokine responses. TIM-1 engagement with RMT1-10 and 1H8.2 mAb on T cells preferentially induces production of Th2 cytokines, whereas high-affinity mTIM-1 mAb such as 3B3 induces secretion of Th1/Th17 cytokines (IFN-γ and IL-17) (Sizing et al. 2007; Xiao et al. 2007). The basis for these conflicting findings is currently unclear and may be related to differing binding affinities, ability to block interaction of TIM-1 with phosphatidylserine on apoptotic cells, and/or differences in various disease models.

Initial studies in a murine cardiac transplant model showed TIM-1 is not only essential for the regulation of Th1 and Th2 immune responses but is also able to regulate Th17 and regulatory T cells (Ueno et al. 2008). In vivo administration of the anti-TIM-1 mAb RMT1-10 significantly prolonged allograft survival in a fully mismatched model and when used synergistically with rapamycin was able to induce indefinite survival (Ueno et al. 2008). Graft prolongation in both instances was associated with inhibition of alloreactive Th1 cells but preservation/promotion of alloreactive Th2 response. This protective effect of RMT1-10 was dependent on the presence of CD4 + CD25+ regulatory T cells. Moreover, in a model of Tbet deficiency, RMT1-10 specifically inhibited IL-17-producing CD8+ T cells, a subset thought to mediate resistance to CD28 blockade and tolerance induction (Yuan et al. 2009b). These findings were corroborated in an islet transplant model, where use of an agonistic anti-TIM-1 antibody 3B3 fostered commitment to Th1/Th17 phenotype, hindered the development of Tregs, and negated the tolerance-promoting effect of anti-CD40L therapy (Degauque et al. 2008). While initial studies on TIM-1 in transplant models focused on T-cell-mediated responses, a growing body of literature demonstrates its importance in B-cell-mediated tolerance (Ding et al. 2011; Yeung et al. 2015). Further complicating matters is the finding that while the anti-TIM-1 mAb clone RMT1-10 has been described as "antagonistic" and capable of blocking TIM-1 signals on T cells, it appears to promote TIM-1 signaling in B cells and confer enhanced suppressive activity of Bregs (Ding et al. 2011; Yeung et al. 2015). The relative importance of TIM-1 signaling in T cells vs B cells in mediating allograft survival, and better characterization of these mAbs, remains to be further elucidated.

The role of TIM-1 has also been examined in models of liver and renal ischemia-reperfusion injury. Treatment with "antagonistic" TIM-1 mAb (RMT1-10) improved the hepatocellular function and diminished TLR4-dependent inflammation in both warm and cold liver IRI models (Uchida et al. 2010; Zhang et al. 2013b). Analysis of CD4 T cells in these mice showed blocking TIM-1 signaling reduced Th1 transcription factor Tbet and IFN-γ mRNA levels while enhancing expression of Th2-related IL-4/IL-10 and Treg transcription factor Foxp3. Disruption of TIM-1 signaling also suppressed neutrophil and macrophage activation and recruitment to ischemic damaged livers. To exclude the predominant roles of TIM-1 on other cell subsets such as NKT and B cells, liver IRI was induced in RAG$-/-$ mice that were reconstituted with purified syngeneic spleen CD4+ T cells. RAG$-/-$ recipients that were then treated with antagonistic TIM-1 mAb demonstrated less hepatocellular damage compared to control-treated recipients. Additionally, pre-activated TIM-1^{Hi} but not TIM-1^{Lo} CD4 T cells were able to trigger significant liver damage in otherwise IR-resistant RAG$^{-/-}$ mice, implying a crucial role of TIM-1+ CD4 T cells in the mechanism of liver IRI. Of note, TIM-1 blockade not only suppressed total macrophage recruitment but preferentially suppressed infiltration of macrophages that expressed TIM-4 (CD68 + TIM-4+ cells). Similarly, use of RMT1-10 preserved renal function and protected against acute tubular necrosis in a model of kidney ischemia-reperfusion injury (Rong et al. 2011). Kidneys from mice treated with RMT1-10 showed decreased recruitment of leukocytes (neutrophils, macrophages, and CD4+ T cells) and reduced local production of pro-inflammatory cytokines. However, the beneficial effects of RMT1-10 after IRI did not appear to be related to a Th2 cytokine shift in this model. Systemic and local Th2 cytokine levels decreased in a similar manner as Th1 cytokine levels did, likely reflecting an overall decrease in T-cell activation. Similar to the liver IRI model, there was a reduction in leukocyte recruitment into the damaged kidney, consistent with reports in autoimmunity showing TIM-1 binds P-selectin and mediates T-cell trafficking (Angiari et al. 2014).

10.4.2 Tim-4

TIM-4 is primarily expressed on APCs, including CD11c[+] dendritic cells, macrophages, and peritoneal B-1 B cells (Meyers et al. 2005) (Rodriguez-Manzanet et al. 2008). Although it was initially identified as the ligand for TIM-1, it is now unclear whether direct interaction occurs and may occur via bridging exosomes (Kobayashi et al. 2007). TIM-4 does act a phosphatidylserine (PS) receptor, capable of binding and engulfing apoptotic bodies (Kobayashi et al. 2007), but it may also have other ligand pairs that have yet to be identified. Studies utilizing TIM-4-Ig fusion proteins, especially in in vitro systems, have demonstrated conflicting results. Effects of TIM-4-Ig may also be dependent on the activation status of T cells. Treatment of naïve T cells with soluble TIM-4 fusion protein has been shown to both activate (Rodriguez-Manzanet et al. 2008) and inhibit (Mizui et al. 2008) T-cell activation, whereas treatment of pre-activated T cells enhanced activation (Mizui et al. 2008).

In a skin transplant model, blockade of TIM-4 using the mAb RMT4-53 resulted in significant prolongation of graft survival characterized by reduction in T effector responses and dependent upon the induction of regulatory T cells (Yeung et al. 2013). Supporting in vitro studies demonstrated it was blockade of DC-expressed TIM-4 that led to differentiation of naïve T cells into Foxp3+ Tregs, through suppression of Th2 differentiation. In contrast, in islet transplantation, the use of RMT4-53 appeared to promote Th2 responses and in a Th1-mediated model was capable of enhancing islet allograft survival by a Th1 to Th2 skewing of the immune response (Vergani et al. 2015). However, when tested in a model where islet graft rejection is mediated through Th2 mechanisms, blockade of TIM-4 precipitated rejection by further enhancing the Th2 response (Vergani et al. 2015). In both models, these effects were dependent on B cells, as the depletion of this population abolished the effect of TIM-4 targeting. A subsequent study has confirmed the importance of TIM-4 on B cells, specifically demonstrating its expression on the IFN-γ-producing effector B-cell subset (Beff) (Ding et al. 2017). Specifically, TIM-4+ Beff cells accelerated rejection in an IFN-γ-dependent manner and promoted pro-inflammatory Th1 responses while decreasing IL-4, IL-10, and Foxp3 expression by CD4[+] T cells. Although these latter studies underscore the importance of B-cell TIM-4 responses, they do not preclude a role for its other functions, such as apoptotic cell uptake or function on DCs, since anti-TIM-4 mAb was able to prolong GS, even in the absence of TIM-4+ B cells. Additionally, TIM-4 appears to be highly expressed on CD169[+] macrophages, a major subset of tissue-resident macrophages that exhibit an immunoregulatory and hypostimulatory phenotype and favor preferential induction of antigen-stimulated Tregs (Thornley et al. 2014). The absence of TIM-4 on these cells appeared to enhance their survival, and TIM4[−/−] heart allografts survived much longer and were more easily tolerized compared with heart allografts from WT mice.

Targeting of TIM-4 has also been explored in liver ischemia-reperfusion injury (Ji et al. 2014). Recipients with disrupted TIM-4 signaling (treated with antagonistic TIM-4 mAb or use of TIM-4KO recipients) were resistant to liver IRI, because of reduced macrophage migration, phagocytosis, and activation. These results appeared to be dependent on macrophage-specific TIM-4 signaling rather than T-cell costimulation. As is the case with TIM-1, further studies are needed to fully characterize the role of TIM-4 on various immune cell subsets before therapeutic targeting can move toward clinical application.

10.4.3 TIM-3/Galectin-9

TIM-3 was initially identified on Th1-differentiated cells but is now known to be present on a variety of immune cells, including constitutive expression on dendritic cells, macrophages, and mast cells (Freeman et al. 2010). On T cells, it is expressed on many fully activated effector T cells and a marker of T cells undergoing exhaustion. Its ligand, galectin-9, is an S-type lectin expressed on T cells including Tregs, B cells, and mast cells, as well as on a variety of non-immune cells. Interaction between TIM-3 on T effector cells and galectin-9 on Tregs results in the selective death of the TIM-3+ cell (Zhu et al. 2005), thereby restraining the Th1/Th17 response. Finally, as with the other TIM family members, TIM-3 is known to be a phosphatidylserine receptor, capable of mediating cross-presentation of antigens associated with dying cells (Nakayama et al. 2009).

Regulatory T cells play a crucial role in the induction and maintenance of donor-specific transplant tolerance (Wood and Sakaguchi 2003; Yeung and Sayegh 2009), and interaction between galectin-9 and TIM-3 appears to be key to the process. Blockade of the TIM-3 pathway abrogated islet allograft tolerance, induced through the tolerizing regimen of DST plus anti-CD40L, by dampening the immunosuppressive function of Tregs (Sanchez-Fueyo et al. 2003). Furthermore, TIM-3-deficient mice rapidly rejected their grafts despite treatment with this tolerizing regimen, which in WT recipients induces indefinite graft survival.

In a cardiac allograft model, blockade of TIM-3/galectin-9 signaling using an anti-TIM-3 mAb (RMT 3-23) also led to accelerated rejection. This was characterized by an increase in Th1 and Th17 responses, suppression of Treg induction, and promotion of donor-specific alloantibody production (Boenisch et al. 2010). Conversely, treatment with exogenous galectin-9 to promote signaling through this pathway promoted graft survival in both murine skin and cardiac transplant recipients through similar mechanisms (Wang et al. 2008; He et al. 2009). Additionally, this pathway has also been shown to negatively regulate alloreactive CD8+ T cells, leading to prolongation of skin allograft survival (Wang et al. 2007a).

To date, human studies in transplantation have largely focused upon using TIM-3 as a marker of Th1 activation and rejection. TIM-3 mRNA has been detected within rejecting allografts at significantly higher levels than in control protocol biopsy samples, with strong correlations between intragraft TIM-3 and IFN-γ levels (Ponciano et al. 2007). Curiously, rejection episodes that were refractory to treatment showed lower levels of TIM-3 than those that responded well. A subsequent murine study found the population of CD4[+]Foxp3+ TIM-3[+]PD-1[+] Tregs increased in frequency and heavily infiltrated the skin allograft as the alloimmune response proceeded (Gupta et al. 2012). Importantly, these Tregs possessed potent regulatory capacity, which may be why the intragraft expression of TIM-3 was shown to correlate with treatment response.

10.5 Conclusion

Costimulation blockade continues to be a promising therapeutic strategy, capable of modulating alloimmune responses and promoting graft tolerance. This is evidence by the success of belatacept, a first-in-class CTLA-4 fusion protein now clinically used in the prevention of transplant rejection. However, it remains clear that we have only scratched the surface in understanding the complexities of how costimulatory pathways modulate the immune system. Our initial assumption that positive costimulatory molecules activate effector T cells and prevent tolerance, while negative costimulatory pathways inhibit effector T cells and promote tolerance, is clearly an oversimplified view. The intricate role of these molecules in controlling regulatory T-cell responses, their importance at various stages in the alloimmune response, and their potential to cross-interact with one another all require further study. Targeting one molecule alone is likely to be insufficient, but in the coming years, we may be able to selectively modulate various costimulatory pathways to achieve transplant tolerance in humans.

References

Adams AB, Larsen CP, Pearson TC, Newell KA (2002) The role of TNF receptor and TNF super-family molecules in organ transplantation. Am J Transplant 2:12–18

Adams AB, Williams MA, Jones TR, Shirasugi N, Durham MM, Kaech SM, Wherry EJ, Onami T, Lanier JG, Kokko KE, Pearson TC, Ahmed R, Larsen CP (2003) Heterologous immunity provides a potent barrier to transplantation tolerance. J Clin Invest 111:1887–1895

Akalin E, Dikman S, Murphy B, Bromberg JS, Hancock WW (2003) Glomerular infiltration by CXCR3+ ICOS+ activated T cells in chronic allograft nephropathy with transplant glomerulopathy. Am J Transplant 3:1116–1120

Akbari O, Freeman GJ, Meyer EH, Greenfield EA, Chang TT, Sharpe AH, Berry G, DeKruyff RH, Umetsu DT (2002) Antigen-specific regulatory T cells develop via the ICOS-ICOS-ligand pathway and inhibit allergen-induced airway hyperreactivity. Nat Med 8:1024–1032

Akhmetzyanova I, Zelinskyy G, Littwitz-Salomon E, Malyshkina A, Dietze KK, Streeck H, Brandau S, Dittmer U (2016) CD137 agonist therapy can reprogram regulatory T cells into cytotoxic CD4+ T cells with antitumor activity. J Immunol 196:484–492

Akiba H, Takeda K, Kojima Y, Usui Y, Harada N, Yamazaki T, Ma J, Tezuka K, Yagita H, Okumura K (2005) The role of ICOS in the CXCR5+ follicular B helper T cell maintenance in vivo. J Immunol 175:2340–2348

Alegre ML, Najafian N (2006) Costimulatory molecules as targets for the induction of transplantation tolerance. Curr Mol Med 6:843–857

Alegre ML, Noel PJ, Eisfelder BJ, Chuang E, Clark MR, Reiner SL, Thompson CB (1996) Regulation of surface and intracellular expression of CTLA4 on mouse T cells. J Immunol 157:4762–4770

Angiari S, Donnarumma T, Rossi B, Dusi S, Pietronigro E, Zenaro E, Della Bianca V, Toffali L, Piacentino G, Budui S, Rennert P, Xiao S, Laudanna C, Casasnovas JM, Kuchroo VK, Constantin G (2014) TIM-1 glycoprotein binds the adhesion receptor P-selectin and mediates T cell trafficking during inflammation and autoimmunity. Immunity 40:542–553

Archdeacon P, Dixon C, Belen O, Albrecht R, Meyer J (2012) Summary of the US FDA approval of belatacept. Am J Transplant 12:554–562

Astellas Pharma Global Development, Inc., Limited Kyowa Hakko Kirin Company, and Astellas Pharma Inc (2013) A study to assess the efficacy and safety of ASKP1240 in de novo kidney transplant recipients. https://ClinicalTrials.gov/show/NCT01780844

Azimzadeh AM, Pfeiffer S, Wu G, Schroder C, Zorn GL 3rd, Kelishadi SS, Ozkaynak E, Kehry M, Atkinson JB, Miller GG, Pierson RN 3rd. (2006) Alloimmunity in primate heart recipients with CD154 blockade: evidence for alternative costimulation mechanisms. Transplantation 81:255–264

Binne LL, Scott ML, Rennert PD (2007) Human TIM-1 associates with the TCR complex and up-regulates T cell activation signals. J Immunol 178:4342–4350

Blattman JN, Antia R, Sourdive DJ, Wang X, Kaech SM, Murali-Krishna K, Altman JD, Ahmed R (2002) Estimating the precursor frequency of naive antigen-specific CD8 T cells. J Exp Med 195:657–664

Bluestone JA, Liu W, Yabu JM, Laszik ZG, Putnam A, Belingheri M, Gross DM, Townsend RM, Vincenti F (2008) The effect of costimulatory and interleukin 2 receptor blockade on regulatory T cells in renal transplantation. Am J Transplant 8:2086–2096

Boenisch O, Sayegh MH, Najafian N (2008) Negative T-cell costimulatory pathways: their role in regulating alloimmune responses. Curr Opin Organ Transplant 13:373–378

Boenisch O, D'Addio F, Watanabe T, Elyaman W, Magee CN, Yeung MY, Padera RF, Rodig SJ, Murayama T, Tanaka K, Yuan X, Ueno T, Jurisch A, Mfarrej B, Akiba H, Yagita H, Najafian N (2010) TIM-3: a novel regulatory molecule of alloimmune activation. J Immunol 185:5806–5819

Brooks CR, Yeung MY, Brooks YS, Chen H, Ichimura T, Henderson JM, Bonventre JV (2015) KIM-1-/TIM-1-mediated phagocytosis links ATG5-/ULK1-dependent clearance of apoptotic cells to antigen presentation. EMBO J 34:2441–2464

Burrell BE, Csencsits K, Lu G, Grabauskiene S, Bishop DK (2008) CD8+ Th17 mediate costimulation blockade-resistant allograft rejection in T-bet-deficient mice. J Immunol 181:3906–3914

Burrell BE, Lu G, Li XC, Bishop DK (2009) OX40 costimulation prevents allograft acceptance induced by CD40-CD40L blockade. J Immunol 182:379–390

Bushell A, Wood K (2007) GITR ligation blocks allograft protection by induced CD25+CD4+ regulatory T cells without enhancing effector T-cell function. Am J Transplant 7:759–768

Butte MJ, Keir ME, Phamduy TB, Sharpe AH, Freeman GJ (2007) Programmed death-1 ligand 1 interacts specifically with the B7-1 costimulatory molecule to inhibit T cell responses. Immunity 27:111–122

Castriconi R, Dondero A, Augugliaro R, Cantoni C, Carnemolla B, Sementa AR, Negri F, Conte R, Corrias MV, Moretta L, Moretta A, Bottino C (2004) Identification of 4Ig-B7-H3 as a neuroblastoma-associated molecule that exerts a protective role from an NK cell-mediated lysis. Proc Natl Acad Sci U S A 101:12640–12645

Chapoval AI, Ni J, Lau JS, Wilcox RA, Flies DB, Liu D, Dong H, Sica GL, Zhu G, Tamada K, Chen L (2001) B7-H3: a costimulatory molecule for T cell activation and IFN-gamma production. Nat Immunol 2:269–274

Chen AI, McAdam AJ, Buhlmann JE, Scott S, Lupher ML Jr, Greenfield EA, Baum PR, Fanslow WC, Calderhead DM, Freeman GJ, Sharpe AH (1999) Ox40-ligand has a critical costimulatory role in dendritic cell:T cell interactions. Immunity 11:689–698

Chen L, Hussien Y, Hwang KW, Wang Y, Zhou P, Alegre ML (2008a) Overexpression of program death-1 in T cells has mild impact on allograft survival. Transpl Int 21:21–29

Chen M, Xiao X, Demirci G, Li XC (2008b) OX40 controls islet allograft tolerance in CD154 deficient mice by regulating FoxP3+ Tregs. Transplantation 85:1659–1662

Cho HR, Kwon B, Yagita H, La S, Lee EA, Kim JE, Akiba H, Kim J, Suh JH, Vinay DS, Ju SA, Kim BS, Mittler RS, Okumura K, Kwon BS (2004) Blockade of 4-1BB (CD137)/4-1BB ligand interactions increases allograft survival. Transpl Int 17:351–361

Claus C, Riether C, Schurch C, Matter MS, Hilmenyuk T, Ochsenbein AF (2012) CD27 signaling increases the frequency of regulatory T cells and promotes tumor growth. Cancer Res 72:3664–3676

Cordoba F, Wieczorek G, Audet M, Roth L, Schneider MA, Kunkler A, Stuber N, Erard M, Ceci M, Baumgartner R, Apolloni R, Cattini A, Robert G, Ristig D, Munz J, Haeberli L, Grau R, Sickert D, Heusser C, Espie P, Bruns C, Patel D, Rush JS (2015) A novel, blocking, Fc-silent anti-CD40 monoclonal antibody prolongs nonhuman primate renal allograft survival in the absence of B cell depletion. Am J Transplant 15:2825–2836

D'Addio F, Yuan X, Habicht A, Williams J, Ruzek M, Iacomini J, Turka LA, Sayegh MH, Najafian N, Ansari MJ (2010) A novel clinically relevant approach to tip the balance toward regulation in stringent transplant model. Transplantation 90:260–269

Degauque N, Mariat C, Kenny J, Zhang D, Gao W, Vu MD, Alexopoulos S, Oukka M, Umetsu DT, DeKruyff RH, Kuchroo V, Zheng XX, Strom TB (2008) Immunostimulatory Tim-1-specific antibody deprograms Tregs and prevents transplant tolerance in mice. J Clin Invest 118:735–741

del Rio ML, Buhler L, Gibbons C, Tian J, Rodriguez-Barbosa JI (2008) PD-1/PD-L1, PD-1/PD-L2, and other co-inhibitory signaling pathways in transplantation. Transpl Int 21:1015–1028

Demirci G, Li XC (2008) Novel roles of OX40 in the allograft response. Curr Opin Organ Transplant 13:26–30

Demirci G, Amanullah F, Kewalaramani R, Yagita H, Strom TB, Sayegh MH, Li XC (2004) Critical role of OX40 in CD28 and CD154-independent rejection. J Immunol 172:1691–1698

Dengler TJ, Szabo G, Sido B, Nottmeyer W, Zimmerman R, Vahl CF, Hunig T, Meuer SC (1999) Prolonged allograft survival but no tolerance induction by modulating CD28 antibody JJ319 after high-responder rat heart transplantation. Transplantation 67:392–398

Ding Q, Yeung M, Camirand G, Zeng Q, Akiba H, Yagita H, Chalasani G, Sayegh MH, Najafian N, Rothstein DM (2011) Regulatory B cells are identified by expression of TIM-1 and can be induced through TIM-1 ligation to promote tolerance in mice. J Clin Invest 121:3645–3656

Ding Q, Mohib K, Kuchroo VK, Rothstein DM (2017) TIM-4 identifies IFN-gamma-expressing Proinflammatory B effector 1 cells that promote tumor and allograft rejection. J Immunol 199:2585–2595

Dong VM, Yuan X, Coito AJ, Waaga AM, Sayegh MH, Chandraker A (2002) Mechanisms of targeting CD28 by a signaling monoclonal antibody in acute and chronic allograft rejection. Transplantation 73:1310–1317

Dudler J, Li J, Pagnotta M, Pascual M, von Segesser LK, Vassalli G (2006) Gene transfer of programmed death ligand-1.Ig prolongs cardiac allograft survival. Transplantation 82:1733–1737

Durrbach A, Pestana JM, Pearson T, Vincenti F, Garcia VD, Campistol J, Rial Mdel C, Florman S, Block A, Di Russo G, Xing J, Garg P, Grinyo J (2010) A phase III study of belatacept versus cyclosporine in kidney transplants from extended criteria donors (BENEFIT-EXT study). Am J Transplant 10:547–557

Durrbach A, Pestana JM, Florman S, Del Carmen Rial M, Rostaing L, Kuypers D, Matas A, Wekerle T, Polinsky M, Meier-Kriesche HU, Munier S, Grinyo JM (2016) Long-term outcomes in Belatacept- versus cyclosporine-treated recipients of extended criteria donor kidneys: final results from BENEFIT-EXT, a phase III randomized study. Am J Transplant 16:3192–3201

Echbarthi M, Zonca M, Mellwig R, Schwab Y, Kaplan G, DeKruyff RH, Roda-Navarro P, Casasnovas JM (2015) Distinct trafficking of cell surface and endosomal TIM-1 to the immune synapse. Traffic 16:1193–1207

Espinosa J, Herr F, Tharp G, Bosinger S, Song M, Farris AB 3rd, George R, Cheeseman J, Stempora L, Townsend R, Durrbach A, Kirk AD (2016) CD57(+) CD4 T cells underlie Belatacept-resistant allograft rejection. Am J Transplant 16:1102–1112

Fallarino F, Grohmann U, Hwang KW, Orabona C, Vacca C, Bianchi R, Belladonna ML, Fioretti MC, Alegre ML, Puccetti P (2003) Modulation of tryptophan catabolism by regulatory T cells. Nat Immunol 4:1206–1212

Ferguson R, Grinyo J, Vincenti F, Kaufman DB, Woodle ES, Marder BA, Citterio F, Marks WH, Agarwal M, Wu D, Dong Y, Garg P (2011) Immunosuppression with belatacept-based, corticosteroid-avoiding regimens in de novo kidney transplant recipients. Am J Transplant 11:66–76

Ford ML, Koehn BH, Wagener ME, Jiang W, Gangappa S, Pearson TC, Larsen CP (2007) Antigen-specific precursor frequency impacts T cell proliferation, differentiation, and requirement for costimulation. J Exp Med 204:299–309

Freeman GJ, Casasnovas JM, Umetsu DT, DeKruyff RH (2010) TIM genes: a family of cell surface phosphatidylserine receptors that regulate innate and adaptive immunity. Immunol Rev 235:172–189

Fu S, Yang Y, Xiao B, Li Y, Yi CG, Xia W, Guo SZ (2010) Use of genetically modified allograft to deliver local immunomodulatory molecule with minimal systemic toxicity in a rat model of allogeneic skin flap transplantation. Transplant Proc 42:3815–3819

Futagawa T, Akiba H, Kodama T, Takeda K, Hosoda Y, Yagita H, Okumura K (2002) Expression and function of 4-1BB and 4-1BB ligand on murine dendritic cells. Int Immunol 14:275–286

Gao W, Demirci G, Strom TB, Li XC (2003) Stimulating PD-1-negative signals concurrent with blocking CD154 co-stimulation induces long-term islet allograft survival. Transplantation 76:994–999

Ge W, Jiang J, Liu W, Lian D, Saito A, Garcia B, Li XC, Wang H (2010) Regulatory T cells are critical to tolerance induction in presensitized mouse transplant recipients through targeting memory T cells. Am J Transplant 10:1760–1773

Goldrath AW, Bogatzki LY, Bevan MJ (2000) Naive T cells transiently acquire a memory-like phenotype during homeostasis-driven proliferation. J Exp Med 192:557–564

Goldwater R, Keirns J, Blahunka P, First R, Sawamoto T, Zhang W, Kowalski D, Kaibara A, Holman J (2013) A phase 1, randomized ascending single-dose study of antagonist anti-human CD40 ASKP1240 in healthy subjects. Am J Transplant Off J Am Soc Transplant Am Soc Transplant Surg 13:1040–1046

Greenwald RJ, Freeman GJ, Sharpe AH (2005) The B7 family Revisited. Annu Rev Immunol 23:515–548

Grohmann U, Orabona C, Fallarino F, Vacca C, Calcinaro F, Falorni A, Candeloro P, Belladonna ML, Bianchi R, Fioretti MC, Puccetti P (2002) CTLA-4-Ig regulates tryptophan catabolism in vivo. Nat Immunol 3:1097–1101

Guiducci C, Valzasina B, Dislich H, Colombo MP (2005) CD40/CD40L interaction regulates CD4+CD25+ T reg homeostasis through dendritic cell-produced IL-2. Eur J Immunol 35:557–567

Guillonneau C, Seveno C, Dugast AS, Li XL, Renaudin K, Haspot F, Usal C, Veziers J, Anegon I, Vanhove B (2007) Anti-CD28 antibodies modify regulatory mechanisms and reinforce tolerance in CD40Ig-treated heart allograft recipients. J Immunol 179:8164–8171

Gupta S, Thornley TB, Gao W, Larocca R, Turka LA, Kuchroo VK, Strom TB (2012) Allograft rejection is restrained by short-lived TIM-3+PD-1+Foxp3+ Tregs. J Clin Invest 122:2395–2404

Halstead ES, Mueller YM, Altman JD, Katsikis PD (2002) In vivo stimulation of CD137 broadens primary antiviral CD8+ T cell responses. Nat Immunol 3:536–541

Hamann D, Baars PA, Rep MHG, Hooibrink B, Kerkhof-Garde SR, Klein MR, van Lier RAW (1997) Phenotypic and functional separation of memory and effector human CD8+ T cells. J Exp Med 186:1407–1418

Harada H, Salama AD, Sho M, Izawa A, Sandner SE, Ito T, Akiba H, Yagita H, Sharpe AH, Freeman GJ, Sayegh MH (2003) The role of the ICOS-B7h T cell costimulatory pathway in transplantation immunity. J Clin Invest 112:234–243

Hashiguchi M, Kobori H, Ritprajak P, Kamimura Y, Kozono H, Azuma M (2008) Triggering receptor expressed on myeloid cell-like transcript 2 (TLT-2) is a counter-receptor for B7-H3 and enhances T cell responses. Proc Natl Acad Sci U S A 105:10495–10500

He W, Fang Z, Wang F, Wu K, Xu Y, Zhou H, Du D, Gao Y, Zhang WN, Niki T, Hirashima M, Yuan J, Chen ZK (2009) Galectin-9 significantly prolongs the survival of fully mismatched cardiac allografts in mice. Transplantation 88:782–790

Hunig T, Dennehy K (2005) CD28 superagonists: mode of action and therapeutic potential. Immunol Lett 100:21–28

Hurtado JC, Kim YJ, Kwon BS (1997) Signals through 4-1BB are costimulatory to previously activated splenic T cells and inhibit activation-induced cell death. J Immunol 158:2600–2609

Hutloff A, Dittrich AM, Beier KC, Eljaschewitsch B, Kraft R, Anagnostopoulos I, Kroczek RA (1999) ICOS is an inducible T-cell co-stimulator structurally and functionally related to CD28. Nature 397:263–266

Imai A, Suzuki T, Sugitani A, Itoh T, Ueki S, Aoyagi T, Yamashita K, Taniguchi M, Takahashi N, Miura T, Shimamura T, Furukawa H, Todo S (2007) A novel fully human anti-CD40 monoclonal antibody, 4D11, for kidney transplantation in cynomolgus monkeys. Transplantation 84:1020–1028

Ji H, Liu Y, Zhang Y, Shen XD, Gao F, Busuttil RW, Kuchroo VK, Kupiec-Weglinski JW (2014) T-cell immunoglobulin and mucin domain 4 (TIM-4) signaling in innate immune-mediated liver ischemia-reperfusion injury. Hepatology 60:2052–2064

Judge TA, Wu Z, Zheng XG, Sharpe AH, Sayegh MH, Turka LA (1999) The role of CD80, CD86, and CTLA4 in alloimmune responses and the induction of long-term allograft survival. J Immunol 162:1947–1951

Kanamaru F, Youngnak P, Hashiguchi M, Nishioka T, Takahashi T, Sakaguchi S, Ishikawa I, Azuma M (2004) Costimulation via glucocorticoid-induced TNF receptor in both conventional and CD25+ regulatory CD4+ T cells. J Immunol 172:7306–7314

Kane LP (2010) T cell Ig and mucin domain proteins and immunity. J Immunol 184:2743–2749

Kanmaz T, Fechner JJ Jr, Torrealba J, Kim HT, Dong Y, Oberley TD, Schultz JM, Bloom DD, Katayama M, Dar W, Markovits J, Schuler W, Hu H, Hamawy MM, Knechtle SJ (2004) Monotherapy with the novel human anti-CD154 monoclonal antibody ABI793 in rhesus monkey renal transplantation model. Transplantation 77:914–920

Kashizuka H, Sho M, Nomi T, Ikeda N, Kuzumoto Y, Akashi S, Tsurui Y, Mizuno T, Kanehiro H, Yagita H, Nakajima Y, Sayegh MH (2005) Role of the ICOS-B7h costimulatory pathway in the pathophysiology of chronic allograft rejection. Transplantation 79:1045–1050

Kawai T, Andrews D, Colvin RB, Sachs DH, Cosimi AB (2000) Thromboembolic complications after treatment with monoclonal antibody against CD40 ligand. Nat Med 6:114

Kean LS, Turka LA, Blazar BR (2017) Advances in targeting co-inhibitory and co-stimulatory pathways in transplantation settings: the Yin to the Yang of cancer immunotherapy. Immunol Rev 276:192–212

Khayyamian S, Hutloff A, Buchner K, Grafe M, Henn V, Kroczek RA, Mages HW (2002) ICOS-ligand, expressed on human endothelial cells, costimulates Th1 and Th2 cytokine secretion by memory CD4+ T cells. Proc Natl Acad Sci U S A 99:6198–6203

Khoury SJ, Akalin E, Chandraker A, Turka LA, Linsley PS, Sayegh MH, Hancock WW (1995) CD28-B7 costimulatory blockade by CTLA4Ig prevents actively induced experimental autoimmune encephalomyelitis and inhibits Th1 but spares Th2 cytokines in the central nervous system. J Immunol 155:4521–4524

Kim JI, Sonawane SB, Lee MK, Lee SH, Duff PE, Moore DJ, O'Connor MR, Lian MM, Deng S, Choi Y, Yeh H, Caton AJ, Markmann JF (2010) Blockade of GITR-GITRL interaction maintains Treg function to prolong allograft survival. Eur J Immunol 40:1369–1374

Kinnear G, Wood KJ, Marshall D, Jones ND (2010) Anti-OX40 prevents effector T-cell accumulation and CD8+ T-cell mediated skin allograft rejection. Transplantation 90:1265–1271

Kinnear G, Wood KJ, Fallah-Arani F, Jones ND (2013) A diametric role for OX40 in the response of effector/memory CD4+ T cells and regulatory T cells to alloantigen. J Immunol 191:1465–1475

Kirk AD, Harlan DM, Armstrong NN, Davis TA, Dong Y, Gray GS, Hong X, Thomas D, Fechner JH Jr, Knechtle SJ (1997) CTLA4-Ig and anti-CD40 ligand prevent renal allograft rejection in primates. Proc Natl Acad Sci U S A 94:8789–8794

Kirk AD, Burkly LC, Batty DS, Baumgartner RE, Berning JD, Buchanan K, Fechner JH Jr, Germond RL, Kampen RL, Patterson NB, Swanson SJ, Tadaki DK, TenHoor CN, White L, Knechtle SJ, Harlan DM (1999) Treatment with humanized monoclonal antibody against CD154 prevents acute renal allograft rejection in nonhuman primates. Nat Med 5:686–693

Kirk AD, Tadaki DK, Abbie C, Scott Batty D, Berning JD, Colonna JO, Cruzata F, Elster EA, Gray GS, Kampen RL, Patterson NB, Szklut P, Swanson J, Xu H, Harlan DM (2001) Induction therapy with monoclonal antibodies specific for Cd80 and Cd86 delays the onset of acute renal allograft rejection in non-human Primates1. Transplantation 72:377–384

Kobayashi N, Karisola P, Pena-Cruz V, Dorfman DM, Jinushi M, Umetsu SE, Butte MJ, Nagumo H, Chernova I, Zhu B, Sharpe AH, Ito S, Dranoff G, Kaplan GG, Casasnovas JM, Umetsu DT, Dekruyff RH, Freeman GJ (2007) TIM-1 and TIM-4 glycoproteins bind phosphatidylserine and mediate uptake of apoptotic cells. Immunity 27:927–940

Kopf M, Ruedl C, Schmitz N, Gallimore A, Lefrang K, Ecabert B, Odermatt B, Bachmann MF (1999) OX40-deficient mice are defective in Th cell proliferation but are competent in generating B cell and CTL responses after virus infection. Immunity 11:699–708

Kosuge H, Suzuki J, Gotoh R, Koga N, Ito H, Isobe M, Inobe M, Uede T (2003) Induction of immunologic tolerance to cardiac allograft by simultaneous blockade of inducible co-stimulator and cytotoxic T-lymphocyte antigen 4 pathway. Transplantation 75:1374–1379

Kremer JM, Westhovens R, Leon M, Di Giorgio E, Alten R, Steinfeld S, Russell A, Dougados M, Emery P, Nuamah IF, Rhys Williams G, Becker J-C, Hagerty DT, Moreland LW (2003) Treatment of rheumatoid arthritis by selective inhibition of T-cell activation with fusion protein CTLA4Ig. N Engl J Med 349:1907–1915

Kryczek I, Wei S, Zou L, Zhu G, Mottram P, Xu H, Chen L, Zou W (2006) Cutting edge: induction of B7-H4 on APCs through IL-10: novel suppressive mode for regulatory T cells. J Immunol 177:40–44

Kuchroo VK, Das MP, Brown JA, Ranger AM, Zamvil SS, Sobel RA, Weiner HL, Nabavi N, Glimcher LH (1995) B7-1 and B7-2 costimulatory molecules activate differentially the Th1/Th2 developmental pathways: application to autoimmune disease therapy. Cell 80:707–718

Kwon BS, Weissman SM (1989) cDNA sequences of two inducible T-cell genes. Proc Natl Acad Sci U S A 86:1963–1967

Kwon B, Yu KY, Ni J, Yu GL, Jang IK, Kim YJ, Xing L, Liu D, Wang SX, Kwon BS (1999) Identification of a novel activation-inducible protein of the tumor necrosis factor receptor superfamily and its ligand. J Biol Chem 274:6056–6061

Langstein J, Michel J, Fritsche J, Kreutz M, Andreesen R, Schwarz H (1998) CD137 (ILA/4-1BB), a member of the TNF receptor family, induces monocyte activation via bidirectional signaling. J Immunol 160:2488–2494

Larsen CP, Alexander DZ, Hollenbaugh D, Elwood ET, Ritchie SC, Aruffo A, Hendrix R, Pearson TC (1996) CD40-gp39 interactions play a critical role during allograft rejection. Suppression of allograft rejection by blockade of the CD40-gp39 pathway. Transplantation 61:4–9

Larsen CP, Pearson TC, Adams AB, Tso P, Shirasugi N, Strobert E, Anderson D, Cowan S, Price K, Naemura J, Emswiler J, Greene J, Turk LA, Bajorath J, Townsend R, Hagerty D, Linsley PS, Peach RJ (2005) Rational development of LEA29Y (belatacept), a high-affinity variant of CTLA4-Ig with potent immunosuppressive properties. Am J Transplant 5:443–453

Lechler RI, Garden OA, Turka LA (2003) The complementary roles of deletion and regulation in transplantation tolerance. Nat Rev Immunol 3:147–158

Leitner J, Klauser C, Pickl WF, Stockl J, Majdic O, Bardet AF, Kreil DP, Dong C, Yamazaki T, Zlabinger G, Pfistershammer K, Steinberger P (2009) B7-H3 is a potent inhibitor of human T-cell activation: no evidence for B7-H3 and TREML2 interaction. Eur J Immunol 39:1754–1764

Lenschow DJ, Zeng Y, Thistlethwaite JR, Montag A, Brady W, Gibson MG, Linsley PS, Bluestone JA (1992) Long-term survival of xenogeneic pancreatic islet grafts induced by CTLA4Ig. Science 257:789–792

Lenschow DJ, Ho SC, Sattar H, Rhee L, Gray G, Nabavi N, Herold KC, Bluestone JA (1995a) Differential effects of anti-B7-1 and anti-B7-2 monoclonal antibody treatment on the development of diabetes in the nonobese diabetic mouse. J Exp Med 181:1145–1155

Lenschow DJ, Zeng Y, Hathcock KS, Zuckerman LA, Freeman G, Thistlethwaite JR, Gray GS, Hodes RJ, Bluestone JA (1995b) Inhibition of transplant rejection following treatment with anti-B7-2 and anti-B7-1 antibodies. Transplantation 60:1171–1178

Lenschow DJ, Herold KC, Rhee L, Patel B, Koons A, Qin H-Y, Fuchs E, Singh B, Thompson CB, Bluestone JA (1996) CD28/B7 regulation of Th1 and Th2 subsets in the development of autoimmune diabetes. Immunity 5:285–293

Levisetti MG, Padrid PA, Szot GL, Mittal N, Meehan SM, Wardrip CL, Gray GS, Bruce DS, Thistlethwaite JR Jr, Bluestone JA (1997) Immunosuppressive effects of human CTLA4Ig in a non-human primate model of allogeneic pancreatic islet transplantation'. J Immunol (Baltimore, Md: 1950) 159:5187–5191

Li W (2001) Costimulation blockade promotes the apoptotic death of graft-infiltrating T cells and prolongs survival of hepatic allografts from FLT3L-treated donors. Transplantation 78:1423–1432

Li Y, Li XC, Zheng XX, Wells AD, Turka LA, Strom TB (1999) Blocking both signal 1 and signal 2 of T-cell activation prevents apoptosis of alloreactive T cells and induction of peripheral allograft tolerance. Nat Med 5:1298–1302

Li XC, Rothstein DM, Sayegh MH (2009) Costimulatory pathways in transplantation: challenges and new developments. Immunol Rev 229:271–293

Li T, Ma R, Zhu J, Wang F, Huang L, Leng X (2014) Blockade of the OX40/OX40L pathway and induction of PD-L1 synergistically protects mouse islet allografts from rejection. Chin Med J 127:2686–2692

Li T, Ma R, Zhu JY, Wang FS, Huang L, Leng XS (2015) PD-1/PD-L1 costimulatory pathway-induced mouse islet transplantation immune tolerance. Transplant Proc 47:165–170

Linsley PS, Greene JL, Brady W, Bajorath J, Ledbetter JA, Peach R (1994) Human B7-1 (CD80) and B7-2 (CD86) bind with similar avidities but distinct kinetics to CD28 and CTLA-4 receptors. Immunity 1:793–801

Lo DJ, Anderson DJ, Weaver TA, Leopardi F, Song M, Farris AB, Strobert EA, Jenkins J, Turgeon NA, Mehta AK, Larsen CP, Kirk AD (2013) Belatacept and sirolimus prolong nonhuman primate renal allograft survival without a requirement for memory T cell depletion. Am J Transplant 13:320–328

Lo DJ, Anderson DJ, Song M, Leopardi F, Farris AB, Strobert E, Chapin S, Devens B, Karrer E, Kirk AD (2015) A pilot trial targeting the ICOS-ICOS-L pathway in nonhuman primate kidney transplantation. Am J Transplant 15:984–992

Lohning M, Hutloff A, Kallinich T, Mages HW, Bonhagen K, Radbruch A, Hamelmann E, Kroczek RA (2003) Expression of ICOS in vivo defines CD4+ effector T cells with high inflammatory potential and a strong bias for secretion of interleukin 10. J Exp Med 197:181–193

Luhder F, Huang Y, Dennehy KM, Guntermann C, Muller I, Winkler E, Kerkau T, Ikemizu S, Davis SJ, Hanke T, Hunig T (2003) Topological requirements and signaling properties of T cell-activating, anti-CD28 antibody superagonists. J Exp Med 197:955–966

Luo L, Chapoval AI, Flies DB, Zhu G, Hirano F, Wang S, Lau JS, Dong H, Tamada K, Flies AS, Liu Y, Chen L (2004) B7-H3 enhances tumor immunity in vivo by costimulating rapid clonal expansion of antigen-specific CD8+ cytolytic T cells. J Immunol 173:5445–5450

Ma D, Duan W, Li Y, Wang Z, Li S, Gong N, Chen G, Chen Z, Wan C, Yang J (2016) PD-L1 deficiency within islets reduces allograft survival in mice. PLoS One 11:e0152087

Mai G, del Rio ML, Tian J, Ramirez P, Buhler L, Rodriguez-Barbosa JI (2007) Blockade of the PD-1/PD-1L pathway reverses the protective effect of anti-CD40L therapy in a rat to mouse concordant islet xenotransplantation model. Xenotransplantation 14:243–248

Malvezzi P, Jouve T, Rostaing L (2016) Costimulation blockade in kidney transplantation: an update. Transplantation 100:2315–2323

McAdam AJ, Greenwald RJ, Levin MA, Chernova T, Malenkovich N, Ling V, Freeman GJ, Sharpe AH (2001) ICOS is critical for CD40-mediated antibody class switching. Nature 409:102–105

Mease P, Genovese MC, Gladstein G, Kivitz AJ, Ritchlin C, Tak PP, Wollenhaupt J, Bahary O, Becker J-C, Kelly S, Sigal L, Teng J, Gladman D (2011) Abatacept in the treatment of patients with psoriatic arthritis: results of a six-month, multicenter, randomized, double-blind, placebo-controlled, phase II trial. Arthritis Rheum 63:939–948

Mellor AL, Munn DH (2004) IDO expression by dendritic cells: tolerance and tryptophan catabolism. Nat Rev Immunol 4:762–774

Meyers JH, Chakravarti S, Schlesinger D, Illes Z, Waldner H, Umetsu SE, Kenny J, Zheng XX, Umetsu DT, DeKruyff RH, Strom TB, Kuchroo VK (2005) TIM-4 is the ligand for TIM-1, and the TIM-1-TIM-4 interaction regulates T cell proliferation. Nat Immunol 6:455–464

Mizui M, Shikina T, Arase H, Suzuki K, Yasui T, Rennert PD, Kumanogoh A, Kikutani H (2008) Bimodal regulation of T cell-mediated immune responses by TIM-4. Int Immunol 20:695–708

Morita M, Fujino M, Jiang G, Kitazawa Y, Xie L, Azuma M, Yagita H, Nagao S, Sugioka A, Kurosawa Y, Takahara S, Fung J, Qian S, Lu L, Li XK (2010) PD-1/B7-H1 interaction contribute to the spontaneous acceptance of mouse liver allograft. Am J Transplant 10:40–46

Moxham VF, Karegli J, Phillips RE, Brown KL, Tapmeier TT, Hangartner R, Sacks SH, Wong W (2008) Homeostatic proliferation of lymphocytes results in augmented memory-like function and accelerated allograft rejection. J Immunol 180:3910–3918

Nadazdin O, Boskovic S, Murakami T, Tocco G, Smith RN, Colvin RB, Sachs DH, Allan J, Madsen JC, Kawai T, Cosimi AB, Benichou G (2011) Host alloreactive memory T cells influence tolerance to kidney allografts in nonhuman primates. Sci Transl Med 3:86ra51

Nakayama M, Akiba H, Takeda K, Kojima Y, Hashiguchi M, Azuma M, Yagita H, Okumura K (2009) Tim-3 mediates phagocytosis of apoptotic cells and cross-presentation. Blood 113:3821–3830

Nanji SA, Hancock WW, Anderson CC, Adams AB, Luo B, Schur CD, Pawlick RL, Wang L, Coyle AJ, Larsen CP, Shapiro AM (2004) Multiple combination therapies involving blockade of ICOS/B7RP-1 costimulation facilitate long-term islet allograft survival. Am J Transplant 4:526–536

Nanji SA, Hancock WW, Luo B, Schur CD, Pawlick RL, Zhu LF, Anderson CC, Shapiro AM (2006) Costimulation blockade of both inducible costimulator and CD40 ligand induces dominant tolerance to islet allografts and prevents spontaneous autoimmune diabetes in the NOD mouse. Diabetes 55:27–33

Oura T, Yamashita K, Suzuki T, Fukumori D, Watanabe M, Hirokata G, Wakayama K, Taniguchi M, Shimamura T, Miura T, Okimura K, Maeta K, Haga H, Kubota K, Shimizu A, Sakai F, Furukawa H, Todo S (2012) Long-term hepatic allograft acceptance based on CD40 blockade by ASKP1240 in nonhuman primates. Am J Transplant 12:1740–1754

Ozkaynak E, Gao W, Shemmeri N, Wang C, Gutierrez-Ramos JC, Amaral J, Qin S, Rottman JB, Coyle AJ, Hancock WW (2001) Importance of ICOS-B7RP-1 costimulation in acute and chronic allograft rejection. Nat Immunol 2:591–596

Ozkaynak E, Wang L, Goodearl A, McDonald K, Qin S, O'Keefe T, Duong T, Smith T, Gutierrez-Ramos JC, Rottman JB, Coyle AJ, Hancock WW (2002) Programmed death-1 targeting can promote allograft survival. J Immunol 169:6546–6553

Pantenburg B, Heinzel F, Das L, Heeger PS, Valujskikh A (2002) T cells primed by Leishmania major infection cross-react with alloantigens and alter the course of allograft rejection. J Immunol 169:3686–3693

Parker DC, Greiner DL, Phillips NE, Appel MC, Steele AW, Durie FH, Noelle RJ, Mordes JP, Rossini AA (1995) Survival of mouse pancreatic islet allografts in recipients treated with allogeneic small lymphocytes and antibody to CD40 ligand. Proc Natl Acad Sci U S A 92:9560–9564

Pauly S, Broll K, Wittmann M, Giegerich G, Schwarz H (2002) CD137 is expressed by follicular dendritic cells and costimulates B lymphocyte activation in germinal centers. J Leukoc Biol 72:35–42

Pawar RD, Goilav B, Xia Y, Herlitz L, Doerner J, Chalmers S, Ghosh K, Zang X, Putterman C (2015) B7x/B7-H4 modulates the adaptive immune response and ameliorates renal injury in antibody-mediated nephritis. Clin Exp Immunol 179:329–343

Peach RJ, Bajorath J, Brady W, Leytze G, Greene J, Naemura J, Linsley PS (1994) Complementarity determining region 1 (CDR1)- and CDR3-analogous regions in CTLA-4 and CD28 determine the binding to B7-1. J Exp Med 180:2049–2058

Pearson TC, Alexander DZ, Hendrix R, Elwood ET, Linsley PS, Winn KJ, Larsen CP (1996) CTLA4-Ig plus bone marrow induces long-term allograft survival and donor-specific unresponsiveness in the murine model: evidence for hematopoietic chimerism1. Transplantation 61:997–1004

Pearson TC, Alexander DZ, Corbascio M, Hendrix R, Ritchie SC, Linsley PS, Faherty D, Larsen CP (1997) Analysis of the B7 costimulatory pathway in allograft rejection. Transplantation 63:1463–1469

Pearson TC, Trambley J, Odom K, Anderson DC, Cowan S, Bray R, Lin A, Hollenbaugh D, Aruffo A, Siadak AW, Strobert E, Hennigar R, Larsen CP (2002) Anti-CD40 therapy extends renal allograft survival in rhesus macaques. Transplantation 74:933–940

Pentcheva-Hoang T, Egen JG, Wojnoonski K, Allison JP (2004) B7-1 and B7-2 selectively recruit CTLA-4 and CD28 to the immunological synapse. Immunity 21:401–413

Perez VL (1997) Induction of peripheral T cell tolerance in vivo requires CTLA-4 engagement. Immunity 6:411–417

Pfeiffer S, Iii GL, Azimzadeh AM, Atkinson J, Newman R, Pierson RN (2001) Monotherapy with anti-CD40 ligand antibody (IDEC 131) for non-human primate allograft heart transplantation. J Heart Lung Transplant 20:250

Podojil JR, Liu LN, Marshall SA, Chiang MY, Goings GE, Chen L, Langermann S, Miller SD (2013) B7-H4Ig inhibits mouse and human T-cell function and treats EAE via IL-10/Treg-dependent mechanisms. J Autoimmun 44:71–81

Poirier N, Azimzadeh AM, Zhang T, Dilek N, Mary C, Nguyen B, Tillou X, Wu G, Reneaudin K, Hervouet J, Martinet B, Coulon F, Allain-Launay E, Karam G, Soulillou JP, Pierson RN 3rd, Blancho G, Vanhove B (2010) Inducing CTLA-4-dependent immune regulation by selective CD28 blockade promotes regulatory T cells in organ transplantation. Sci Transl Med 2:17ra10

Poirier N, Blancho G, Hiance M, Mary C, Van Assche T, Lempoels J, Ramael S, Wang W, Thepenier V, Braudeau C, Salabert N, Josien R, Anderson I, Gourley I, Soulillou JP, Coquoz D, Vanhove B (2016) First-in-human study in healthy subjects with FR104, a Pegylated monoclonal antibody fragment antagonist of CD28. J Immunol 197:4593–4602

Ponciano VC, Renesto PG, Nogueira E, Rangel EB, Cenedeze MA, Franco MF, Camara NO, Pacheco-Silva A (2007) Tim-3 expression in human kidney allografts. Transpl Immunol 17:215–222

Prasad DV, Richards S, Mai XM, Dong C (2003) B7S1, a novel B7 family member that negatively regulates T cell activation. Immunity 18:863–873

Prasad DVR, Nguyen T, Li Z, Yang Y, Duong J, Wang Y, Dong C (2004) Murine B7-H3 is a negative regulator of T cells. J Immunol 173:2500–2506

Qian Y, Hong B, Shen L, Wu Z, Yao H, Zhang L (2013) B7-H4 enhances oncogenicity and inhibits apoptosis in pancreatic cancer cells. Cell Tissue Res 353:139–151

Riella LV, Watanabe T, Sage PT, Yang J, Yeung M, Azzi J, Vanguri V, Chandraker A, Sharpe AH, Sayegh MH, Najafian N (2011) Essential role of PDL1 expression on nonhematopoietic donor cells in acquired tolerance to vascularized cardiac allografts. Am J Transplant 11:832–840

Riella LV, Liu T, Yang J, Chock S, Shimizu T, Mfarrej B, Batal I, Xiao X, Sayegh MH, Chandraker A (2012a) Deleterious effect of CTLA4-Ig on a Treg-dependent transplant model. Am J Transplant 12:846–855

Riella LV, Paterson AM, Sharpe AH, Chandraker A (2012b) Role of the PD-1 pathway in the immune response. Am J Transplant 12:2575–2587

Robles-Carrillo L, Meyer T, Hatfield M, Desai H, Davila M, Langer F, Amaya M, Garber E, Francis JL, Hsu YM, Amirkhosravi A (2010) Anti-CD40L immune complexes potently activate platelets in vitro and cause thrombosis in FCGR2A transgenic mice. J Immunol 185:1577–1583

Rodriguez-Manzanet R, Meyers JH, Balasubramanian S, Slavik J, Kassam N, Dardalhon V, Greenfield EA, Anderson AC, Sobel RA, Hafler DA, Strom TB, Kuchroo VK (2008) TIM-4 expressed on APCs induces T cell expansion and survival. J Immunol 180:4706–4713

Rodriguez-Manzanet R, DeKruyff R, Kuchroo VK, Umetsu DT (2009) The costimulatory role of TIM molecules. Immunol Rev 229:259–270

Ronchese F, Hausmann B, Hubele S, Lane P (1994) Mice transgenic for a soluble form of murine CTLA-4 show enhanced expansion of antigen-specific CD4+ T cells and defective antibody production in vivo. J Exp Med 179:809–817

Rong S, Park JK, Kirsch T, Yagita H, Akiba H, Boenisch O, Haller H, Najafian N, Habicht A (2011) The TIM-1:TIM-4 pathway enhances renal ischemia-reperfusion injury. J Am Soc Nephrol 22:484–495

Rudd CE (2008) The reverse stop-signal model for CTLA4 function. Nat Rev Immunol 8:153–160

Rudd CE, Taylor A, Schneider H (2009) CD28 and CTLA-4 coreceptor expression and signal transduction. Immunol Rev 229:12–26

Salama AD, Yuan X, Nayer A, Chandraker A, Inobe M, Uede T, Sayegh MH (2003) Interaction between ICOS-B7RP1 and B7-CD28 costimulatory pathways in alloimmune responses in vivo. Am J Transplant 3:390–395

Salomon B, Bluestone JA (2001) Complexities of CD28/B7: CTLA-4 costimulatory pathways in autoimmunity and transplantation. Annu Rev Immunol 19:225–252

Sanchez-Fueyo A, Tian J, Picarella D, Domenig C, Zheng XX, Sabatos CA, Manlongat N, Bender O, Kamradt T, Kuchroo VK, Gutierrez-Ramos JC, Coyle AJ, Strom TB (2003) Tim-3 inhibits T helper type 1-mediated auto- and alloimmune responses and promotes immunological tolerance. Nat Immunol 4:1093–1101

Saoulli K, Lee SY, Cannons JL, Yeh WC, Santana A, Goldstein MD, Bangia N, DeBenedette MA, Mak TW, Choi Y, Watts TH (1998) CD28-independent, TRAF2-dependent costimulation of resting T cells by 4-1BB ligand. J Exp Med 187:1849–1862

Sayegh MH, Akalin E, Hancock WW, Russell ME, Carpenter CB, Linsley PS, Turka LA (1995) CD28-B7 blockade after alloantigenic challenge in vivo inhibits Th1 cytokines but spares Th2. J Exp Med 181:1869–1874

Schenk S, Kish DD, He C, El-Sawy T, Chiffoleau E, Chen C, Wu Z, Sandner S, Gorbachev AV, Fukamachi K, Heeger PS, Sayegh MH, Turka LA, Fairchild RL (2005) Alloreactive T cell responses and acute rejection of single class II MHC-disparate heart allografts are under strict regulation by CD4 +CD25+ T cells. J Immunol 174:3741–3748

Schenk AD, Gorbacheva V, Rabant M, Fairchild RL, Valujskikh A (2009) Effector functions of donor-reactive CD8 memory T cells are dependent on ICOS induced during division in cardiac grafts. Am J Transplant 9:64–73

Schuler W, Bigaud M, Brinkmann V, Di Padova F, Geisse S, Gram H, Hungerford V, Kleuser B, Kristofic C, Menninger K, Tees R, Wieczorek G, Wilt C, Wioland C, Zurini M (2004) Efficacy and safety of ABI793, a novel human anti-human CD154 monoclonal antibody, in cynomolgus monkey renal allotransplantation. Transplantation 77:717–726

Seo SK, Park HY, Choi JH, Kim WY, Kim YH, Jung HW, Kwon B, Lee HW, Kwon BS (2003) Blocking 4-1BB/4-1BB ligand interactions prevents herpetic stromal keratitis. J Immunol 171:576–583

Shao W, Chen J, Dai H, Peng Y, Wang F, Xia J, Thorlacius H, Zhu Q, Qi Z (2011a) Combination of monoclonal antibodies with DST inhibits accelerated rejection mediated by memory T cells to induce long-lived heart allograft acceptance in mice. Immunol Lett 138:122–128

Shao W, Yan G, Lin Y, Chen J, Dai H, Wang F, Xi Y, Thorlacius H, Qi Z (2011b) CD44/CD70 blockade and anti-CD154/LFA-1 treatment synergistically suppress accelerated rejection and prolong cardiac allograft survival in mice. Scand J Immunol 74:430–437

Shariff H, Tanriver Y, Brown KL, Meader L, Greenlaw R, Mamode N, Jurcevic S (2010) Intermittent antibody-based combination therapy removes alloantibodies and achieves indefinite heart transplant survival in presensitized recipients. Transplantation 90:270–278

Shi Y, Hu S, Song Q, Yu S, Zhou X, Yin J, Qin L, Qian H (2013) Gene silencing of 4-1BB by RNA interference inhibits acute rejection in rats with liver transplantation. Biomed Res Int 2013:192738

Shi R, Honczarenko M, Zhang S, Fleener C, Mora J, Lee SK, Wang R, Liu X, Shevell DE, Yang Z, Wang H, Murthy B (2017) Pharmacokinetic, Pharmacodynamic, and safety profile of a novel anti-CD28 domain antibody antagonist in healthy subjects. J Clin Pharmacol 57:161–172

Shimizu J, Yamazaki S, Takahashi T, Ishida Y, Sakaguchi S (2002) Stimulation of CD25(+)CD4(+) regulatory T cells through GITR breaks immunological self-tolerance. Nat Immunol 3:135–142

Sica GL, Choi IH, Zhu G, Tamada K, Wang SD, Tamura H, Chapoval AI, Flies DB, Bajorath J, Chen L (2003) B7-H4, a molecule of the B7 family, negatively regulates T cell immunity. Immunity 18:849–861

Sizing ID, Bailly V, McCoon P, Chang W, Rao S, Pablo L, Rennard R, Walsh M, Li Z, Zafari M, Dobles M, Tarilonte L, Miklasz S, Majeau G, Godbout K, Scott ML, Rennert PD (2007) Epitope-dependent effect of anti-murine TIM-1 monoclonal antibodies on T cell activity and lung immune responses. J Immunol 178:2249–2261

Sonawane SB, Kim JI, Lee MK, Lee SH, Duff PE, Moore DJ, Lian MM, Deng S, Choi Y, Yeh H, Caton AJ, Markmann JF (2009) GITR blockade facilitates Treg mediated allograft survival. Transplantation 88:1169–1177

Stapler D, Lee ED, Selvaraj SA, Evans AG, Kean LS, Speck SH, Larsen CP, Gangappa S (2008) Expansion of effector memory TCR Vbeta4+ CD8+ T cells is associated with latent infection-mediated resistance to transplantation tolerance. J Immunol 180:3190–3200

Suchard SJ, Davis PM, Kansal S, Stetsko DK, Brosius R, Tamura J, Schneeweis L, Bryson J, Salcedo T, Wang H, Yang Z, Fleener CA, Ignatovich O, Plummer C, Grant S, Nadler SG (2013) A monovalent anti-human CD28 domain antibody antagonist: preclinical efficacy and safety. J Immunol 191:4599–4610

Suchin EJ, Langmuir PB, Palmer E, Sayegh MH, Wells AD, Turka LA (2001) Quantifying the frequency of alloreactive T cells in vivo: new answers to an old question. J Immunol 166:973–981

Suh WK, Gajewska BU, Okada H, Gronski MA, Bertram EM, Dawicki W, Duncan GS, Bukczynski J, Plyte S, Elia A, Wakeham A, Itie A, Chung S, Da Costa J, Arya S, Horan T, Campbell P, Gaida K, Ohashi PS, Watts TH, Yoshinaga SK, Bray MR, Jordana M, Mak TW (2003) The B7 family member B7-H3 preferentially down-regulates T helper type 1-mediated immune responses. Nat Immunol 4:899–906

Suh WK, Wang SX, Jheon AH, Moreno L, Yoshinaga SK, Ganss B, Sodek J, Grynpas MD, Mak TW (2004) The immune regulatory protein B7-H3 promotes osteoblast differentiation and bone mineralization. Proc Natl Acad Sci U S A 101:12969–12973

Suntharalingam G, Perry MR, Ward S, Brett SJ, Castello-Cortes A, Brunner MD, Panoskaltsis N (2006) Cytokine storm in a phase 1 trial of the anti-CD28 monoclonal antibody TGN1412. N Engl J Med 355:1018–1028

Swallow MM, Wallin JJ, Sha WC (1999) B7h, a novel costimulatory homolog of B7.1 and B7.2, is induced by TNFalpha. Immunity 11:423–432

Tafuri A, Shahinian A, Bladt F, Yoshinaga SK, Jordana M, Wakeham A, Boucher LM, Bouchard D, Chan VS, Duncan G, Odermatt B, Ho A, Itie A, Horan T, Whoriskey JS, Pawson T, Penninger JM, Ohashi PS, Mak TW (2001) ICOS is essential for effective T-helper-cell responses. Nature 409:105–109

Takahashi T, Tagami T, Yamazaki S, Uede T, Shimizu J, Sakaguchi N, Mak TW, Sakaguchi S (2000) Immunologic self-tolerance maintained by CD25(+)CD4(+) regulatory T cells constitutively expressing cytotoxic T lymphocyte-associated antigen 4. J Exp Med 192:303–310

Tan P, Anasetti C, Hansen JA, Melrose J, Brunvand M, Bradshaw J, Ledbetter JA, Linsley PS (1993) Induction of alloantigen-specific hyporesponsiveness in human T lymphocytes by blocking interaction of CD28 with its natural ligand B7/BB1. J Exp Med 177:165–173

Tan JT, Ha J, Cho HR, Tucker-Burden C, Hendrix RC, Mittler RS, Pearson TC, Larsen CP (2000) Analysis of expression and function of the costimulatory molecule 4-1BB in alloimmune responses. Transplantation 70:175–183

Tang Q, Henriksen KJ, Boden EK, Tooley AJ, Ye J, Subudhi SK, Zheng XX, Strom TB, Bluestone JA (2003) Cutting edge: CD28 controls peripheral homeostasis of CD4+CD25+ regulatory T cells. J Immunol 171:3348–3352

Tesselaar K, Xiao Y, Arens R, van Schijndel GM, Schuurhuis DH, Mebius RE, Borst J, van Lier RA (2003) Expression of the murine CD27 ligand CD70 in vitro and in vivo. J Immunol 170:33–40

Thangavelu G, Murphy KM, Yagita H, Boon L, Anderson CC (2011) The role of co-inhibitory signals in spontaneous tolerance of weakly mismatched transplants. Immunobiology 216:918–924

Thornley TB, Fang Z, Balasubramanian S, Larocca RA, Gong W, Gupta S, Csizmadia E, Degauque N, Kim BS, Koulmanda M, Kuchroo VK, Strom TB (2014) Fragile TIM-4-expressing tissue resident macrophages are migratory and immunoregulatory. J Clin Invest 124:3443–3454

Tivol EA, Borriello F, Schweitzer AN, Lynch WP, Bluestone JA, Sharpe AH (1995) Loss of CTLA-4 leads to massive lymphoproliferation and fatal multiorgan tissue destruction, revealing a critical negative regulatory role of CTLA-4. Immunity 3:541–547

Tone M, Tone Y, Adams E, Yates SF, Frewin MR, Cobbold SP, Waldmann H (2003) Mouse glucocorticoid-induced tumor necrosis factor receptor ligand is costimulatory for T cells. Proc Natl Acad Sci U S A 100:15059–15064

Tsai M-K, Ho H-N, Chien H-F, Ou-Yang P, Lee C-J, Lee P-H (2004) The role of b7 ligands (cd80 and cd86) in cd152-mediated allograft tolerance: a crosscheck hypothesis. Transplantation 77:48–54

Turka LA (1992) T-cell activation by the CD28 ligand B7 is required for cardiac allograft rejection in vivo. Proc Natl Acad Sci U S A 89:11102–11105

Uchida Y, Ke B, Freitas MC, Ji H, Zhao D, Benjamin ER, Najafian N, Yagita H, Akiba H, Busuttil RW, Kupiec-Weglinski JW (2010) The emerging role of T cell immunoglobulin mucin-1 in the mechanism of liver ischemia and reperfusion injury in the mouse. Hepatology 51:1363–1372

Ueda H (2003) Association of the T-cell regulatory gene CTLA4 with susceptibility to autoimmune disease. Nature 423:506–511

Ueno T, Habicht A, Clarkson MR, Albin MJ, Yamaura K, Boenisch O, Popoola J, Wang Y, Yagita H, Hisaya A, Ansari MJ, Yang J, Turka LA, Rothstein DM, Padera RF, Najafian N, Sayegh MH (2008) The emerging role of T cell Ig mucin 1 in alloimmune responses in an experimental mouse transplant model. J Clin Invest 118:742–751

Ueno T, Yeung MY, McGrath M, Yang S, Zaman N, Snawder B, Padera RF, Magee CN, Gorbatov R, Hashiguchi M, Azuma M, Freeman GJ, Sayegh MH, Najafian N (2012) Intact B7-H3 signaling promotes allograft prolongation through preferential suppression of Th1 effector responses. Eur J Immunol 42:2343–2353

Valujskikh A, Pantenburg B, Heeger PS (2002) Primed allospecific T cells prevent the effects of costimulatory blockade on prolonged cardiac allograft survival in mice. Am J Transplant 2:501–509

Vanhove B, Laflamme G, Coulon F, Mougin M, Vusio P, Haspot F, Tiollier J, Soulillou JP (2003) Selective blockade of CD28 and not CTLA-4 with a single-chain Fv-alpha1-antitrypsin fusion antibody. Blood 102:564–570

Vasu C, Prabhakar BS, Holterman MJ (2004) Targeted CTLA-4 engagement induces CD4+CD25+CTLA-4high T regulatory cells with target (allo)antigen specificity. J Immunol 173:2866–2876

Vergani A, Gatti F, Lee KM, D'Addio F, Tezza S, Chin M, Bassi R, Tian Z, Wu E, Maffi P, Nasr MB, Kim JI, Secchi A, Markmann JF, Rothstein DM, Turka LA, Sayegh MH, Fiorina P (2015) TIM4 regulates the anti-islet Th2 alloimmune response. Cell Transplant 24:1599–1614

Ville S, Poirier N, Branchereau J, Charpy V, Pengam S, Nerriere-Daguin V, Le Bas-Bernardet S, Coulon F, Mary C, Chenouard A, Hervouet J, Minault D, Nedellec S, Renaudin K, Vanhove B, Blancho G (2016) Anti-CD28 antibody and Belatacept exert differential effects on mechanisms of renal allograft rejection. J Am Soc Nephrol 27:3577–3588

Vincenti F, Charpentier B, Vanrenterghem Y, Rostaing L, Bresnahan B, Darji P, Massari P, Mondragon-Ramirez GA, Agarwal M, Di Russo G, Lin CS, Garg P, Larsen CP (2010) A phase III study of belatacept-based immunosuppression regimens versus cyclosporine in renal transplant recipients (BENEFIT study). Am J Transplant 10:535–546

Vincenti F, Dritselis A, Kirkpatrick P (2011) Belatacept. Nat Rev Drug Discov 10:655–656

Vincenti F, Rostaing L, Grinyo J, Rice K, Steinberg S, Gaite L, Moal MC, Mondragon-Ramirez GA, Kothari J, Polinsky MS, Meier-Kriesche HU, Larsen CP (2016) Belatacept and long-term outcomes in kidney transplantation. N Engl J Med 374:333–343

Vu MD, Clarkson MR, Yagita H, Turka LA, Sayegh MH, Li XC (2006) Critical, but conditional, role of OX40 in memory T cell-mediated rejection. J Immunol 176:1394–1401

Vu MD, Xiao X, Gao W, Degauque N, Chen M, Kroemer A, Killeen N, Ishii N, Li XC (2007) OX40 costimulation turns off Foxp3+ Tregs. Blood 110:2501–2510

Walunas TL, Bakker CY, Bluestone JA (1996) CTLA-4 ligation blocks CD28-dependent T cell activation. J Exp Med 183:2541–2550

Wang J, Guo Z, Dong Y, Kim O, Hart J, Adams A, Larsen CP, Mittler RS, Newell KA (2003) Role of 4-1BB in allograft rejection mediated by CD8+ T cells. Am J Transplant 3:543–551

Wang G, Feng Y, Hao J, Li A, Gao X, Xie S (2005a) Induction of xenogeneic islet transplantation tolerance by simultaneously blocking CD28-B7 and OX40-OX40L co-stimulatory pathways. Sci China C Life Sci 48:515–522

Wang L, Fraser CC, Kikly K, Wells AD, Han R, Coyle AJ, Chen L, Hancock WW (2005b) B7-H3 promotes acute and chronic allograft rejection. Eur J Immunol 35:428–438

Wang F, He W, Zhou H, Yuan J, Wu K, Xu L, Chen ZK (2007a) The Tim-3 ligand galectin-9 negatively regulates CD8+ alloreactive T cell and prolongs survival of skin graft. Cell Immunol 250:68–74

Wang L, Han R, Hancock WW (2007b) Programmed cell death 1 (PD-1) and its ligand PD-L1 are required for allograft tolerance. Eur J Immunol 37:2983–2990

Wang F, He W, Yuan J, Wu K, Zhou H, Zhang W, Chen ZK (2008) Activation of Tim-3-Galectin-9 pathway improves survival of fully allogeneic skin grafts. Transpl Immunol 19:12–19

Wang X, Hao J, Metzger DL, Mui A, Ao Z, Verchere CB, Chen L, Ou D, Warnock GL (2009) Local expression of B7-H4 by recombinant adenovirus transduction in mouse islets prolongs allograft survival. Transplantation 87:482–490

Wang X, Hao J, Metzger DL, Mui A, Ao Z, Akhoundsadegh N, Langermann S, Liu L, Chen L, Ou D, Verchere CB, Warnock GL (2011) Early treatment of NOD mice with B7-H4 reduces the incidence of autoimmune diabetes. Diabetes 60:3246–3255

Wang X, Hao J, Metzger DL, Mui A, Ao Z, Verchere CB, Chen L, Ou D, Warnock GL (2012) B7-H4 induces donor-specific tolerance in mouse islet allografts. Cell Transplant 21:99–111

Wang H, Zhang Z, Tian W, Liu T, Han H, Garcia B, Li XC, Du C (2014) Memory T cells mediate cardiac allograft vasculopathy and are inactivated by anti-OX40L monoclonal antibody. Cardiovasc Drugs Ther 28:115–122

Waterhouse P, Penninger JM, Timms E, Wakeham A, Shahinian A, Lee KP, Thompson CB, Griesser H, Mak TW (1995) Lymphoproliferative disorders with early lethality in mice deficient in Ctla-4. Science 270:985–988

Watts TH (2005) TNF/TNFR family members in costimulation of T cell responses. Annu Rev Immunol 23:23–68

Williams MA, Trambley J, Ha J, Adams AB, Durham MM, Rees P, Cowan SR, Pearson TC, Larsen CP (2000) Genetic characterization of strain differences in the ability to mediate CD40/CD28-independent rejection of skin allografts. J Immunol 165:6849–6857

Wing K, Onishi Y, Prieto-Martin P, Yamaguchi T, Miyara M, Fehervari Z, Nomura T, Sakaguchi S (2008) CTLA-4 control over Foxp3+ regulatory T cell function. Science 322:271–275

Wojciechowski D, Vincenti F (2016) Current status of costimulatory blockade in renal transplantation. Curr Opin Nephrol Hypertens 25:583–590

Wood KJ, Sakaguchi S (2003) Regulatory T cells in transplantation tolerance. Nat Rev Immunol 3:199–210

Wood KJ, Bushell A, Hester J (2012) Regulatory immune cells in transplantation. Nat Rev Immunol 12:417–430

Wu Z, Bensinger SJ, Zhang J, Chen C, Yuan X, Huang X, Markmann JF, Kassaee A, Rosengard BR, Hancock WW, Sayegh MH, Turka LA (2004) Homeostatic proliferation is a barrier to transplantation tolerance. Nat Med 10:87–92

Xia J, Chen J, Shao W, Lan T, Wang Y, Xie B, Thorlacius H, Tian F, Huang R, Qi Z (2010) Suppressing memory T cell activation induces islet allograft tolerance in alloantigen-primed mice. Transpl Int 23:1154–1163

Xiao S, Najafian N, Reddy J, Albin M, Zhu C, Jensen E, Imitola J, Korn T, Anderson AC, Zhang Z, Gutierrez C, Moll T, Sobel RA, Umetsu DT, Yagita H, Akiba H, Strom T, Sayegh MH, DeKruyff RH, Khoury SJ, Kuchroo VK (2007) Differential engagement of Tim-1 during activation can positively or negatively costimulate T cell expansion and effector function. J Exp Med 204:1691–1702

Xiao S, Brooks CR, Zhu C, Wu C, Sweere JM, Petecka S, Yeste A, Quintana FJ, Ichimura T, Sobel RA, Bonventre JV, Kuchroo VK (2012) Defect in regulatory B-cell function and development of systemic autoimmunity in T-cell Ig mucin 1 (Tim-1) mucin domain-mutant mice. Proc Natl Acad Sci U S A 109:12105–12110

Xu H, Montgomery SP, Preston EH, Tadaki DK, Hale DA, Harlan DM, Kirk AD (2003) Studies investigating pretransplant donor-specific blood transfusion, rapamycin, and the CD154-specific antibody IDEC-131 in a nonhuman primate model of skin allotransplantation. J Immunol 170:2776–2782

Yamada A, Kishimoto K, Dong VM, Sho M, Salama AD, Anosova NG, Benichou G, Mandelbrot DA, Sharpe AH, Turka LA, Auchincloss H Jr, Sayegh MH (2001) CD28-independent costimulation of T cells in alloimmune responses. J Immunol 167:140–146

Yamada A, Salama AD, Sho M, Najafian N, Ito T, Forman JP, Kewalramani R, Sandner S, Harada H, Clarkson MR, Mandelbrot DA, Sharpe AH, Oshima H, Yagita H, Chalasani G, Lakkis FG, Auchincloss H Jr, Sayegh MH (2005) CD70 signaling is critical for CD28-independent CD8+ T cell-mediated alloimmune responses in vivo. J Immunol 174:1357–1364

Yamaura K, Watanabe T, Boenisch O, Yeung M, Yang S, Magee CN, Padera R, Datta S, Schatton T, Kamimura Y, Azuma M, Najafian N (2010) In vivo function of immune inhibitory molecule B7-H4 in alloimmune responses. Am J Transplant 10:2355–2362

Yang J, Popoola J, Khandwala S, Vadivel N, Vanguri V, Yuan X, Dada S, Guleria I, Tian C, Ansari MJ, Shin T, Yagita H, Azuma M, Sayegh MH, Chandraker A (2008) Critical role of donor tissue expression of programmed death ligand-1 in regulating cardiac allograft rejection and vasculopathy. Circulation 117:660–669

Yang J, Riella LV, Boenisch O, Popoola J, Robles S, Watanabe T, Vanguri V, Yuan X, Guleria I, Turka LA, Sayegh MH, Chandraker A (2009) Paradoxical functions of B7: CD28 costimulation in a MHC class II-mismatched cardiac transplant model. Am J Transplant 9:2837–2844

Yang J, Riella LV, Chock S, Liu T, Zhao X, Yuan X, Paterson AM, Watanabe T, Vanguri V, Yagita H, Azuma M, Blazar BR, Freeman GJ, Rodig SJ, Sharpe AH, Chandraker A, Sayegh MH (2011) The novel costimulatory programmed death ligand 1/B7.1 pathway is functional in inhibiting alloimmune responses in vivo. J Immunol 187:1113–1119

Yang Z, Wang H, Salcedo TW, Suchard SJ, Xie JH, Schneeweis LA, Fleener CA, Calore JD, Shi R, Zhang SX, Rodrigues AD, Car BD, Marathe PH, Nadler SG (2015) Integrated pharmacokinetic/

10 Costimulation Blockade in Transplantation

Pharmacodynamic analysis for determining the minimal anticipated biological effect level of a novel anti-CD28 receptor antagonist BMS-931699. J Pharmacol Exp Ther 355:506–515

Yeung MY, Sayegh MH (2009) Regulatory T cells in transplantation: what we know and what we do not know. Transplant Proc 41:S21–S26

Yeung MY, McGrath MM, Nakayama M, Shimizu T, Boenisch O, Magee CN, Abdoli R, Akiba H, Ueno T, Turka LA, Najafian N (2013) Interruption of dendritic cell-mediated TIM-4 signaling induces regulatory T cells and promotes skin allograft survival. J Immunol 191:4447–4455

Yeung MY, Najafian N, Sayegh MH (2014) Targeting CD28 to prevent transplant rejection. Expert Opin Ther Targets 18:225–242

Yeung MY, Ding Q, Brooks CR, Xiao S, Workman CJ, Vignali DAA, Ueno T, Padera RF, Kuchroo VK, Najafian N, Rothstein DM (2015) TIM-1 signaling is required for maintenance and induction of regulatory B cells. Am J Transplant Off J Am Soc Transplant Am Soc Transplant Surg 15:942–953

Yoshinaga SK, Whoriskey JS, Khare SD, Sarmiento U, Guo J, Horan T, Shih G, Zhang M, Coccia MA, Kohno T, Tafuri-Bladt A, Brankow D, Campbell P, Chang D, Chiu L, Dai T, Duncan G, Elliott GS, Hui A, McCabe SM, Scully S, Shahinian A, Shaklee CL, Van G, Mak TW, Senaldi G (1999) T-cell co-stimulation through B7RP-1 and ICOS. Nature 402:827–832

Yuan X, Salama AD, Dong V, Schmitt I, Najafian N, Chandraker A, Akiba H, Yagita H, Sayegh MH (2003) The role of the CD134-CD134 ligand costimulatory pathway in alloimmune responses in vivo. J Immunol 170:2949–2955

Yuan X, Paez-Cortez J, Schmitt-Knosalla I, D'Addio F, Mfarrej B, Donnarumma M, Habicht A, Clarkson MR, Iacomini J, Glimcher LH, Sayegh MH, Ansari MJ (2008) A novel role of CD4 Th17 cells in mediating cardiac allograft rejection and vasculopathy. J Exp Med 205:3133–3144

Yuan CL, Xu JF, Tong J, Yang H, He FR, Gong Q, Xiong P, Duan L, Fang M, Tan Z, Xu Y, Chen YF, Zheng F, Gong FL (2009a) B7-H4 transfection prolongs beta-cell graft survival. Transpl Immunol 21:143–149

Yuan X, Ansari MJ, D'Addio F, Paez-Cortez J, Schmitt I, Donnarumma M, Boenisch O, Zhao X, Popoola J, Clarkson MR, Yagita H, Akiba H, Freeman GJ, Iacomini J, Turka LA, Glimcher LH, Sayegh MH (2009b) Targeting Tim-1 to overcome resistance to transplantation tolerance mediated by CD8 T17 cells. Proc Natl Acad Sci U S A 106:10734–10739

Zaitsu M, Issa F, Hester J, Vanhove B, Wood KJ (2017) Selective blockade of CD28 on human T cells facilitates regulation of alloimmune responses. JCI Insight 2:pii: 89381

Zang X, Loke P, Kim J, Murphy K, Waitz R, Allison JP (2003) B7x: a widely expressed B7 family member that inhibits T cell activation. Proc Natl Acad Sci U S A 100:10388–10392

Zhang G, Hou J, Shi J, Yu G, Lu B, Zhang X (2008) Soluble CD276 (B7-H3) is released from monocytes, dendritic cells and activated T cells and is detectable in normal human serum. Immunology 123:538–546

Zhang T, Fresnay S, Welty E, Sangrampurkar N, Rybak E, Zhou H, Cheng XF, Feng Q, Avon C, Laaris A, Whitters M, Nagelin AM, O'Hara RM Jr, Azimzadeh AM (2011) Selective CD28 blockade attenuates acute and chronic rejection of murine cardiac allografts in a CTLA-4-dependent manner. Am J Transplant 11:1599–1609

Zhang L, Wu H, Lu D, Li G, Sun C, Song H, Li J, Zhai T, Huang L, Hou C, Wang W, Zhou B, Chen S, Lu B, Zhang X (2013a) The costimulatory molecule B7-H4 promote tumor progression and cell proliferation through translocating into nucleus. Oncogene 32:5347–5358

Zhang Y, Ji H, Shen X, Cai J, Gao F, Koenig KM, Batikian CM, Busuttil RW, Kupiec-Weglinski JW (2013b) Targeting TIM-1 on CD4 T cells depresses macrophage activation and overcomes ischemia-reperfusion injury in mouse orthotopic liver transplantation. Am J Transplant 13:56–66

Zhang T, Pierson RN 3rd, Azimzadeh AM (2015) Update on CD40 and CD154 blockade in transplant models. Immunotherapy 7:899–911

Zheng XX, Markees TG, Hancock WW, Li Y, Greiner DL, Li XC, Mordes JP, Sayegh MH, Rossini AA, Strom TB (1999) CTLA4 signals are required to optimally induce allograft tolerance with combined donor-specific transfusion and anti-CD154 monoclonal antibody treatment. J Immunol 162:4983–4990

Zheng XX, Sanchez-Fueyo A, Sho M, Domenig C, Sayegh MH, Strom TB (2003) Favorably tipping the balance between cytopathic and regulatory T cells to create transplantation tolerance. Immunity 19:503–514

Zhu C, Anderson AC, Schubart A, Xiong H, Imitola J, Khoury SJ, Zheng XX, Strom TB, Kuchroo VK (2005) The Tim-3 ligand galectin-9 negatively regulates T helper type 1 immunity. Nat Immunol 6:1245–1252

Chapter 11
Cancer Immunotherapy Targeting Co-signal Molecules

Masao Nakajima and Koji Tamada

Abstract Great success of immune checkpoint blockade represented by anti-PD-1 monoclonal antibodies (mAbs) has changed a landscape of cancer immunotherapy. There is no doubt about an importance of co-signal molecules as one of the most promising targets in anti-cancer drugs. However, it should be noted that the proportion of patients who have objective and durable responses to immune checkpoint blockade remains less than 30% in majority of cancers. Thus, in addition to refine the usage of existing drugs for checkpoint blockade, identification and characterization of novel checkpoint molecules other than CTLA-4 and PD-1 is a highly anticipated research subject. In addition, agonists of stimulatory co-signal molecules have a potential to further improve anti-tumor effects, rendering them attractive in research and drug development. In this chapter, functions of co-signal molecules in anti-tumor immunity in terms of pre-clinical animal models as well as clinical trials are described.

Keywords Inhibitory co-signals · Immune checkpoint blockade · T cell exhaustion · Stimulatory co-signals · Agonistic antibody

11.1 Introduction

In recent years, immune checkpoint blockade which interferes with inhibitory co-signals has demonstrated substantial advances and a striking success as a novel strategy in cancer immunotherapy. Anti-CTLA-4 antibody (Ab) and anti-PD-1 Ab represent approaches of immune checkpoint blockade, which have been approved by FDA as drugs for various types of cancers including melanoma, non-small cell lung cancer (NSCLC), renal cell carcinoma (RCC), classical Hodgkin lymphoma

---

M. Nakajima · K. Tamada (✉)
Department of Immunology, Yamaguchi University Graduate School of Medicine,
Yamaguchi, Japan
e-mail: ktamada@yamaguchi-u.ac.jp

© Springer Nature Singapore Pte Ltd. 2019
M. Azuma, H. Yagita (eds.), *Co-signal Molecules in T Cell Activation*,
Advances in Experimental Medicine and Biology 1189,
https://doi.org/10.1007/978-981-32-9717-3_11

(cHL), etc. Currently, application of immune checkpoint blockade is expanding into combinations with other approaches of immunotherapies, e.g., tumor vaccine using neo-antigens, and adoptive T cell transfer such as chimeric antigen receptor (CAR) T cells, as well as non-immunotherapies including chemotherapeutic drugs, kinase inhibitors, and irradiation. At the same time, further efforts have been made to identify novel checkpoint molecules besides CTLA-4 and PD-1 and manipulate them for therapeutic purposes. In addition, agonistic Abs which deliver stimulatory co-signals to activate anti-tumor T cell responses have been also developed and tested in clinical trials as novel cancer immunotherapies. In this chapter, we introduce inhibitory and stimulatory co-signal molecules which have been investigated to develop anti-tumor drugs.

11.2 Immune Checkpoint Molecules Transmitting Inhibitory Co-signals

As definition of immune checkpoint molecules, they typically possess unique intracellular motifs, such as ITIM (immunoreceptor tyrosine-based inhibitory motif) and ITSM (immunoreceptor tyrosine-based switch motif), so as to deliver inhibitory co-signals into T cells and negatively regulate T cell responses for preventing immune-mediated tissue damage caused by excess amount of T cell activation. While they are expressed on T cells either constitutively on naïve status or inducibly in response to activation, the highest expression is often detected on non-functional status including exhausted T cells, especially at the chronic viral infection and tumor-bearing status. Depending on the cells expressing ligands of checkpoint molecules, its blockade mediates the effect at two potential phases of T cell response, i.e., priming phase and effector phase. For instance, since CD80/CD86, ligands of CTLA-4, are expressed on professional APC including dendritic cells (DC), blockade of CTLA-4 enhances initial activation of the naïve T cells at the priming phase. On the other hand, PD-L1 (B7-H1), a ligand of PD-1, is mainly expressed in the tumor microenvironment, e.g., tumor cells and tumor stromal cells, indicating that PD-1 blockade potentiates T cell cytotoxic functions against cancer cells at the effector phase. Collectively, attenuation of immune checkpoint is capable of preventing and restoring the T cell unresponsiveness against tumor antigens, supporting the rationale for applying checkpoint blockade to cancer immunotherapy.

11.2.1 Blockade of CTLA-4 Inhibitory Co-signal

Cytotoxic T lymphocyte antigen 4 (CTLA-4) was discovered as a surface antigen on cytotoxic T lymphocytes (CTL) in 1987 (Brunet et al. 1987). CTLA-4 is inducibly and transiently expressed on the activated T cells, while it is constitutively detected on regulatory T cells (Treg). The fatal autoimmune phenotype observed in CTLA-4-deficient mice revealed its critical role in immune inhibition to induce and/or maintain tolerance condition (Waterhouse et al. 1995). Regarding inhibitory mechanisms, CTLA-4 transmits inhibitory co-signals through its binding with CD80/86 (Waterhouse et al. 1995). This interaction simultaneously decreases CD28-dependent stimulatory co-signals, as CTLA-4 binds CD80/86 at much higher affinity than CD28 in a competitive manner (Collins et al. 2002). In addition, it has been reported that CTLA-4 interaction induces downregulation and trans-endocytosis of CD80/86 on APC, resulted in a decreased CD28 signal into T cells (Wing et al. 2008; Qureshi et al. 2011). On the other hand, CTLA-4 expressed on Treg plays a critical role to sustain their suppressive functions (Wing et al. 2008).

Based on discovery of CTLA-4 as immune inhibitory molecules, attenuation of CTLA-4 functions by antagonistic Ab has been investigated as immunotherapeutic approach against cancer and found to be effective in various pre-clinical animal models (Leach et al. 1996). Although the precise mechanisms remain to be fully clarified, anti-CTLA-4 Ab induces anti-tumor effects by at least several distinct mechanisms, i.e., blockade of inhibitory signal in T cells (Chambers and Allison 1999), restoration of CD80/86 availability on APC (Wing et al. 2008; Qureshi et al. 2011), and depletion of Treg in the tumor microenvironment by Fc receptor-mediated Ab-dependent cellular cytotoxicity (ADCC)(Selby et al. 2013).

Clinical efficacy of CTLA-4 blockade in cancer therapy was revealed by ipilimumab, a fully human IgG$_1$-type anti-CTLA-4 antagonistic Ab (Keler et al. 2003). Two landmark studies highlighted clinical benefits of ipilimumab over vaccination therapy or ipilimumab plus chemotherapy over chemotherapy alone in patients with metastatic melanoma (Hodi et al. 2010; Robert et al. 2011). As a result, ipilimumab was approved for metastatic melanoma in the USA in 2011 as the first drug of immune checkpoint inhibitor (Table 11.1). At present, ipilimumab is also approved for the adjuvant treatment of patients who had resected regional lymph node-positive, stage III melanoma with a high risk of recurrence (Eggermont et al. 2015).

11.2.2 Blockade of PD-1 Inhibitory Co-signal

Programmed cell death-1 (PD-1) was discovered in 1992 as a protein detected in lymphocytes undergoing activation-induced cell death (Ishida et al. 1992). Subsequent studies revealed that PD-1 is expressed on activated or exhausted T cells and negatively regulates the activation of T lymphocytes by dephosphorylating TCR or CD28 signaling molecules via association with SHP2 (Src homology 2 domain-containing tyrosine phosphatase 2) (Hui et al. 2017; Yokosuka et al. 2012). The non-lethal autoimmune phenotype of PD-1-deficient mice indicated that PD-1 regulates peripheral tolerance in a distinct manner compared to CTLA-4 (Parry et al. 2005; Nishimura et al. 2001). PD-1 has two ligands, programmed cell death-ligand 1 (PD-L1, also known as B7-H1) and programmed cell death-ligand 2 (PD-L2, also known as B7-DC) (Latchman et al. 2001; Freeman et al. 2000). PD-L1 is widely

Table 11.1 FDA-approved immune checkpoint inhibitors (as of the end of 2017)

Target	Generic name	Trade name	Antibody class	Company	Indications
CTLA4	Ipilimumab	Yervoy	Human IgG1k	Bristol-Myers Squibb Co.	Stage III/IV melanoma
PD-1	Nivolumab	Opdivo	Human IgG4	Bristol-Myers Squibb Co.	Metastatic melanoma, NSCLC, RCC, cHL, SCCHN, urothelial carcinoma, MSI-H CRC and hepatocellular carcinoma
	Pembrolizumab	Keytruda	Humanized IgG4	Merck and Co. Inc.	Metastatic melanoma, NSCLC, SCCHN, cHL, urothelial carcinoma, MSI-H cancers and gastric cancer
PD-L1	Atezolizumab	Tecentriq	Humanized IgG1	Genentech Inc.	Urothelial carcinoma and NSCLC
	Durvalumab	Imfinzi	Human IgG1k	AstraZeneca UK Limited	Urothelial carcinoma
	Avelumab	Bavencio	Human IgG1	EMD Serono Inc.	Merkel cell carcinoma and urothelial carcinoma

NSCLC non-small cell lung cancer, *RCC* renal cell carcinoma, *cHL* classical Hodgkin lymphoma, *SCCHN* squamous cell carcinoma of the head and neck, *MSI-H CRC* microsatellite instability-high metastatic colorectal cancer

expressed in various tissues, including cancer cells and stromal cells in the tumor microenvironment, and upregulated in response to pro-inflammatory cytokines (Dong et al. 2002). PD-L2 is mainly expressed on DC and macrophages, while its expression in tumor tissues was also reported (Yearley et al. 2017). In addition to PD-1, PD-L1 has an ability to interact with CD80, which is considered to be important for induction and maintenance of peripheral T cell tolerance (Park et al. 2010).

When PD-L1 expression is induced in the tumor microenvironment in response to pro-inflammatory cytokines secreted from infiltrating tumor-reactive CTL, binding of PD-L1 to PD-1 on CTL could downregulate anti-tumor immunity. Therefore, blockade of PD-L1/PD-1 pathway is an ideal therapeutic approach to restore and augment anti-tumor immune responses. In pre-clinical models, anti-PD-1 Ab and anti-PD-L1 Ab demonstrated anti-tumor effects in various tumor models, especially those using immunogenic tumors, by enhancing tumor antigen-specific T cell responses including cytokine production, survival, cellular motility, and glycolysis (Chang et al. 2015; Zinselmeyer et al. 2013; Okazaki et al. 2013).

In the clinical trials, anti-PD-1 Abs represented by nivolumab and pembrolizumab have been investigated for treatment of various advanced cancers. Early studies reported a clinical efficacy of nivolumab in metastatic melanoma, NSCLC, and RCC (Topalian et al. 2012). Based on this, nivolumab was first approved as a drug for metastatic melanoma in Japan and the USA in 2014. Based on favorable outcomes in subsequent clinical trials, nivolumab has been approved for NSCLC,

RCC, classical Hodgkin lymphoma (cHL), squamous cell carcinoma of the head and neck (SCCHN), urothelial carcinoma, microsatellite instability-high (MSI-H) metastatic colorectal cancer (CRC), and hepatocellular carcinoma in the USA as of the end of 2017 (Table 11.1). Nivolumab was also approved for gastric cancer in Japan. As to pembrolizumab, its clinical efficacy was demonstrated in various clinical trials, resulted in FDA approval for metastatic melanoma, NSCLC, SCCHN, cHL, urothelial carcinoma, MSI-H cancers, and gastric cancer (Table 11.1). Regarding anti-PD-L1 Ab, atezolizumab, avelumab, and durvalumab have been developed, although they came onto the market later than anti-PD-1 Ab. As of 2017, atezolizumab is approved for urothelial carcinoma and NSCLC, avelumab is approved for Merkel cell carcinoma and urothelial carcinoma, and durvalumab is approved for urothelial carcinoma in the USA (Table 11.1).

11.2.3 Clinical Efficacy of Checkpoint Blockade and Combination Immunotherapies

It has been reported that clinical responses caused by immune checkpoint blockade exhibit features distinct to those observed by conventional anti-cancer drugs such as chemotherapy and molecular target therapy. As immunotherapy mediates anti-tumor effects via upregulation of tumor-reactive immunity but not direct killing of tumor cells, clinical responses would emerge slowly compared to the conventional therapies. Thus, tumor regression following a transient progression, referred to as pseudo-progression, is observed in some cases treated with immune checkpoint blockade (Chiou and Burotto 2015). In this context, novel criteria to evaluate clinical efficacy of cancer immunotherapy are demanded, in which irRC, irRECIST, and iRECIST have been proposed (Hodi et al. 2016).

While immune checkpoint blockade could yield durable therapeutic benefits in various cancers, its response rate remains less than 30% when given as a monotherapy. To further increase the clinical efficacy, importance of combining multiple immune checkpoint blockades or administration together with existing anti-tumor therapeutic modalities has been emphasized. As CTLA-4 and PD-1 inhibit T cell functions in the distinct immune conditions, i.e., priming vs. effector phase, it is reasonable to utilize anti-CTLA-4 Ab and anti-PD-1 Ab as a combination therapy (Parry et al. 2005). Clinical trials using these Abs induced favorable clinical benefits in metastatic melanoma, which were superior to those observed by monotherapy of each drug (Postow et al. 2015), resulted in FDA approval of this combination therapy in 2015. As of 2017, several clinical trials of anti-CTLA-4 Ab plus anti-PD-1 Ab combination therapy are under progress in solid cancers including NSCLC and RCC. As for combination of immune checkpoint blockade with existing therapeutic modalities, such as chemotherapy, kinase inhibitors, and radiation therapy, numbers of clinical trials have been tested and currently under investigation. So far, FDA approved pembrolizumab for use in combination with pemetrexed plus carboplatin as a frontline treatment for patients with metastatic or advanced NSCLC (Langer et al. 2016). There is no doubt that various combination therapies together with immune checkpoint blockade will come onto the market in very near future.

11.2.4 Adverse Events Associated with Immune Checkpoint Blockade Therapy

Immune checkpoint blockade therapy could cause unique adverse effects through immune-mediated tissue damage by auto-reactive T cells, known as immune-related adverse events (irAE). irAE are defined as immunopathological features in various organ systems, including the gastrointestinal tract, liver, lung, endocrine glands, eye, nerve system, and hematopoietic systems. The incidence of irAE of any grades reaches around 60% of patients receiving checkpoint blockade therapy, while the incidence of grade 3–4 irAE were reported to be 20–30% by anti-CTLA-4 Ab, 10–15% by anti-PD-1 Ab, and 5–10% by anti-PD-L1 Ab (Robert et al. 2015). Although irAE could be severe and sometimes even fatal, the majority of patients are manageable with prompt recognition of irAE and precise treatments including discontinuation of checkpoint blockade and immunosuppression with steroid administration and/or anti-tumor necrosis factor Ab therapy.

11.2.5 Novel Targets of Immune Checkpoint Molecules

As the success of anti-PD-1/PD-L1 Ab and anti-CTLA-4 Ab fueled the research and development of cancer immunotherapy, the search for novel checkpoint molecules as next targets has been accelerating. Although numbers of candidates have been reported, those for therapeutic targets should meet, at least in part, the following criteria: (1) capacity of delivering inhibitory signal to cause T cell unresponsiveness, (2) blockade of its functions to activate T cells by abrogating unresponsiveness, and (3) its expression on non-functional (e.g., exhausted) T cells and its ligand expression on APC or in the tumor microenvironment. LAG-3, TIM-3, and TIGIT are among the promising and novel checkpoint molecules which meet these criteria.

11.2.5.1 LAG-3 (Lymphocyte Activation Gene-3, CD223)

LAG-3, a molecule belonging to immunoglobulin superfamily, is structurally homologous to CD4 and expressed on activated T cells, B cells, NK cells, and DC (Huard et al. 1994; Baixeras et al. 1992). LAG-3 binds MHC class II with an affinity higher than that of CD4 (Huard et al. 1994) and mediates immune-regulatory functions via various mechanisms as follows: (1) transmission of inhibitory signals through the intracellular KIEELE motif (Workman et al. 2002), (2) enhancement of immunosuppressive functions of regulatory T cells (Huang et al. 2004), and (3) maturation and activation of DC by signaling through MHC class II molecule (Andreae et al. 2002). As a cell surface marker, LAG-3 expression is associated with T cell exhaustion caused by chronic infection (Blackburn et al. 2009). Recent studies further indicated that functionally impaired T cells in cancer patients also express LAG-3 simultaneously with PD-1 (Matsuzaki et al. 2010).

Therapeutic application regulating LAG-3 functions for cancer immunotherapy has been attempted by LAG-3-Ig fusion proteins and anti-LAG-3 Ab. Administration of LAG-3-Ig induces the activation of DC via signaling through MHC class II and upregulates tumor-reactive immune responses, leading to growth retardation and regression of various types of tumor in mouse models (Prigent et al. 1999). Combined usage of LAG-3-Ig with poly(I:C) as an adjuvant of tumor vaccine was reported to induce potent and durable anti-tumor effects (Kano et al. 2016). In clinical studies, LAG-3-Ig has been developed as IMP321 and tested against several solid tumors as monotherapy or in combination with chemotherapy or other immunotherapies (Romano et al. 2014; Brignone et al. 2010; Brignone et al. 2009). As of 2017, a clinical trial of IMP321 combined with anti-PD-1 Ab (pembrolizumab) in melanoma patients is ongoing, and favorable results were reported. Besides LAG-3-Ig, antagonistic anti-LAG-3 Ab has been shown to restore T cell exhaustion in mouse tumor model (Goding et al. 2013). Accordingly, several clinical trials of anti-LAG-3 Ab alone or combined with anti-PD-1 Ab in solid cancers and hematological malignancies are in progress.

11.2.5.2 TIM-3 (T Cell Immunoglobulin and Mucin-Containing Protein-3, CD366)

TIM-3 is a type I transmembrane protein which is expressed on multiple T cell populations, NK cells, NKT cells, and APC (McIntire et al. 2001). TIM-3 binds multiple ligands, including galectin-9, phosphatidylserine, HMGB-1, and CEACAM-1 (Huang et al. 2016; Chiba et al. 2012; Freeman et al. 2010; Zhu et al. 2005), and plays an important role in termination of inflammatory T cell responses and subsequent induction of T cell tolerance, while detailed mechanisms have yet to be fully understood (Rangachari et al. 2012; Sánchez-Fueyo et al. 2003; Monney et al. 2002).

TIM-3 would be an attractive target for cancer immunotherapy, since its expression is detected on tumor-infiltrating lymphocytes (TIL), similar to PD-1, in various types of cancer, and is associated with T cell exhaustion (Sakuishi et al. 2010). It should be noted that T cells expressing both PD-1 and TIM-3 represent the most deeply exhausted phenotype, in terms of proliferation and cytokine production of IL-2, TNF-α, and IFN-γ (Sakuishi et al. 2010). Based on this finding, combined blockade of TIM-3 and PD-1 was examined and found to restore T cell functions and to inhibit tumor growth at an efficacy superior to a single blockade of either molecule (Zhou et al. 2011). Besides direct effects on anti-tumor T cells, TIM-3 has been reported to promote granulocytic myeloid-derived suppressor cells (MDSC) via cognate interaction with galectin-9, which is expressed on CD11b[+] Ly6G[+] cells (Dardalhon et al. 2010). As MDSC expand in tumor-bearing hosts and mediate immunosuppression at tumor microenvironment, blockade of TIM-3 could also indirectly stimulate anti-tumor immunity by attenuating MDSC functions. As of 2017, clinical trials of anti-TIM-3 Ab alone or with anti-PD-1 Ab in advanced malignancies are in progress.

11.2.5.3   TIGIT (T Cell Immunoreceptor with Ig and ITIM Domains)

TIGIT, a molecule belonging to the immunoglobulin superfamily, is expressed on activated or exhausted T cells and NK cells (Yu et al. 2009). TIGIT binds poliovirus receptor (PVR, CD155) and Nectin-2 (CD112) and exerts the inhibitory function via several distinct mechanisms (Pauken and Wherry 2014; Martinet and Smyth 2015). First, TIGIT inhibits T cell responses directly by transmitting inhibitory signals through intracellular ITIM. Second, interaction of TIGIT with CD155 competitively inhibits CD155 binding with CD226, a receptor delivering a stimulatory co-signal in T cells. Third, TIGIT prevents homodimerization of CD226 and inhibits CD226-mediated T cell activation (Johnston et al. 2014). Finally, TIGIT binding with CD155 on DC induces tolerogenic conversion of DC characterized by promoting IL-10 production while diminishing IL-12 production (Yu et al. 2009; Johnston et al. 2014).

The pre-clinical models for evaluating the efficacy of anti-TIGIT Ab revealed that the combination therapy of anti-TIGIT Ab with anti-PD-L1 Ab showed the durable therapeutic effect against murine solid tumors (Johnston et al. 2014). Moreover, it has been reported that PD-1 and TIGIT were highly expressed on TIL from patients with melanoma, while combined blockade by anti-TIGIT Ab and anti-PD-1 Ab reinvigorated the function of TIL (Chauvin et al. 2015). Based on these findings, several clinical trials using anti-TIGIT Ab alone or with anti-PD-1/PD-L1 Ab against solid cancers are under investigation as of 2017.

11.3   Stimulatory Co-signal Molecules as Targets for Cancer Immunotherapy

Quality and quantity of T cell responses are determined by a fine balance between stimulatory and inhibitory co-signals. When stimulatory co-signals surpass inhibitory co-signals, T cells are activated and rendered to make productive responses. On the other hand, when inhibitory co-signals are dominant, T cells undergo dysfunctional state, such as anergy and exhaustion, leading to a termination of immune responses. Thus, in order to accelerate anti-tumor immunity, triggering stimulatory co-signals, in addition to blockade of immune checkpoint, could be an important strategy. Accordingly, agonistic Abs against stimulatory co-signal molecules have been developed, and some of them are currently under clinical investigation. Abs against 4-1BB, OX-40, and GITR are among the most promising and advanced reagents in this strategy.

11.3.1 4-1BB (CD137)

4-1BB, a molecule of TNF receptor superfamily, is inducibly expressed on T cells along with their activation. Interaction with its ligand, 4-1BBL, triggers 4-1BB stimulatory co-signal, which activates NF-κB and MAPK via recruitment of TRAF (Wang et al. 2009). 4-1BB signal enhances T cell activation and cytokine production and promotes their survival by inducing anti-apoptotic molecules such as Bcl-X_L, especially in effector memory CD8$^+$ T cells (Pulle et al. 2006; Lee et al. 2002). Expression of 4-1BB is also detected on NK cells and DC, and stimulatory effects of 4-1BB on these cells have been also reported (Wilcox et al. 2002a; Wilcox et al. 2002b).

In mouse tumor models, triggering 4-1BB stimulatory co-signal by agonistic Ab or 4-1BBL gene expression upregulated anti-tumor immune responses and induced tumor regression (Ye et al. 2002; Melero et al. 1997). Moreover, combination therapies of anti-4-1BB Ab and anti-PD-1 Ab prolonged mouse survival against poorly immunogenic tumors (Chen et al. 2015). Based on these studies, fully human anti-4-1BB Ab with agonistic capacity has been developed and tested as monotherapy or in combination with anti-PD-1 Ab against advanced solid cancers in clinical trials. While favorable safety profile and therapeutic effects were reported (Tolcher et al. 2017), its advantage over anti-PD-1 Ab monotherapy or conventional therapies has yet to be established, thus requiring further clinical investigations.

11.3.2 OX-40 (CD134)

OX-40 is a member of TNF receptor superfamily and originally identified as an activation marker on rat CD4$^+$ T cells (Mallett et al. 1990). Subsequent studies revealed that OX-40 is expressed on both CD4$^+$ and CD8$^+$ T cells upon activation, as well as NK cells, and OX-40 signal promotes proliferation, cytokine production, migration, and effector functions of these cells (Gramaglia et al. 1998). Mice deficient of OX-40 or OX-40 L, a ligand of OX-40, exhibited impaired T cell responses in vivo, indicating a role of this pathway in providing a stimulatory co-signal to T cells (Chen et al. 1999; Kopf et al. 1999). In animal experiments, administration of

OX-40 agonists prolonged the mouse survival in various tumor models (Weinberg et al. 2000). In addition to direct effects in stimulating T cell activation, there is also evidence that OX-40 agonists dampen suppressive function of Treg, thus indirectly facilitating anti-tumor immunity (Piconese et al. 2008; Vu et al. 2007). In cancer patients, the existence of OX-40-positive T cells in TIL and tumor-draining lymph nodes has been reported (Vetto et al. 1997). Phase I clinical trial using anti-OX-40 Ab demonstrated a favorable safety profile, induction of T cell proliferation, and tumor shrinkage in some patients (Curti et al. 2013). In addition to monotherapy, combination therapies of anti-OX-40 Ab with immune checkpoint blockade are also under investigation. These studies, however, should be carefully designed and interpreted, since a possibility of dampening the effect of anti-OX-40 Ab by addition of anti-PD-1 Ab has been reported (Shrimali et al. 2017).

11.3.3 GITR (Glucocorticoid-Induced Tumor Necrosis Factor Receptor, CD357)

GITR is expressed on various immune cells including activated T cells. GITR signal delivers stimulatory co-signal into T cells and enhances their proliferation, cytokine production, and survival (Tone et al. 2003). In addition, it has been reported that GITR is constitutively expressed on Treg at high levels and that GITR signal abrogates the suppressive functions of Treg (Shimizu et al. 2002). Consistent with these studies, treatment with anti-GITR agonistic Ab caused tumor regression in preclinical mouse models through T cell activation and induction of Treg instability and depletion (Cohen et al. 2010). Several phase I/II clinical trials using humanized anti-GITR agonistic Ab alone or combination with other immunotherapies against solid cancers are currently under investigation.

11.4 Summary

Recent development of anti-CTLA-4 Ab and anti-PD-1 Ab represents magnificent success in caner immunotherapy. Accordingly, approaches to manipulate inhibitory or stimulatory co-signal functions are considered to be the most promising approaches in the field, and identification of novel targets with a potent therapeutic potential is eagerly anticipated. While this chapter focuses on several well-known molecules which are among the most explored in clinical translation, there are many other intriguing targets which are not described here. Development of novel reagents to regulate co-signal molecules as monotherapy or combined immunotherapy with other medical interventions including chemotherapy, kinase inhibitors, radiotherapy, and surgery will establish next generation of cancer treatment.

References

Andreae S, Piras F, Burdin N, Triebel F (2002) Maturation and activation of dendritic cells induced by lymphocyte activation gene-3 (CD223). J Immunol 168:3874–3880

Baixeras E et al (1992) Characterization of the lymphocyte activation gene 3-encoded protein. A new ligand for human leukocyte antigen class II antigens. J Exp Med 176:327–337

Blackburn SD et al (2009) Coregulation of CD8+ T cell exhaustion by multiple inhibitory receptors during chronic viral infection. Nat Publ Group 10:29–37

Brignone C, Escudier B, Grygar C, Marcu M, Triebel F (2009) A phase I pharmacokinetic and biological correlative study of IMP321, a novel MHC class II agonist, in patients with advanced renal cell carcinoma. Clin Cancer Res 15:6225–6231

Brignone C et al (2010) First-line chemoimmunotherapy in metastatic breast carcinoma: combination of paclitaxel and IMP321 (LAG-3Ig) enhances immune responses and antitumor activity. J Transl Med 8:71

Brunet JF et al (1987) A new member of the immunoglobulin superfamily--CTLA-4. Nat Int Weekly J Sci 328:267–270

Chambers CA, Allison JP (1999) Costimulatory regulation of T cell function. Curr Opin Cell Biol 11:203–210

Chang C-H et al (2015) Metabolic competition in the tumor microenvironment is a driver of cancer progression. Cell 162:1229–1241

Chauvin J-M et al (2015) TIGIT and PD-1 impair tumor antigen-specific CD8+ T cells in melanoma patients. J Clin Invest 125:2046–2058

Chen AI et al (1999) Ox40-ligand has a critical costimulatory role in dendritic cell:T cell interactions. Immunity 11:689–698

Chen S et al (2015) Combination of 4-1BB agonist and PD-1 antagonist promotes antitumor effector/memory CD8 T cells in a poorly immunogenic tumor model. Cancer Immunol Res 3:149–160

Chiba S et al (2012) Tumor-infiltrating DCs suppress nucleic acid-mediated innate immune responses through interactions between the receptor TIM-3 and the alarmin HMGB1. Nat Publ Group 13:832–842

Chiou VL, Burotto M (2015) Pseudoprogression and immune-related response in solid tumors. J Clin Oncol 33:3541–3543

Cohen AD et al (2010) Agonist anti-GITR monoclonal antibody induces melanoma tumor immunity in mice by altering regulatory T cell stability and intra-tumor accumulation. PLoS One 5:e10436

Collins AV et al (2002) The interaction properties of costimulatory molecules revisited. Immunity 17:201–210

Curti BD et al (2013) OX40 is a potent immune-stimulating target in late-stage cancer patients. Cancer Res 73:7189–7198

Dardalhon V et al (2010) Tim-3/galectin-9 pathway: regulation of Th1 immunity through promotion of CD11b+Ly-6G+ myeloid cells. J Immunol 185:1383–1392

Dong H et al (2002) Tumor-associated B7-H1 promotes T-cell apoptosis: a potential mechanism of immune evasion. Nat Med 8:793–800

Eggermont AMM et al (2015) Adjuvant ipilimumab versus placebo after complete resection of high-risk stage III melanoma (EORTC 18071): a randomised, double-blind, phase 3 trial. Lancet Oncol 16:522–530

Freeman GJ et al (2000) Engagement of the PD-1 immunoinhibitory receptor by a novel B7 family member leads to negative regulation of lymphocyte activation. J Exp Med 192:1027–1034

Freeman GJ, Casasnovas JM, Umetsu DT, DeKruyff RH (2010) TIM genes: a family of cell surface phosphatidylserine receptors that regulate innate and adaptive immunity. Immunol Rev 235:172–189

Goding SR et al (2013) Restoring immune function of tumor-specific CD4+ T cells during recurrence of melanoma. J Immunol 190:4899–4909

Gramaglia I, Weinberg AD, Lemon M, Croft M (1998) Ox-40 ligand: a potent costimulatory molecule for sustaining primary CD4 T cell responses. J Immunol 161:6510–6517

Hodi FS et al (2010) Improved survival with ipilimumab in patients with metastatic melanoma. N Engl J Med 363:711–723

Hodi FS et al (2016) Evaluation of immune-related response criteria and RECIST v1.1 in patients with Advanced melanoma treated with pembrolizumab. J Clin Oncol 34:1510–1517

Huang C-T et al (2004) Role of LAG-3 in regulatory T cells. Immunity 21:503–513

Huang Y-H et al (2016) Corrigendum: CEACAM1 regulates TIM-3-mediated tolerance and exhaustion. Nature 536:359–359

Huard B, Gaulard P, Faure F, Hercend T, Triebel F (1994) Cellular expression and tissue distribution of the human LAG-3-encoded protein, an MHC class II ligand. Immunogenetics 39:213–217

Hui E et al (2017) T cell costimulatory receptor CD28 is a primary target for PD-1-mediated inhibition. Science 355:1428–1433

Ishida Y, Agata Y, Shibahara K, Honjo T (1992) Induced expression of PD-1, a novel member of the immunoglobulin gene superfamily, upon programmed cell death. EMBO J 11:3887–3895

Johnston RJ et al (2014) The immunoreceptor TIGIT regulates antitumor and antiviral CD8(+) T cell effector function. Cancer Cell 26:923–937

Kano Y et al (2016) Combined adjuvants of poly(I:C) plus LAG-3-Ig improve antitumor effects of tumor-specific T cells, preventing their exhaustion. Cancer Sci 107:398–406

Keler T et al (2003) Activity and safety of CTLA-4 blockade combined with vaccines in cynomolgus macaques. J Immunol 171:6251–6259

Kopf M et al (1999) OX40-deficient mice are defective in Th cell proliferation but are competent in generating B cell and CTL responses after virus infection. Immunity 11:699–708

Langer CJ et al (2016) Carboplatin and pemetrexed with or without pembrolizumab for advanced, non-squamous non-small-cell lung cancer: a randomised, phase 2 cohort of the open-label KEYNOTE-021 study. Lancet Oncol 17:1497–1508

Latchman Y et al (2001) PD-L2 is a second ligand for PD-1 and inhibits T cell activation. Nat Immunol 2:261–268

Leach DR, Krummel MF, Allison JP (1996) Enhancement of antitumor immunity by CTLA-4 blockade. Science 271:1734–1736

Lee H-W et al (2002) 4-1BB promotes the survival of CD8+ T lymphocytes by increasing expression of Bcl-xL and Bfl-1. J Immunol 169:4882–4888

Mallett S, Fossum S, Barclay AN (1990) Characterization of the MRC OX40 antigen of activated CD4 positive T lymphocytes--a molecule related to nerve growth factor receptor. EMBO J 9:1063–1068

Martinet L, Smyth MJ (2015) Balancing natural killer cell activation through paired receptors. Nat Rev Immunol 15:243–254

Matsuzaki J et al (2010) Tumor-infiltrating NY-ESO-1-specific CD8+ T cells are negatively regulated by LAG-3 and PD-1 in human ovarian cancer. Proc Natl Acad Sci U S A 107:7875–7880

McIntire JJ et al (2001) Identification of Tapr (an airway hyperreactivity regulatory locus) and the linked Tim gene family. Nat Immunol 2:1109–1116

Melero I et al (1997) Monoclonal antibodies against the 4-1BB T-cell activation molecule eradicate established tumors. Nat Med 3:682–685

Monney L et al (2002) Th1-specific cell surface protein Tim-3 regulates macrophage activation and severity of an autoimmune disease. Nat Int Weekly J Sci 415:536–541

Nishimura H et al (2001) Autoimmune dilated cardiomyopathy in PD-1 receptor-deficient mice. Science 291:319–322

Okazaki T, Chikuma S, Iwai Y, Fagarasan S, Honjo T (2013) A rheostat for immune responses: the unique properties of PD-1 and their advantages for clinical application. Nat Publ Group 14:1212–1218

Park J-J et al (2010) B7-H1/CD80 interaction is required for the induction and maintenance of peripheral T-cell tolerance. Blood 116:1291–1298

Parry RV et al (2005) CTLA-4 and PD-1 receptors inhibit T-cell activation by distinct mechanisms. Mol Cell Biol 25:9543–9553

Pauken KE, Wherry EJ (2014) TIGIT and CD226: tipping the balance between costimulatory and coinhibitory molecules to augment the cancer immunotherapy toolkit. Cancer Cell 26:785–787

Piconese S, Valzasina B, Colombo MP (2008) OX40 triggering blocks suppression by regulatory T cells and facilitates tumor rejection. J Exp Med 205:825–839

Postow MA et al (2015) Nivolumab and ipilimumab versus ipilimumab in untreated melanoma. N Engl J Med 372:2006–2017

Prigent P, El mir S, Dréano M, Triebel F (1999) Lymphocyte activation gene-3 induces tumor regression and antitumor immune responses. Eur J Immunol 29:3867–3876

Pulle G, Vidric M, Watts TH (2006) IL-15-dependent induction of 4-1BB promotes antigen-independent CD8 memory T cell survival. J Immunol 176:2739–2748

Qureshi OS et al (2011) Trans-endocytosis of CD80 and CD86: a molecular basis for the cell-extrinsic function of CTLA-4. Science 332:600–603

Rangachari M et al (2012) Bat3 promotes T cell responses and autoimmunity by repressing Tim-3–mediated cell death and exhaustion. Nat Med 18:1394–1400

Robert C et al (2011) Ipilimumab plus dacarbazine for previously untreated metastatic melanoma. N Engl J Med 364:2517–2526

Robert C et al (2015) Pembrolizumab versus Ipilimumab in Advanced Melanoma. N Engl J Med 372:2521–2532

Romano E et al (2014) MART-1 peptide vaccination plus IMP321 (LAG-3Ig fusion protein) in patients receiving autologous PBMCs after lymphodepletion: results of a phase I trial. J Transl Med 12:97

Sakuishi K et al (2010) Targeting Tim-3 and PD-1 pathways to reverse T cell exhaustion and restore anti-tumor immunity. J Exp Med 207:2187–2194

Sánchez-Fueyo A et al (2003) Tim-3 inhibits T helper type 1-mediated auto- and alloimmune responses and promotes immunological tolerance. Nat Immunol 4:1093–1101

Selby MJ et al (2013) Anti-CTLA-4 antibodies of IgG2a isotype enhance antitumor activity through reduction of intratumoral regulatory T cells. Cancer Immunol Res 1:32–42

Shimizu J, Yamazaki S, Takahashi T, Ishida Y, Sakaguchi S (2002) Stimulation of CD25(+)CD4(+) regulatory T cells through GITR breaks immunological self-tolerance. Nat Immunol 3:135–142

Shrimali RK et al (2017) Concurrent PD-1 blockade negates the effects of OX40 agonist antibody in combination immunotherapy through inducing T-cell apoptosis. Cancer Immunol Res 5:755–766

Tolcher AW et al (2017) Phase Ib study of Utomilumab (PF-05082566), a 4-1BB/CD137 agonist, in combination with Pembrolizumab (MK-3475) in patients with advanced solid tumors. Clin Cancer Res 23:5349–5357

Tone M et al (2003) Mouse glucocorticoid-induced tumor necrosis factor receptor ligand is costimulatory for T cells. PNAS 100:15059–15064

Topalian SL et al (2012) Safety, activity, and immune correlates of anti-PD-1 antibody in cancer. N Engl J Med 366:2443–2454

Vetto JT et al (1997) Presence of the T-cell activation marker OX-40 on tumor infiltrating lymphocytes and draining lymph node cells from patients with melanoma and head and neck cancers. AJS 174:258–265

Vu MD et al (2007) OX40 costimulation turns off Foxp3+ Tregs. Blood 110:2501–2510

Wang C, Lin GHY, McPherson AJ, Watts TH (2009) Immune regulation by 4-1BB and 4-1BBL: complexities and challenges. Immunol Rev 229:192–215

Waterhouse P et al (1995) Lymphoproliferative disorders with early lethality in mice deficient in Ctla-4. Science 270:985–988

Weinberg AD et al (2000) Engagement of the OX-40 receptor in vivo enhances antitumor immunity. J Immunol 164:2160–2169

Wilcox RA, Tamada K, Strome SE, Chen L (2002a) Signaling through NK cell-associated CD137 promotes both helper function for CD8+ cytolytic T cells and responsiveness to IL-2 but not cytolytic activity. J Immunol 169:4230–4236

Wilcox RA et al (2002b) Cutting edge: expression of functional CD137 receptor by dendritic cells. J Immunol 168:4262–4267

Wing K et al (2008) CTLA-4 control over Foxp3+ regulatory T cell function. Science 322:271–275

Workman CJ, Dugger KJ, Vignali DAA (2002) Cutting edge: molecular analysis of the negative regulatory function of lymphocyte activation gene-3. J Immunol 169:5392–5395

Ye Z et al (2002) Gene therapy for cancer using single-chain Fv fragments specific for 4-1BB. Nat Med 8:343–348

Yearley JH et al (2017) PD-L2 expression in human tumors: relevance to anti-PD-1 therapy in Cancer. Clin Cancer Res 23:3158–3167

Yokosuka T et al (2012) Programmed cell death 1 forms negative costimulatory microclusters that directly inhibit T cell receptor signaling by recruiting phosphatase SHP2. J Exp Med 209:1201–1217

Yu X et al (2009) The surface protein TIGIT suppresses T cell activation by promoting the generation of mature immunoregulatory dendritic cells. Nat Publ Group 10:48–57

Zhou Q et al (2011) Coexpression of Tim-3 and PD-1 identifies a CD8+ T-cell exhaustion phenotype in mice with disseminated acute myelogenous leukemia. Blood 117:4501–4510

Zhu C et al (2005) The Tim-3 ligand galectin-9 negatively regulates T helper type 1 immunity. Nat Immunol 6:1245–1252

Zinselmeyer BH et al (2013) PD-1 promotes immune exhaustion by inducing antiviral T cell motility paralysis. J Exp Med 210:757–774

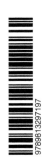